U0203714

Diagnostics of Traditional
Chinese Medicine
and Treatment
for Some Common Diseases

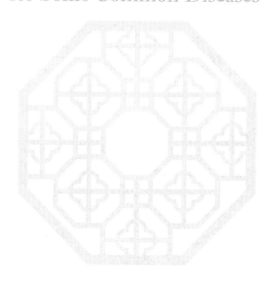

与
常见病治疗

中医诊断

（汉英对照）

(Chinese-English Edition)

毛德西 编著

张玉红 禄保平 译

Compiler Mao Dexi

Translators Zhang Yuhong Lu Baoping

河南科学技术出版社

·郑州·

⊙ 本著作受国家中医药管理局"全国名中医传承工作室建设项目"资助。

图书在版编目（CIP）数据

中医诊断与常见病治疗：汉英对照/毛德西编著；张玉红，禄保平译.
郑州：河南科学技术出版社，2020.6
ISBN 978-7-5349-9829-4

Ⅰ.①中…　Ⅱ.①毛…　②张…　③禄…　Ⅲ.①中医诊断学-汉、英
②中医治疗学-汉、英　Ⅳ.①R24

中国版本图书馆 CIP 数据核字（2020）第 013962 号

出版发行：河南科学技术出版社
　　　　　地址：郑州市郑东新区祥盛街 27 号　　邮编：450016
　　　　　电话：(0371) 65788613　　65788625
　　　　　网址：www.hnstp.cn
策划编辑：武丹丹
责任编辑：武丹丹
责任校对：牛艳春
封面设计：张　伟
责任印制：张艳芳
印　　刷：河南博雅彩印有限公司
经　　销：全国新华书店
开　　本：787 mm×1 092 mm　1/16　印张：29.5　字数：680 千字
版　　次：2020 年 6 月第 1 版　　2020 年 6 月第 1 次印刷
定　　价：198.00 元

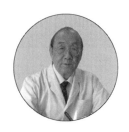

毛德西简介
Brief Introduction to Professor Mao Dexi

* * *

毛德西，男，生于 1940 年 10 月，中国河南省巩义市人。河南省中医院中医内科主任医师、教授、研究生导师，全国名中医，全国老中医药专家学术经验继承工作指导老师，中医药科普专家，河南省中医事业终身成就奖获得者。

从事中医临床工作 60 余年，医德高尚，心系百姓；谙熟经典，通贯各家；对心脑血管疾病、消化系统疾病及疑难杂病临床经验丰富，颇多独到见解；善用经方，不弃时方，并不断吸取民间验方，临床效果多佳，受到百姓称赞。

发表学术论文 120 余篇，出版学术专著 20 余部。退休之后，仍坚持不懈地为病人把脉看病，带教后学，传承经验。工作之余，致力于中医养生学的研究，出版中医养生学著作 4 部，并获全国中医药科学普及金话筒奖。

Professor Mao Dexi, was born in Gongyi of Henan Province in October, 1940. He has been chief physician of internal medicine of TCM, postgraduate tutor in Henan Province Hospital of Traditional Chinese Medicine, National Prominent and Experienced TCM Doctor, Supervisor of National Famous TCM Doctor Workshop of Inheritance Project and expert of TCM science popularization. He is also the winner of the Prize of Life-long Career Achievement for TCM Cause of Henan Province.

Professor Mao has engaged in TCM clinical practice for over 6 decades. He consistently cares for his patients with lofty medical ethics and benevolence. With profound academic accomplishment by mastering many medical classics and various medical sects, he has his own unique insights and analysis in treating cardio-cerebrovascular, digestive and some other difficult miscellaneous diseases with his rich clinical experience. He is also a great expert in integrating classical with modern prescriptions. Besides, he keeps on assimilating the advantages of folk remedies. The excellent clinical effect earns him plenty of compliments and acclaim widely from his patients.

Academically, Professor Mao has attained great achievements, too. Up to now, more than 120 of his academic papers and 20 monographs have been published. Even in his retirement, he persists in treating his patients by taking pulse himself and passing his expertise and experience on to other doctors and students through clinical teaching. In his spare time, he is committed to the study of TCM health maintenance. So far, his four monographs in this field have been published and he has been awarded the Prize of Golden Microphone for TCM Science Popularization.

译者简介
Translator's profile

* * *

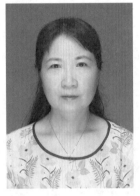

张玉红（1970—），女，英语语言文学硕士，河南中医药大学副教授。主要从事外国语言学与应用语言学及中医英语翻译等教学与研究工作。近年来主持或参与省厅级科研项目 12 项，获省厅级教学、科研奖励 6 项，先后在国内多家期刊发表论文近 20 篇，参与翻译《中医方剂学》、参编教材《涉外医疗英语》等著作。

Zhang Yuhong（1970 - ），female，is a master majoring in English linguistics and English literature，an associate professor in Henan University of Chinese Medicine. Engaging herself in teaching foreign linguistics and applied linguistics as well as the research of TCM English translation. She has presided and participated in 12 provincial and municipal-level scientific research projects，winning 6 teaching and research awards. So far，almost 20 of her academic papers have been published in some famous Chinese journals，and she has taken part in the translation and compilation of several books such as *Formula of Chinese Medicine*，*Foreign Medical English*，etc.

* * *

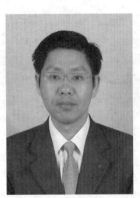

禄保平（1971—），男，医学博士，河南中医药大学教授、硕士生导师。系河南省学术技术带头人、国家中医药管理局重点学科后备学科带头人、河南省高校青年骨干教师、河南省高校科技创新人才；兼任河南省中医药学会肝病分会副主任委员、河南省中西医结合学会消化病分会副主任委员、河南中医药大学肝病研究所所长等职。

主持或参与省部级以上科研课题 12 项，获省级科研和教学奖励 5 项，发表学术论文 60 余篇，出版著作 7 部。

Lu Baoping（1971-），male，is a medical doctor，professor and tutor of postgraduates in Henan University of Chinese Medicine. For his outstanding achievements，he has been awarded the following honors such as "Academic and Technological Leader of Henan Province" "Reserve-discipline Leader of National Administration of Traditional Chinese Medicine" "Young Backbone Teacher" and "Talent of Scientific and Technological Innovation" of Henan Provincial Higher Education Institution，etc. Besides，he is Vice Chairman of Hepatopathy Society of Henan Association of TCM，Deputy Director of Digestive Disease Branch of Henan Association of Integration of TCM and Western Medicine as well as Director of Hepatopathy Institute of Henan University of Chinese Medicine.

Academically，as the author of over 60 academic papers and 7 books and the winner of 5 provincial-level scientific research and teaching awards，he has presided and participated in 12 research projects above provincial level.

东方的思维模式是综合的，西方的思维模式是分析的。用一个更通俗的说法来表达一下，西方是头痛医头，脚痛医脚，头痛医脚，脚痛医头，只见树木，不见森林，而东方则是头痛医脚，脚痛医头，既见树木，又见森林，说得再抽象一点，东方综合思维模式的特点是整体概念，普遍联系，而西方分析思维模式正相反。

季羡林自选集《谈国学》

毛德西

毛德西教授手书季羡林《谈国学》

Professor Mao's presentation of Ji Xianlin's *On Chinese Studies* in calligraphy

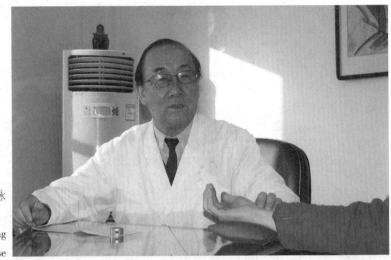

毛德西教授为病人把脉
诊病
Professor Mao is diagnosing
by taking a patient's pulse

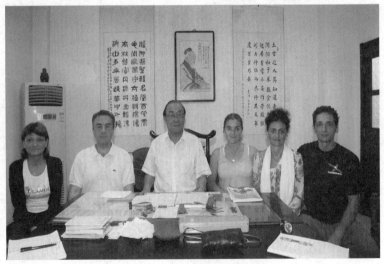

毛德西教授（左三）与
意大利进修医师毕路朝
（左二）等合影
A picture of Professor Mao
（left 3） sitting with 5
Italian doctors headed by
Lucio Pippa （left 2） who
have received training from
him for several years

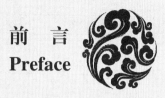
在世界历史的长河中，灿烂的东方文化闪耀着永恒的生命火花，这朵火花至今还在世界各地发挥着光和热，它给中国人民和世界各国人民带来了温暖与快乐，带来了健康与圆满，它就是中国的传统医学——中医药学。

In the long course of the world's history, the splendid oriental culture shines with its eternal "sparkle of life", radiant with its permanent brilliance all over the world and bringing warmth, happiness and health to China and the other nations as well. An indispensable part of the culture, which has contributed remarkably to the wellbeing and prosperity of mankind of the world, is TCM—traditional Chinese medicine.

改革开放给中医药学带来了极大的发展动力，许多国家和地区的朋友怀揣着敬慕的心情、探索和学习的目的来到中国，学习汉语、中医药学、针灸、太极拳等。有幸的是，我接触到几位来自意大利的朋友，他们中有几位在意大利国内还是有点名气的中医师。他们在中国各地考察了几家中医院，经朋友介绍最后来到了河南省中医院（河南中医药大学第二附属医院）。几经了解，他们发现这家中医院中医特色突出，没有过多的西医元素，颇有"纯中医"的味道。于是，2009 年他们决定在这里"安营扎寨"，学习中医。

The reform and opening-up policy of China has brought enormous impetus to the development of TCM, which has been widely recognized for its unique characteristics and marvelous curative effect. Therefore, quite a lot of foreign friends, with great curiosity and admiration, come to China to explore Chinese culture including Chinese language, medicine, acupuncture and moxibustion, Taijiquan and so on. In 2009, a group of Italians came to China to study TCM, a few of them were popular TCM practitioners in their home country. After careful observation across China, they found Henan Province Hospital of Traditional Chinese Medicine (The Second Affiliated Hospital of Henan University of Traditional Chinese Medicine) special in its "pure TCM characteristics", without mixing with some Western medicine elements. Then in 2009, they arrived at the hospital and determined to settle down, making it the ideal place where they could learn TCM.

　　时光荏苒，转眼四年过去了。虽然每年他们跟随我学习的时间仅仅一个月，但他们那种认真好学、孜孜不倦的精神也在感动着我和我周围的青年学子。2012年夏，学习告一段落的时候，他们希望我能写一本讲解中医诊断与常见病辨证论治的书。他们的渴望真诚而直率，我当即应允了下来，并于当年冬季开始编写《中医诊断与常见病治疗》这本书。此书的编写，根据他们的中医水平，本着通俗易懂、语言简练、科学实用的原则，以高校的本科教材为框架，以中医基本理论为指导，以密切联系临床为基点，采用白话直叙的方式。我花费半年多的时间，完成了初稿。后将初稿（中英文对照）交予他们阅读，看看是否合乎他们的口味。他们看了以后，翘起大拇指说：很好！看到他们那高兴劲儿，听到他们对中国传统医学的赞扬，作为一名年过七旬的老中医，我从内心里感到骄傲、荣幸，这种骄傲与荣幸来自对东方文化的热爱，来自对中国传统医学的坚持！

　　How time flies! Four years have elapsed since then. Although every year they can only stay here to learn TCM under my guidance for a month, their hard work and serious attitude greatly impressed me and some young Chinese students. As they finished their study in the summer of 2012, they told me that they wished that I could write a book about TCM diagnostics and treatments of common diseases for them. I felt quite moved by their eagerness, sincerity and frankness, and promised them at once and started to write this book in the winter of that year. Aiming at meeting their needs, the book, in "the language of popular, easy-to-understand and concise", is based on "the scientific and practical principle". Under the guidance of elementary TCM theory, it adopts the framework of college textbook and bases itself on connecting closely with clinical practice. Six months later, it is completed in a plain and straightforward style. After reading the English version of the first manuscript last summer, they spoke highly of it. As a TCM practitioner who is over 70 years old, on seeing their delight and hearing their praise of Chinese medicine, how proud and honored I felt! The pride comes from my love for Chinese culture as well as my persistent pursuit of TCM for so many years!

这本书的英译部分，是由河南中医药大学张玉红、禄保平完成的。在本书即将付梓的时候，我由衷地感谢他们在百忙中的辛勤劳动！

The book is translated by ZhangYuhong and Lu Baoping from Henan University of Chinese Medicine. As it is to be published, I would like to extend my heartfelt thanks for their hard work!

初次撰写这种中外交流的书，在谨慎之中难免有这样或那样的缺憾，希望朋友们提出自己的看法，以便本书再版时加以修正。

This is the first time that I do some writing on TCM for foreign friends. Though with every effort in the process of writing, there are still some errors or defects in the book. Therefore, I sincerely welcome valuable suggestions from friends and experts of this field to revise the book in the future.

The compiler: Mao Dexi

目　录
Contents

总　论
An Overview of TCM

一 / I

中医学是中华民族在长期的医疗、生活实践中，不断积累、反复总结而逐渐形成的具有独特理论风格的医学体系。正是由于它具有独特的理论，所以在世界传统医学发展史中，是唯一保存完整且有着强大生命力的传统医学。

Traditional Chinese medicine (TCM) is a medical system with unique theoretical characteristics summarized and developed by Chinese people in their long-term living and medical practice against diseases. It is precisely because of its special theory that in the history of world'traditional medicine, TCM is the only one that could get preserved intactly with its strong vitality.

中医学的基本理论形成于两千多年前的战国时期，代表著作是《黄帝内经》，它奠定了中医学的理论基础；而东汉时期张仲景的《伤寒杂病论》则是中医临床学的奠基之作，至今仍具有临床指导意义。

The formation of the basic theoretical framework of TCM can be traced back to the Warring States over two thousand years ago, represented by the coming-out *of Huangdi Neijing* (*Huangdi's Internal Classic*) which lays the groundwork for TCM theory. *Shanghan Zabing Lun* (*Treatise on Cold-induced and Miscellaneous Diseases*), compiled by Zhang Zhongjing, an outstanding medical practitioner in the Eastern Han Dynasty, is regarded as the foundation of clinical study on TCM and it has been exerting an enormous influence on guiding TCM clinical practice up to now.

中医学发展到金元时期，医学家根据当时社会环境与医学发展的状况，以及个人的临床经验，提出了各自的学术观点，相继出现了刘河间的"火热论"，张子和的"实邪论"，李东垣的"气虚论"和朱丹溪的"阴常不足论"等。他们的理论与实践经验至今还有应用价值。

During the period of the Jin and Yuan Dynasties, TCM theoretical system developed continuously. Medical practitioners or experts at that time put forward their viewpoints based on the developing situation of medicine, the social environment as well as their personal clinical practice. One academic doctrine succeeded the other, such as Liu Hejian's remark on "fire heat", Zhang Zihe's statement about "sthenic pathogens" "qi asthenia" of Li Dongyuan and Zhu Danxi's opinion about "universal deficiency of yin". Their theoretical and practical experience has still been of great value to clinical practice nowadays.

明清时期，是中医学的又一个发展高峰，温病（包括瘟疫）学说相继兴起，医学流派又出现了温补、疏肝、清解等多家学说。特别是清代的叶天士、薛生白、吴鞠通、王孟英等，对温病的辨证论治提出了新的观点，使中医学治疗温热病的水平向前推进了一大步。

The Ming and Qing Dynasties witnessed another peak of the development of TCM. The theories about seasonal febrile disease (including pestilences or plagues) appeared successively. Many theoretical schools on medicine sprang up, for instance, tonifying and warming, soothing the liver, clearing away heat and relieving toxin, etc. In particular, in the Qing Dynasty, scholars such as Ye Tianshi, Xue Shengbai, Wu Jutong and Wang Mengying proposed a new perspective, "treating febrile disease based on syndrome differentiation", which pushes the TCM therapeutic methods for febrile disease a big step further.

中华人民共和国成立以后，中医学摆脱了"各自为政"的束缚，国家支持中医学的发展，相继成立了中医药高等院校、研究院所、中医院、中医药学术团体，并且走出了国门，中医药学传播到了世界各地，成为造福于全人类的世界性传统医学。

After the founding of People's Republic of China, TCM developed vigorously for it got rid of the previous shackle of "various schools isolating themselves from one another". The government attached great importance to its development, and a great number of TCM institutions of higher learning, research institutes, TCM hospitals and academic groups were established successively. Nowadays, TCM has spread to all parts of the world and become a universal traditional medicine, making great contributions to the wellbeing of mankind in the world.

二 / Ⅱ

在中医学发展过程中，也出现了一些违背事实的声音，就是将中医学与西医学对立起来，认为中医学"不科学"，甚至有人提出要取消中医，想使这门已有数千年历史、为中华民族的繁衍昌盛做出巨大贡献的传统医学从地球上消失。这种论调时隐时现，但它阻碍不了中医学的发展，因为中医学的治疗效果是被广大群众所肯定的；中医学的经典之作是历史留下来的科学理论，是古代东方文明的巨大财富。

In the process of developing TCM, there are some voices going against the truth, namely, the opinions that put TCM and Western medicine at the opposite ends, regarding TCM "unscientific". Even some propose to cancel traditional Chinese medicine, the one that enjoys a history of thousands of years and has made tremendous contributions to the prosperity of

Chinese nation. The arguments appear from time to time, but they can't hinder it from further developing, for its therapeutic effect has convinced the public. And its classic, as a scientific theory left by history, is an indispensable part of ancient oriental civilization.

至于中医学与西医学的差别，是客观存在的，关键是怎样去理解。在这里我引用国学大师季羡林的一段话来阐明，季羡林先生在《谈国学》中说："东方的思维模式是综合的，西方的思维模式是分析的。勉强打一个比方，我们可以说：西方是'一分为二'，而东方则是'合二为一'。再用一个更通俗的说法来表达一下：西方是'头痛医头，脚痛医脚''只见树木，不见森林'，而东方则是'头痛医脚，脚痛医头''既见树木，又见森林'。说得再抽象一点：东方综合思维模式的特点是，整体概念，普遍联系；而西方分析思维模式正相反。"季先生在这里谈到一个思维模式问题，也就是思路问题。这一段话可以借用看待中医与西医的区别，这对理解中医学理论与临床非常重要。那些不懂中医而对中医指手画脚的人，应该坐下来认真读一读中医经典，亲身感受一下中医的效应，然后再发表看法，包括批评的意见，只要是善意的，中医同道都是会乐意接受的，而且也会加以改进和提高。

As to the difference between Chinese medicine and Western medicine, it does exist objectively. Therefore, the key is how to understand it correctly. Here I would like to illustrate it by quoting the statement from Ji Xianlin, a great master of traditional Chinese culture. In his book *On Studies of Ancient Chinese Civilization*, Ji points out, "Eastern thinking mode is comprehensive, while in western countries, analytical thinking is highly popular. For instance, Westerners tend to understand a thing in a way of cutting it into different pieces and analyzing them one by one, while Eastern people focus on comprehensive thinking and take it as a whole. To put it more popularly, in clinical practice, western doctors tend to analyze and study the exact region where a disease is or to take stopgap measures, however, Chinese medical workers will take the overall condition of a patient into consideration and make an overall analysis based on the comprehensive inspection, not just by examining and analyzing the specific region of the disease. Abstractly speaking, oriental comprehensive thinking mode is featured by the concept of holism on the basis of universal connection among things, while western analytical thinking is just the opposite." Professor Ji here talks about the issue of thinking mode, which is also a question of way of thinking. His words can be used to look at the difference between TCM and Western medicine, which is very important to understand the theory of TCM and its clinical practice. Those who do not understand TCM tend to criticize it. The correct way for them is to sit down to read a little more carefully about TCM and experience its curative effect themselves before they express their opinions, including criticism. As long as they are well-meant, TCM practitioners would be happy to accept, and they would even make some improvement according to the critical suggestions.

三 / III

中医对疾病的认识是从整体观念出发的。整体观念是一种哲学理念，认为人与大自然是息息相通的，人的生理、病理受到大自然的制约，当然也得到大自然的滋养与恩赐。另外，人的内环境也是息息相通的，脏腑经络之间互为利用、互为制约，维持着生理的相对平衡。如果某一脏腑有了病，它必然影响到其他脏器，例如肺热咳嗽，不单单是肺脏的病变，很可能是肝经燥热刑罚于肺产生的，中医名为"木火刑金"；也可能是大肠燥热引起的，因为肺与大肠相表里，由此而发作咳嗽，中医名为"腑病及脏"。而一年四季所发生的感冒，中医还要与四季的气候变化联系起来，中医将一年四季气候的变化称为"五运六气"，只有明了五运六气的变化，才能对不同季节的感冒提出正确的治疗方案。如果脱离了整体观念，孤零零地去"看病"，那只能是"头痛医头，脚痛医脚"了。

According to TCM, the recognition of a particular disease is based on a philosophy concept, holism, which holds that human being and the nature are closely connected, the physiological and pathological conditions of a person's body are regulated by the nature, therefore, he, in turn, is nurtured by it. Besides, all parts of a person's internal environment are closely connected, too. The zang-fu organs, meridians and collaterals are mutually utilized and restricted, maintaining a relative physiological balance. If there is something wrong with a patient's zang or fu organ, other viscera will inevitably be affected. For instance, lung heat may give rise to cough. However, it is not only some pathological changes of the lung, it is more likely caused by dryness and heat in liver meridian impairing the lung, which is known as "wood-fire (fire in the liver) impairing metal (the lung)" in TCM terminology. Or maybe the disease is due to dryness and heat in the large intestine, for the lung and large intestine are external-internally connected, accordingly, cough with the above pathogenesis is named as "fu-disease involving zang viscus". When a patient catches colds in different seasons of a year, TCM practitioners should connect the causes with seasonal climate changes, which are known as "five phases' motion and six natural factors" in TCM. Only by grasping their regular changes, can a TCM doctor acquire the correct treating plan. If his diagnosis and treating plan are not based on the concept of holism, that is, if a doctor does not relate a patient's symptoms to the changes of natural climate, his prescription would be partial, incorrect and lack of overall analysis.

由上可以知道，中医对疾病的认识，是从三个方面去考虑的，即天、地、人，古人称为"三才"。就是以"人"为中心，并考虑到天时、地利，以及疾病谱的变化，这种将人放在大自然中去考虑的医学，就是整体的、动态的、辩证的。所以中医对某一疾病的治疗，多数是一人一方，一证一方，而不是用一个方子去治疗多个人的疾病。这就是中医学"因人而异""因时而异""因地而异"的三因学说。

From the above analysis, a conclusion can be reached that the understanding of a particular disease in terms of TCM is based upon an overall consideration of three aspects, i. e., the heaven, the earth and man (the "three talents" named by ancient Chinese). Among them, man is the focus, and changes in climate, geographical position as well as disease spectrum should be taken into account. The medicine that place man in the nature is overall, dynamic and dialectic. Therefore, in most cases, due to the particular disease conditions as well as individual feature of different patients, a TCM practitioner's treatment of a certain disease in one patient differs from that of the disease in another. Exactly speaking, one treating plan is in accordance with one patient, or with one specific syndrome. It is absolutely impossible for a doctor to use one prescription to cure many patients' diseases. This is the so-called principle of three categories of etiologic factors, namely, "applying proper therapeutic methods based on individuality, time, as well as regions of a disease".

四 / IV

中医对疾病的治疗，非常重视"三因学说"，尤其重视"因人而异"。所谓"因人而异"，就是重视人的个体化，包括人的性别、年龄、体型、性格、职业、家庭环境、文化水平、饮食习惯、个人爱好等，这些因素综合起来叫作"体质"因素，它对疾病的发生与转化都有直接或间接的影响，同时，对疾病治疗的效果也有一定的影响。

As far as TCM therapeutic measure is concerned, great importance is attached to "the principle of three categories of etiologic factors", with particular emphasis on "applying proper therapeutic methods based on individuality", which means, in treating a patient's disease, special attention should be paid to his individuality, including his gender, age, physical build, personality, profession, family background, education, dietary habits, hobbies and so on. These are collectively called "physique" factor. Directly or indirectly, it affects the occurrence, development and changes of a disease. Simultaneously, it will definitely exert an influence on the curative effect for a disease to some extent.

《黄帝内经》对于人的体质与性格的划分就有 25 种之多。经过中医学家多年的研究，现在对中国人体质的划分提出了新的观点和划分方法，这就是王琦教授的"九种体质划分法"，即平和体质、阳虚体质、阴虚体质、气虚体质、痰湿体质、湿热体质、血瘀体质、气郁体质、特禀体质等。

According to *Huangdi Neijng*, constitution and character of mankind can be divided into 25 types. Recently, after many years of research, some Chinese medical scholars have proposed a new point of view on the division of Chinese people's physique, which is Professor Wang Qi's "classification of nine types of basic constitutions", namely, yin-yang balance, yang asthenia, yin asthenia, qi asthenia, phlegm-dampness, damp-heat, blood stasis, qi stagnation and allergic constitution.

王琦教授通过对全国 2 万多例调查结果的分析，发现各种体质均与亚健康状态关系密切。疼痛型亚健康状态与阳虚体质、湿热体质、血瘀体质呈正相关，早衰型亚健康状态与阳虚体质、痰湿体质呈正相关，疲劳型亚健康状态与气虚体质、湿热体质、气郁体质呈正相关，心理型亚健康状态与气虚体质、阴虚体质、气郁体质呈正相关。

Through analyzing the survey result of 20 000 cases across the country, Professor Wang

Qi's research shows that various types of body constitution are closely related to the states of sub-health. Exactly speaking, state of sub-health of pain is positively related to the types of constitution of yang asthenia, damp-heat and blood stasis. State of sub-health of premature senility has a positive correlation to the types of physique of yang asthenia and phlegm-dampness. State of sub-health due to fatigue is positively connected with constitution of qi asthenia, damp-heat and qi stagnation and psychological sub-health state is positively associated with qi asthenia, yin asthenia, and qi stagnation constitution.

这些研究说明，体质不同，所表现的体征与症状也不相同，这就为治疗提供了很重要的一个前提。例如同样患高血压病，一个人是痰湿体质，一个人是阴虚体质，他们所呈现出的症候就决然不会一样，医生所拟定的治疗措施也是有区别的，前者宜祛湿化痰，后者宜滋阴补肾，但他们的治疗结果是殊途同归的。如果医生在治疗的时候，对病人的体质不管不问，只看重药物的效应，那么治疗结果就可能会南辕北辙，达不到预期的效果，这是被无数事实所证明了的。

The study indicates that diversity in patients' physical conditions and manifestations is attributed to difference in their constitution, which provides an important prerequisite for treating diseases. For instance, there are two patients suffering from hypertension, one has the constitution of phlegm-dampness, while the other's physique is yin asthenia. The syndrome and symptoms that the former manifests is definitely different from those of the latter, accordingly their doctor should take different therapeutic measures. To the former, he can adopt eliminating dampness and resolving phlegm, while the prescription to the latter should be nourishing yin and replenishing kidney. The same treating result can be achieved by using different prescriptions. In the process of treating, if a doctor only takes the curative effect of medication, rather than his patients' individual constitution into account, the results would be the opposite, and the expected curative effect couldn't be achieved, which has been proved by numerous medical cases.

五 / V

中医是否排斥西医呢？中医历来都是开放性的，中医不但不排斥西医，而且还吸取西医的科学部分，充实自己的理论与临床。许多中医医生在坚持中医理论与临床技能的基础上，从微观上用现代科学检查手段来为临床服务，诸如生化检查、CT、核磁共振、彩超等；有些难以治疗的疾病，还请西医医生会诊；在理论上也重视微观方面的诊断方法。中医专业或科普著作中，也不断地吸取着现代科学新技术。

Does TCM repulse Western medicine? The answer is definitely no. TCM has been open-minded since its beginning. It does not repel Western medicine, instead, it absorbs the reasonable and scientific parts of Western medicine to enrich its own theoretical system and guide its clinical practice. On the basis of adhering to the theory and clinical skills of TCM, to help them make clinical diagnosis and treatment, quite a lot of TCM practitioners make use of modern and scientific inspecting methods at the microscopic level, such as biochemical examination, CT, NMR imaging (nuclear magnetic resonance examination) and Color Doppler Ultrasonography. Sometimes, to some diseases that are difficult to treat, they will probably invite some of his colleagues specialized in Western medicine to hold a consultation. Theoretically, great importance has been attached to diagnostic methods at microscopic level. What's more, the advanced knowledge of science and technology has been absorbed in a great number of TCM works and books of science popularization.

中国的卫生事业发展方针是中医、西医、中西医结合并重，这说明这三种医学都有其长，但也各有其短。在发展过程中，只有吸取其他医学的长处，弥补自己的不足，才能使三者有所进步，有所发展，才能满足人民群众的需要。

The guideline for developing Chinese medical cause is "to integrate TCM with Western medicine" and to "attach equal stress to TCM and Western medicine, and integration of TCM with Western medicine", which shows that the three have their own advantages as well as disadvantages. In promoting the development of TCM, only by learning the strengths of other medicine, can Chinese medical practitioners make up the weakness of TCM. And only in this way could great progress be made in the three fields and the medical needs of the public could be truly met.

自改革开放以来，许多外国人来我国学习中医药知识，他们同时也带来了多样的文化与文明，带来了新的科学技术手段，带来了新的思维方式，为中医药科学技术注入了新的活力。

Since the reform and opening-up, countless foreign scholars come to China to learn Chinese medicine. With them, they have brought their own splendid culture and civilization, advanced scientific technology and new thinking modes. In the meantime, they have injected new vigor and vitality into Chinese medical science and technology.

作为一位中医医生，我愿意将自己数十年的临床经验和中医基本知识奉献给世界各国朋友，希望他们在学习的过程中，从中得到启发和受益，共同为人类的卫生保健事业做出贡献！

As a professional TCM practitioner, I would like to dedicate my knowledge on TCM and clinical experience collected over decades to friends from all over the world in the hope that they could get some inspiration and benefit from their learning and make their devotion to the medical cause and well-beings of mankind！

上篇　中医诊断

Section A　Diagnostics of TCM

第一章 四诊

1 Four diagnostic methods of TCM

一、望诊

1.1 Inspection

望诊是诊断的第一步。当医生与病人接触时，首先看到的是病人的神色与形态的反常变化，从而可以获得一些疾病的初步印象。望诊的范围包括病人的形体、动态、神气、色泽，以及排泄物与分泌物等。特别是面部的神色与舌苔的变化，在诊断上具有非常重要的意义。

Inspection is the first of the four diagnostic methods of TCM. When a doctor meets a patient, he examines the abnormal manifestation of the patient's facial expression and body shape so as to acquire the preliminary condition about the patient's illness. Generally speaking, inspection includes body shape, behavior, spirit, as well as the color, texture of excreta and secretion. It is of great importance for a doctor to examine change of a patient's complexion and that of tongue fur to ensure a correct and proper diagnosis of a disease.

（一）全身望诊

1.1.1 Inspection of the whole body

1. 望神气

1.1.1.1 Inspection of spirit

神，是指神气、神志。从神的盛衰，可以看出病情的轻重和预后的好坏。"得神者昌，失神者亡"。

安静：病在阴（血）。

爽朗：病在阳（气）。

烦躁不安：见于热性病或神气将要消亡之时。

呆钝郁闷：见于情志病或抑郁症。

恍惚：神识似清非清，似明非明，难以捉摸，为气血津液亏亡之象。

疲惫：见于大病后，或心肾亏虚，或胃虚不纳。

昏聩：神识不清，心中闷乱，为热邪传入心包之象。

Spirit refers to the state and manner of a person's mental activities. By examining spirit, a doctor can conclude whether the healthy qi of his patient is exuberant or deficient, the pathological condition is serious or unserious and the prognosis is benign or malignant. That is the so-called "he whose spirit is present can be cured, and he who lacks of spirit is incurable and bound to die".

Tranquil or quiet state of a patient suggests diseases are of yin nature (involving blood).

Frank or cheerful state of a patient indicates diseases are of yang nature (involving qi).

Agitated state or restlessness usually indicates a heat syndrome, or depletion of vitality.

Dull and retarded or depressed state shows emotional upset or melancholia.

State of trance indicates that a patient is now mentally conscious and then unconsciousness, suggesting consumption or depletion of qi, blood, and body fluid.

Fatigue usually occurs after a serious disease, or caused by asthenia of the heart and kidney or by failure of asthenic stomach to receive.

Confused mentality refers to unconsciousness and depression, a sign of pathogenic invasion of heat into the pericardium.

2. 望形态

1.1.1.2 Inspection of body shape

形态是指病人体质的强弱与病人的动态，这对了解病人的抗病能力与预测疾病的转归非常重要。

肥胖：肥胖形体多有湿邪，多气虚，易患中风。

消瘦：消瘦形体多阴血不足，易见虚火症状，多患劳嗽。

项强：为太阳经病，或痉病，落枕。

偏枯：即半身不遂，为中风后遗症。

瘛疭：手足相引，一伸一缩，多见于惊风或痉病。

震颤：为气血亏虚，经络不通之象。

浮肿：为心肾阳气虚弱、水湿停聚证。

瘰疬：为肝胆气滞血瘀、痰湿内结之兆。

瘿瘤：多为肝火伤及血脉，气血不能通畅所致。

口眼㖞斜：为中风常见症状。

（其他形体望诊在以下有关章节叙述。）

Body shape refers to the physical constitution and posture of a patient, which are particularly important to learn about the patient's disease resistance and sequelae of a disease.

Obesity indicates pathogenic dampness, qi asthenia and susceptibility to apoplexia.

Emaciation is due to deficiency of yin and blood, usually seen in the syndrome of internal exuberance of asthenic fire, with susceptibility to over-strained cough.

Stiff neck is a syndrome of taiyang meridian, or convulsive disease, or caused by improper sleeping postures.

Hemiplegia is also named "paralysis of half of the body", a sequelae of apoplexia.

Convulsive limbs refer to hand-foot coupling, or spasm of hands and feet. It is frequently seen in the syndrome of infantile convulsion or convulsive disease.

Tremor of limbs indicates deficiency of qi and blood, caused by obstruction of meridians and collaterals.

Facial dropsy is caused by deficient yang qi of the heart and kidney, a sign of internal retention of dampness.

Scrofula is usually caused by qi stagnation and blood stasis in the liver and gallbladder, a sign of internal accumulation of phlegmatic dampness.

Gall nodule is due to stagnation of qi and blood which gives rise to liver fire impairing blood vessels.

Facial paralysis is a common syndrome of apoplexia.

(Other symptoms will be introduced in the following chapters.)

（二）局部望诊
1.1.2 Inspection of regional body parts

1. 望头面
1.1.2.1 Inspection of head and face

（1）部位
阳明（胃与肠）主面部，额属心，左颊属肝，右颊属肺，鼻属脾，颏属肾。

（1）About regions
Yangming meridian (the stomach meridian of foot yangming and the large intestine meridian of hand yangming converge at the face and the head) travels through the face and head. Therefore, the forehead pertains to the heart, the left cheek to the liver, the right cheek to the lung, the nose to the spleen, and the chin to the kidney.

（2）形状
肿大：热毒攻面，如大头瘟、疔疮走黄、肾水肿、急性风水浮肿等。
囟凸：督脉火邪上攻。
囟凹：先天不足，脾肾气血虚弱。
囟门不合：肾气与脑髓不足。
摇头：年轻体壮者，为风火上攻；年老体弱之人，多为气血亏虚。

（2）About shapes of the head

Swollen head is due to heat toxicity attacking the face, which causes swellings and redness of some parts of the face, carbuncle complicated by septicemia, renal edema, and acute edema due to wind and dampness.

Protrusion of fontanel indicates pathogenic fire in the governor meridian attacking upwards to the head.

Sunken fontanel is caused by congenital insufficiency of brain marrow or asthenia of blood and qi in the spleen and kidney.

Non-closure of fontanel indicates congenital insufficiency of kidney qi and deficiency of brain marrow.

Involuntary shaking of head suggests up-attack of pathogenic wind and fire factors in young and strong patients, and deficiency of qi and blood in old and weak patients.

（3）面色

白色：为胃寒体质，主虚寒及气脱。如面有白点或白斑，为消化不良或腹中有虫积。

黄色：为湿，为热，为脾虚。色鲜明为热，色暗滞为湿伤脾胃，黄而枯瘦为胃火，黄而肥胖为胃中湿热。

赤色：面色缘缘而赤，为阳气怫郁在表；面色如醉，为胃热；午后颧赤，为阴虚火旺；面赤如妆，嫩红带白，为戴阳证（即浮阳上越）。

青色：为风，为寒，为痛，为气滞血瘀。小儿为惊风。胸胁腹痛，为肝气犯胃。小腹寒痛，男子为疝气，女子为痛经。

黑色：为寒，为痛，为瘀血。黑而带黄，为痰饮；鼃黑为女劳疸；苍黑而瘦，为五脏虚火。

（3）About complexion

Whitish complexion is due to constitutional asthenia and cold, indicating syndromes of asthenia and cold, as well as qi collapse, while white spots or leukasmus is caused by indigestion or parasitic infestation.

Yellowish complexion indicates syndromes of dampness, heat and asthenia of the spleen. Brightness suggests heat syndrome; dark and dull yellowish complexion reveals dampness impairing the spleen and stomach; sallow and emaciated complexion is due to stomach fire; yellow and facial edema is caused by dampness and heat in the stomach.

Flushed complexion signifies that yangming meridian runs through the face, causing stagnation of yang qi on the superficial, therefore, the complexion is flushed. Flushed complexion like drunkard's face is indicative of heat of the stomach; appearance of flushed zygomatic regions in the afternoon suggests exuberant fire resulting from yin asthenia; pale face with occasional migratory reddish luster like wearing makeup is the syndrome of "real cold and false heat" due to up-floating of yang.

Cyanotic complexion indicates wind, cold, pain, and syndrome of qi stagnation and blood stasis. Cyanotic complexion in infants is a syndrome of convulsion. Cyanotic complexion coupled with pain in the chest, hypochondrium and abdomen shows hyperactive liver qi invading the stomach. Cyanotic complexion with cold and pain over lower abdomen, in male patients, is a sign of hernia, and the complexion in female indicates dysmenorrhea (painful menstruation).

Blackish complexion indicates syndrome of cold, pain and blood stasis. Yellowish and blackish complexion is usually caused by retention of phlegm and fluid; darkish complexion is a sign of jaundice due to sexual intemperance; thin face with pale blackish complexion is due to asthenic fire in viscera.

2. 望毛发
1.1.2.2   Inspection of hair

（1）头发

发美润长：气血旺盛。

发白而落：气血俱亏。

发枯憔悴：气血衰竭。

发落如败絮：内热伤津。

发润如洗，头汗不止：并见喘症者，为肺气将脱之兆，病危。

（1）hair

Dense and lustrous hair suggests exuberance of qi and blood.

White and sparse hair indicates insufficiency of qi and blood.

Yellow, withered and brittle hair is a sign of exhaustion of qi and blood.

Sparse and even loss of hair like patches of worn-out cotton wadding of quilt shows that endogenous heat impairing body fluid.

Moistened hair like being washed with non-stopping sweating on the forehead, coupled with asthma is a precursor of collapse of lung qi, a critical and even dying pathological condition.

（2）髭须

生于上唇为髭，生于下颌者为须，生于两侧腮部者为髯。

髯美而长，黑如重漆：男子气血旺盛。

髭须转为黄白：气血衰少。

（2）Moustache and beard

Moustache is above the upper lip, while beard is in chin and in both cheeks.

Lustrous, dense and long beard like black paint shows exuberance of qi and blood in male.

Yellowish and whitish moustache and beard indicate declination of qi and blood.

（3）眉毛

忽生长毛：肝胆中血分有热。

眉毛脱落：为疠风的特征。

（3）Eyebrows

Sudden appearance of long eyebrow indicates pathogenic heat factors in blood phase of the liver and gallbladder.

Loss of eyebrow is a sign of pestilential wind （leprosy）.

（4）毫毛

毫毛乃指身体细小的体毛。

肥人毛疏，瘦人毛密。

毛色憔悴：肺气虚弱，津枯血少。

毫毛脱落：为疠风之兆。

下肢毫毛脱落：下肢将成肿胀之患。

（4）Vellus hair

Vellus hair refers to the soft hair on the surface of body.

Vellus hair in obese people is sparse, while thin people have thick vellus hair.

Dry and withered vellus hair is an indication of deficiency of lung qi and depletion of body fluid and scanty blood.

Loss of vellus hair is also a sign of leprosy.

Loss of vellus hair in lower limbs suggests swollen legs.

3. 望目

1.1.2.3　Inspection of the eyes

目为肝之窍，为五脏精华所注。目又为五脏分属之所，赤眦属心，白珠属肺，黑珠属肝，瞳子属肾，目胞属脾。

The eyes are the orifices connected with the liver, and all the visceral essence flows into eyes. An Eye is divided into five parts corresponding to the five-zang organs, namely, canthus pertains to the heart, the white of the eye to the lung, the black of the eye to the liver, pupil to the kidney, and eyelids to the spleen.

（1）神色

神光充足：为有神气。

神无光彩：为神气衰败。

白珠发黄：为黄疸病。

目赤肿痛：为肺肝热结。

目暗黑色：为内有干血。

（1）Color and spirit of the eyes

Abundant vitality and flexible expression of the eyes signify the presence of spirit and energy.

Dull and spiritless expression means declination of spirit and energy.

The white part of eyes changes into yellow color is a sign of jaundice.

Flushing and painful swelling of a whole eye shows stagnation of heat in the lung and liver.

Darkish eyes are caused by internal dry blood.

（2）形态

眼胞浮肿：为脾虚，或湿火上攻。

眦红而痛：为心与小肠经火邪上攻。

多泪：为肝经风热。

天吊：为肝风上扰。

睛定：为不治之症。若目睛微定，移时而动者，为痰浊内闭。

目瞑：眼睛不想睁开，为阴虚阳脱或将衄之兆。

直视：为热病惊风之象。

羞明：为肝经有余之热。

目斜视：主病惊风。

目窠浮肿：为脾经气虚，水病之始。

目开不合：为卒中病，为肝经绝。

瞳孔散大：为卒中病，主肾水不足。

（2）Shapes and postures of the eyes

Dropsy of the eyelids is a sign of spleen asthenia or up-attack of pathogenic dampness and fire.

Flushed and painful canthus（eye-corner）shows up-attack of pathogenic fire in heart and small intestine meridians.

Delacrimation is usually due to up-disturbance of wind and heat in liver meridian.

Up-straight and oblique staring posture of the eye is a sign of up-disturbance of liver wind.

Immobile and straight staring posture of the eye is indicative of incurable and fatal disease; slight fixation of the vision is usually caused by internal blockage of turbid phlegm.

Unwillingness to open the eyes is due to yin asthenia and yang collapse or a sign of nose bleeding.

Straight staring posture is a sign of convulsion due to heat syndrome.

Photophobia（abnormal fear of light or painful sensitiveness to light）shows surplus heat in liver meridian.

Oblique staring posture is connected with convulsion.

Dropsy of eye socket is caused by qi asthenia in spleen meridian, a precursor of edema.

Failure to close eyes is indicative of apoplexy（blood stroke）, a sign of declination of liver meridian.

Platycoria is also a sign of blood stroke resulting from insufficiency of kidney yin fluid.

4. 望鼻

1.1.2.4　Inspection of the nose

（1）色泽

鼻头色青：腹中痛，为寒证，特别怕冷者预后不良。

鼻头色黄：为大肠传导功能减退，大便艰难。

鼻色红赤：为风热。

鼻头色白：气虚或失血。

鼻头色黑：为虚劳，微黑有水气。

鼻色鲜明：体内有留饮。

鼻如烟煤：为阳毒热深。

（1）Color

Cyanotic nose tip is a syndrome of cold indicating abdominal pain, and severe cold sensation suggests a bad prognosis.

Yellowish nose tip usually indicates hypofunction of the large intestine in transportation, giving rise to difficulty in defecation.

Reddish nose is a sign of pathogenic wind and heat.

Whitish nose tip indicates qi asthenia or loss of blood.

Blackish nose tip is usually caused by a consumptive disease, while slight blackish nose tip is a sign of edema.

Brightness of the nose indicates prolonged fluid retention.

Nose with the color like bitumastic coal is a sign of yang toxin and superabundant heat.

（2）形态

鼻头肿大：邪气偏盛。

鼻翼煽动：肺热之甚。

鼻头坍陷：疠气所伤，或梅毒。

鼻流清涕：外感风寒。

鼻流浊涕：外感风热。

鼻头弯曲：中风，或鼻中隔偏曲。

鼻衄：热伤阳经之络。

（2）Shapes of nose

Swollen and enlarged nose tip indicates exuberance of pathogenic qi.

Flapping wings of nose is caused by exuberance of heat in the lung.

Sunken nose tip is caused by impairment of epidemic pathogenic factor or syphilis.

Stuffy nose with clear snivel is due to exogenous wind cold.

Stuffy nose with turbid snivel is due to exogenous wind heat.

Curved nose tip is indicative of wind stroke or deviated nasal septum.

Nasal hemorrhage（nose bleeding）suggests pathogenic heat impairing the collaterals of yang meridians.

5. 望耳

1.1.2.5 Inspection of the ears

（1）色泽

耳轮黄赤：为热病、风病。

耳轮青白：为虚寒证候。

耳轮黑色：为肾水亏虚。

耳轮青黑：为痛候。

耳轮枯润：耳轮焦干为下消；耳轮甲错为肠痈；耳轮枯燥无光者危，耳轮红润者生；耳轮薄黑者肾败。

（1）Color

Yellowish and reddish ears indicate heat and pathogenic wind syndrome.

Cyanotic and whitish ears are a syndrome of asthenia and cold.

Blackish ears indicate deficiency of kidney yin fluid.

Cyanotic and blackish ears are often seen in pain syndrome.

Dry and scorching ears signify lower consumptive thirst（diabetes involving the lower energizer）; squamous ears suggest acute appendicitis; dull, dry and lusterless ears are a precursor of death; reddish ears with moist luster signify health and vitality; thin and blackish ears suggest exhaustion of kidney essence.

（2）外形

聤耳：耳内分泌物增多，为热邪乘虚而入所致。

脓耳：多为手少阳三焦经、足厥阴肝经血虚，风热乘虚而入所致。

耳漏：是继发于聤耳的肝胆湿热证。

肿大：风热客于手少阳经所致。

萎缩：为营养不良候，或为恶候之兆。

（2）Shapes

Otopyorrhea is due to increased secretion of ears, caused by invasion of pathogenic heat because of asthenia.

Purulent ear indicates blood asthenia in triple energizer meridian of hand-shaoyang and liver meridian of foot-jueyin which causes invasion of pathogenic wind and heat.

Otorrhea is caused by damp heat in the liver and gallbladder resulting from prolonged otopyorrhea.

Swollen ears are caused by wind heat attacking hand-shaoyang meridian.

Atrophy of ears indicates malnutrition, or a premonitory sign of critical disease.

6. 望口唇

1.1.2.6　Inspection of lips

（1）色泽

口唇色白：为血虚，为肺病。

口唇红紫：为热病，为血瘀。

口唇红赤：为心病，为血热。

口唇青紫：为肝病，为阳虚寒凝。

口唇焦干：为脾热，为疳积。

口唇干裂：为血燥，为血亏。

口唇红润：为血气旺盛。

（1）Color and luster

Pale lips indicate blood asthenia, as well as lung disease.

Reddish and purple lips signify blood stasis and heat syndrome.

Flushed lips indicate heart disease and blood heat.

Cyanotic lips suggest liver disease, caused by deficiency of yang and coagulation of cold.

Parching or dry lips indicate heat of the spleen or malnutrition and indigestion.

Dry and fissured lips indicate dryness of blood or asthenia of blood.

Flushed and moist lips suggest blood exuberance in healthy people.

（2）形态

口噤不开：为中风，为痉厥。

口张不合：为中风心绝，为痉病神昏状，为中暑热极症。

撮口：小儿口撮如囊，不能吃乳，为脐风症状之一，为胎热所致。

口糜：口腔糜烂，为心脾湿热所致。

唇肿：为脾热所致，一般见于温热病。

唇揭：唇皮揭起，多因过食酸性食物所致，或久寒而致。

唇裂：温燥病引起。

唇瞤动：唇口蠕动不禁，多为风病或脾虚不能收敛所致。

口疮：为心脾积热。

口歪：中风症状之一。

鹅口：满口白斑如雪片，为胎中热毒。

（2）Shapes

Difficulty in opening mouth is seen in apoplexy or syncope with convulsion.

Failure to close mouth indicates heart exhaustion due to apoplexy, or loss of consciousness due to convulsion, or summer-heat stroke.

Failure to suck milk in infants is locked jaw, a syndrome of neonatal tetanus, caused by fetal fever.

Aphthous stomatitis is often caused by accumulation of dampness and heat in the heart and spleen.

Swollen lips are often seen in warm（seasonal febrile）disease due to heat in the spleen.

Torn-off lips refer to lips that are like being torn off，caused by excess intake of acid food or by prolonged cold.

Harelip（cleft lip）is caused by warm-dryness disease.

Lip muscular twitching indicates wind syndrome，or failure of asthenic spleen to astringe the lips.

Aphtha or sore of the mouth is caused by accumulated heat in the heart and spleen.

Deviated mouth is one of the syndromes of apoplexy.

Infantile thrush（white patches on the buccal mucosa and tongue）is caused by heat toxin during the fetal stage.

7. 望齿与齿龈
1.1.2.7 Inspection of teeth and gums

（1）色泽
齿黑：肾热之极。
齿如枯骨：肾阴涸竭。
齿龈色浅：失血过多。
齿龈色紫：热毒偏盛。
齿龈色青：为铅毒之象。
齿龈焦枯：阴液亏虚。
齿龈有垢：肾虚火旺。
齿龈无津：上齿龈无津为胃络热极，下齿龈燥为肠络热极。前板齿燥为胃热或中暑。

（1）Color and luster

Blackish teeth are caused by superabundance of heat in the kidney.

Dull pale teeth like withered bone indicate consumption of kidney yin.

Pale gums are indicative of excess loss of blood.

Purplish gums are caused by exuberant heat toxin.

Cyanotic gums indicate lead poisoning.

Dry and withered gums are caused by deficient yin fluid.

Stained gums suggest hyperactive fire due to kidney asthenia.

Upper gums without saliva indicate extreme heat in stomach collaterals；lower gums without saliva are indicative of extreme heat in bowel collaterals；dryness of the front dental plate is a sign of heat in the stomach or heat stroke.

（2）形态
龄齿：即齿相击噤。为风痰阻络，热化作痉证，但虫积、胃虚、阴虚亦可见到。

齿龈红肿：主胃热。

龋齿：初期牙龈肿痛，遇风痛甚，继而牙龈腐孔，时出臭脓，久则龈齿宣露。多为风热客于胃肠，或小儿疳积所致。

牙疳：即见牙床腐烂，牙齿脱落，口臭血出，穿腮蚀唇，多因温热积滞，宿食久停，或小儿元气虚弱，火邪上腐，或是痘疹余毒所致。

牙龈出血：红肿而痛者为胃火，不红肿而齿痛者为肾火。

（2）Shapes

Grinding of teeth indicates obstruction of wind-phlegm in collaterals, a syndrome of transformation of pathogenic heat into convulsion. It can also be caused by malnutrition due to parasitic infestation, or by stomach asthenia, or by yin asthenia.

Reddish and swollen gums are caused by stomach heat.

Dental caries (or decayed teeth) refer to a syndrome, which, at the beginning, gums are swollen and painful, more painful when exposed in wind, gingival rotten holes arise with frequent foul pus, over time, gums and teeth are unconnected. It is often caused by pathogenic wind-heat invading the stomach and intestines, or by infantile malnutrition and indigestion.

Gingival malnutrition is a syndrome with symptoms as decayed gums, loss of teeth, halitosis and bleeding, and rotten cheeks and erosion of lips. It is caused by accumulation of epidemic febrile pathogens, prolonged food retention, or by deficiency of primordial qi in infants, which causes up-attack of pathogenic fire, or by remained toxicity of vaccinid.

Swollen and painful bleeding gums indicate stomach fire; painful bleeding gums without swelling are a sign of fire in the kidney.

8. 望咽喉
1.1.2.8　Inspection of the throat

（1）色泽

色殷红：为实热。

色粉淡：为虚寒。

（1）Color

Dark reddish throat is a syndrome of sthenia and heat.

Light pinkish throat is a syndrome of asthenia and cold.

（2）形态

红肿高凸：为实热。

红肿不甚：为虚寒。

乳蛾：即咽部两侧肉肿起（扁桃体肿大），为火热内蕴。

白腐：见于白喉。

（2）Shapes

Reddish swollen and protruding throat is caused by sthenic heat.

Light reddish throat with slight swellings is a syndrome of asthenic cold.

Bilateral reddish lumps like mastoid process (namely, swelling tonsil) are due to internal retention of pathogenic fire and heat.

Whitish membrane or rot on the throat is a syndrome seen in diphtheria.

9. 望舌
1.1.2.9 Inspection of tongue body (figure)

（1）部位

舌尖属心，舌边（四畔）属脾，舌根属肾，舌两旁属肝胆（左边属肝，右边属胆），舌心属胃。

（1）Area

The tip of the tongue pertains to the heart (so it can reflect pathogenic changes of the heart); the margins (the four banks) of the tongue pertain to the spleen (so it can reflect pathogenic changes of the spleen); the root of the tongue is connected with the kidney (so it can reflect pathogenic changes of the kidney); the left edge of the tongue corresponds to the liver (so it can reflect pathological changes of the liver), and the right edge corresponds to the gallbladder (therefore, it can reflect pathological changes of the gallbladder); and the center of the tongue corresponds to the stomach (so it can reflect pathological changes of the stomach).

（2）舌质

（2）Color

1）红舌质

淡红无苔：心脾气血亏虚。

舌质鲜红：外感病为热盛，虚劳病为阴虚火旺。

舌尖独红：心火上炎。

舌边红赤：肝热。

舌心干红：阴虚内热。

舌光红无津（镜面舌）：阴液内耗之象。

舌红中间有紫斑：温病发斑之兆。

1）Reddish tongue

Pale reddish tongue without tongue fur is a sign of deficiency of qi and blood in the heart and spleen.

Bright reddish tongue suggests superabundant heat due to exogenous pathogenic factors, or consumptive disease due to yin asthenia and hyperactivity of fire.

Reddish tongue tip indicates up-flaring of heart fire.

Flushed tongue margins indicate heat in the liver.

Dry and reddish color in the centre of the tongue is a sign of yin asthenia due to endogenous heat.

Reddish tongue without fluid (also known as "mirror-like tongue") is a sign of consumption of yin-fluid.

Reddish tongue with purplish spots in the center is indicative of generation of suggillation because of seasonal febrile disease.

2）紫舌质

舌紫而肿大：因嗜酒而酒毒冲心。

舌紫晦暗：内有瘀血蓄积。

舌紫而中心有白苔：酒后伤寒。

青紫滑润：属阴证，为寒邪直中肝肾。

舌紫而苔黄干燥：脏腑蕴热，脾胃尤甚。

2）Purplish tongue

Purplish and swollen tongue is caused by alcoholic toxin attacking the heart.

Dark purplish tongue is a sign of internal accumulation of blood stasis.

Purplish tongue with whitish tongue fur in the center suggests exogenous febrile disease after drinking.

Cyanotic, purplish and slippery tongue with moist fur is a yin syndrome, caused by invasion of pathogenic cold into the liver and kidney.

Purplish tongue with dry and yellowish fur is due to heat accumulation in the viscera, in particular, in the spleen and stomach.

3）绛舌质

绛舌：热病传营。

绛舌兼黄白苔：邪热入营，但未完全脱离气分。

舌质纯绛而润泽：包络受邪。

舌绛而中心干燥：心胃火燔，津液被灼。

舌尖独绛：心火独盛。

舌绛而附有垢腻：营分蕴热而中夹秽浊之气。

舌绛而有大红点：为热毒乘心。

舌绛而光亮：胃阴已亡。

舌绛，干枯而萎：肾阴已涸。

舌绛，有散在的黄白苔：生疳之兆。

舌绛，望之干而扪之有津：为津亏而湿热熏蒸，将成痰浊蒙蔽心窍之象。

3）Deep-reddish tongue

Deep-reddish tongue indicates transmission of pathogenic febrile factors into nutrient phase.

Deep-reddish tongue with yellow and white fur indicates pathogenic febrile factors invading nutrient phase, but they have not been free from qi phase completely.

Pure deep-reddish tongue with moisture indicates pathogenic febrile factors invading collaterals of the pericardium.

Deep-reddish tongue with dryness in the center indicates exuberant fire in the heart and stomach scorching yin fluid.

Deep-reddish tongue tip is a sign of hyperactive fire in the heart.

Deep-reddish tongue with greasy dirt indicates accumulation of heat in nutrient phase coupled with foul and turbid qi.

Deep-reddish tongue with big and reddish spots suggests heat toxin attacking the heart.

Deep-reddish tongue with bright luster is a sign of depletion of stomach yin.

Dry and withered deep-reddish tongue indicates consumption of kidney yin.

Deep-reddish tongue with scattered yellow and white tongue fur is a sign of malnutrition.

Dry deep-reddish tongue with fluid when pressing indicates fumigation of damp heat as well as fluid consumption, a sign of turbid phlegm blocking the orifice of the heart.

4）蓝舌质

舌蓝生苔：脏腑损伤未甚。

舌蓝无苔：属气血亏极，难以治疗。

舌苔白腻中见蓝色：阴邪化热。

舌蓝较微：为湿热不解，或为湿痰作祟。

4）Bluish tongue

Bluish tongue with fur shows slight impairment of zang-fu organs.

Bluish tongue without fur indicates depletion of qi and blood, an incurable syndrome.

Bluish tongue with white greasy fur is caused by transformation of heat from pathogenic yin factors.

Light bluish tongue is a sign of unrelieved stagnation of dampness and heat, or caused by damp phlegm.

5）青舌质

舌面如水牛之舌：阴寒邪盛，阳气郁滞，血脉凝滞。

全舌青者：寒邪直中肝肾，阳郁不宣。

舌边青者：口燥漱水不欲咽，是内有瘀血。

5）Cyanotic tongue

The surface of the tongue like that of a water buffalo suggests exuberance of pathogenic yin cold, giving rise to stagnation of yang qi and obstructed blood vessel.

Cyanotic coloration over the whole tongue is a sign of pathogenic cold invading the liver and kidney, resulting in failure to disperse stagnated yang qi.

Cyanotic tongue margins with no desire to drink, though the mouth is dry indicates internal blood stasis, causing the patient to have a sensation of gargling.

（3）舌形

老嫩：舌形坚敛苍老，纹理粗糙，为实证；舌形浮胖娇嫩，纹理细腻，为虚证。

肿胀：舌体肿大，自觉盈口满嘴，多为痰浊、水湿或湿热上蕴。

薄瘦：多因气血阴液不足，或阴虚火旺所致。

胖大：属于气虚湿阻证。

芒刺：舌生芒刺为热邪内结。

重舌：舌下血络肿起，好像生一小舌，为重舌。为心火旺盛而致。

卷缩：舌卷囊缩，病入厥阴，为危候。

僵硬：为中风主要症状之一。

齿痕：为脾虚湿盛之象。

伸长：伸长而偏，为中风偏枯；伸缩无力，为元气大虚；时欲将舌伸出口外，为内热惊风之象。

弄舌吐舌：多见于小儿，为心脾热结。

舌体抖颤：舌体颤动不已，为肝风；舌颤难以说话者，为心脾气虚。

舌下络脉：将舌翘起，舌系带两侧可见隐隐络脉（即舌下静脉），当金津玉液处。正常情况下，络脉不粗，两侧无明显分支或球状脉络。若络脉青紫，或有许多颗粒状脉络球，即为心脉瘀阻、气滞血瘀的征象。

（3）Shapes of the tongue

Rough tongue marked by rough or curved texture is sthenia syndrome; while tender, bulgy tongue with fine texture indicates asthenia syndrome.

Swollen tongue with a sensation of filling up the whole mouth is caused by turbid phlegm, dampness or up-invasion of dampness-heat.

Thin and emaciated tongue is caused by insufficiency of qi, blood, and yin fluid, or yin asthenia and exuberant fire.

Enlarged tongue suggests qi asthenia and retention of dampness.

Prickly tongue is caused by internal accumulation of pathogenic heat.

Double tongue refers to swelling of sublingual vessels which feels like another little tongue. It is caused by exuberance of heart fire.

Contracted tongue refers to curled or shrunk tongue body, indicating the disease is in jueyin meridian, a very critical condition.

Stiffness of the tongue is a leading symptom of apoplexy.

Teeth-marked tongue is a sign of spleen asthenia and exuberant dampness.

Protruding tongue which deviates sideways is a sign of hemiplegia due to apoplexy; weak and flaccid tongue is due to failure of weak primordial qi to stretch the tongue and draw it back; the condition that the tongue frequently protrudes out indicates convulsion due to endogenous heat.

Protruding and wagging tongue is often seen in infants, caused by heat accumulation in the heart and spleen.

Involuntary shivering tongue indicates endogenous liver wind; frequent shivering tongue causes difficulty to speak, suggesting qi asthenia in the heart and spleen.

The condition of collaterals beneath the tongue: When lifting up the tongue, just in position of the points of Jinjin and Yuye, sublingual veins on both side of the lingual frenum could be seen unclearly. Thin collaterals without obvious branches nor spherical blood vessels signify normal tongue. Cyanotic and purplish collaterals, or with lots of granular spherical blood vessels suggest obstruction of heart vessels, or an indication of qi stagnation and blood stasis.

（4）舌苔

（4）Inspection of tongue fur

1）白苔

白苔病在卫分、气分，主病为表、为湿、为寒。

薄白而滑：外感风寒。

白滑黏腻：内有痰湿。

白中带黄：邪将传里。

白苔绛底：湿遏热伏。

白苔边红：风温犯肺。

白如积粉：温毒秽浊。

白苔如碱：胃中有宿滞，夹有秽浊郁伏。

尖白根黄：邪已入里，表证未罢。

苔白而厚，无津而燥：脾胃实热。

苔白嫩滑，刮之明净：为虚寒证。

1）Whitish tongue fur

Whitish tongue fur suggests that the disease is in qi phase and defensive phase, indicative of external, damp and cold syndrome.

Thin whitish and slippery tongue fur indicates the syndrome of exogenous wind cold.

Slippery sticky and greasy whitish tongue fur indicates internal damp phlegm.

Whitish and yellowish tongue fur suggests pathogenic factors are transmitting from the exterior to the interior.

Whitish tongue fur with deep-reddish color on the bottom of the tongue suggests retention of heat and blockage of dampness.

Whitish tongue fur with red margins suggests pathogenic wind and febrile factors invading the lung.

Powder-like thick and whitish tongue fur is caused by mixture of exogenous fetid pathogenic factors with warm toxin.

Whitish tongue fur like alkali suggests dyspepsia in the stomach, accompanied with retention of exogenous fetid pathogenic factors.

Whitish tongue tip with yellow tongue root indicates transmission of pathogenic factors from the exterior to the interior, however, the external syndrome is unrelieved.

Thick dry and whitish tongue fur without fluids is a sign of sthenic heat in the spleen and stomach.

Tender, slippery and whitish tongue fur which can be easily removed, indicates syndrome of asthenic cold.

2）黄苔

黄苔病在气分，主里病、热病、实证。

苔薄黄而润：表邪入里。

苔黄而干：内火炽盛。

苔黄而厚：阳明（胃肠）实热证。

舌苔微黄而不燥：邪将传里之象。

舌苔深黄而滑腻：湿热蕴结于中。

舌苔黄燥而生芒刺：里热已极，气阴耗竭。

苔黄而燥，舌质红赤：温毒已入营分。

2）Yellowish tongue fur

Yellowish tongue fur indicates internal, heat and sthenia syndrome, and the disease is in qi phase.

Moist, thin and yellowish tongue fur suggests transmission of pathogenic factors from the exterior into the interior.

Dry and yellowish tongue fur indicates exuberance of endogenous fire.

Thick and yellowish tongue fur indicates sthenic heat in yangming meridian (the stomach meridian of foot-yangming and the large intestine of hand-yangming).

Slight yellowish tongue fur without dryness shows transmission of pathogenic factors from the exterior into the interior.

Slippery and greasy dark-yellowish tongue fur indicates the internal accumulation of damp-heat.

Dry, yellowish and prickly tongue fur indicates extreme endogenous heat and consumption of qi and yin.

Reddish tongue with dry and yellowish tongue fur indicates transmission of epidemic febrile toxin into nutrient phase.

3）灰苔

灰苔主湿，但亦有热象。

苔灰黑而干：为热证、实证。

苔灰黑而滑润：为寒水侮土，脾经中寒证。

苔灰而润，中有点状墨汁苔：邪热传里而夹有宿食。

3）Grayish tongue fur

Grayish tongue fur indicates dampness, but sometimes it is also complicated with a sign of heat syndrome.

Dry and grayish and blackish tongue fur suggests heat and sthenia syndrome.

Greasy, moist, grayish and blackish tongue fur signifies splenic cold syndrome due to cold water (cold in the kidney) reversely restricting earth (the spleen).

Moist and grayish tongue fur with patches like dark ink in center indicates transmission of external pathogenic factors into the interior complicated with food retention.

4）黑苔

黑苔主湿病、热病和寒病。

白苔中心变黑：伤寒邪热传里。

红苔中心变黑：湿热瘟疫传里，坏病之兆。

舌苔黑而燥裂：温热病邪热炽盛，热灼津液。

舌苔黑而滑润：阳虚而阴寒盛。

苔根黑而燥：实热结于下焦，为急下存阴证。

苔黑滑润而腻：痰湿寒饮伤脾。

4）Blackish tongue fur

Blackish tongue fur suggests damp, heat as well as cold syndrome.

White tongue fur with its center changing into black shows transmission of pathogenic heat caused by exogenous febrile disease into the interior.

Reddish tongue fur with its center changing into black shows transmission of exogenous dampness and heat pathogens into the interior, a precursor of an increasingly worsening disease.

Dry, fissured and blackish tongue fur indicates pathogenic heat scorching body fluids due to transmission of superabundant exogenous febrile pathogen into the interior.

Slippery, moist and blackish tongue fur indicates exuberance of yin cold caused by yang asthenia.

Dry and blackish root of tongue fur indicates accumulation of sthenic heat in lower energizer (the zang-fu organs below the abdomen), a syndrome of emergent purgation to preserve yin.

Slippery, moist, greasy and blackish tongue fur suggests retention of cold and fluid due to damp phlegm which impairs the spleen.

（5）形态

厚苔：痰湿停滞。

薄苔：表邪未解。

腻苔：三焦秽浊之邪未化。

滑苔：停滞中焦。

滑润：津液未伤。

干燥：津液已伤。

腐腻：白腐为肺湿热熏蒸，黄腐为胃湿热熏蒸。

黏腻：湿热内结或痰浊停滞之象。

舌裂：为正气虚或阴津受伤。

白霉：满口糜烂发白，为腐浊之邪太重，难治。

花剥：舌苔一块一块地剥落，胃气难复。

（5）Shapes of tongue fur

Thick tongue fur indicates retention of damp phlegm.

Thin tongue fur is a sign of unrelieved superficial pathogenic factors.

Greasy tongue fur suggests failure to transform exogenous fetid pathogenic factors in triple energizers.

Slippery tongue fur suggests retention of damp phlegm in middle energizers.

Slippery and moist tongue fur indicates that body fluid has not been impaired.

Dry tongue fur is a sign of impairment of body fluid.

Whitish, putrid and greasy tongue fur is caused by fumigation of dampness and heat in the lung; while yellowish, putrid and greasy fur is caused by fumigation of dampness and heat in the stomach.

Sticky, greasy tongue fur is caused by internal accumulation of damp-heat or stagnation of turbid phlegm.

Fissured tongue is caused by asthenia of healthy qi or impairment of yin fluid.

Erosive tongue with white mold all over the mouth is caused by excess pathogenic erosive and turbid factors, a sign of incurable syndrome.

Patchy-peeled tongue fur indicates difficulty in restoring stomach qi.

10. 望痰

1.1.2.10 Inspection of sputum

痰是由肺与气道排出的黏液，其稠而浊者为痰，清而稀者为饮。

Sputum is sticky fluid excreted from the lung and the trachea. The thick and turbid sputum is called "phlegm", while the thin and clear sputum is "fluid".

（1）颜色

色黄：主热病。色黄而稠，主火；色黄而干燥，主热病伤阴。

色白：主寒湿病。色白而润，主湿病；色白而清稀，主水饮。

痰中带血：急性病为热伤肺络，火有余；慢性病为虚火内炎，阴不足。

（1）Color of sputum

Yellowish sputum indicates heat syndrome. Yellowish and sticky sputum is caused by pathogenic fire, while the yellowish and dry sputum indicates pathogenic heat factors impairing yin.

Whitish sputum indicates syndrome of cold and dampness. White and moist sputum indicates dampness syndrome; white, thin and clear sputum suggests fluid retention.

Sputum mingled with blood in acute diseases means heat impairing pulmonary collaterals due to exuberant fire; in chronic diseases, it means asthenic fire flaming internally due to insufficiency of yin.

（2）痰量

痰量多者为实证，痰量少者为虚证。

（2）Volume of sputum

Profuse sputum is a sign of sthenia syndrome, while scanty sputum is a sign of asthenia syndrome.

（3）形状

稠痰：稠黏而呈块状的，为热痰。

稀痰：稀白而呈液状的，为寒痰。

块状痰：痰呈块状胶结难化的，为热痰；色黄呈块状的，为热结；色白呈块状的，为湿痰。

泡沫痰：稀薄而有水泡沫样的，为风痰。

脓血痰：血痰为肺热，脓痰为肺痈。

（3）Shapes of sputum

Thick, sticky and coagulated sputum indicates heat phlegm.

Whitish, thin and uncoagulated sputum is cold phlegm.

Hard and coagulated sputum with difficulty to resolve indicates heat phlegm, yellowish and coagulated sputum is accumulation of heat, while whitish and coagulated sputum is indicative of damp phlegm.

Thin and frothy sputum is due to wind phlegm.

Sputum mingled with blood results from lung heat, while purulent sputum indicates pulmonary abscess.

11. 望涎与唾

1.1.2.11 Inspection of saliva and spittle

口流清涎：脾冷。

口吐黏液：脾经湿热。

口角流涎，睡则更甚：脾虚不能收摄；亦见于小儿胃热虫积。

口吐唾沫：胃中有寒，亦见于肾寒。

Thin and clear saliva from the mouth indicates cold in the spleen.

Sticky saliva suggests dampness and heat in spleen meridian.

More saliva drooling from the corner of the mouth during sleep is due to failure of asthenic spleen to control fluid, or due to heat in the stomach or parasitic malnutrition in infants.

Frothy spittle from the mouth suggests cold in the stomach or cold in the kidney.

12. 望呕吐物
1.1.2.12 Inspection of vomitus

呕吐物有饮食物、清水、痰涎或脓血。多为胃气上逆所致。

呕吐物清稀无味：胃寒所致。

呕吐物秽浊酸臭：胃热所致。夹杂有不消化食物，为食积。

呕吐清水痰涎：为痰饮。

呕吐黄绿苦水：多为肝胆湿热或郁热。

呕吐鲜血或紫暗血块：为胃有积热或肝火犯胃。

呕吐脓血：多为胃痈。

Vomitus includes food dregs, clear fluid, sputum, saliva or pus as well as blood. It is caused by adverse flow of stomach qi.

Thin vomitus without foul smell is caused by cold in the stomach.

Foul, turbid and sour vomitus is caused by heat in the stomach; vomitus mingled with indigested food is caused by retention of food.

Vomiting of clear fluid, sputum and saliva is due to phlegm retention in the stomach.

Vomiting of yellowish or greenish bitter fluid is due to accumulation of damp heat or stagnation of heat in the liver and gallbladder.

Vomiting of fresh blood or purplish blood clot is often due to accumulation of heat in the stomach or liver fire attacking the stomach.

Vomitus with pus and blood indicates abscess in the stomach.

13. 望大便
1.1.2.13 Inspection of stool

（1）性状

稀薄便：肠中有寒。

酱色便：肠中有热。

粗稠便：津液已伤。

干结便：肠液干涸，若如羊矢者为噎膈病晚期。

便如蟹沫：为气滞。

大便溏黏：为湿热。

完谷不化：为里寒或中阳不足。

（1）Texture of stool

Thin and loose stool is caused by pathogenic cold in the intestines.

Dark reddish stool is caused by pathogenic heat in the intestines.

Thick stool means impairment of body fluid.

Dry feces with constipation mean consumption of intestinal fluid; stool like sheep dung indicates advanced dysphagia (cancer of the esophagus).

Stool like froths from the crab's mouth indicates qi stagnation.

Sticky and loose stool is caused by damp heat.

Stool mingled with undigested food is caused by endogenous cold or insufficiency of yang qi in middle energizer (the spleen and stomach).

（2）颜色

黄色便：为热。

白色便：为湿寒。

色红如酱：为血热。

色黑如漆：为瘀血内积。

婴儿绿便：为消化不良。

红色血便：为痢疾。

鱼脑便：为湿热痢、疫痢。

痢下白色：病在气分。

痢下红色：病在血分。

（2）Color of stool

Yellowish stool is heat syndrome.

Whitish stool is caused by dampness and cold.

Dark reddish brown stool indicates heat in blood.

Stool like black paint is caused by blood stasis.

Infantile greenish stool indicates indigestion.

Red stool with blood is a sign of dysentery.

Stool like brain of fish is a sign of ekiri caused by dampness and heat

Whitish dysentery suggests the disease is in qi phase.

Reddish dysentery suggests the disease is in blood phase.

14. 望小便

1.1.2.14 Inspection of urination

（1）性状

清长过多：属于寒。

混浊短涩：属于热。

血尿：热结膀胱。

小儿尿如米泔：多数食滞。

尿中有细石者：为石淋。

尿浊如膏：为膏淋。

尿有余沥：为气淋。

（1）Texture of urine

Profuse and clear urine indicates cold syndrome.

Reduced turbid urine with difficulty in urination indicates heat syndrome.

Urine with blood indicates coagulation of heat in the bladder.

Rice-water infantile urine is usually caused by dyspeptic retention.

Urolithic stranguria refers to urine mingled with fine stones.

Turbid paste-like urine is stranguria marked by chyluria.

Dripping urination is qi strangury caused by disorder of qi.

（2）颜色

淡黄：平人无病。亦显示肾经虚热。

尿白清长：为寒，无热。

尿黄而红：为肝经实热，黄浊不清为湿热。

尿色澄黄，有油状物漂浮：为下消病。

尿红如苏木色：为血热。

尿如酱色：为肾病、水气病。

（2）Color of urine

Pale yellowish urine indicates normal urine of healthy people without any disease, it is also a sign of asthenic heat in kidney meridian.

Clear, profuse and whitish urine shows cold syndrome without heat.

Yellowish and reddish urine is caused by sthenic heat in liver meridian, turbid yellowish urine is caused by dampness and heat.

Clear yellowish urine with substances like oil floating in it is a sign of lower consumptive thirst（diabetes involving the lower energizer）.

Reddish urine like the color of Sumu（*Lignum Sappan*）suggests blood heat.

Dark reddish urine suggests diseases of the kidney, or edema.

（3）尿量

量多：有消渴病之疑。

尿少：为水肿病，多为肾虚。

夜尿多：青年人为下焦湿热，老年人为肾气亏虚。

（3）Volume of urine

Profuse urine is susceptibility to diabetes.

Reduced urine is a sign of edema, usually due to kidney asthenia.

Frequent urination during sleep in young people is caused by dampness and heat in lower energizer; in aging people is caused by deficiency of kidney qi.

15. 望鱼际络脉
1.1.2.15 Inspection of Yuji vein

鱼际是指拇指本节后肌肉丰满处。鱼际为手太阴肺经之部。望鱼际与独取寸口脉象一样，可以查知胃气的盛衰和肺气的充盈与否。

鱼际脉络色青：主寒，主痛。

鱼际脉络色赤：主热病。

鱼际脉络青暗：主胃寒与气滞。

鱼际脉络红赤：主胃热。

鱼际脉络色黑：主久痹。

Yuji refers to the point located at the prominent muscular flexor of pollicis in the palm. It belongs to lung meridian of hand-taiyin. To examine Yuji is of the same importance as to inspect Cunkou vein. Exuberance or deficiency of stomach qi and abundance or weakness of lung qi can be ascertained in inspecting Yuji vein.

Bluish Yuji vein suggests cold syndrome and pain syndrome.

Reddish Yuji vein signifies heat syndrome.

Dark cyanotic Yuji vein indicates cold in the stomach and qi stagnation.

Reddish Yuji vein indicates heat in the stomach.

Blackish Yuji vein indicates prolonged rheumatism syndrome.

16. 望指甲
1.1.2.16 Inspection of fingernail

（1）形态

指甲凹陷：主气血亏虚，心中胆怯。

指甲高凸：甲癣。

指甲变形：多风湿病。

指甲弯曲：体弱骨软。

指甲刚柔：刚者体壮，胆气充实；柔者体弱，胆气虚怯。

指甲纹理：纵纹多者为阴虚血瘀，横纹多者为气虚血亏。

杵状指：指尖如鼓槌状，多为心肺慢性疾病。

（1）Shapes and texture

Sunken fingernail indicates timidity in nature and deficiency of qi and blood.

Protruding fingernail is a sign of mycosis ungualis.

Deformed fingernail is a sign of rheumatism.

Curved fingernail indicates weakness and osteomalacia.

Hard fingernail indicates strong body and abundance of qi in the gallbladder; while soft fingernail indicates weakness, timidity and lack of courage due to deficiency of qi in the gallbladder.

Fingernail with lots of vertical lines indicates yin asthenia and blood stasis, while fingernail with lots of transverse lines indicates qi asthenia and blood depletion.

Clubbed finger tip like drumsticks is often seen in chronic diseases of the heart and lung.

（2）颜色

指甲红润：为健康之人。

指甲鲜红：为血热。

指甲色淡：为内脏虚寒。

指甲色黄：为黄疸。

指甲色青：为阳衰血虚之极，病危。

指压病人指甲：按之白而放之红者，为气血畅通之象，可治；按之白放之不复者，为气血瘀滞之证，难治。

（2）Color

Ruddy fingernail indicates health.

Bright reddish fingernail indicates blood heat.

Pale fingernail suggests cold and asthenia syndrome in the viscera.

Yellowish fingernail indicates jaundice.

Cyanotic fingernail is a sign of extreme yang declination and blood asthenia, critical or dying condition.

When being pressed, fingernail will turn white, yet it will turn red if set free, which is a sign of smooth circulation of qi and blood and the patient can be cured; if fingernail turns white while the color will not turn red when set free, it is a syndrome of qi stagnation and blood stasis, which is incurable.

17. 望指纹

1.1.2.17　Inspection of index finger vein

指纹是指两手示指内侧的脉纹，它与寸口同为一脉所出。为诊断 3 岁以下小儿疾病的独特诊法。

Inspection of index finger veins refers to examining the superficial veins on the palmar side of the index finger, which originates from the same artery as cunkou. It is a special diagnostic method for infants under 3 years.

以手掌示指向指尖推算，初节为风关，次节为气关，三节为命关（见图 1）。纹在风关为病轻，纹达气关为病重，若透过命关为病重难治。

Index finger vein can be divided into three parts: wind pass (the first stem of the index finger), qi pass (the second stem of the index finger) and life pass (the third stem of the index finger) (Fig. 1). Appearance of index finger veins in wind pass means mild disease; if it extends to qi pass, it indicates that the disease is serious; if it extends to life pass, it means a critical syndrome and incurable condition.

（1）颜色

淡红隐隐：为虚寒。

正红纹：为伤寒。

深红纹：为热盛。

紫红纹：为热极。

青色纹：食伤或痰气上逆。

青而兼黑：为痰、食与热互结。

淡白色：为脾胃气虚。

青黄色纹：为肺脾俱败之象。

（1）Color

Pale reddish color with indistinct index finger vein indicates asthenia and cold syndromes.

Reddish vein indicates exogenous febrile disease.

Deep-reddish vein shows exuberance of heat.

Purplish vein is a sign of excess heat.

Cyanotic vein is caused by indigestion or adverse flow of phlegm and qi.

Cyanotic and blackish vein indicates coagulation of dyspeptic food intermingled with phlegm and heat.

Pale whitish vein indicates qi asthenia in the spleen and stomach.

Cyanotic and yellowish vein suggests qi declination in the lung and spleen.

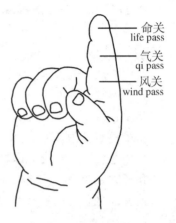

图1 小儿示指指纹

Fig. 1 Infantile index finger vein

（2）形态

指纹显露于外：为表证。

指纹沉没：为病邪入里。

指纹向内弯：为风寒。

指纹向外弯：为痰、食或热积。

指纹入掌中：为腹痛。

透关射甲：为病重。

青筋一条：为危候。

（2）Shapes

Obvious appearance of index finger vein on the superficies is an external syndrome.

Deep and invisible vein means transmission of pathogenic factors into the interior.

Vein twisting inward indicates exogenous wind and cold pathogen.

Vein twisting outward indicates indigestion due to retention of phlegm and food, or heat accumulation.

Vein stretching into the palm suggests abdominal pain.

Vein stretching directly to the tip of the finger and can be seen from there signifies critical condition of a disease and unfavorable prognosis.

One single cyanotic index finger vein indicates dying condition.

18. 望皮肤
1.1.2.18 Inspection of the skin

皮肤望诊是中医四诊的重要内容，它包括望皮肤之色泽、形态、痘疹、痈疖等。

Inspection of the skin is an important part of four diagnostic methods of TCM. It involves inspecting color, shape, and pathogenic changes of the skin, as well as macula, eruptions, abscess and furuncle on it.

（1）色泽

皮肤发赤：如染脂涂丹，为丹毒；如红色云片，游走不定，为赤游丹毒；如局部红赤，为流火；如下肢红肿，为湿热下注。

皮肤发黄：为黄疸。阳黄鲜明如橘子色，多为肝胆湿热所致；阴黄晦暗如烟煤，多为脾胃湿寒所困。

皮肤发黑：皮肤黄中显黑，黑而晦暗，称"黑疸"，为黄疸之一种，多由黄疸转变而来。

（1）Color

Reddish skin like wearing make-up indicates erysipelas (an inflammatory disease with redness of skin); reddish skin like wandering red clouds is infantile erysipelas; regional reddish skin is usually connected with erysipelas; swollen lower limbs are caused by downward migration of dampness and heat.

Yellowish skin indicates jaundice. Bright yellowish skin like tangerine peel is caused by dampness and heat in the liver and gallbladder; dark yellowish and tarnished skin like the color of bituminous coal usually results from stagnation of dampness and cold in the spleen and stomach.

Blackish and sallow skin is called "black jaundice", one type of the jaundice disease, usually transformed from jaundice.

（2）形态

皮肤湿润：脾经湿气太盛。

皮肤枯槁：脾肺气衰。

皮肤如鱼鳞：即肌肤甲错，是肺痿的表现。

皮焦毛落：肺损之极。

皮肤若蛇皮：多属疠风之皮病。

皮肤肿胀：气肿，皮厚色苍；水肿，皮薄色明。阳水，一身尽肿，皮色黄赤；阴水，遍身俱肿，皮色苍黄。

（2）Shape and texture

Moist skin indicates exuberant dampness in spleen meridian.

Dry and lusterless skin is a sign of declination of qi in the spleen and lung.

Squamous and lustrous skin like fish scale is indication of atrophic lung disease.

Withered skin with glandular hair falling off is due to depletion of lung qi.

Skin like that of snakes is a sign of dermatosis due to leprosy.

Dropsy with thick skin and pale color is a sign of emphysema; thin skin with bright color signifies edema; dropsy all over the body with yellowish brownish skin is called yang edema; dropsy all through the body with pale yellowish skin belongs to yin edema.

（3）痘疹

水痘：四周无红圈，根脚内所含水液发亮，无发热灌浆阶段，一般无危险性。

麻疹：皮肤上出现极小红点，如粟状，抚之不碍手者为疹；如果形大如芝麻，抚之刺指者为麻。

风疹：疹形细小稀疏，稍稍隆起，其色淡红，瘙痒不已，时发时止，一般不影响食欲与工作。多由风热而致。

瘾疹：其疹时隐时现，发作时皮肤瘙痒，高于皮肤，搔之连片如云，色淡红带白。多由风邪中于经络所致。

（3）Exanthema variolosum

Chicken pox refers to vesicular rash of spots, with no red circles on its external edge but with brightness in its root, and no outbreak of fever in the forming stage of vesicles. In general, chicken pox is not dangerous.

Measles and morbilli: The extremely small and reddish spots on the skin like millet which cannot be felt by hands are called measles; the spots that are as big as sesame and can be felt like thorny pricks are called morbilli.

Rubella is thin and small in size, sparsely distributed, slightly hunching in shape, pale red in color and continuous itchy sensation. Rubella occasionally breaks out and disappears, but it does not affect appetite and work. It is usually caused by pathogenic wind and heat.

Urticaria is caused by invasion of pathogenic wind into meridians and collaterals, marked by occasional outbreak and disappearance, protruding over the skin, appearing in patches after being scratched with light reddish and whitish color. Its outbreak is accompanied with itchy sensation of the skin.

（4）斑疹

斑疹由血热而发，多见于温热病。大者为斑，小者为疹；色鲜红而松浮于皮面者为轻，色紫红稠密而紧束有根者为重。

（4）Macule

Macule is caused by blood heat, usually seen in pathogenic febrile disease. The bigger in size is macule, and the smaller is measles. Macule and measles with bright reddish color and loosened surface indicate an unserious disease; while purplish color, tense root and densely distributed macule and measles signify a critical disease.

（5）痈疽疔疖

痈：红肿高大，为阳证。多由湿热火毒内蕴，气血瘀滞，热盛肉腐而成痈。

疽：不红平塌，为阴证。多由气血虚亏、寒痰凝滞，或脏腑积热，攻于肌肉，内陷筋骨所致。

疔：如米如粟，根脚坚硬，顶白而痛者为疔。多由疫气毒邪袭于皮肤，传注经络，以致阴阳二气不得宣通，气血凝滞而成。

疖：起于浅表部位，形小而圆，红肿热痛不甚，容易化脓，脓溃即愈。多由暑湿阻于肌肤，或脏腑蕴积湿热所致。

（5）Carbuncle, phlegmon, malignant boil and furuncle

Carbuncle refers to regional swellings protruding over the skin, indicating yang syndrome and caused by internal accumulation of damp heat and virulent fire, stagnation of qi and blood, as well as exuberance of heat which causes decay of muscles.

Phlegmon refers to even patches on the skin with no change of color. It is a yin syndrome and usually caused by asthenia of qi and blood and stagnation of cold and phlegm, or by invasion of accumulated heat of zang-fu organs into muscles, leading to sinking of tendons and bones.

Malignant boil appears like millet with hard root, white top and painful sensation. It is caused by invasion of pestilent pathogens and virulence onto the skin, which transmits and migrates in meridians and collaterals, resulting in failure of yang qi and yin qi to be dispersed as well as stagnation of qi and blood.

Furuncle appears on the superficial skin, small and round in size, slight swelling, pyrexia and painful sensation. It is susceptible to suppuration and ulceration, with liability to healing after disappearance of purulence. It is caused by obstruction of summer damp heat on the skin, or by accumulation of dampness and heat in zang-fu organs.

（6）白㾦

白㾦是温热病（暑湿、湿温）出现在皮肤上的一种白色小颗粒。多由湿郁汗出不透所致。白㾦有顺证与逆证。

顺证：色白而细，形如粟，明亮滋润像水晶样，称晶㾦，为顺证，是湿邪外泄之象。

逆证：色干枯者，是津液枯竭之象，为逆证，危候。

（6）Miliaria alba

Miliaria alba refers to small whitish blisters, a manifestation of pathogenic febrile disease (including summer heat dampness and damp febrile disease) on the skin. It is often caused by stagnation of exogenous dampness on the surface of skin which inhibits sweating.

Crystal miliaria alba refers to millet-like miliaria alba in size, as bright and transparent as crystal. It is a sign of out eruption of pathogenic dampness, indicating a favorable prognosis.

Dry and lusterless miliaria alba is indicative of consumption of body fluid, an unfavorable prognosis and a critical syndrome.

（7）湿疹

湿疹又称浸淫疮，表现多种多样。多由风、湿、热留于肌肤，或病久耗血，以致血虚生风化燥，肌肤失养而成。湿疹初期为红斑，迅速形成肿胀、丘疹或水疱，继而水疱破裂、渗液，出现红色湿润糜烂，以后干燥结痂，痂脱后留有痕迹，日久可自行消退。

（7）Eczema

Eczema, also known as acute eczema, is caused by retention of exogenous wind, dampness as well as heat on the skin, or by generation of wind because of blood asthenia and malnutrition of the skin, resulting from prolonged disease consuming large amount of blood. At the initial stage of eczema, red patches appear on the skin, then they rapidly turn into swellings, papulae or blisters. As they are broken, fluid oozes from the inside, and the superficial skin becomes red and moist with erosion. Later, the skin turns dry and scabs. With disappearance of the scabs, the wound is healed leaving no marks.

19. 望胸
1.1.2.19　Inspection of the chest

鸡胸：小儿因胸部发育畸形所致。成人乃因风热相搏，以致肺气胀满，攻于胸膈而致。

扁平胸：先天肺气虚，肺活量不足，易患肺痨。

桶状胸：多因慢性呼吸系疾病所致，或为畸形。

凸或凹胸：多为畸形或肺胀、肺痿所致。

Chicken breast is often seen in infants because of developmental malformation of chest bones. The disease in adults is caused by struggle between pathogenic wind and heat, giving rise to attack of distention of lung qi in the chest and diaphragm.

Flat chest is caused by congenital asthenia of lung qi and insufficient vital capacity of the lung. These patients have susceptibility to tuberculosis.

Barrel chest is caused by chronic respiratory diseases or congenital deformity.

Protruding chest is caused by congenital deformity or lung distention, while concaved chest is caused by atrophic lung disease.

20. 望腹
1.1.2.20　Inspection of the abdomen

腹大：皮厚色苍为气虚或气滞，皮薄色亮为水为湿。

水肿：皮肤黄亮者为阳水，皮肤白亮者为阴水。

臌胀：胸腹胀满，四肢消瘦，为气臌；腹部青筋暴露，或手足有红丝赤缕，为血臌；腹皮大而绷紧，皮色苍黄，为水臌。

脐凸：小儿脐凸为脐疝，成人脐凸为水肿恶候。

脐凹：胃肠干瘪，气虚之极，为难治。

Big abdomen：Thick and pale color of abdominal wall suggests qi asthenia or stagnation of qi, while thin and bright color of abdominal wall is a sign of edema or retention of dampness.

Edema with bright yellowish skin is yang edema. Edema with bright whitish colored skin is a sign of yin edema.

Bulged abdomen：Distension and fullness in chest and abdomen and emaciated limbs are qi tympanites due to internal retention of stagnated qi. Exposed cyanotic veins on abdominal wall or appearance of thin red blood vessels in the skin of feet and hands are signs of tympanites due to blood stasis. Big, tense, hard and full abdomen with pale yellowish skin is tympanites due to internal retention of body fluid.

Navel protrusion in infants is due to hernia, protrusion of navel in adults is a manifestation of edema, signifying critical and unfavorable prognosis.

Sunken navel is caused by shriveled stomach and intestines due to extreme qi asthenia, suggesting incurable disease.

21. 望背

1.1.2.21　Inspection of the back

龟背：或因先天肾气亏虚，督脉失养所致；或因后天坐姿不当所引起；或因大病之后，肾精损耗，不能充养脊髓而致。

反张：反张者，脊背向后牵拉，不能正常坐位。此疾多由高热伤及脊髓所致，多见于破伤风、痉病、脐风、脑病等。

背平：正常背部应中央督脉处略洼陷，两肩胛处隆起。背平者，中央无洼陷，此乃肾气衰败之征。

脊椎畸形：除先天发育形成外，多由风寒湿流注关节所致。

Humpback is due to congenital asthenia of kidney qi and malnutrition of governor meridian; or due to improper sitting posture; or due to consumption of kidney essence after serious diseases, which fails to nourish spinal marrow.

Opisthotonus of spinal column refers to reverse bending of spinal column leading to abnormal sitting posture. It is caused by impairment of spinal marrow due to high fever, usually seen in tetanus, convulsive disease, tetanus neonatorum, cerebropathy, and so on.

Flat back：Normal back sinks in the region of central governor meridian, and hunches from the blade bones of the shoulders. Flat back refers to the back doesn't sink in the middle, a syndrome of declination of kidney qi.

Deformity of spinal column：Besides the congenital deformity of spinal column, deformed spinal column is caused by discharge of pathogenic wind, cold or dampness into the joints.

（三） 望诊注意事项
1.1.3 Tips for inspection

①望诊时，应注意光线对病人面色与舌苔的影响。还要注意饮食与药物对舌苔的影响。

②望诊时，应注意心理情绪及运动对病人形体、形态的影响。

③望诊时，医患均应保持镇定，医者应仔细观察，甚至从不同角度去观察，不可匆忙了事。

a. Attention should be paid to the effect of light on a patient's complexion as well as that on tongue fur. In addition, food and medication could also affect on tongue fur, which should not be neglected.

b. Attention should be paid to the effect of state of mind, mood as well as sports exercises on a patient's body physique and shape.

c. During inspection, both the doctor and the patient should keep calm. And the doctor should examine carefully, even from different angles. Carelessness and hasty action should be avoided.

二、闻诊
1.2 Listening and olfaction

闻诊包括听声音、嗅气味两个方面。

听声音可以测知五脏气血的盛衰以及病变的动态，嗅气味则可分辨病变的虚实寒热，两者也是不可忽视的诊察方法。

Listening and olfaction include the diagnostic methods of listening to various sounds and noises made by a patient and smelling the odor and excreta of the body of a patient.

By means of listening, sufficiency or deficient condition of qi and blood in viscera as well as pathological changes of the viscera could be detected. Likewise, conditions of visceral pathological changes such as asthenia, sthenia, cold or heat can be diagnosed with the help of olfaction. Therefore, both diagnostic methods cannot be ignored.

（一）听声音
1. 2. 1 Listening to the voice

1. 语言
1.2.1.1 Speech

语声重浊，高厉有力：为实证。

语声轻清，出音低怯：为虚证。

烦而多言：为热证。

静而少言：为寒证。

谵语狂言，骂詈不避亲属：为热盛神昏。

语言若续若断：为中气虚弱。

语无伦次，先后不相呼应：为神志失常。

语声低微，细语喃喃：多为虚证。

语言謇塞：为中风之疾。

睡中呢喃，醒时错语：为心气亏损，神志不守。

Deep, heavy and sonorous voice indicates sthenia syndrome.

Weak, low and feeble voice suggests asthenia syndrome.

Polylogia with irritancy is due to heat syndrome.

Oligologia with quietness is due to cold syndrome.

Delirious speech, ravings as well as manic shouting even in the presence of relatives indicates heat exuberance and unconsciousness.

Disjointed voice is caused by deficiency and weakness of qi in middle energizer.

Incoherent and confused speech suggests mental disorder.

Low weak murmuring indicates asthenia syndrome.

Slurred speech is usually due to apoplexia.

Murmuring speech during sleep but paraphasia when waking up is due to consumption and insufficiency of heart qi as well as malnutrition of the heart and mind.

2. 呼吸
1.2.1.2 Respiration

气短：气若有所室，语言不能接续，有因留饮者，有因肺气虚者。

气喘：有虚实之分。实喘胸闷气粗，出气不爽，以呼出为快，病在肺；虚喘吸长呼短，入气有声，其病在肾。

哮喘：呼吸急促，喉中痰鸣。由痰饮内伏，偶感外寒，寒邪束表，引动伏饮而发。或久卧湿地，或过食辛辣、糖果、生冷之物，促发此病。亦有病根深固，频发频止，缠绵终身者。

肩息：气管窒塞，吸气费力，且以抬肩助呼吸者。这是肾不纳气的表现。

Shortness of breath refers to incontinuous breath as if it has been choked and accompanied with disjointed voice. It is usually due to prolonged retention of phlegm, or asthenic lung qi.

Dyspnea is either sthenia syndrome or asthenia syndrome. Sthenic dyspnea is marked by chest oppression, deep breath, unsmooth gasping as well as quick exhalation, signifying that pathogenic factors are in the lung; asthenic dyspnea is featured by long inhalation with voice and short exhalation, indicating that pathogenic factors are in the kidney.

Asthma is marked by rapid breath accompanied with stridor in the throat, usually caused by internal retention of phlegm complicated by attack of exogenous pathogenic cold factor, which encumbers the superficies and stirs up the latent retention of phlegm. Or it is caused by prolonged staying in wetland, or by excessive intake of pungent food, candies as well as raw and cold food. There exist other reasons for the syndrome, such as deep-rooted diseases, repeated relapse and recovery as well as lingering illness with difficulty to heal.

Dyspnea with elevated shoulders is featured by choked respiratory tract and strenuous inhalation which causes patients to raise shoulders to improve breath, indicating failure of the kidney to receive qi.

3. 咳嗽
1.2.1.3　Cough

咳声重浊，痰清色白：外感风寒。
咳痰不爽，痰稠色黄：热伤于肺。
干咳无痰，咽喉瘙痒：燥伤肺阴。
暴咳声哑：多为肺实。
微咳声怯：中气不足。
顿咳：常见于小儿百日咳。
呛咳：见于百日咳、咯血。
哑咳：咳嗽声音嘶哑，多见于内有蕴热，外有风寒。
因咳而有痰：病在肺，脾为次。
因痰而咳：病在脾，肺为次。

Deep and heavy cough with clear whitish sputum is due to exogenous wind and cold pathogens.

Difficulty in expectoration with thick sticky yellowish sputum is due to heat impairing the lung.

Dry cough without sputum and itching throat are caused by pathogenic dryness impairing lung yin.

Sudden cough with hoarse voice is due to pulmonary sthenia.

Weak cough with low and feeble voice is due to insufficient qi in middle energizer.

Whooping cough is usually seen in infantile pertussis.

Bucking cough is often seen in infantile pertussis and hemoptysis.

Cough with low hoarse voice is due to accumulation of endogenous heat as well as invasion of exogenous wind cold.

Sputum caused by cough indicates pathological change is mainly in the lung as well as in the spleen.

Cough caused by sputum indicates pathological change is mainly in the spleen as well as in the lung.

4. 呕吐
1.2.1.4　Vomiting

吐势猛烈，声音壮厉：为实热证。
吐势徐缓，声音低微：为虚寒证。
朝食暮吐，暮食朝吐：脾胃气虚。
呕而胁痛，情志抑郁：肝气犯胃。

A violent rapid vomiting with a loud and strong noise is due to sthenic heat syndrome.

A slow vomiting with a low voice is asthenic cold syndrome.

Eating in the morning but vomiting in the evening or vomiting in the morning what is eaten at previous dinner indicates qi asthenia in the stomach and spleen.

Vomiting accompanied with hypochondriac pain and emotional depression is caused by liver qi attacking the stomach.

5. 呃逆
1.2.1.5　Hiccup

呃逆连声有力：为实热证。
呃逆声音低怯：为气虚证。

Constant hiccup with powerful voice signifies sthenic heat syndrome.

Hiccup with low and feeble voice indicates qi asthenia.

6. 嗳气
1.2.1.6　Belching

嗳腐吞酸，脘腹胀满：宿食不化。
嗳气响亮，频频发作：肝气犯胃。
嗳气低沉，纳谷不馨：脾胃虚弱。
病后嗳气，心下痞硬：胃弱不和。

Belching with fetid odor, acid regurgitation as well as abdominal distention is due to indigestion.

Frequent belching with loud noise is due to liver qi attacking the stomach.

Belching with low noise and poor appetite is caused by weakness and asthenia of the stomach and spleen.

Belching after illness and epigastric fullness and hardened sensation suggest weakness of the stomach in descending qi.

7. 嚏欠
1.2.1.7 Sneezing and yawning

喷嚏：阳气和利之象。中寒阳虚者，不能作嚏；病久无嚏忽得之属阳回，是将愈之佳兆。

欠：阳弱阴盛之象。失睡之人多欠，体虚和疲劳者常喜呵欠；病者善欠，为阳衰气虚之证。

Sneezing is a sign of smooth and orderly circulation of yang qi. Cold and yang asthenia in middle energizer lead to failure to sneeze; occasional outbreak of sneezing in a protracted illness without sneeze indicates recovery of yang qi and a favorable prognosis.

Yawning signifies deficiency of yang and exuberance of yin. Those patients who suffer from insomnia yawn frequently, and yawning is accompanied with weak constitution and overstrain; frequent yawning during illness is a manifestation of yang declination and qi asthenia.

8. 呻吟
1.2.1.8 Groaning

声高而急：证属有余，偏于邪实。
声低而缓：证属不足，偏于正虚。
呻吟不能转侧：其痛在腰。
呻吟不能行走：其痛在脚。
呻吟而摇头攒眉：为头痛。
呻吟而以手扪腮：为牙齿痛。

Loud and rapid groaning indicates a syndrome of sthenia, especially excessive pathogenic factors.

Low and slow groaning indicates a syndrome of deficiency, especially asthenia of healthy qi.

Groaning with inability to turn sidewards suggests pathogenic factors in the loins.

Groaning with inability to walk indicates pathological change in the feet.

Groaning with head shaking as well as frowning suggests severe headache.

Groaning with hand cupping cheeks is a sign of toothache.

9. 肠鸣

1.2.1.9　Borborygmus

声在脘部，振动有声，其声漉漉下行：为痰饮留聚于胃。
声在脘腹，得温、得食则缓，饿时加重：为脾胃气虚。
腹中肠鸣如雷，大便濡泻：为风寒湿邪聚于脘腹，寒甚则肢厥。

Borborygmus in the epigastrium with a tendency to moving downward indicates retention of phlegm and fluid in the stomach.

Borborygmus in the epigastrium and abdomen, alleviation with warmth and intake of food, and aggravation with hunger suggests qi asthenia in the stomach and spleen.

Borborygmus in the intestines like thunder with loose stool or diarrhea indicates accumulation of pathogenic wind, cold, and dampness factors in the epigastrium and abdomen, and cold limbs could be caused by severe cold pathogens.

10. 小儿哭啼

1.2.1.10　Infant cry

声大响亮，左顾右盼：为发脾气。
声高而尖：因痛而哭。
声高有力：为邪实。
声低而怯：为正虚。
哭声绵长无力：因饥饿而哭。
哭声嘶哑，呼吸不利：为咽喉痛。

Crying with sonorous voice accompanied with the posture of looking around indicates losing temper.

Crying with loud and sharp voice is due to pain.

Crying with loud and strong voice indicates sthenic pathogen.

Crying with low and feeble voice is caused by asthenia of healthy qi.

Crying with a weak voice and lasting a long time is due to hunger.

Crying with a hoarse voice with unsmooth breath is due to sore throat.

（二）嗅气味
1.2.2　Olfaction

1. 口气

1.2.2.1　Odor of mouth

口臭：多属消化不良，或有龋齿，或口腔不洁。

口酸臭：为内有宿食。

口腐臭：多有溃疡、疮疡。

口香：消渴病人病情加重时有果香味。

Foul odor of the mouth is caused by indigestion, or decayed teeth, or unclean oral cavity.

Acid foul odor of the mouth indicates internal food retention.

Putrid odor is due to ulcer or abscess.

Fragrant fruit odor is a symptom of aggravation of diabetes.

2. 汗气
1.2.2.2　Odor of sweat

汗臭：热病后衣被不洁，或风湿热病的汗出。

Smelly odor of sweat is caused by wearing unclean clothes or sweat fumigation after fever due to pathogenic wind and dampness factors.

3. 痰臭
1.2.2.3　Smelly odor of sputum

痰臭为肺痈。

Smelly odor of sputum is due to pulmonary abscess.

4. 鼻臭
1.2.2.4　Fetor narium

鼻臭为鼻渊、脑漏（即鼻渊日久，流黄稠涕而头痛者）。

Fetor narium is nasosinusitis, or nasal sinusitis (namely, prolonged nasosinusitis, discharge of foul and thick yellowish snivel, causing headache).

5. 大便
1.2.2.5　Odor of feces

大便酸臭：肠中有食积。

大便腥臭：为大肠湿寒证。

Sour and foul odor of stool is due to food retention in the intestines.

Stinking odor of stool indicates damp and cold syndromes in the large intestine.

6. 小便

1.2.2.6　Odor of urine

小便臊浊：膀胱有热。

小便甜：消渴之重症。

Turbid urine with stinking odor suggests heat in the bladder.

Urine with sweet odor indicates severe diabetes.

7. 月经

1.2.2.7　Odor of menstruation

月经秽臭：湿热蕴结日久。

月经腥臭：寒邪内蕴日久。

Foul odor of menstrual blood indicates prolonged internal accumulation of dampness and heat.

Menstruation with stinking smell is due to prolonged internal accumulation of pathogenic cold factors.

8. 带下

1.2.2.8　Odor of leucorrhea

带下秽臭：下焦湿热。

带下腥臭：下焦虚寒。

Foul odor of leucorrhea is due to dampness and heat in lower energizer.

Stinking odor of leucorrhea indicates asthenic cold in lower energizer.

三、问诊

1.3　Inquiry

问诊是四诊中的一项重要内容。通过问诊，可以了解疾病的发生、发展、治疗经过、现在症状，以及与疾病相关的信息。

问诊要围绕病人的主要痛苦进行，既要突出重点，又不可有所偏颇。在注重病人主要痛苦的同时，还要问及其家庭环境、饮食喜恶、起居状况、平素体质、有何嗜好等，为正确地辨证收集相关的资料。

问诊是一种技巧，也是一种心态。问诊者必须以关怀的心态，耐心、和蔼地询问。使病人感受到体贴、温馨，从而乐意诉说自己的痛苦。切忌主观地引导病人向某一方面倾诉，而丢掉他内心真正想说的内容。若遇到不能自述病情的病人，要从其家属那里尽量多地询问病人的发病经过、主要痛苦、最近治疗情况等，以便较快地做出决定，为治疗提供可靠的依据。

Inquiry is an important part among the four diagnostic methods. By means of inquiry, onset and development of a disease, treating process, present manifestations as well as related information about the disease can be acquired.

Inquiry should be centred on a patient's chief complaints. However, in addition to the key problems, details should not be neglected. In order to ensure correct diagnosis, besides a patient's chief symptoms, inquiry should involve family background, living habits such as diets, preferences, sleep, congenital constitution as well as interests or hobbies, and so on.

Inquiry is more than a skill, it can indicate a doctor's state of mind. Therefore, during an inquiry, a doctor must show his kindness, patience as well as his considerate attitude to make his patient feel the concern and warmth from the doctor, so that he could be content to tell about his sufferings. It is forbidden to induce the patient to talk about some unimportant information and give up his main complaint. As to some patient who cannot express himself, the doctor should acquire from his family members the information concerning the course of the illness, its main symptoms, the previous diagnosis and treatment in order to ensure a quick diagnosis and to provide reliable evidence for further treatment.

（一）一般问诊
1.3.1 General inquiry

①问病人的姓名、年龄、性别、民族、婚否、职业、籍贯、现住址等。

②问病人就诊时的主要痛苦。

③问病人的发病日期，以及病情发展的经过。

④问引起本病的发病原因以及有关事项。

⑤问疾病的治疗情况、用药反应。

⑥问病人的生活环境，性格如何，有什么嗜好。

⑦问家族史。

a. The patient's name, age, gender, nationality, marital status, profession, place of origin, present address, and so on.

b. Chief complaint of the patient on visiting the doctor.

c. The date of onset and development of a disease.

d. Main causes of the disease as well as relevant information.

e. Previous treatment of the disease and reaction or side effects after taking medicines.

f. Family surroundings, character, interests or hobbies of the patient.

g. Family history of diseases.

（二）具体问诊
1.3.2　Detailed inquiry

1. 问寒热

1.3.2.1　Inquiry about fever and cold

（1）发热时间

发热无定时：多为外感热病。

早晨发热：多为气虚。

下午发热：为湿温、阴虚、虚劳发热之状。

日晡发热：病在胃肠。

夜间热重：阴虚、血虚，或食滞。

隔日发热：间日疟。

三日一发热：三日疟。

（1）Time of outbreak of fever

Outbreak of fever without fixed time indicates exogenous febrile disease.

Outbreak of fever in the morning is due to qi asthenia.

Outbreak of fever in the afternoon is due to retention of dampness and heat, yin asthenia, deficient-fever.

Continuous fever from 15 to 17 o'clock in the afternoon indicates pathogenic factors are in the stomach and intestines.

Aggravation of fever at night suggests yin asthenia, blood asthenia or food retention.

Outbreak of fever every other day is tertian malaria.

Regular outbreak of fever every three days is due to malaria quartana.

（2）发热状况

寒热往来：病在半表半里。

但热不寒：病发于阳经。

但寒不热：病发于阴经。

发热恶寒：为外感发热。

热多于寒：阳胜于阴。

寒多于热：阴胜于阳。

寒热有汗：表虚。

寒热无汗：表实。

烦热：里热。

壮热：里有实热。

骨蒸劳热：多见于阴虚证。

久热不退：多为阴虚。

（2）Types of fever

Alternation of cold and fever indicates pathological change in the semi-external and semi-internal region.

Fever without cold shows pathological change arising from yang meridians.

Cold without fever signifies pathological change in yin meridians.

Fever with aversion to cold is due to exogenous pathogenic heat factors.

Severe fever and mild aversion to cold indicate exuberant yang overcoming yin.

Severe aversion to cold and mild fever indicate excessive yin overcoming yang.

Aversion to cold, fever and hidrosis indicate external asthenia.

Aversion to cold, fever and anhidrosis indicate external sthenia.

Fever with dysphoria is due to interior heat syndrome.

High fever is due to internal sthenic heat.

Bone-steaming and consumptive fever is usually seen in the syndrome of yin asthenia.

Prolonged fever is due to yin asthenia.

（3）发热部位

热在手足：热性病的表现。

寒在手足：阳气不足，或热深厥深。

热在胸腹：里有积热。

寒在胸腹：里有沉寒。

寒在背部：阳气不足。

热在面部：多为阳明经实热。

全身恶寒发热：多为外感病。

（3）Location of fever

Fever sensation over hands and feet is a sign of heat syndrome.

Cold sensation over hands and feet indicates insufficiency of yang qi or excessive heat causing cold.

Fever sensation over the chest and abdomen indicates internal accumulation of heat.

Cold in the chest and abdomen suggests internal retention of cold.

Cold in the back is due to insufficiency of yang qi.

Fever sensation over the face is due to sthenic heat in yangming meridian.

Fever sensation over the whole body and aversion to cold indicate exogenous disease.

2. 问汗
1.3.2.2　Inquiry about sweating

（1）出汗时间

醒时出汗：为自汗，多属阳气虚。

睡时出汗：为盗汗，多属阴虚。

高热后出汗、身凉：为邪解之兆。

（1）Time of sweating

Sweating in waking state indicates spontaneous sweating due to asthenia of yang qi.

Sweating during sleep indicates night sweating due to yin asthenia.

Sweating following high fever coupled with cold sensation over the body indicates that pathogenic factors have been relieved.

（2）汗出情况

大汗：热在阳明经，或过服发表剂所致。

微汗：外感病表虚证。

冷汗：阳虚。

热汗：阳气亢盛。

黄汗：为黄疸或历节病。

黏汗：汗出如油，多见于大汗亡阳。

战汗：身体战抖而汗出，多为正气来复，汗后脉静身凉为顺，汗后神昏烦躁为逆。

汗后肢冷：为阳气衰微。

汗后身热：邪热不解。

（2）Condition of sweating

Profuse sweating suggests heat in yangming meridian, or excessive intake of superficies-relieving medicine.

Mild sweating indicates external asthenia due to exogenous disease.

Cold sweat is due to yang asthenia.

Feverish sweating is due to hyperactivity of yang qi.

Yellowish sweat indicates jaundice or severe and migratory arthralgia.

Profuse and sticky sweat like oil is usually seen in yang depletion syndrome.

Sweating following shivering is due to recovery of healthy qi, sweating followed by pulse calming down and body turning cold is a favorable prognosis; sweating followed by coma and irritancy is an unfavorable prognosis.

Cold sensation of the limbs after sweating is a sign of yang qi exhaustion.

Sweating followed by feverish sensation over the body indicates unrelieved pathogenic heat factor.

（3）汗出部位

头汗出：为表虚、胃热、湿热上蒸等。

心胸出汗：多为心阴不足。

左右半身出汗：多为气血偏虚，为中风之先兆。

手足出汗：多为脾胃湿热证，或阳明里实证。

（3）Regions of sweating

Sweating over the head suggests external asthenia, stomach heat and up-steaming of damp heat.

Sweating over the chest indicates insufficiency of heart yin.

Sweating either over the left or the right half of body is due to deficiency of qi and blood, indicating wind stroke.

Sweating over the palms and soles is a syndrome of damp heat in the spleen and stomach, or yangming internal sthenia syndrome.

3. 问头痛
1.3.2.3 Inquiry about headache

（1）头痛时间

上午头痛：多为气虚。

午后头痛：多为阴虚。

昼日头痛：多为阳虚。

夜间头痛：多为阴虚。

（1）Time

Onset of headache in the morning is due to qi asthenia.

Onset of headache in the afternoon is due to yin asthenia.

Headache during the day indicates yang asthenia.

Headache at night indicates yin asthenia.

（2）头痛状况

痛无休止：多为外感热病。

时痛时止：多为内伤。

感风而痛：为风邪头痛。

感寒而痛：为寒邪头痛。

感热而痛：为热病头痛。

头痛如裹：为湿病头痛。

烦恼而痛剧：多为血虚头痛。

头痛而沉闷：多为痰湿。

劳累而痛剧：多为气虚。

（2）Conditions of headache

Non-stop headache is due to exogenous febrile disease.

Frequent headache is due to internal impairment.

Headache due to exogenous pathogenic wind is pathogenic-wind headache.

Headache due to exogenous pathogenic cold is pathogenic-cold headache.

Headache due to exogenous heat pathogen is pathogenic-heat headache.

Headache with the sensation like being wrapped is due to pathogenic damp factors.

Worsening headache with vexation is usually caused by blood asthenia.

Headache with oppressed sensation is usually due to phlegm dampness.

Worsening headache with overstrain is caused by qi asthenia.

（3）头痛部位

偏头痛：为少阳经头痛。

前额及眉棱骨痛：为阳明经头痛。

头枕部连及项痛：为太阳经头痛。

头顶疼痛：为厥阴经或太阳经头痛。

全头作痛：外感风寒之邪伤及三阳经。

（3）Region of headache

Hemicrania is related to shaoyang meridian.

Pain over the forehead and supraorbital bone is associated with yangming meridian.

Pain in occipital region involving the neck indicates a syndrome of taiyang meridian.

Pain on top of the head is connected with jueyin meridian or taiyang meridian.

Pain over the whole head suggests exogenous wind and cold pathogens impairing the three yang meridians.

4. 问眩晕

1.3.2.4　Inquiry about vertigo

暴眩：多为实证。

久眩：多为虚证。

头晕目昏：多为肝肾阴虚。

头响鸣：多为阴虚肝旺。

眩晕而呕：多为痰湿夹肝风作祟。

Sudden vertigo indicates a syndrome of sthenia.

Prolonged vertigo suggests a syndrome of asthenia.

Vertigo with blurred vision indicates yin asthenia of the liver and kidney.

Sonorous noise in the head is due to yin asthenia and fire hyperactivity in the liver.

Vertigo with vomiting is caused by damp phlegm coupled with endogenous liver wind.

5. 问面部

1.3.2.5　Inquiry about the face

面部发热：多为阳明经热。

面部发痒：风、湿、热邪均可导致。

面部疼痛：多为气滞血瘀。

面部麻木：多为气血虚亏，或风邪中络所致。

Feverish sensation of the face indicates heat in yangming meridian.

Itching sensation of the face is caused by pathogenic wind, dampness and heat factors.

Painful sensation of the face is due to qi stagnation and blood stasis.

Numb sensation of the face is caused by qi and blood deficiency, or by invasion of pathogenic wind factor into the collaterals.

6. 问眼部
1.3.2.6　Inquiry about the eyes

目赤肿痛：多为风热实证。

目痒：为风热所致。

两目干涩：为肝血不足或肾阴不足。

两眼羞明：红肿为实证，仅羞明而无异常者为阴血不足。

视物如蒙：多为气血不足。

视物如双：为肝肾亏虚。

小儿睡露睛：多为脾虚慢惊之候。

雀目（夜盲）：肝血不足。

Reddish and swollen eyes with painful sensation indicate sthenia syndrome of wind and heat.

Itching sensation of the eyes is caused by pathogenic wind and heat factors.

Dry and astringent sensation of the eyes indicates liver blood insufficiency or deficiency of kidney yin.

Flushed and swollen eye suggest sthenia syndrome, while only photophobia of the eyes without abnormal sensation indicates insufficiency of yin and blood.

Blurred vision is due to insufficiency of qi and blood.

Diplopia is caused by asthenia of the liver and kidney.

Sleep with eyes half-closed is a sign of spleen asthenia and chronic infantile convulsion.

Night blindness is due to insufficiency of liver blood.

7. 问鼻
1.3.2.7　Inquiry about the nose

鼻臭：为湿热内蒸之候，或内生疮疡。

鼻干燥：多为肺胃热盛。

鼻痛：肺火所致。

鼻痒：风热或虫积所致。

鼻涕稀薄：外感风寒。

鼻涕黏稠：外感风热。

鼻衄：外感热毒犯肺，或肝火犯肺所致。

鼻塞：外感多见。

Foul breath of the nose is a syndrome of internal steaming of dampness and heat or sores generated internally.

Dryness of the nose is due to heat superabundance in the lung and stomach.

Pain in the nose is caused by lung fire.

Itchy nose is caused by wind-heat or parasitic infestation.

Thin and clear snivel of the nose is caused by exogenous wind cold.

Thick and sticky snivel is due to exogenous wind heat.

Nasal hemorrhage is caused by invasion of exogenous heat toxin into the lung, or by liver fire attacking the lung.

Stuffy nose is usually due to exogenous diseases.

8. 问耳
1.3.2.8 Inquiry about the ears

耳鸣：多为肝肾不足所引起，或为少阳风热所致。
耳聋：外感风寒，或温热病，或肾气不足所致。
耳痛：为少阳热病。
重听：多为肾虚风邪干扰所致。

Tinnitus is usually caused by insufficiency of the liver and kidney, or wind heat pathogens in shaoyang meridian.

Deafness is due to exogenous wind cold, or pathogenic febrile disease, or insufficiency of kidney qi.

Pain in the ears indicates shaoyang heat syndrome.

Diplacusis is caused by disturbance of wind pathogen due to asthenia of the kidney.

9. 问口
1.3.2.9 Inquiry about taste and the mouth

口咸：多为肾热。
口淡：属气虚与湿邪不化。
口甜：多属脾湿夹热。
口苦：多为实热。
口酸：多为宿食或肝热。
口辛（辣）：多属肺热。
口臭：胃有实热。
口香：消渴病重症。
口干：阴津不足，或内有热蒸。
口黏：多为湿热。

Salty taste of the mouth is due to heat stagnation in the kidney.

Bland taste is caused by qi asthenia and failure to resolve pathogenic dampness.

Sweet taste is due to dampness in the spleen coupled with heat accumulation.

Bitter taste is due to sthenic heat.

Sour taste indicates food retention or heat stagnation in the liver.

Pungent taste is due to heat stagnation in the lung.

Foul odor of the mouth indicates sthenic heat in the stomach.

Fragrant odor of the mouth indicates worsening diabetes.

Dry mouth indicates insufficiency of yin fluid, or internal steaming of heat.

Sticky mouth is due to damp heat stagnation.

10. 问唇
1.3.2.10　Inquiry about lips

唇痒：多为火热病。
唇麻：多为气血瘀滞。
唇木：多为血虚不荣所致。

Itching lips are usually fire-heat syndrome.

Numb lips indicate qi stagnation and blood stasis.

Severe numb sensation of the lips is caused by failure of asthenic blood to nourish the lips.

11. 问饮
1.3.2.11　Inquiry about drinking of water

口渴消水：消渴病或热病入于气分。
不思饮：多为里寒证或湿邪内蕴。
喜冷饮：为里热证。
喜热饮：为里寒证。
口渴不欲饮：可见于阴亏、湿热瘀阻、津液不升，或蓄血证。
烦渴：为里热证。

Thirst with profuse drinking of water is indicative of consumptive disease（diabetes）or invasion of exogenous febrile factors into qi phase.

No desire for drinking water indicates internal cold syndrome or internal accumulation of pathogenic damp factors.

Thirst with preference for cold drinks is a sign of internal heat syndrome.

Thirst with preference for hot drinks suggests internal cold syndrome.

Thirst but without desire to drink water suggests yin deficiency, internal obstruction of dampness and heat, failure of body fluid to flow upwards or syndrome of blood amassment.

Polydipsia suggests internal heat syndrome.

12. 问食

1.3.2.12　Inquiry about appetite

不思食：胃肠有滞或肝胃不和。

饥而不欲食：为脾不运化，或痰火内闭。

多食易饥：为消渴病或胃热所致。

食后胀饱：脾不运化，或食滞。

嗜偏食：多为虫积。

食量正常：病向愈。

食量减少：病向恶。

Anorexia indicates food retention in the stomach and intestines, or disharmony of the liver and stomach.

Hunger but with no desire to eat indicates failure of the spleen to transport and transform food or internal blockage of phlegmatic fire.

Excessive eating and frequent hunger are caused by consumptive disease (diabetes), or heat accumulation in the stomach.

Full sensation in the stomach after meals is due to failure of the spleen to transport and transform food, or food retention.

Dietary bias indicates malnutrition due to parasitic infestation.

Normal repast indicates disease with a tendency to being healed.

Reduced repast indicates unfavorable prognosis of a disease.

13. 问呕吐

1.3.2.13　Inquiry about vomitus

呕吐食物酸味：内有食滞。

呕吐清水：内有停水。

呕吐痰涎：内有痰饮。

呕吐血液：胃有积热，或怒气伤肝。

呕吐酸水：为肝气犯胃。

呕吐苦水：为肝胆气逆。

欲吐不吐：为干霍乱症。

呕吐腹痛：为虫积或食物中毒。

吐后思饮：吐后伤阴，或内有停饮。

吐后思热饮：多属胃寒。

食已即吐：多为阳明经实热证。

朝食暮吐：多为胃虚寒证。

Vomitus with acid and putrid odor indicates internal food retention.

Clear and thin vomitus is due to internal fluid retention.

Vomiting of sputum and saliva indicates internal retention of phlegm and fluid.

Vomiting of blood suggests heat accumulation in the stomach or rage impairing the liver.

Vomiting of sour fluid signifies liver qi attacking the stomach.

Vomiting of bitter fluid suggests adverse flow of qi in the liver and gallbladder.

Retching without any vomitus indicates dry cholera.

Vomiting accompanied with abdominal pain is due to parasitic malnutrition or food poisoning.

Desire for drinking water after vomiting indicates yin impairment after vomiting or internal retention of fluid.

Desire for hot drinks after vomiting is due to cold syndrome in the stomach.

Vomiting of food just after eating is a syndrome of sthenic heat in yangming meridian.

Evening vomiting of food eaten at breakfast is a syndrome of asthenic cold in the stomach.

14. 问咳喘

1.3.2.14　Inquiry about cough and dyspnea

咳喘不得卧：暴咳不得卧为肺胀，为水饮内停；久咳不得卧，汗出不止，为肺气欲绝之象。

咳喘不得卧且呼吸困难：痰饮内阻，肾不纳气。

憋气难忍：痰浊闭于肺经，不得肃降所致。

短气：留饮、肺虚皆可有之。

Rapid cough leading to sleeplessness indicates distention of lung qi in the lung due to internal fluid retention. Sleeplessness resulting from persistent cough with endless sweating suggests depletion of lung qi.

Sleeplessness caused by cough and dyspnea is due to internal obstruction of phlegm and fluid, and failure of the kidney to receive qi.

Unbearable oppressed breath is caused by failure of turbid phlegm obstructed in lung meridian to be dispersed.

Short breath is caused either by fluid retention or by lung asthenia.

15. 问痰饮

1.3.2.15　Inquiry about sputum and fluid

黏稠色白：为湿痰。

黏稠而黄：为热痰。

清稀色白：为寒饮。

泡沫痰：为风痰。

痰中有血丝：热伤肺络。

Thick, sticky and whitish sputum indicates damp phlegm.

Thick, sticky and yellowish sputum suggests heat phlegm.

Thin, clear and whitish sputum suggests cold fluid retention.

Frothy sputum indicates wind phlegm.

Sputum mingled with blood is due to heat impairing lung collaterals.

16. 问胸胁
1.3.2.16　Inquiry about the chest and hypochondrium

胁痛：由肝郁、肝火、肝血虚、痰饮等不同因素所致。

胸胁刺痛：为气滞血瘀。

胸胁窜痛：为肝气不舒。

Pain in the hypochondrium is caused by various factors such as liver qi stagnation, liver fire, liver blood asthenia as well as retention of phlegm and fluid.

Piercing pain in the chest and hypochondrium is due to qi stagnation and blood stasis.

Wandering pain in the chest and hypochondrium is caused by qi depression in the liver.

17. 问心悸动
1.3.2.17　Inquiry about the heart

心悸：有气虚、血亏、痰饮、瘀血等不同。

心慌：心内气虚所致。

心烦：内热，包括虚热和实热。

心中懊恼：心中烦乱不安，为虚热所致。

Palpitation indicates qi asthenia, blood deficiency, retention of fluid and phlegm, as well as blood stasis.

Palpitation with flustered and nervous sensation is caused by qi asthenia in the heart.

Dysphoria is due to accumulation of endogenous heat including asthenic heat and sthenic heat.

Vexation and restlessness are caused by asthenic heat.

18. 问胃脘
1.3.2.18　Inquiry about the epigastrium

胃脘痛：有虚、实、寒、热之辨。痛而喜按为虚，痛而拒按为实；痛而喜热为寒，痛而喜凉为热。

攻刺胀痛：为气滞血瘀。

痞满痛：为胃气滞，有湿热、肝郁、食滞之不同。

Pain in the epigastrium can be differentiated from the following aspects such as asthenia, sthenia, cold and heat. Pain with preference for pressure indicates asthenia, while unpalpable pain indicates sthenia syndrome. Pain with preference for warmth is cold, pain with preference for cold is heat syndrome.

Piercing and distending pain in the epigastrium is due to qi stagnation and blood stasis.

Distending pain and fullness in the epigastrium are due to stagnation of stomach qi, which can be differentiated by various pathogenic factors such as damp heat, liver qi depression and food retention.

19. 问腹部
1.3.2.19   Inquiry about the abdomen

腹胀满：有虚实之分。拒按、喜冷、便秘，为实；喜按、喜温、便稀，为虚。

痞块：多为瘀血、痰阻、气滞所致。

隐隐痛：多为气虚证。

小腹痛：蓄血证，或水停膀胱。

少腹痛：肝气不和，或脾肠瘀滞，或妇科病等。

脐腹痛：脾经虚寒，或虫积，或内有燥结。

肠鸣腹痛：内有水湿停滞，或肠内有寒气，或湿热淤积等。

腹痛下坠：痢疾，或内脏下垂。

Distention and fullness in the abdomen can fall into sthenia syndrome which involves unpalpable pain, preference for cold as well as constipation, and asthenia syndrome including pain, preference for pressure and warmth as well as diarrhea.

Lumps in the abdomen are caused by blood stasis, phlegm obstruction and qi stagnation.

Dull pain in the abdomen suggests qi asthenia.

Pain in the lower abdomen is due to blood amassment, or fluid retention in the bladder.

Pain over bilateral parts of lower abdomen suggests disorder of liver qi or qi stagnation in the spleen and intestines, or gynaecological disease.

Pain over peri-navel region is due to asthenic cold in spleen meridian, or parasitic infestation, or internal accumulation of dryness.

Abdominal pain with borborygmus indicates internal stagnation of dampness, or cold qi in the intestines, or coagulation of dampness and heat.

Abdominal pain with tenesmus is due to dysentery, or due to prolapse of viscera.

20. 问腰
1.3.2.20   Inquiry about the loins

腰酸痛：多为肾虚。

腰沉痛：多为寒湿。

腰刺痛：多为瘀血。

活动后痛减：为气滞血瘀。

喜按、喜热敷：为虚寒。

Aching and pain in the loins are due to kidney asthenia.

Heavy pain in the loins is due to dampness and cold syndrome.

Stabbing pain in the loins indicates blood stasis.

Alleviation of pain after movement is due to qi stagnation and blood stasis.

Discomfort in the loins with preference for pressure and hot compression suggests asthenic cold syndrome.

21. 问全身、四肢
1.3.2.21 Inquiry about the body and limbs

寒热身痛：为外感风寒。
身热而痛：为外感风热。
身体沉痛：为湿邪困扰。
身体酸痛：或为外感，或为内伤。
身体困倦：为气虚血亏，或湿浊淤阻。
痛无定处：多为风邪，或肝气窜痛。
痛有定处：多为寒湿、瘀血所致。
四肢抽痛：多为肝虚血不荣筋所致。
产后身痛：多为血虚或瘀血滞于经络。

Aversion to cold, fever and painful sensation of the body are due to exogenous wind cold.

Fever and painful sensation of the body indicate exogenous wind heat.

Heavy sensation and pain over the body is due to obstruction of pathogenic dampness.

Aching and pain over the body indicate exogenous disease or internal impairment.

Fatigue is due to qi asthenia and blood deficiency, or stagnation of turbid dampness obstructing qi flow.

Wandering pain is caused by wind pathogen or wandering of liver qi.

Fixed pain is caused by cold and dampness obstruction and blood stasis.

Dragging pain over limbs is caused by failure of blood to nourish the tendons due to liver asthenia.

Painful sensation of the body after childbirth indicates blood asthenia or obstruction of blood stasis in meridians and collaterals.

22. 问睡眠
1.3.2.22 Inquiry about sleep

多寐：多因阳虚阴盛，痰湿困遏。
少寐：有心肾不交、血不养心、肝肾阴虚、痰火扰心等不同。
易醒：多为心胆气怯，心火旺盛。

早醒：多见于老年人，为气虚所致。

夜卧不安：多为饮食过饱，胃气不和所致。

入睡困难：多为心气虚弱，或心情不安，或阴虚火旺。

嗜卧欲寐：多属少阴病（心肾亏虚），多见于老年人。

Somnolence indicates yang asthenia and yin exuberance as well as obstruction of damp phlegm.

Insomnia can be attributed to the factors such as imbalance between the heart and the kidney, failure of blood to nourish the heart, yin asthenia of the liver and the kidney, disturbance of phlegmatic fire and so on.

Disturbed sleep with susceptibility to being waken up is caused by fright due to qi asthenia in the heart and gallbladder and exuberance of heart fire.

Waking up from sleep before the normal time is caused by qi asthenia, usually seen in aging people.

Restless sleep at night is due to excessive intake of food and disorder of stomach qi.

Falling asleep with difficulty is due to deficiency and weakness of heart qi, or dysphoria, or yin asthenia because of exuberance of fire.

Preference for lying with tendency to sleep indicates shaoyin syndrome (deficiency of the heart and kidney), usually seen in aging people.

23. 问精神

1.3.2.23 Inquiry about spirit

健忘：有心肾不交、心脾亏虚、心气不足、瘀血内阻等不同因素。

怔忡：心有跳动不安的感觉。惊恐之后，心血不足，阴虚火旺，均可见此症。

烦躁：多为阴虚证候。

抑郁：多为肝气不舒所致。

精神失常：如癫、狂、痫、脏躁等。

Amnesia is due to imbalance between the heart and kidney, deficiency of the heart and spleen, insufficiency of heart qi as well as internal obstruction of blood stasis.

Palpitation refers to the symptoms such as unease heartbreak, usually caused by being terrified due to insufficiency of heart blood, or exuberant fire resulting from yin asthenia.

Restlessness indicates yin asthenia.

Depression is caused by stagnation of liver qi.

Derangement suggests insanity, craziness, epilepsy and hysteria, etc.

24. 问大便

1.3.2.24　Inquiry about defecation

（1）便秘

伴有身热口臭、尿赤、腹满：热性便秘。

伴有喜热怕冷、脉迟、唇淡：寒性便秘。

伴有胸胁苦满、嗳气频作：气滞便秘。

伴有形体消瘦、口干盗汗：血枯便秘。

伴有气短吁吁、自汗头晕：气虚便秘。

（1）Constipation

Constipation accompanied with fever and foul odor of the mouth, reddish urine and abdominal fullness is due to heat syndrome.

Constipation accompanied with preference for warmth, aversion to cold, slow pulse and pale lips indicates cold syndrome.

Constipation with fullness and discomfort in the chest and hypochondrium and frequent ructation is due to qi stagnation.

Constipation accompanied with emaciation, dry mouth and night sweating indicates blood depletion.

Constipation with shortness of breath, panting, spontaneous sweating as well as dizziness suggests qi asthenia.

（2）便泄

腹痛即泄、便色黄褐：热性便泄。

腹痛绵绵、便泄清稀：寒性便泄。

泄下急迫、肛门灼热：暴泄为热。

五更作泄、泄下清稀：阳虚泄泻。

大便稀薄、隐隐腹痛：虚寒泄泻。

完谷不化：脾肾虚寒。

先干后溏：脾虚有湿。

便溏不爽：多属湿热。

（2）Diarrhea

Diarrhea marked by abdominal pain and brownish discharge of stool is heat syndrome.

Lingering abdominal pain with clear thin discharge indicates syndrome of cold.

Acute discharge with scorching sensation over the anus indicates heat syndrome.

Diarrhea before dawn with loose clear discharge of stool indicates yang asthenia.

Thin and loose stool with dull abdominal pain is due to asthenic cold.

Diarrhea with indigested food indicates asthenic cold in the spleen and kidney.

Dry feces followed by loose stool are due to spleen asthenia with dampness.

Unsmooth defecation of loose stool suggests dampness and heat syndromes.

（3）血便

先血后便、下血鲜红：热伤血络，为肠风。

先便后血、血色暗淡：脾不统血，为远血。

（3）Stool mingled with blood

Bleeding followed by stool with fresh blood is known as hemorrhoidal hemorrhage due to heat impairing blood vessels.

Stool followed by bleeding with pale darkish blood is known as distant anal bleeding, caused by failure of the spleen to control blood.

（4）大便颜色

色白：黄疸病或大肠虚寒。

色红：赤痢、便血。

色黑：蓄血。

色绿：肝郁克脾。

如鱼脑：热性痢疾。

（4）Color of stool

Whitish stool indicates jaundice or asthenic cold in the large intestine.

Reddish stool indicates red dysentery or stool mingled with blood.

Blackish stool is due to blood retention.

Greenish stool is due to stagnation of liver qi restraining the spleen.

Stool like fish brain indicates dysentery due to heat stagnation.

25. 问小便

1.3.2.25 Inquiry about urination

（1）排尿

小便闭：三焦气化失常。

小便难：热盛伤津。

小便涩难：多属淋病。

小便混浊：多属膀胱湿热。

小便不禁：气虚下陷。

遗尿：膀胱虚寒，肾气虚惫。

臊气重：膀胱有热。

小便数：次数多而痛，为下焦湿热；次数多而不痛，为阳虚；多饮多尿，为消渴。

（1）Conditions of urination

Obstruction in urination is due to disordered transformation of qi in triple energizer.

Urination with difficulty indicates exuberant heat impairing body fluid.

Obstructive urination with difficulty is usually seen in stranguria.

Turbid urine is due to stagnation of damp heat in the bladder.

Failure to control urination is caused by qi collapse due to qi asthenia.

Urinary incontinence during sleep indicates asthenia and cold in the bladder, and insufficiency and exhaustion of kidney qi.

Urine with foul smell suggests heat retention in the bladder.

Frequent urination with pain is due to dampness and heat in lower energizer; frequent urination without pain is due to yang asthenia; frequent urination as well as frequent drinking indicates diabetes.

（2）颜色

小便清白：多为虚寒。

小便黄赤：多为热象。

小便有白色黏液：多属淋浊。

小便有白色砂粒：多为石淋。

血尿：房劳伤肾。涩痛者为血淋，不痛者为尿血。

（2）Color of urine

Clear whitish urine indicates asthenic cold.

Yellowish and brownish urine suggests heat syndrome.

Sticky whitish urine indicates stranguria with turbid discharge.

Urine with whitish sand signifies urolithiasis.

Urine mingled with blood is due to intemperance of sexual life, which impairs the kidney. The syndrome with obstruction and pain is stranguria due to hematuria, while the syndrome without pain is hematuria.

26. 问前阴

1.3.2.26　Inquiry about external genitalia

（1）形态

阴肿：湿热下注或生有疮疡。

阳痿：肾阳衰竭，或肝郁遏阳。

强中：肾阴枯竭，阳气浮越。

囊缩：阴囊收缩，病属肝绝。

疝气：凡湿热、气滞、热壅等，均可引起。

（1）Shapes

Swollen external genitalia is caused by downward migration of damp heat or ulcer on the external genitalia.

Sexual impotence is due to exhaustion of kidney yang or liver depression which restrains yang qi.

Persistent erection of external genitalia is due to depletion of kidney yin, which results in out floating of deficient yang qi.

Sunken scrotum is due to liver qi declination.

Hernia is caused by damp heat, qi stagnation and heat obstruction, etc.

（2）症状

阴痒：多因湿热下聚所致。

抽搐：多因肝经受寒所致。

阴吹：多因谷气下泄，或因饮而致。

早泄：多因肾气虚，精不内固所致。

遗精：有梦而遗为心肾不交，无梦而遗为精关不固。

（2）Symptoms

Pruritus vulvae are due to downward accumulation of damp heat.

Twitching external genitalia is caused by invasion of cold into liver meridian.

Flatus vaginalis is due to downward discharge of essence derived from food, or caused by fluid retention.

Premature ejaculation is caused by asthenia of kidney qi and failure to store sperm.

Seminal emission during dreaming is due to imbalance of the heart and kidney; seminal emission without dreams is due to failure of the kidney in storing sperms.

27. 问后阴
1.3.2.27　Inquiry about anus

肛痒：湿热下注，或蛲虫干扰。

肛痛：痔疮，为湿热下迫所致。

脱肛：为中气下陷，或久利湿热下注，或产后元气未复等。

痔漏：为大肠风热，或阴虚火旺，或湿热郁结，或脾肾燥火而致。

Itchy anus is due to downward migration of damp heat or disturbance of pinworms.

Pain over the anus indicates haemorrhoids, caused by tenesmus of damp heat.

Archoptoma is due to qi sinking in middle energizer, or migration of damp heat resulting from persistent dysentery, or failure to regain primordial qi after delivery.

Fistula is due to accumulation of pathogenic wind and heat factors in the large intestine, or exuberant endogenous fire because of yin asthenia, or stagnancy of damp heat, or dryness and fire in the spleen and kidney.

28. 问月经

1.3.2.28 Inquiry about menstruation

（1）问经期

月经先期：多属血热。

月经后期：多属血瘀或虚寒。

月经前后无定期：肝气郁结，或心脾气虚。

(1) Duration of menstruation

Menstruation in advance of the normal date indicates blood heat.

Delayed menstruation is due to blood stasis or asthenic cold.

Unfixed time of menstruation suggests liver qi depression or qi asthenia in the heart and spleen.

（2）问血量

血量过多：多因血热，或气虚不摄。

血量涩少：多因血虚或血瘀，或痰阻。

血量时多时少：多因肝郁。

(2) Amount of menstrual blood

Profuse menstrual blood is usually caused by blood heat or failure of qi asthenia to control blood.

Scanty menstrual blood is due to blood asthenia or blood stasis, or phlegmatic obstruction.

Irregular amount of menstrual blood is due to liver depression.

（3）问颜色

血色鲜红：多为血热。

血色淡红：多为气虚，或血虚。

血色紫暗：多为气滞血瘀，或热结所致。

(3) Color of menstrual blood

Bright reddish blood indicates blood heat.

Pale reddish blood suggests qi asthenia or blood asthenia.

Dark purplish blood is due to qi stagnation and blood stasis, or heat accumulation.

（4）问腹痛

经前腹痛：多为气滞血瘀，寒凝。

经后腹痛：多为血弱气滞。

(4) Abdominal pain

Abdominal pain before menstruation is usually due to qi stagnation, blood stasis as well as cold coagulation.

Abdominal pain after menstruation is due to blood deficiency and qi stasis.

（5）问崩漏

血色清淡，气短恶寒：为气虚血崩。

血色鲜红，五心烦热：为虚热血崩。

血色紫红，腥秽黏稠：湿热下注。

血色紫暗，腹痛有块：为血瘀。

血色紫暗，精神抑郁：为气郁血崩。

（5）Profuse and sudden uterine bleeding

Uterine bleeding with thin and pale blood accompanied with short breath as well as aversion to cold is due to qi asthenia.

Uterine bleeding with fresh reddish blood combined with feverish sensation over five centers （the palms, soles and chest） is due to asthenic heat.

Thick sticky and purplish blood with stinking and filthy odor indicates downward migration of dampness and heat.

Dark purplish blood with fixed region of abdominal pain is due to blood stasis.

Purplish blood with depressed spirit is due to qi depression.

（6）问经闭

形体消瘦，气短乏力：为血枯经闭。

皮肤干糙，少腹拘急而痛：为血瘀经闭。

形寒肢冷，面色青白：为寒凝经闭。

形体肥胖，舌苔厚腻：为痰湿经闭。

精神郁闷，胸胁苦满：为气郁经闭。

（6）Amenorrhea

Amenorrhea with emaciated body, short breath as well as lassitude is due to blood depletion.

Amenorrhea with dry skin, spasm and pain over lower abdomen indicate blood stasis.

Amenorrhea with cold body and limbs as well as pale and cyanotic complexion is due to cold coagulation.

Amenorrhea with portly body as well as thick greasy tongue fur is due to phlegmatic dampness.

Amenorrhea with depressed emotion as well as distention and fullness of the chest and hypochondrium is due to qi depression.

29. 问带下

1.3.2.29   Inquiry about leucorrhea

白带：多属脾虚或肝郁。

黄带：多属湿热。

青带：多属肝经湿热。

赤白带：多属湿热留恋而腐化所致。

带下腥稀：多属寒湿。

带下稠臭：多属湿热。

Whitish leucorrhea is due to spleen asthenia or qi depression in the liver.

Leukorrhagia with yellowish discharge suggests dampness and heat.

Leukorrhagia with cyanotic discharge is due to dampness and heat in liver meridian.

Whitish leucorrhea mingled with blood indicates retained dampness an heat and turning putrid.

Thin leucorrhea with stinking odor is due to dampness and cold.

Thick leucorrhea with foul odor is due to dampness and heat.

（三）问诊注意事项
1.3.3 Notes for inquiry

①问诊时，医生应当严肃认真，和蔼可亲，不应轻浮嬉笑。

②问诊时，要有同情心，耐心地询问，不可急躁从事。

③问诊时，要结合病人的主诉有序地询问，不可东一句西一句，不着边际地乱问。

④对于不能自述病情的，可以询问病人的家属；小儿可由家长代述。

⑤对于患有精神病者，要注意病人的表情变化及举动，以防出现意外情况，影响其他病人的就诊环境。

a. Doctors should be strict, careful as well as kind. They should not let out frivolous laughs at patients.

b. Doctors should show sympathy for the patients and inquire about the information about the disease carefully and patiently. Restlessness and hasty action must be avoided.

c. Inquiry should be based on patient's chief complaint. Information irrelevant to the patient's illness must be avoided.

d. For patients who cannot describe their own illness, the doctor should ask their relatives. With regard to infants or children, doctor should ask their parents for details of the illnesses.

e. In order not to affect other patients, attention should be paid to the changes in expressions, emotions as well as manners in those who suffer from mental disorder in case of accidents.

四、切诊

1.4 Pulse-taking and palpation

切诊是中医独特的诊断手段之一。它包括切脉与按诊两大部分。它与西医的摸脉和身体各部位的触诊有着明显不同。

Different from feeling pulse and tactus of certain regions of human body in Western medicine, pulse-taking, as one special diagnostic method of TCM, includes taking pulse and palpation.

（一）切脉
1.4.1 Pulse-taking

切脉是中医独有的诊断方法。医生以自己的手指触觉来体验脉搏的动态，从中分辨出脉搏的浮沉迟数、滑涩虚实等脉象，再参合其他诊断所收集到的资料信息，综合分析其中的真伪与主次，从而为疾病做出正确的病证诊断。

As a unique diagnosis of TCM, pulse-taking is the method by which a doctor examines the states of a patient's pulse with the help of touching sense of his or her hand to distinguish features of various types of pulse such as floating, sunken, slow, fast, slippery, astringent, weak as well as powerful pulse. Different pulse conditions combined with the information collected through other diagnostic methods can help a doctor to make a comprehensive analysis and draw a conclusion about the true or false information so as to ensure a correct diagnosis.

1. 切脉时间
1.4.1.1 Time of pulse-taking

《黄帝内经》非常重视切脉，该书指出切脉的时间应当是"常以平旦，阴气未动，阳气未散，饮食未进，经脉未盛，络脉调匀，气血未乱，故乃可诊有过之脉"。"平旦"是清晨。清晨时间病人饮食未进，气血未乱，体内外的环境比较安静，还未受到饮食与起居活动的影响，所以容易诊断出病态的脉象。但社会发展到今天，诊脉不可能都放在清晨。这是强调切脉时要有一个安静的内外环境，使切脉尽量不受到客观因素的影响。

Huangdi Neijing (*Huangdi's Internal Classic*) attaches much stress to pulse-taking, in which, the best time for taking pulse has been mentioned. "Usually, pulse-taking is at pingdan (dawn), the time when yin qi has not been disturbed, yang qi has not been consumed, food is not taken, meridians are not vigorous, collaterals are in balance, and qi and blood are circulating in order. So changes of abnormal pulse can be detected." "Pingdan" refers to dawn when internal and external environment of human body are relatively quiet, for they are not affected by food and movements after getting up. Consequently, abnormal changes of pulse can be easily detected. However, it is impossible to take pulse only in the early morning nowadays. Therefore, it is essential to keep a quiet internal-external environment of human body so as to ensure that pulse-taking should not be affected by some outside objective factors if possible.

2. 切脉部位
1.4.1.2　Region for pulse-taking

切脉的部位有寸口切脉法、跌阳切脉法、太溪切脉法、太冲切脉法等。

寸口切脉法：寸口又称气口、脉口，其位置在腕后桡动脉所在部位。

跌阳切脉法：跌阳在足背的最高处，动脉应手处即是。

太溪切脉法：太溪在足内踝后，跟骨之上。

太冲切脉法：太冲在足大趾本节后 1 寸许，动脉应手处。

The regions for pulse-taking include Cunkou, Fuyang, Taixi, Taichong, and so on.

Cunkou, known as Qikou (opening of qi), or Maikou (opening of pulse), is located in the radial artery in the wrist.

Fuyang is located in the highest position of foot dorsum, on the pulsation of the artery.

Taixi is behind malleolus medialis, above calcaneus.

Taichong is about one cun (thumb cun) from proximal phalanx of hallux toe. It is also on the pulsation of the artery.

本书主要叙述寸口切脉法。寸口切脉的部位如下（见图2）。

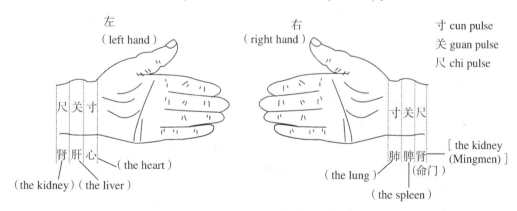

图2　寸口切脉法

Fig. 2　Pulse-taking method over Cunkou

左寸，主心、心包。

左关，主肝、胆。

左尺，主肾、膀胱、小肠。

右寸，主肺、胸中。

右关，主脾、胃。

右尺，主肾（命门）、大肠。

（以上是采用李时珍《濒湖脉学》的定位法。）

This book focuses on Cunkou—the usual pulse-taking method. The following are the regions of taking pulse from Cunkou（Fig. 2）：

The left cun pulse and its corresponding viscera：the heart and the pericardium.

The left guan pulse and its corresponding viscera：the liver and the gallbladder.

The left chi pulse and its corresponding viscera：the kidney, the bladder and the small intestine.

The right cun pulse and its corresponding viscera：the lung and the thorax.

The right guan pulse and its corresponding viscera：the spleen and the stomach.

The right chi pulse and its corresponding viscera：the kidney（Mingmen）and the large intestine.

（The above method is excerpted from Li Shizhen's *Binhu's Sphygmology*.）

3. 切脉方法

1.4.1.3   The method for taking pulse

病人端坐后，休息片刻，然后让其伸臂，将手腕部放在脉枕上，手掌向上放平。医生先用中指定其关位，继下示指以定寸位，再以无名指定尺位。如病人身材修长，则医生的三指排列可稍宽一些；如病人的身材比较矮胖，医生的三指排列可稍紧一些。但不论病人高、矮、胖、瘦，医生三指的排列要整齐，不能紧松不一。

切脉时手指轻放轻起。接触及肌肤的程度分浮取、中取、沉取三种力度。轻触皮肤为浮取，又名"举"；若用力触按为中取，又名"寻"；重按则为沉取，又名"按"。诊脉时，医生应在寸、关、尺三部分别用浮取、中取、沉取的方法进行脉诊，这种方法就是常用的"三部九候法"。

After a patient sits erectly and rests for a while to adjust his breath, he can stretch out one forearm and put the wrist on the pulse-taking pillow with the palm up and flat. The doctor should press his middle finger on the guan pulse, with his index finger on the cun pulse, ring finger on the chi pulse. Position of the fingers can be adjusted based on a patient's figure. If a patient is tall and thin, the doctor should place his three fingers a little wider. If a patient is stout and short, the doctor can put his three fingers a little closer. Regardless of the figure of a patient, the doctor's three fingers should be put at the same level orderly.

In the process of taking pulse, the fingers should be put and lifted lightly. Lifting, pressing and searching refer to the degree of pressure on the pulse. Light pressure means "lifting", moderate pressure means "searching", while heavy pressure means "pressing". The doctor should take pulse at chi, guan, cun, the three portions of Cunkou, which is also known as "three portions and nine pulse-takings".

4. 正常脉象

1.4.1.4 Normal pulse condition

　　正常人的脉象在静止状态下是可以摸到的，它不快不慢，不大不小，不软不硬，一呼一吸之间 4~5 次。如果脉象在至数、硬度、形态上发生变化，那就是病态脉象。

　　正常脉象，俗称"平脉"，平脉具有胃、神、根三个特点。

　　胃：胃为水谷之海，气血生化之源，胃气的有无决定着疾病的进退，所以经云"有胃气则生，无胃气则死"。平人的脉象不浮不沉，不快不慢，从容缓和，节律一致，是为有胃气。否则，是胃气衰弱的脉象。

　　神：脉来有力谓之神。脉的有力是否，与心脏的主血脉与心脏的"神气"有关。心神健旺则脉来有力，心气衰弱则脉来无力，所以古代医学家说："得神者昌，失神者亡。"

　　根：脉来有根是指沉取应指，尤其是尺部脉应指更为重要。尺部脉候肾脏的阴阳，好像树根一样，尺部脉缓和有力是有根之脉，否则是无根之脉。

Normal pulse condition refers to the pulse condition of healthy people taken in a motionless state, neither fast nor slow, neither soft nor hard, moderate in size, and usually beating 4 ~ 5 times in a cycle of breath (the duration between an exhalation and an inhalation). If normal pulse condition changes in rhythm, strength and pattern, morbid pulse conditions will appear.

The normal pulse condition is characterized by existence of stomach qi, vitality and root.

Existence of stomach qi: The stomach is the reservoir of water and cereals, and the source of qi and blood. The healing or development of a disease depends on existence of stomach qi, which is in accord with the saying "Life depends on the existence of stomach qi, and death occurs with absence of stomach qi". With stomach qi, the pulse condition of a healthy person is marked by neither floating nor sunken, regular in beating, gentle and orderly in rhythm. The contrary pulse condition indicates deficiency of stomach qi.

Existence of vitality means that the normal pulse has vitality (power), which indicates the close relationship between the statements "the heart is the residence of mind" and "the heart has the function of dominating blood vessels". Powerful pulse suggests that the heart is full of vigor and vitality. And deficiency of heart qi suggests weak pulse. Therefore, ancient TCM practitioners come to a conclusion that "existence of vitality indicates recovery from a disease, and absence of vitality is a sign of death."

Existence of root refers to powerful and constant beating of normal pulse under heavy pressure, and it is particularly important for taking pulse on chi portion. Chi pulse is corresponding to kidney yin and yang, which is like root of a tree. If chi pulse is moderate and powerful, it signifies the pulse has got root, otherwise, powerless pulsation indicates the pulse does not get root.

5. 四季脉象

1.4.1.5 Pulse conditions in the four seasons

由于受到气候的影响，四季的脉象亦有所不同，即春季脉弦，夏季脉洪，秋季脉浮，冬季脉沉。在春、夏、秋、冬依次见到上述脉象，乃是正常的脉象。如《濒湖脉学》中的浮脉"三秋得令知无恙"，洪脉"满指滔滔应夏时"等，都是季节性正常脉象。

Pulse conditions may vary with different seasons. Generally speaking, pulse tends to be slightly taut in spring, full in summer, floating in autumn and sunken in winter. The above pulse conditions appear in turn during four seasons, so they are the normal pulses. The following descriptions about floating pulse and full pulse quoted from *Binhu's Sphygmology* suggest they are seasonal normal pulses. For instance, "appearance of floating pulse in autumn is normal, it is not an indication of diseases", and "full and powerful pulse indicates the pulse condition appears in summer".

6. 常态脉象

1.4.1.6 Common pulse conditions

所谓常态脉象，是指不同体形、不同年龄、不同地域、不同性别、不同心态、不同生活习惯等形成的脉象。这些人的不同脉象，并不是病态脉象，而是由于内外因素不同所出现的正常脉象。常见的有以下几种。

①胖瘦之别：肥胖之人的脉象常带沉象，瘦薄之人的脉象常带浮象。

②老少之别：老年人脉多虚弱，少年人脉多实大，儿童的脉多数象。

③地域之别：北方之人多强实，南方之人多柔弱。

④劳逸之别：剧烈活动之后脉多洪数，久卧之人脉多沉迟。

⑤饮食之别：饮酒后脉多急数，久饿之人脉多迟缓。

⑥情绪之别：抑郁之人脉多濡弱，恬淡之人脉多平和，兴奋时脉多数，惊恐之时脉多动数。

Common pulse conditions refer to factors such as body figure, age, regions, gender, state of mind as well as life style may give rise to a particular pulse condition. The fact that pulse condition varies from person to person does not mean some people have got morbid pulse conditions. They fall into the normal pulse conditions due to their specific internal and external factors. Common pulse conditions are as follows:

a. (about differences between obese and thin figure) Sunken pulse is usually seen in obese people, floating pulse in thin people.

b. (about different ages) Weak pulse in aging people, powerful and large pulse in young people and fast pulse in children.

c. (about differences in geographical factor) Powerful pulse in northern people, soft and weak pulse in southern people.

d. (about differences between the state of ease and overstrain) Full and fast pulse after intense movements, sunken and slow pulse in people staying in bed with illness.

e. (about differences in dietary habits) Rapid and fast pulse appears after drinking alcohol, slow and moderate pulse in hungry people.

f. (about differences in emotions) Soft and feeble pulse seen in depressed people, even and soft pulse in people with peaceful state of mind; fast pulse in excited people and tremulous and fast pulse in terrified people.

7. 病态脉象
1.4.1.7　Abnormal pulse conditions

脉诊在中医诊断学上是必不可少的方法之一。多数疾病在脉象上都有显示，特别在八纲辨证上显示得更为明确。但脉象的诊断价值必须与其他诊断资料相参合，不可仅凭脉象一项就匆忙下诊断，而要四诊参合，客观地进行分析，这样才能做出正确的诊断，为治疗提供可靠的前提。这里将常见中的二十八脉详列于后，供大家在临床实践中参考使用。

Pulse-taking is an essential diagnostic method of TCM. Most diseases have certain manifestations in pulse condition, more obvious in syndrome differentiation of eight principles in particular. However, combined with the other three diagnostic methods, pulse-taking can be more valuable and correct diagnosis could be achieved by analyzing all information derived from four diagnostic methods synthetically and objectively, for they can ensure a correct treatment. Otherwise, hasty and partial diagnosis could possibly be made by the sole means of pulse-taking. The following are 28 common pulse conditions.

（1）浮脉

脉象：浮取即得，如水漂木，举之泛泛有余。

主病：表证，亦主虚证。

说明：浮脉主表，说明病邪在经络肌表的位置。外邪侵犯肌表，卫阳抵抗外邪，脉气鼓动于肌表，其脉应指而浮。但久病正气虚弱，亦可见到浮脉，但这种浮脉浮而无力，不作外邪论治。

（1）Floating pulse

Feature of pulse condition：Sensible under light pressure, feeling like the floating wood in water, so it is easy to "lift".

Clinical significance：Indicating external syndrome and asthenia syndrome.

Analysis：Floating pulse indicates external syndrome, it shows that pathogenic factors are in meridians and collaterals of the superficial skin and muscles. When exogenous pathogens attack the superficies, defensive yang qi combats them, qi in the vessels rises to the superficial muscles. As a result, floating pulse appears. Floating and weak pulse due to deficiency of healthy qi in chronic diseases should not be regarded as a syndrome of exogenous pathogen.

（2）沉脉

脉象：重取乃得，如石投水，轻取则无。

主病：里证，有力为里实证，无力为里虚证。

说明：邪气郁于里，气血内困，则脉象沉而有力；若气血虚弱，阳气下陷，不能升举，气血无鼓动之力，故脉象沉而无力。

（2）Sunken pulse

Feature of pulse condition：Sensible under heavy pressure, feeling like stone thrown into water.

Clinical significance：Indicating internal syndrome, sunken and powerful pulse signifies sthenic internal syndrome, while sunken and weak pulse indicates asthenic internal syndrome.

Analysis：Sunken and powerful pulse suggests internal stagnation of pathogenic factors and internal obstruction of qi and blood; sunken and weak pulse indicates asthenia of qi and blood, yang qi sinking down and failing to rise, so qi and blood lack strength to rise. Thus, sunken and weak pulse appears.

（3）迟脉

脉象：脉来迟缓，一息（一呼一吸）不足4次（相当于每分钟脉搏60次以下）。

主病：寒证。有力为寒积，无力为虚寒。

说明：寒气凝滞，阳气虚弱，鼓动无力，故脉呈迟象。迟而有力为冷寒积滞，迟而无力为虚寒之象。但脏腑郁热内结，阻塞气血不行，亦可见到迟脉，如伤寒病阳明经的腑实证等。

（3）Slow pulse

Feature of pulse condition：No more than 4 beats in a cycle of breath（equivalent to less than 60 times of sphygmus within one minute, <60/min）.

Clinical significance：Indicating cold syndrome. Slow and powerful pulse signifies internal cold accumulation; slow and weak pulse indicates asthenic cold syndrome.

Analysis：Slow pulse is due to cold stagnation and deficiency of yang qi, giving rise to failure of qi to rise. Slow and powerful pulse is due to cold accumulation; slow and weak pulse indicates asthenic cold. However, slow pulse could also be caused by internal heat stagnation in zang-fu organs, which obstructs qi and blood to circulate. This pulse condition can be seen in yangming fu sthenia syndrome of exogenous febrile disease.

（4）数脉

脉象：一息脉来5次以上（相当于每分钟脉搏90次以上）。

主病：热证。有力为实热，无力为虚热。

说明：邪热内炽，气血运行加速，故见数脉，且数而有力；阴虚内热，亦可见到数脉，必数而无力。若阳虚外浮，脉象则数大无力，按之中空。

（4）Fast pulse

Feature of pulse condition：More than 5 beats in a cycle of breath（equivalent to more than 90 times of sphygmus within one minute，>90/min）.

Clinical significance：Indicating heat syndrome. Fast and powerful pulse indicates sthenic heat，while fast and weak pulse indicates asthenic heat.

Analysis：Fast and powerful pulse is caused by superabundance of pathogenic heat factor，which leads to speeding up of qi and blood circulation；fast and weak pulse can also be seen in syndrome of endogenous heat due to yin asthenia. Fast，large，weak and hollow pulse under pressure is due to asthenic yang floating outwards.

（5）滑脉

脉象：往来流利，如珠走盘，应指圆滑。

主病：痰饮、实热、食滞，妇女怀孕后也会见到滑脉。

说明：实邪壅滞于体内，加之正气不弱，气盛血涌，故脉来滑利。营卫充实的人也会出现滑脉，当视为平脉。妊娠出现滑脉是气血充盛之象。

（5）Slippery pulse

Features of pulse condition：Beating freely and smoothly like the movement of beads on a plate.

Clinical significance：Indicating retention of phlegm and fluid，sthenic heat and food indigestion，sometimes it is seen in pregnant women.

Analysis：Slippery pulse is caused by internal accumulation of sthenia pathogenic factors together with sufficient healthy qi，which result in exuberance of qi and blood，thus giving rise to slippery pulse. Sthenia and sufficiency of nutrient qi and defensive qi can give rise to slippery pulse，too，which can be seen as normal pulse condition. Slippery pulse in pregnancy is a sign of qi and blood sufficiency.

（6）涩脉

脉象：脉来细而迟，往来难。

主病：血少，精少，反胃，亡阳，寒湿血痹。

说明：精亏血少，不能充盈血脉，血行不畅，往来艰难，故见涩脉。另外，湿阻、食积亦可见到涩脉，这是邪实阻塞血脉的脉象。

（6）Astringent pulse

Feature of pulse condition：Slow and thin，beating in an inhibited way.

Clinical significance：Indicating scanty blood and essence，nausea with regurgitation，yang depletion，dampness and cold syndromes as well as arthralgia due to blood obstruction.

Analysis：Astringent pulse is due to failure of scanty blood and essence to fill up the vessels，which，gives rise to inhibited or unsmooth blood circulation. In addition，astringent pulse can also be seen in syndromes such as obstruction of dampness and food retention，so it is a pulse condition indicating obstruction of sthenic pathogenic factors in blood vessels.

（7）虚脉

脉象：迟大而软，按之无力。

主病：虚证，伤暑。浮而无力是气虚，沉而无力是血虚，迟而无力是阳虚，数而无力是阴虚。

说明：虚脉是气血与脏腑俱虚均可见到的脉象。气血俱不足，自然脉搏显得无力虚弱。

（7）Weak pulse

Features of pulse condition：Slow， large and soft pulse， weak beating under pressure.

Clinical significance：Indicating asthenia and sun stroke. Floating and weak pulse indicates qi asthenia， sunken and weak pulse suggests blood asthenia， slow and weak pulse signifies yang asthenia， while fast and weak pulse is a sign of yin asthenia.

Analysis：Weak pulse is a sign of qi and blood asthenia as well as deficiency of zang-fu organs. Insufficiency of qi and blood definitely gives rise to weak pulsation.

（8）实脉

脉象：浮沉皆可触及，脉大而长。

主病：一切实证。

说明：实脉为邪气亢盛，正气不虚，正邪交争，气血涌盛，脉道充实，故见实象。

（8）Powerful pulse

Features of pulse condition：Large and long pulse can be combined with floating or sunken pulse.

Clinical significance：Indicating sthenia syndrome.

Analysis：Powerful pulse indicates struggle between hyperactive pathogenic qi and sufficient healthy qi， which leads to exuberant qi and blood as well as full-filled vessels. Therefore， the pulse is powerful.

（9）长脉

脉象：不大不小，首尾端直，超过本位。

主病：阳明热深，或肝阳有余，或阳毒癫痫。

说明：若长脉缓和，不急不迟，是为和缓之象，故曰"长则气治"。若长而弦硬，是为病脉，主有余之疾。

（9）Long pulse

Features of pulse condition：Neither large nor small， straight from the beginning to the end， stretching beyond the range of the cun， guan and chi portions.

Clinical significance：Indicating superabundance of heat in yangming meridian， or hyperactivity of yang in the liver， or epilepsy due to yang toxin.

Analysis：Long pulse coupled with moderate beating， neither rapid or slow， is known as "Long pulse is a sign that qi has been regulated" . Long pulse coupled with taut and hard sensation under pressure is morbid pulse, signifying syndrome of sufficiency.

（10）短脉

脉象：不及本位，应指不能满布。

主病：短脉主气不足之病。短而有力为气郁，短而无力为气虚。

说明：短脉为应指不及之象。由于气分不足，不能正常地鼓动血脉流行，故应指短而无力。但亦有气滞血瘀，或痰食积滞，阻塞脉道，以致脉气不能伸展，此短脉有力，不可作虚证看。

（10）Short pulse

Features of pulse condition：Shorter than the normal range of cun, guan and chi portions.

Clinical significance：Indicating syndrome of insufficient qi. Short and powerful pulse indicates qi stagnation, while short and weak pulse suggests qi asthenia.

Analysis：Short pulse means that the pulse is shorter than normal range of cun, guan and chi portions. Short and weak pulse is due to deficiency of qi, which causes failure to rise in blood vessels as usual. However, other factors such as qi stagnation, blood stasis, or obstruction of phlegm or food retention in blood vessels could also cause failure of qi in blood vessels to extend and flow. Short and powerful pulse can not be regarded as asthenia syndrome.

（11）洪脉

脉象：脉搏极大，如波涛汹涌，来盛去衰。

主病：气分热盛。

说明：体内热极，脉管扩张，气血涌盛，故见洪脉。若久病见到洪脉，是邪盛正衰的危候。

（11）Full pulse

Features of pulse condition：Large pulse beating like surging waves with sudden flowing and ebbing.

Clinical significance：Indicating superabundance of heat in qi phase.

Analysis：Exuberant heat causes expansion of blood vessels and surging and exuberance of qi and blood, which results in full pulse. Full pulse in chronic diseases is a critical sign suggesting hyperactivity of pathogenic factors and declination of healthy qi.

（12）微脉

脉象：极细极软，按之欲绝，若有若无。

主病：阴阳气血诸虚，尤以阳气虚为主。

说明：阴阳气血诸不足，故见微脉。轻取似无是阳气衰，重按似无是阴气衰，久病脉微是阳气欲绝，新病脉微是阳气暴脱，均为不佳之脉。

（12）Indistinct pulse

Features of pulse condition：Extremely thin and soft, almost insensible under pressure.

Clinical significance：Indicating asthenia syndromes of yin, yang, qi and blood, in particular, asthenia of yang qi.

Analysis：Indistinct pulse is due to insufficiency of yin, yang, qi and blood. Nearly insensible pulse when lifting indicates yang qi declination; nearly insensible pulse under pressure suggests declination of yin qi. Indistinct pulse due to chronic disease signifies exhaustion of yang qi, indistinct pulse in new disease is yang qi collapse. The above pulse conditions indicate unfavorable prognosis.

（13）紧脉

脉象：往来绷紧，如牵绳转索。

主病：寒、宿食、疼痛。

说明：寒邪阻遏阳气，阳气不能温通脉道，以致脉道紧张而拘急。寒邪在表，脉象浮紧；寒邪在里，脉象沉紧。另外，宿食、拘急疼痛亦可见到紧脉。

（13）Tense pulse

Features of pulse condition：Tense pulse appears like the pulling of a rope.

Clinical significance：Indicating cold syndrome, pain syndrome and food retention.

Analysis：Pathogenic cold factors obstructing yang qi causes failure of yang qi to warm the vessels, which results in tense and contracting pulse. Floating and tense pulse indicates pathogenic cold factors retaining in the superficies, while sunken and tense pulse is due to pathogenic cold factors in the interior. Besides, tense pulse can also be seen in food retention, spasm as well as pain syndrome.

（14）缓脉

脉象：一息四至，如丝在经，应指和缓。

主病：脾胃虚弱，湿病。

说明：脾胃虚弱，中气不足，故脉来和缓。湿邪黏滞，容易阻遏气机，使脉来无力，故亦可见缓脉。若平人脉象不急不迟，均匀和缓，则为常脉。

（14）Moderate pulse

Features of pulse condition：Beating 4 times in a cycle of breath. It is like thread in vessels with a soft and moderate sensation.

Clinical significance：Indicating asthenic spleen and stomach, and dampness syndrome.

Analysis：Asthenic spleen and stomach results in insufficient qi in middle energizer, which gives rise to moderate pulse. Stagnation of sticky dampness pathogens in blood vessels which is susceptible to inhibiting qi circulation, can give rise to weak and moderate pulse, too. Even and moderate pulse, not fast nor slow, is a sign of normal pulse of healthy people.

（15）芤脉

脉象：浮大中空，如按葱管。

主病：失血，伤阴。

说明：由于失血过多，使脉道中的血液骤然减少，阳气无所依附，浮在于外，故脉见于上下两旁，而中间却无。

（15）Hollow pulse

Features of pulse condition：Floating, large, and hollow in the middle, like the leaf of scallion.

Clinical significance：Indicating hemorrhage and impairment of yin.

Analysis：Sudden loss of blood in the vessels due to hemorrhage leads to yang qi floating outward. As a result, pulse could only be felt on both sides but hollow in the middle of vessels.

（16）弦脉

脉象：端直而长，如按琴弦。

主病：肝胆疾患、痰饮、疼痛、疟疾等。

说明：弦脉是血管紧张而不柔和的一种脉象。与肝胆气机不舒有密切关系。肝胆之气宜舒达不宜拘急，宜柔和不宜紧张。若肝胆气机失和，脉管失和就会出现弦脉。另外，痰饮、疼痛会影响气机的畅达，也会有弦脉出现。"疟脉自弦"，疟疾发于少阳，少阳者胆也，胆气失束，发为疟疾，故见弦脉。

（16）Taut pulse

Features of pulse condition：Straight and long pulse, like pressing the string of a violin.

Clinical significance：Indicating disorders of the liver and gallbladder, phlegm and fluid retention, pain as well as malaria.

Analysis：Taut pulse is a condition of pulse with tense and hard blood vessels, closely related to inhibited qi flow or qi stagnancy in the liver and gallbladder. Normally, qi in the liver and gallbladder is in a free, soft and uninhibited state. Inhibited qi flow in the liver and gallbladder and disordered vessels may give rise to taut pulse. In addition, inhibited qi flow due to phlegm and fluid retention as well as pain could also bring about taut pulse. "The pulse that suggests malaria is obviously taut." Malaria usually occurs in shaoyang meridian which is associated with the gallbladder, uncontrolled qi in the gallbladder would result in malaria, so taut pulse appears.

（17）革脉

脉象：外坚中空，如按鼓皮。

主病：亡血、失精、半产、漏下。

说明：革脉犹如按紧绷的鼓皮，由于阴精不能内藏，阳气无所附而浮越于外，所以见中空外坚的革脉，如亡血、失精、半产、漏下，多见革脉。

（17）Tympanic pulse

Features of pulse condition：Hard in the superficies and hollow in the middle. It feels like pressing the drum skin.

Clinical significance：Indicating bleeding depletion, consumption of essence, abortion as well as metrostaxis.

Analysis: The pulse feels like a tightly fastened drum skin. Failure to store yin essence internally results in yang qi floating outward because it could not be attached to yin, thus, giving rise to tympanic pulse, which is usually seen in syndromes such as hemorrhage bleeding, consumption of essence, abortion as well as metrostaxis.

（18）牢脉

脉象：沉取实大而长。

主病：寒积、腹痛、癥瘕。

说明：牢脉浮取、中取均不应，唯有沉取方可触及。多因病气牢固，沉积于里，如寒积、腹痛、癥瘕等，多为有形之邪内结的脉象，为危重之候。

（18）Firm pulse

Features of pulse condition: Powerful, large, and long pulse under heavy pressure.

Clinical significance: Indicating cold stagnation, abdominal pain as well as abdominal mass.

Analysis: Insensible under light pressure and moderate pressure, only sensible under heavy pressure. Firm pulse is usually due to internal accumulation of immobile pathogenic factors, such as cold stagnation, abdominal pain as well as abdominal mass. It is mainly the pulse condition of internal accumulation of tangible pathogenic factors, suggesting a critical syndrome with unfavorable prognosis.

（19）濡脉

脉象：浮而柔细，如帛在水中漂浮，一按即无。

主病：气虚、湿病，包括寒湿、湿温、伤暑。

说明：气分虚于表，脉管因虚而不敛，有松弛之势，故见濡脉。湿邪使正气无力鼓动脉搏，亦见濡脉。

（19）Soft pulse

Features of pulse condition: Superficial, soft and thin, like silk floating on the surface of water, and disappearing under heavy pressure.

Clinical significance: Indicating qi asthenia and dampness syndrome including damp cold, damp heat as well as sunstroke.

Analysis: Qi phase syndrome results in external asthenia, which causes failure of blood vessels to astringe as well as a loose and slack tendency, bringing about soft pulse. Furthermore, soft pulse can also arise as healthy qi fails to rise up the pulse because of pathogenic damp factor.

（20）弱脉

脉象：沉细而软，沉取乃得。

主病：气血不足。

说明：气不足则鼓动无力，血不足则脉不充盈，气血俱不足则脉象萎弱不振，所以脉象呈沉细而软。

（20）Feeble pulse

Features of pulse condition：Deep and thin, only sensible under heavy pressure.

Clinical significance：Indicating qi and blood deficiency.

Analysis：Qi deficiency results in weakness to beat due to lack of strength; blood insufficiency causes failure to fill up the vessels; asthenia of qi and blood causes weak and sluggish pulsation, therefore, the pulse is deep, thin and feeble.

（21）散脉

脉象：浮大散乱，至数不齐，按之即无，来去不明。

主病：气血涣散，阴阳脱离，将危之兆。

说明：散是无有规律无有约束之象，"散似杨花散漫飞"。由于气血涣散，脉管中的气血无有规律的流动，因此，脉搏也会无规律。但孕妇临盆之时会出现散脉，不为病脉。

（21）Scattered pulse

Features of pulse condition：Floating, large and scattered, arrhythmic, disappearing under pressure, and unobvious beating.

Clinical significance：Indicating scattered and unregulated state of qi and blood and disassociation of yin and yang, a sign of critical disease and prognosis of death.

Analysis：Scattered pulse suggests irregular and unrestrained condition, like scattered poplar filaments flying freely in the sky. Scattered and unregulated state of qi and blood results in irregular flow of qi and blood in blood vessels, causing irregular pulsation. However, scattered pulse that occurs in pregnant women at delivery is not a morbid pulse condition.

（22）细脉

脉象：脉细如线，但应指可以触到。

主病：气血亏虚，诸虚劳损，并见于湿邪侵凝腰肾。

说明：细脉为气血俱虚之象。但湿邪阻滞脉道，亦可见到细脉。细脉并非触及不到，而是"应指沉沉无绝期"。

（22）Thin pulse

Feature of pulse condition：As thin as thread, quite sensible under pressure.

Clinical significance：Indicating deficiency of qi and blood in all asthenia syndromes due to overstrain and consumption as well as invasion and coagulation of pathogenic damp factor in the loins and kidney.

Analysis：Thin pulse indicates qi asthenia and blood asthenia. However, it can also be seen when pathogenic damp factors obstruct and stagnate in blood vessels. Thin pulse is not insensible but "deep and constantly sensible under pressure".

（23）伏脉

脉象：重按至骨，隐约得之。

主病：邪闭于内，或厥证，也主痛极。

说明：伏为气闭于内。邪气闭于内，气机不得宣通，故脉沉至于骨，为危重之候。

（23）Deep-sited pulse

Features of pulse condition：Faintly sensible only under heavy and forceful pressure on the bone.

Clinical significance：Indicating internal blockage of pathogenic factors, or syndrome of syncope as well as severe pain.

Analysis：Deep-sited pulse indicates internal blockage of pathogenic factors, giving rise to failure of qi to be dispersed, thus, pulse sinks into the bones, a critical sign and unfavorable prognosis.

（24）动脉

脉象：滑数如豆，厥厥动摇，见于关上下。

主病：疼痛，惊恐，阴虚，阳虚。

说明：疼痛、惊恐可见动脉；阳虚则汗出，阴虚则发热，阴阳相搏则脉数如豆。凡脉象滑数有力，但有不宁之势，皆属于动脉。

（24）Tremulous pulse

Features of pulse condition：The pulse is fast and slippery, like rolling beans with short and sudden leaps, usually seen at guan portion.

Clinical significance：Indicating syndrome of pain, scare, yin asthenia, or yang asthenia.

Analysis：Tremulous pulse is accompanied with scare or panic due to pain. Yang asthenia causes sweating, while yin asthenia gives rise to fever. Tremulous pulse like rolling beans indicates struggle between yin and yang. Fast, slippery and powerful pulse without stop belongs to tremulous pulse.

（25）促脉

脉象：脉来数而时一止，止无定数。

主病：阳盛实热，痰积、发狂、痈肿等。

说明：阳盛实热，阴不和阳，脉来急促，但有中止。若有痰积、发狂、痈肿等实热之邪，亦可见到脉促有力。

（25）Rapid and intermittent pulse

Features of pulse condition：Beating fast with occasional and irregular intermittence.

Clinical significance：Indicating yang exuberance due to sthenic heat, phlegm retention, deliria, carbuncle well as swellings.

Analysis：Rapid pulse with intermittence is due to yang exuberance with sthenic heat and disharmony of yin and yang. Rapid, intermittent and powerful pulse could also be seen in phlegm retention, deliria, carbuncle well as swellings because of sthenic pathogenic heat factors.

（26）结脉

脉象：脉来缓而时一止，止无定数。

主病：阴盛阳衰，气血凝结，老痰结滞。

说明：阴盛气结，阳不和阴，脉来缓和，但有中止。凡寒痰凝滞，气血郁阻，脉气不通，亦可见到结脉。

（26）Slow and intermittent pulse

Features of pulse condition：Beating slowly with occasional and irregular intermittence.

Clinical significance：Indicating yin exuberance, yang declination, qi stagnation and blood stasis, as well as accumulation of lingering phlegm.

Analysis：Slow and moderate pulse with intermittence is caused by yin exuberance, qi accumulation and disharmony of yin and yang. Slow and intermittent pulse can also be seen in syndromes such as stagnancy of cold phlegm, obstruction of qi and blood, as well as failure of qi in vessels to circulate.

（27）代脉

脉象：脉来一止，止有定数，良久方来。

主病：脏气衰微，泻痢大伤元气，跌打损伤。

说明：脏气衰微，气血亏虚，元气不足，以致脉气不能相接，故中止而有定数。泻痢伤及元气，元气不能充盈，使脉来中止。跌打损伤，伤及气血，使脉气难以接续，亦可见到代脉。

（27）Slow-intermittent-regular pulse

Features of pulse condition：Beating slowly with regular and long intermittence.

Clinical significance：Indicating declination of visceral qi and impairment of primordial qi due to diarrhea with dysentery as well as traumatic injury.

Analysis：Slow-intermittent-regular pulse is due to declination of visceral qi, deficiency of qi and blood, and insufficiency of primordial qi, causing failure of qi in vessels to circulate continuously. Impaired primordial qi, which could not be replenished due to diarrhea with dysentery, brings about intermittent pulse. Impairment of qi and blood due to traumatic injury causes failure of qi in the vessels to be replenished, thus, resulting in slow-intermittent-regular pulse.

（28）疾脉

脉象：脉来数急，一息七八次。

主病：热极阴伤，元气将脱。

说明：疾，是数极的意思。疾脉是阴竭于下，阳浮于上，阴阳将要脱离之象。伤寒与温病在热极阶段，会有疾脉出现。疾而有力是真阴垂危，疾而无力是元阳将脱之兆。

（28）Swift pulse

Features of pulse condition：Beating fast and rapidly about 7 ~ 8 times in a cycle of breath.

Clinical significance：Indicating yin impairment due to extreme heat and collapse of primordial qi.

Analysis：The word "swift" means extremely fast. Swift pulse indicates exhaustion of kidney yin and up-floating of hyperactive yang qi as well as disassociation of yin and yang. Swift pulse may arise at the superabundant heat stage of exogenous febrile disease and epidemic febrile disease. Swift and powerful pulse indicates declination of kidney yin and critical disease；swift but weak pulse is a sign of collapse of yang and primordial qi.

除了上述脉象外，还有其他少见的几种脉象：

In addition to the above pulse conditions，there are other rare types of pulse conditions listed as follow：

七绝脉

雀啄脉：如雀啄连连，止而又作，主肝绝。

鱼翔脉：头定尾摇，如鱼之游，主心绝。

屋漏脉：雨后屋漏，半时一落，主胃绝。

解索脉：乍密乍疏，乱如解索，主脾绝。

釜沸脉：釜沸空浮，毫无跟脚，主肺绝。

弹石脉：弹石沉弦，毫无柔和，主肾绝。

虾游脉：虾游冉冉，忽然一跃，主大肠绝。

Seven dangerous pulse conditions

Bird-pecking pulse is like birds pecking repeatedly with intermittence，indicating liver exhaustion.

Fish-swimming pulse is like fish swimming in water with head fixed and tail flapping, signifying exhaustion of heart qi.

Roof-leaking pulse is like roof leaking water after rain with occasional fall，suggesting gastric exhaustion.

Knot-untying pulse is like untying knots，with occasionally dense beat or occasional sparse-beat pulse，suggesting spleen exhaustion.

Bubble-rising pulse refers to rootless pulse，like rising bubbles in boiling water of a kettle，a sign of lung exhaustion.

Stone-knocking pulse is like stone-knocking and declining string with sharp but not soft sounds，indicating kidney exhaustion.

Shrimp-swimming pulse is like shrimps swimming slowly in water yet abruptly jumping up, suggesting exhaustion of the large intestine.

（二）按诊
1.4.2 Palpation

按诊是切诊的一部分，是四诊中不可缺少的一环。按诊大致可分触、摸、按三类。

触是以手指或手掌轻轻接触病人的患部，如额部、四肢皮肤等，以了解寒热、润燥等情况。摸是以手抚摸患部，如肿胀部位，以探明局部的感觉，以便了解肿物的形态、大小等。按是以手按其患部，如胸腹或肿物部位，以便了解有无压痛，以及肿物的形态、质地、性质、程度等。

今天的医学检查，虽然有彩超、CT 等微观检查手段，但简易的按诊仍然有着临床实用价值，有的按诊是即刻可明确诊断的，也是彩超、CT 不可替代的。

Palpation is an essential part of the four diagnostic methods. The usual techniques are palpation, feeling and slight pressing.

Palpation refers to feeling a patient's discomfort area with fingers or palms, for instance, the forehead, four limbs and the skin, etc, so as to detect whether the part is cold, feverish, moist or dry. Feeling means touching the discomfortable region with hands such as lumps and swellings to detect the shape and size of them. Slight pressing refers to pressing hands over the chest, abdomen as well as swellings to examine existence of pressing pain, shapes, texture, nature as well as degree of swelling parts.

Nowadays, palpation, with its own advantage of simple operation, is of great clinical value though there does exist some advanced medical equipments such as Colour Doppler Ultrasound and CT (Computed Tomography) for micro-level examination. However, with its remarkable curative effect, palpation cannot be replaced by modern equipments.

1. 按肌肤
1.4.2.1 Palpation on the skin

肌肤热为阳盛，肌肤寒为阴盛。

初按热甚，久按热反轻者，为热在表；初按热轻，久按热重者，为热在里。

肌肤柔软喜按为虚证，肌肤硬痛拒按为实证。

轻按即痛病在表，重按方痛病在里。

按之凹陷，不能即起者为水肿；按之凹陷，抬手即起者为气肿。

Feverish sensation on the skin indicates predominance of yang, while cold sensation on the skin suggests yin sufficiency.

Heavy feverish sensation at the beginning but light feverish sensation after prolonged palpation signifies heat in the superficies; light feverish sensation at the beginning but heavy feverish sensation after prolonged palpation indicates internal heat.

Soft skin with preference for palpation indicates syndrome of asthenia; hard and pain sensation in the skin with aversion to palpation indicates sthenia.

Immediate pain sensation after palpating with light pressure indicates disease is in the superficies; pain sensation after palpating with heavy pressure indicates internal disease.

Failure to spring back if the fingers sink into the skin after palpation indicates edema; if sunken skin could spring back immediately after taking the fingers away indicates emphysema.

2. 按手足
1.4.2.2　Palpation on hands and feet

手足俱冷为阳虚阴盛，寒证；手足俱热为阳盛阴虚，热证。
手背发热，为外感发热；手心发热，为内伤发热。
四肢温热，阳气犹存；四肢厥冷，阳气衰亡。
小儿中指独热为外感风寒，中指尖独冷为麻痘将发之象。
头额热甚于手心，为表热；手心热甚于头额，为里热。

Cold sensation over the hands and feet suggests yang asthenia and yin exuberance, a cold syndrome; feverish sensation over the hands and feet indicates yang sthenia and yin asthenia, a heat syndrome.

Feverish sensation over dorsa of hands is caused by exogenous disease; feverish sensation over the palms of hands is caused by internal impairment.

Warm sensation of four limbs indicates existence of yang qi; cold limbs suggest declination of yang qi.

Feverish sensation of the middle finger of an infant is due to exogenous pathogenic wind and cold; cold sensation is a sign of measle and exanthema variolosum.

More obvious feverish sensation over the forehead than the palms indicates external heat; more obvious feverish sensation over the palms than the head and forehead is endogenous heat.

3. 按疮疡
1.4.2.3　Palpation on the area of ulceration

肿硬不热者为寒证，肿处烙手者为热证。
患部坚硬，无脓；顶软边硬，脓已成。
盘根平塌漫肿为虚证，盘根收束高起为实证。

Swollen and hard ulceration without feverish sensation is cold syndrome; swollen ulceration with burning sensation is heat syndrome.

Hard ulceration indicates absence of pus inward; soft sensation on top of the ulceration with hardness at periphery suggests the formation of pus.

Flat and swollen ulceration from the root is asthenia syndrome, while contracted ulceration from the root with protrusion in the centre indicates sthenia syndrome.

4. 按胸腹
1.4.2.4　Palpation on the chest and abdomen

（1）按虚里

虚里在左乳下心尖搏动处，为诸脉所宗。在正常健康状态下，虚里按之应手，动而不紧，缓而不散。若动而不显，为不及，是宗气内虚；若动而应衣，为太过，是宗气外泄；若动而欲绝，为危候，或有痰饮阻塞。

（1）Palpation on the precordium

The precordium refers to the pulsating point of the heart apex below the left breast, where all vessels converge. Normally, pulsation on the precordium is sensible, beating smoothly and moderately but unscatteredly with rhythm. If the pulsation of the part is not obviously sensible, it is a sign of internal deficiency of thoracic qi; if pulsation is so obviously sensible that it vibrates the clothes on the body, it is an indication of hyperactivity of precordial beating, a sign of outburst of thoracic qi; if pulsation feels to be exhausted, it is a critical sign, or obstruction of phlegm and fluid.

（2）按胸胁

前胸高起，按之而喘，为肺胀；胸胁按之胀痛，为痰热气结或水饮内停；右胁胀痛，按之热感，手触之痛甚，为肝痈；左胁下胀痛，按之有痞块者，为疟母。

（2）Palpation on the chest and hypochondrium

Protruding prothorax with asthma when pressing indicates lung distention. Distending pain over the chest and hypochondrium when pressing is caused by phlegmatic heat and accumulation of qi, or by internal fluid retention. Distending pain over the right hypochondrium combined with feverish sensation when pressing and severe pain when touching with hands indicates liver abscess. Distending pain over the left hypochondrium and lump in the abdomen when pressing suggests malarial nodules.

（3）按腹部

腹部触诊的情况比较复杂，反映的病情也比较多变。

辨寒热：腹壁冷喜温手按者，为寒证；腹壁灼热喜冷拒按者，为热证。

辨疼痛：腹痛喜按者，为虚；腹痛拒按者，为实。

辨腹胀：腹部胀满，按之压痛，叩之声重浊者，为实满；腹壁胀满，喜按，无压痛，叩之声空，为虚满。

辨痞满：心下痞满，按之柔软，无压痛，为虚证；按之硬痛，有抵抗感，为实证。

辨结胸：胃脘痞闷，按之而痛，为小结胸；胸脘、腹部硬满疼痛，为大结胸。

辨积聚：痛有定处，按之有形而不移者，为积，病在血分；痛无定处，按之无形，为聚，病在气分。

辨动气：以脐为中心，脐上动气为心气不舒，脐下动气为肾气虚弱，脐左动气为肝气不展，脐右动气为肺气虚弱，脐中动气为脾胃气虚。

（3）Palpation on the abdomen

The cases on palpation on the abdomen are very complex, and it could reflect various diseases.

About cold and heat：Cold sensation over abdominal wall with preference for warmth and pressure indicates cold syndrome；scorching sensation over abdominal wall with preference for cold and aversion to pressure is heat.

About pain：Abdominal pain with preference for pressure indicates asthenia syndrome；abdominal pain with aversion to pressure is due to sthenia syndrome.

About abdominal distention：Abdominal distention and fullness with pain under pressure and heavy and dull sound when tapped indicates sthenic fullness；distention and fullness over abdominal wall, no pain under pressure, with preference for pressure and empty sensation when pressed is asthenic fullness.

About abdominal fullness：Fullness in the epigastrium with soft sensation and no pain under pressure suggests asthenia；epigastric fullness with hard, resisting and painful sensation is due to sthenia.

About accumulation of pathogens in the chest：Fullness and oppression in the epigastrium with pain under pressure is due to accumulation of phlegmatic heat in the chest；fullness, hard and painful sensation in the chest, epigastrium and abdomen indicates large accumulation of phlegmatic heat in the chest.

About abdominal amassment：Immobile lumps with fixed shape and painful sensation under pressure is unmovable mass, indicating diseases in blood phase；intangible lumps with migratory pain sensation under pressure is known as movable amassment, suggesting diseases in qi phase.

About qi throb around the navel：Qi throb above the navel is due to depression of heart qi；qi throb under the navel indicates deficiency of kidney qi；qi throb on the left of the navel is due to depressed liver qi；qi throb on the right of the navel suggests insufficiency of lung qi；qi throb in the centre of navel indicates qi asthenia in the stomach and spleen.

其他还有按腧穴、按肿块等，不在这里一一叙述。

The other palpating regions include acupoints, swelling and distension, and so on, which are omitted here.

结语

Conclusion of the four diagnostic methods

四诊是不可分割的整体，四者不可缺一。医生在诊断取材时，必须以负责的态度，逐一进行。在四诊过程中，态度要和蔼，动作要轻柔，使病人感到温馨而贴切。四诊是为辨证提供可靠的资料，如果是以粗心随意的态度去取材，那些所得到的资料，必定是不可靠的、不全面的，其论治也必然是错误的。所以四诊必须去掉主观意识，全面细致地一一进行，然后将所得到的资料，去伪存真，去粗存精，在中医基本理论的指导下，进行辨证分析，从而为正确的治疗提供可以信赖的信息。

The four diagnostic methods are an inseparable organic whole. Any one of them cannot be neglected, and doctors must take them one by one in order to carefully collect detailed information so as to ensure a comprehensive analysis of a disease. In clinical diagnosis, doctors must be kind in attitude and gentle in action in order that patients could feel at home. Adopting the four diagnostic methods aims at providing reliable information for syndrome differentiation, therefore, data collected carelessly must be unreliable and partial, and treatment based on syndrome differentiation in this unserious way is certainly incorrect. Consequently, subjective judgment should be avoided in diagnosis. In order to ensure accurate treatment, syndrome differentiation must be based on comprehensive and careful analysis and under the guidance of TCM theory to provide reliable data.

第二章 辨证
2 Differentiation of syndromes

一、八纲辨证

2.1   Syndrome differentiation of eight principles

八纲，即阴、阳、表、里、虚、实、寒、热，是辨证论治的基础理论之一。它是通过四诊将所收集的资料进行分析，根据疾病的部位、性质、正气的盛衰等，归纳为八个证候，称为八纲辨证。

八纲辨证，一般以阴阳为总纲，辨表里以明疾病的深浅，辨寒热以明疾病的性质，辨虚实以明正气的强弱。阴阳可以概括其他六纲，即表、热、实证为阳，里、寒、虚证为阴。故阴阳乃是八纲中的总纲。

八纲辨证，在临床中常常是两证互见，或三证互见，如表热证、里寒证、表实证、里虚证等，还有表实热证、里虚寒证等。更有表热与里寒证互见，表实与里虚证互见等。因此在诊察辨证中，应以真实的资料为依据，不要以自己的主观见解而下诊断。单凭经验做出诊断，是临床医生的大忌。

Eight principles, including yin and yang, internal and external aspects, asthenia and sthenia as well as cold and heat, constitute the foundation of treatment and syndrome differentiation. Accordingly, by analyzing collected information with four diagnostic methods, the eight syndromes, summed up on the basis of location, characteristics of a disease as well as sufficiency or deficiency of healthy qi, are known as syndrome differentiation with eight principles.

Among the eight principles, yin and yang are the general principles. Differentiation of external and internal syndromes enables a doctor to learn whether pathogenic factors in a patient's body are internal or on the superficies; differentiation of heat and cold syndromes enables him to detect the nature of pathogenic factors; differentiation of asthenia and sthenia syndromes enables him to find out whether healthy qi is deficient or sufficient. Yin and yang are the general principles used to summarize the other six principles, that is, heat, sthenia and external syndromes pertain to yang, while cold, asthenia and internal syndromes are attributed to yin.

In clinical diagnosis, two or three of the eight principles are usually complicated together. For instance, if external and heat syndromes are complicated together, the syndrome of external heat would appear. Likewise, the notions of internal cold, external sthenia, internal asthenia, external sthenic heat syndromes as well as syndrome of internal asthenia cold, etc, have been developed in this way. What's more, syndrome of external heat complicated with internal cold, and external sthenia complicated with internal asthenia. As a result, clinically, diagnosis should be based on truthfulness of collected data rather than on a doctor's own subjective assumption. Besides, diagnosis based only on a doctor's clinical experience should be avoided too.

（一）阴阳辨证
2.1.1　Syndrome differentiation of yin and yang

从理论上讲，凡表证、实证、热证，均归于阳证，凡里证、虚证、寒证，均归于阴证，但这还不能为治疗提供有针对性的前提。还必须阐明该证的具体症状、舌象与脉搏，然后再结合脏腑辨证，才能明确证候的性质。

In theory, external, sthenia and heat syndromes fall into yang syndrome, while internal, asthenia and cold syndromes belong to yin syndrome, which, however, cannot provide corresponding precondition for clinical treatment. Furthermore, in order to figure out general characteristics of a syndrome, manifestations such as specific symptoms, signs of tongue as well as pulse condition involved in it must be explicitly illustrated by combining its corresponding fu-zang syndrome differentiation.

（1）阴证

精神委顿，乏力，语音低微，面色晦暗，两目无神，动作迟缓，畏寒肢冷，喜暖近衣，口淡乏味，饮食少馨，大便不实，舌苔淡白而滑，脉象沉细无力。治以温阳益气，用金匮肾气丸、右归丸之类。

（1）Yin syndrome

Main clinical manifestations：Dispiritedness with lassitude, lack of energy, low voice, tarnished complexion, dull expression of the eyes, tardy movement of body, aversion to cold, cold limbs, preference for warmth with liability to putting on clothes, bland taste, poor appetite, loose stool, slippery and pale tongue fur as well as sunken, thin and weak pulse.

Prescription：Warm yang and benefit qi.

Formulas：Jingui Shenqi Wan (Pill), as well as Yougui Wan (Pill).

（2）阳证

精神兴奋，甚则烦躁狂言，语声高亢，面红目赤，口渴而饮，呼吸气粗，喜凉去衣，饮食不减，大便燥结，小便短赤，舌苔厚腻，脉象有力或数大。治以清心泻火，用泻心汤之类。

（2）Yang syndrome

Main clinical manifestations：Excited mood, even restlessness with ravings, high voice, flushed complexion and eyes, thirst with preference for drink, hoarse breath, preference for cold with liability to taking off the coat, normal appetite, dry feces, short and brownish urine, thick and greasy tongue fur as well as powerful or fast large pulse.

Prescription：Clear the heart and purge fire.

Formulas：Xiexin Tang（Decoction）.

（3）辨证要点

单纯的阴证与阳证，辨别起来并不困难。但阴证可以转化为阳证，阳证也可以转化为阴证。如寒性腹泻为阴证，若腹泻日久，阴液耗伤，又可转化为阴虚内热证；又如发热恶寒为阳证，但若发热久羁，使阳气耗散，又可转化为单纯恶寒的阴证。另外，在错综复杂的病症中，阴证和阳证还会出现假象，即阳证表现有假寒象，阴证表现有假热象，真真假假，不易分辨。这就要求医者多临床、多实践、多思考，唯此才能明辨真假，抓住病症的本质。

（3）Key points for syndrome analysis

It is not difficult to differentiate single yin syndrome from that of yang. However, yin syndrome can transform into yang, and yang syndrome can transform into yin. For instance, diarrhea due to cold is yin syndrome. However, persistent diarrhea may consume and impair yin fluid, so yin syndrome here may transform into that of endogenous heat due to yin asthenia. Let's take fever with aversion to cold as another example. It is a yang syndrome, however, prolonged fever may cause consumption of yang qi, therefore, it can transform into yin syndrome with the single manifestation of aversion to cold. Additionally, in some complicated cases, both yin and yang syndrome may present false manifestations, that is, yang syndrome may present manifestations of false cold. Likewise, yin syndrome may have signs of false heat, so it would become more difficult to distinguish them. Accordingly, doctors should take more clinical practice and think more. Only in this way, could true features of a syndrome be distinguished from its false presentation, and characteristics of a specific disease be mastered.

（二）表里辨证

2.1.2 Differentiation of internal and external syndromes

表里辨证，是指疾病的发生部位而言。凡是风、寒、暑、湿、燥、火及其他因素侵犯肌表所呈现的病症，即是表证；而由内伤七情、饮食劳倦等因素所致的脏腑病变则是里证。

Differentiation of internal and external syndromes is used to distinguish the location of a disease. External syndrome refers to symptoms caused by invasion of six pathogenic factors namely wind, cold, summer-heat, dampness, dryness and fire together with other factors into the superficies of human body. Internal syndrome refers to the symptoms such as dysfunction of zang-fu organs due to impairment of the organs caused by seven intemperate emotional activities, improper diet as well as overstrain in daily life.

（1）表证
恶寒，发热，头痛，无汗或有汗，脉浮，舌苔薄白。
①表寒证：恶寒重，发热轻，脉浮紧。治以发散风寒，用杏苏散之类。
②表热证：发热重，恶寒轻或不恶寒，脉浮数。治以发散风热，用银翘散之类。
③表虚证：发热恶寒，有汗，脉浮缓。治以调和营卫，用桂枝汤之类。
④表实证：发热恶寒，无汗，脉浮紧。治以发汗解表，用麻黄汤之类。

（1）External syndrome

Main clinical manifestations：Aversion to cold, fever, headache, no sweating or sweating, floating pulse, thin and whitish tongue fur.

a. External cold syndrome：Heavy aversion to cold, light fever as well as floating and tense pulse.

Prescription：Dissipate wind and cold.

Formulas：Xing Su San (Powder).

b. External heat syndrome：High fever, slight aversion to cold or no aversion to cold as well as floating and fast pulse.

Prescription：Expel wind and heat.

Formulas：Yinqiao San (Powder).

c. External asthenia syndrome：Fever, aversion to cold, sweating as well as floating and slow pulse.

Prescription：Regulate nutrient qi and defensive qi.

Formulas：Guizhi Tang (Decoction).

d. External sthenia syndrome：Fever, aversion to cold, no sweating as well as floating and tense pulse.

Prescription：Induce sweating to relieve superficies.

Formulas：Mahuang Tang (Decoction).

（2）里证
高热，神昏，谵语，烦躁，口渴，腹胀，便秘，舌苔厚腻，脉沉。
①里寒证：口不渴，恶心，呕吐，腹痛，腹泻，四肢不温，舌苔白滑，脉象沉迟。治以温里散寒，用理中汤之类。
②里热证：口渴引饮，发热，烦躁，小便黄赤，舌质红赤，舌苔黄腻，脉象数而

有力。治以清热滋阴，用白虎汤或人参白虎汤之类。

③里虚证：精神疲惫，少气懒言，食欲减少，心慌气短，舌质淡红，舌苔薄白，脉象沉弱。治以补益中气，用四君子汤或补中益气汤之类。

④里实证：烦躁不安，大便秘结，腹满腹痛拒按，或有谵语发狂，舌苔黄腻，脉象沉实有力。治以通腑泻实，用承气汤之类。

（2）Internal syndrome

Main clinical manifestations：High fever, coma, delirium, restlessness, thirst, abdominal distension, constipation, thick greasy tongue fur as well as sunken pulse.

a. Internal cold syndrome：No thirst, nausea, vomiting, abdominal pain, diarrhea, cold limbs, slippery whitish tongue fur as well as sunken and slow pulse.

Prescription：Warm the interior and expel cold.

Formulas：Lizhong Tang (Decoction).

b. Internal heat syndrome：Thirst with profuse drinking of water, fever, restlessness, yellowish and brownish urine, reddish tongue with yellowish greasy fur as well as powerful and fast pulse.

Prescription：Clear away heat and nourish yin.

Formulas：Baihu Tang (Decoction), or Renshen Baihu Tang (Decoction).

c. Internal asthenia syndrome：Lassitude, dispiritedness, weak breath with few words, reduced appetite, palpitation with short breath, pale reddish tongue with thin whitish fur as well as weak and sunken pulse.

Prescription：Replenish and benefit qi in middle energizer.

Formulas：Sijunzi Tang (Decoction), or Buzhong Yiqi Tang (Decoction).

d. Internal sthenia syndrome：Irritancy and restlessness, constipation, unpalpable abdominal distention and pain, or accompanied with delirium and ravings, yellowish greasy fur as well as powerful and sunken pulse.

Prescription：Eliminate stagnation in fu organs and purge sthenic heat.

Formulas：Chengqi Tang (Decoction).

（3）辨证要点

单纯的表证与里证，比较容易辨别。但证候是变动不拘的，尤其是表证。表证既可出表而愈，也可入里侵犯脏腑。因此注意表证的动向很重要。温病有"一日三变药三宗"之诚语，即是此意。另外，应当注意表里同病，如表里俱寒、表里俱热、表里俱虚、表里俱实，还有表寒里热、表热里寒、表虚里实、表实里虚等。在表里同病时，还要分清主次，以便为论治确定正确的治疗原则。

（3）Key points for syndrome differentiation

It is not hard to differentiate simple external and internal syndromes. However, diseases are variable, especially of those external syndromes, which can be cured if pathogenic factors are just on the surface, but pathogenic factors may transmit into the interior and attack zang-fu organs. Therefore, it is essential to pay attention to developing direction of external syndrome.

For instance, epidemic febrile disease can "vary three times and treatment for it can change more frequently just in a single day". In addition, much weight should be attached to the fact that external and internal syndromes may have some similar symptoms, for example, cold, fever, asthenia as well as sthenia can appear in external syndrome, and they could also appear in internal syndrome. And other phenomena such as external cold complicated with internal heat, external heat complicated with internal cold, external asthenia coupled with internal sthenia, and external sthenia with internal asthenia should be noticed too. In order to work out correct therapeutic methods, a doctor should distinguish major from minor syndrome in the course of dealing with external and internal syndromes with similar symptoms.

（三）寒热辨证
2.1.3 Differentiation of cold and heat syndromes

寒热辨证，主要是辨别疾病的性质。寒证与热证是机体对致病因素的内在反应，阳气偏盛的表现为热证，阴气偏盛的表现为寒证；反之，阳气偏虚的为寒证，阴津偏虚的则为热证。只是，前者的热证与寒证为实，后者的热证与寒证为虚。正如《素问》说：“阳盛则热，阴盛则寒。”“阳虚则外寒，阴虚则内热。”

Differentiation of cold and heat syndromes refers to distinguishing the features of a disease. Cold syndrome or heat syndrome is the inherent reaction of human body to pathogenic factors causing a disease, for instance, manifestation of exuberant yang qi indicates heat syndrome, while predominance of yin qi signifies cold syndrome. On the contrary, yang qi asthenia belongs to cold syndrome, insufficiency of yin fluid is heat syndrome. The syndromes mentioned above are different in nature, in the former heat and cold syndromes are sthenic, while in the latter, they are asthenic. Just as what is stated in *Suwen* (*Plain Questions*), "Exuberance of yang causes heat, and yin predominance gives rise to cold." "Yang asthenia causes external cold, while yin asthenia brings about endogenous heat."

（1）寒证
手足逆冷，恶寒，面色苍白，口不渴，喜热饮，小便清长，大便稀薄，舌苔白滑，脉象沉迟。治以温阳益气，用理中汤或四逆汤之类。

（1）Cold syndrome
Main clinical manifestations：Cold limbs, aversion to cold, pale complexion, no thirst, preference for hot drink, clear and profuse urine, loose stool, slippery whitish tongue fur as well as sunk and slow pulse.

Prescription：Warm yang and benefit qi.

Formulas：Lizhong Tang (Decoction), or Sini Tang (Decoction).

（2）热证

发热，恶热，口渴，喜冷饮，面赤，烦躁，小便短赤，大便秘结，舌苔厚腻，脉象数而有力。治以清热通腑，用白虎汤或承气汤之类。

（2）Heat syndrome

Main clinical manifestations：Fever, aversion to heat, thirst, preference for cold drink, flushed complexion, restlessness, scanty and brownish urine, constipation, thick and greasy tongue fur as well as powerful and fast pulse.

Prescription：Clear away heat and dredge fu organs.

Formulas：Baihu Tang（Decoction）, or Chengqi Tang（Decoction）.

（3）辨证要点

单纯的寒证与热证比较容易鉴别，在诸多症状中，其口渴与否、四肢冷热、二便状态、舌苔、脉搏等则是辨证的主要依据。但要注意寒热证候的真假，如病人身大热反近衣者，则为假热真寒证；身大寒反不近衣者，则为假寒真热证。另外，还会出现上热下寒证、上寒下热证、表里俱寒证、表里俱热证等。寒热证还可以互相转化，因此在辨证时要注意其主症的动态变化，以便做出正确的证候诊断。

（3）Key points for syndrome differentiation

It is not difficult to distinguish simple cold from heat syndrome. Of many symptoms in heat and cold syndromes, thirst or no thirst, cold or warm limbs, condition of urination and defecation, sign of tongue fur as well as pulse condition are the foundation for syndrome differentiation. However, doctors must make sure whether cold and heat syndromes are false or true. For instance, the case that a patient with high fever would rather put on clothes is a syndrome of false cold and true heat, while the case that a patient with severe cold would rather not put on clothes is regarded as a syndrome of false cold and true heat. Besides, there exist other syndromes such as upper heat and lower cold, upper cold and lower heat, external and internal cold, and external and internal heat syndrome, etc. Since cold and heat syndromes may transform into each other, therefore, during syndrome differentiation, much stress should be attached to the dynamic changes of the main syndrome of some disease so as to ensure a correct diagnosis about a syndrome.

（四）虚实辨证
2.1.4　Syndrome differentiation of asthenia and sthenia

虚实辨证，是对病人体质强弱即抗病能力的综合判断。虚证是指病人的正气虚弱，抗病能力低下；实证是指病人的正气未衰，抗病能力比较强。实证、虚证与病人的体质有密切关系。同样一个致病因素，不同的体质会产生不同的虚证与实证。当然，当致病因素超过人体的抗病能力时，人的抵抗能力也是有限的。这正如《素问》所说："邪气胜则实，精气夺则虚。"

Syndrome differentiation of asthenia and sthenia refers to comprehensive judgment about a patient's constitution of weakness or strength, that is, whether a patient has resistance against a disease. Asthenia means that healthy qi in human body is too deficient to fight against diseases, while sthenia refers to sufficient healthy qi which can resist diseases. Asthenia or sthenia is closely related to a patient's constitution. To the same pathogenic factor, patients with different constitutions can react differently, thus, asthenia or sthenia syndrome appears. Pathogenic factors can overcome the degree that human body could resist, for it is definitely limited. Just as what is stated in *Suwen* (*Plain Questions*), "Predominance of pathogenic qi indicates sthenia, loss of vital essence (healthy qi) suggests asthenia."

（1）虚证

生理功能减退，抗病能力低下，出现精神萎靡，饮食减少，形寒肢冷，自汗出，语音低微，气短乏力，身体酸困，视力听力减退，大便溏薄，小便失禁，舌淡胖嫩，脉象沉细无力。治以补益气血，用四君子汤或四物汤之类。

（1）Asthenia syndrome

Main clinical manifestations：Physiological hypofunction of viscera with failure to resist diseases, with symptoms such as dispiritedness, reduced appetite, cold limbs, spontaneous sweating, low voice, short breath with lassitude, aching and tired sensation, dysfunction of sight and hearing, loose stool, urinary incontinence, pale fat and tender tongue as well as thin weak and sunken pulse.

Prescription：Tonify qi and benefit blood.

Formulas：Sijunzi Tang (Decoction), or Siwu Tang (Decoction).

（2）实证

病邪过盛，生理功能亢进，病邪与正气交争显著，出现发热，腹痛拒按，胸闷烦躁，甚则神昏谵语，呼吸气粗，痰涎涌盛，大便秘结，小便淋漓涩痛，舌质坚老，舌苔厚腻，脉象沉实有力。治以清热破积，用防风通圣散或承气汤之类。

（2）Sthenia syndrome

Main clinical manifestations：Physiological hyperfunction of the viscera due to predominance of pathogenic factors, obvious struggle between pathogenic factors and healthy qi, such as fever, unpalpable pain of abdomen, chest oppression, even coma and delirium, hoarse breath, exuberance of phlegm and saliva, dry feces, inhibited urination with astringent and painful sensation, tough tongue with thick greasy fur as well as powerful and sunken pulse.

Prescription：Clear away heat and break accumulation.

Formulas：Fangfeng Tongsheng San (Powder), or Chengqi Tang (Decoction).

（3）辨证要点

辨别虚实，要认真甄别虚实的真假。真假的辨别要从脉象的有力与无力、语声的高亢与低怯、舌质的胖嫩与坚老，以及体质的状况去分辨。还要注意虚实证候的转化与兼夹，如虚中夹实证，实中夹虚证；实证久居，消耗气阴，可以转化为虚证；虚证缠绵，使气血瘀阻，亦可转化为实证。古代医学家有"大实有羸状，至虚有盛候"证候描述，提示医家在注重实证的时候，不要忘记是否有虚证的存在；在注重虚证的时候，也要注意是否有实证的羁留。另外，在辨别虚实证候的时候，还要分析证候的部位，即何脏虚？何脏实？以便有的放矢地遣方用药。

(3) Key points for syndrome differentiation

Syndrome differentiation between asthenia and sthenia involves careful distinguishing whether a syndrome is false or true of asthenia or sthenia based on weak or powerful pulse, low or high voice, fat tender tongue or rough tongue as well as state of constitution. Besides, attention should be given to transformation between asthenia and sthenia as well as complication of asthenia and sthenia. For instance, asthenia syndrome may be complicated by sthenia, and sthenia syndrome complicated by asthenia. Prolonged sthenia would consume qi and yin, thus, it can transform into asthenia. Likewise, lingering asthenia would cause qi stagnancy and blood stasis, so it may transform into sthenia. The statement of ancient TCM experts that "excessive sthenia may have deficient symptoms, while extreme asthenia can possess sufficient symptoms" reminds doctors that due stress should be placed on the presence of asthenia while emphasizing sthenia. Similarly, they should pay attention to the existence of sthenia syndrome while thinking about asthenia. Additionally, in order to take suitable therapeutical methods for treating a disease, a doctor must make sure "which part the location of asthenia is and where the area of sthenia is" in differentiating asthenia and sthenia as well as in analyzing the location of a disease.

二、六经辨证

2.2　Syndrome differentiation of six meridians

六经辨证，是东汉张仲景在《黄帝内经》理论指导下，结合临床实践总结出来的辨证方法。这种方法，是依据疾病的性质，将其错综复杂、变化多端的症状，归纳为六种有内在联系的症状群，即六种证候，依次为太阳经、阳明经、少阳经、太阴经、少阴经、厥阴经六经病症候群。学习和运用六经辨证，能使我们正确地掌握外感疾病变化发展的规律，从而在治疗上起着重要的指导作用。

Six-meridian syndrome differentiation is a principle summarized by Zhang Zhongjing of the Eastern Han Dynasty under the guidance of the theory in *Huangdi Neijing* (*Huangdi's Internal Classic*). Based on features of different diseases, this principle classifies complicated and changeable symptoms into six groups of syndromes, which are correlated to one another. They are, in turn, taiyang, yangming, shaoyang, taiyin, shaoyin and jueyin syndrome. Learning and using six-meridian syndrome differentiation can help doctors master the developing law of exogenous diseases to guide treatment of various diseases.

（一）太阳病证

2. 2. 1　Taiyang syndrome

太阳病证有经证与腑证之分。太阳经证是指外邪侵犯肌表所呈现的证候；而太阳腑证是表邪传入太阳之腑——膀胱而呈现的证候，有蓄水证与蓄血证之分。

Taiyang syndrome can be divided into meridian as well as fu syndrome. Taiyang meridian syndrome refers to invasion of exogenous pathogenic factors into the superficies, while taiyang fu syndrome refers to transmission of pathogenic factors from the superficies into fu organs of taiyang, the bladder. It can be divided into water-accumulation and blood-accumulation syndrome.

（1）主要脉证

头痛，恶寒发热，脉浮。

①太阳表虚证：除主要脉证外，还有自汗，恶风，脉缓。治以调和营卫，祛风解表，用桂枝汤之类。

②太阳表实证：除主要脉证外，还有无汗，身痛，脉紧。治以发汗解表，用麻黄汤之类。

③太阳蓄水证：除出现太阳经脉证外，同时又有烦躁，口渴欲饮，水入即吐，小便不利等症。治以行气利水，佐以解表，用五苓散之类。

④太阳蓄血证：除有恶寒发热，颈项强痛外，乃以其人如狂，或发狂，少腹急结，小便自利，脉象微沉等为主症。治以活血化瘀，通下郁热，用桃核承气汤之类。

（1）Main clinical manifestations

Headache, aversion to cold, fever as well as floating pulse.

a. Taiyang external asthenia syndrome: Headache, aversion to cold, fever, floating pulse, spontaneous sweating, aversion to wind and moderate pulse.

Prescription: Reconcile nutrient qi and defensive qi, expel wind and relieve superficies.

Formulas: Guizhi Tang (Decoction).

b. Taiyang external sthenia syndrome: Headache, aversion to cold, fever, floating pulse, no sweating, aching sensation of the body and tense pulse.

Prescription: Induce sweating to relieve the superficies.

Formulas: Mahuang Tang (Decoction).

c. Taiyang water-accumulation syndrome: Besides the above symptoms of taiyang meridian syndrome, there exists other symptoms such as restlessness, thirst with desire to drink, immediate vomiting after drinking water, dysuria, etc.

Prescription: Promote qi circulation, induce diuresis and relieve the superficial syndromes.

Formulas：Wuling San（Powder）.

d. Taiyang blood-accumulation：In addition to fever, aversion to cold, stiffness and pain in the neck, its main manifestations are mania, lower abdominal spasm, normal urination as well as indistinct and sunken pulse.

Prescription：Activate blood circulation and dissolve blood stasis, and promote discharge of stagnation of heat.

Formulas：Taohe Chengqi Tang（Decoction）.

（2）辨证要点

①太阳病证以寒热为特点，因此必须分辨寒热的轻重，以及发热的时间，依此来判断寒热的性质，以确定是否为太阳经病。

②有汗与无汗亦是辨别太阳经病的主要症状，有汗为虚，无汗为实，治法有别，在问诊中不可忽视这一项。

（2）Key points for syndrome differentiation

a. Taiyang syndrome is characterized by cold and heat, so doctors must distinguish the extent of cold and heat（whether the cold or heat is slight or severe）, and the time of fever so as to make sure the feature of cold or heat and diagnose whether the disease is taiyang meridian disease or not.

b. Sweating and no sweating are also the main symptoms to distinguish taiyang syndrome. Sweating indicates asthenia, while no sweating indicates sthenia, so the treatment should be differentiated, which cannot be neglected in diagnosis of inquiry.

（二）阳明病证
2.2.2　Yangming syndrome

阳明病证是因太阳病未愈，病邪逐渐亢盛入里所致。它的病变主要表现为里热实证，有经证与腑证之分。在经为热证，在腑为里热实证。

Yangming syndrome is caused by delayed or improper treatment of taiyang disease, resulting in internal transmission of hyperactive pathogenic factors. The syndrome is manifested as internal sthenic heat, which can be divided into yangming meridian disease, indicating heat, and yangming fu disease, indicating an internal sthenic heat.

（1）主要脉证

身热，汗自出，不恶寒，反恶热，脉大。

①经证：身大热，汗大出，烦渴引饮，不恶寒，反恶热，脉洪大。治以清热保津，或兼以益气，用白虎汤或人参白虎汤之类。

②腑证：日晡（下午3~5时）潮热，手足漐然汗出，腹部硬满痛，大便燥结，甚则谵语、狂言，不得眠，舌苔黄燥而厚腻，脉象沉实或滑数有力。治以通腑泻实，攻

坚消痞，用大承气汤、小承气汤、调胃承气汤之类。

（1）Main clinical manifestations

Fever, spontaneous sweating, no aversion to cold but aversion to heat as well as large pulse.

a. Yangming meridian syndrome：High fever, profuse sweating, polydipsia with desire to drink, no aversion to cold but aversion to heat as well as full large pulse.

Prescription：Clear away heat and preserve body fluid, or combined with benefiting qi.

Formulas：Baihu Tang（Decoction）, or Renshen Baihu Tang（Decoction）.

b. Yangming fu syndrome：Afternoon tidal fever（15 ～ 17 o'clock in the afternoon）, continuous sweating over hands and feet, abdominal hardness and fullness with unpalpable pain, dry feces, restlessness, even with delirium and ravings, insomnia, dry thick greasy and yellowish tongue fur as well as sunken powerful pulse or fast, slippery and powerful pulse.

Prescription：Dredge fu organs, purge sthenic heat stagnation, remove dry feces and eliminate abdominal lumps.

Formulas：Large Chengqi Tang（Decoction）, Small Chengqi Tang（Decoction）, as well as Tiaowei Chengqi Tang（Decoction）.

（2）辨证要点
①阳明病是由太阳病或少阳病传变而来。在甄别时，要注意它们之间的关联，是否还有太阳病或少阳病的存在。
②阳明病是阳热亢盛阶段，但也有与湿邪结合的可能，发为黄疸；或瘀血内停，发为狂证。如果辨别有误，误治或延治，就有可能贻误生机。

（2）Key points for syndrome differentiation

a. Yangming syndrome is transformed from taiyang or shaoyang syndrome. In differentiation, attention should be paid to correlation between the two syndromes so as to analyze the existence of lingering taiyang disease or shaoyang disease.

b. Yangming syndrome appears at the hyperactive stage of yang heat, which, however, could be combined with pathogenic damp factors. In that case, jaundice may arise, or manic psychosis can be brought about due to internal retention of blood stasis. Incorrect syndrome differentiation or wrong as well as delayed treatment may endanger the patient's life.

（三）少阳病证
2.2.3　Shaoyang syndrome

少阳病证从疾病的传变来看，是已离太阳之表，未入阳明之里，正处于太阳与阳明之间，即半表半里部位，因而在病证的表现上，既不属于表证，又不属于里证，故称为半表半里证。

Shaoyang syndrome signifies that pathogenic factors have left the superficies where taiyang syndrome is located, yet they haven't transmitted into the interior, the location of yangming syndrome. They are just between the location of taiyang syndrome and that of yangming, namely, the area of semi-interior and semi-exterior. Shaoyang syndrome does not belong to external nor internal syndrome. Therefore, it is a syndrome of semi-interior and semi-exterior.

（1） 主要脉证

口苦，咽干，目眩，往来寒热，胸胁苦满，心烦喜呕，默默不欲饮食，脉弦，苔白或薄黄。治以和解表里，用小柴胡汤之类。

①少阳兼太阳病证：发热，微恶寒，骨节烦痛，微呕，心下支结。前三证为太阳病证，后二证为少阳病证。治以疏解表里，用柴胡桂枝汤之类。

②少阳兼阳明病证：胸胁苦满而呕，日晡潮热，或大便不通，前者为少阳证，后二者为阳明证。治以和解少阳，通里泻实，用大柴胡汤之类。

③少阳兼水饮互结病证：往来寒热，胸胁满微结，小便不利，渴而不呕，头汗出。前二证为少阳病证，中一证为太阳病证，后二证为水饮内结证。治以和解表里，逐饮开结，用柴胡桂枝干姜汤之类。

（1） Main clinical manifestations

Bitter taste of the mouth, dry throat, dizziness, alternate chills and fever, discomfort and fullness in the chest and hypochondrium, vexation with susceptibility to vomiting, no appetite, taut pulse as well as whitish tongue fur or thin yellowish fur.

Prescription：Reconcile and relieve the external and internal syndrome.

Formulas：Small Chaihu Tang （Decoction）.

a. Shaoyang complicated by taiyang syndrome：Fever, slight aversion to cold, restlessness and pain sensation in bones and knuckles （the above symptoms belong to syndrome of taiyang）, slight vomiting, sensation of obstruction in the epigastrium （the latter two symptoms are shaoyang syndrome）.

Prescription：Dissolve the exterior and interior.

Formulas：Chaihu Guizhi Tang （Decoction）.

b. Shaoyang complicated by yangming syndrome：Vomiting due to discomfort and fullness in the chest and hypochondrium （the symptom of shaoyang）, afternoon tidal fever （15～17 o'clock in the afternoon）, or constipation （the latter two symptoms are yangming syndrome）.

Prescription：Reconcile shaoyang, dredge the interior and purge sthenic heat.

Formulas：Large Chaihu Tang （Decoction）.

c. Shaoyang syndrome complicated by fluid retention：Alternate chill and fever, fullness in the chest and hypochondrium with fluid retention, unsmooth urination, thirst but without vomiting, sweating over the head. Of the above five symptoms, the first two belong to shaoyang syndrome, the one in the middle is a symptom of taiyang syndrome, while the last two are the symptoms of internal retention of body fluid.

Prescription：Reconcile the exterior and interior, dispel fluid retention and disperse lumps.

Formulas：Chaihu Guizhi Ganjiang Tang（Decoction）.

（2）辨证要点

①由于少阳病证处于半表半里之间，每有兼表或兼里的病证出现，因此要注意它的动态变化。

②少阳病证在表里中间阶段，其脉证不可能完整地出现。但只要辨析为半表半里证，就可以以少阳病证论治。

（2）Key points for syndrome differentiation

a. The location of shaoyang syndrome is between semi-interior and semi-exterior, therefore, shaoyang syndrome complicated by external or by internal syndrome tends to appear. As a result, weight should be attached to its dynamic transformation.

b. Shaoyang syndrome appears at the intermediate stage of external and internal syndromes, its main manifestations cannot display completely. As long as it is differentiated as semi-interior and semi-exterior syndrome, the disease could be diagnosed and treated as shaoyang syndrome.

（四）太阴病证
2. 2. 4　Taiyin syndrome

太阴病的形成有两个因素：一是阳经疾病传变而来；二是脾胃素虚，外邪直接侵犯太阴。由阳经而来者称为"传经"，外邪直接侵犯者称为"直中"。病变多表现为里虚寒证。

The occurence of taiyin disease is either transmitted from yang meridian syndromes, known as "meridian transmission", or from direct attack of pathogenic factors into taiyin due to prolonged asthenia of the spleen and stomach, which is known as "direct attack". It is usually manifested as internal asthenia cold syndrome.

（1）主要脉证

腹满而吐，食不下，自利益甚，时腹自痛，舌苔白而滑腻，脉象濡弱或迟缓。治以温中散寒，健脾运湿，用理中丸之类。

（1）Main clinical manifestations

Vomiting due to abdominal fullness, poor appetite even with severe diarrhea, frequent abdominal pain, whitish, slippery and greasy tongue fur as well as soft and feeble pulse or slow and moderate pulse.

Prescription：Warm middle energizer, dispel cold and invigorate the spleen to promote transportation of dampness.

Formulas：Lizhong Wan（Pill）.

（2）辨证要点

①太阴与阳明部位相同，互为表里，但病证性质相反，太阴为虚寒证，阳明为实热证。临床上常有相似症状出现，如腹满、呕吐等，须谨慎辨证，方能分辨清晰。

②太阴虽为虚寒证，但病经数日，亦可见大便硬，脉象由弱变长，此是由阴转阳，不可一味地按虚寒治疗。

③太阴病如果见到暴烦下利，这是脾阳将复，欲愈之兆。

（2）Key points for syndrome differentiation

a. The location of taiyin syndrome is the same to that of yangming, so they have formed a mutual external-internal connection. However, the features of both syndromes are just contrary to each other, syndrome of taiyin belongs to asthenic cold, while that of yangming is sthenic heat in the stomach. Clinically, similar symptoms such as abdominal fullness and vomiting could appear, therefore, they must be differentiated carefully and clearly.

b. Taiyin syndrome belongs to asthenic cold. But after several days' disease, dry and hard feces may also appear, and weak pulse may become long pulse, which indicates yang transformed from yin. Therefore, the disease should not be regarded as asthenic cold syndrome all the time.

c. If sudden restlessness and diarrhea occur in taiyin syndrome, it is a sign of recovery of yang qi in the spleen, a tendency to be healed.

（五）少阴病证
2.2.5 Shaoyin syndrome

少阴病，一是由传变而来，一是外邪直接侵犯所致。不管是"传变"，或是"直中"，都是疾病的严重阶段，是心肾功能衰退，抗病能力薄弱的表现。心肾是水火之脏，病证既可寒化，又可热化，所以病至少阴，一般分为虚寒与虚热两种证候。

Shaoyin disease is caused either by viscera transmission, or by direct attack of pathogenic factors, both of them are the serious stage of it, indicating dysfunction of the heart and kidney as well as weakness of resistance of the body. The heart and kidney are taken as the viscera of fire and water (according to five element theory), in which, pathogenic factors can be transformed into heat or cold. Therefore, shaoyin syndrome is classified into asthenic cold and asthenic heat syndrome.

（1）主要脉证

脉微细，但欲寐。

①少阴寒化证：无热恶寒，下利清谷，四肢厥冷，呕不能食，或食而即吐，脉象沉微。治以回阳救逆，用四逆汤之类。

②少阴热化证：心烦不得眠，口燥咽痛，舌尖红赤，脉象细数。治以滋阴清热，用黄连阿胶汤之类。

（1）Main clinical manifestations

Thin and indistinct pulse and tendency to sleep.

a. Shaoyin cold-transformation syndrome：Aversion to cold，no fever，diarrhea with indigested food，cold limbs，vomiting without appetite，or vomiting after eating as well as sunken and indistinct pulse.

Prescription：Recuperate depletion of yang for resuscitation.

Formulas：Sini Tang（Decoction）.

b. Shaoyin heat-transformation syndrome：Insomnia with vexation，dry mouth and pain in throat，reddish tongue tip and thin fast pulse.

Prescription：Nourish yin and clear away heat.

Formulas：Huanglian Ejiao Tang（Decoction）.

（2）辨证要点

①四肢厥冷是少阴寒化证之一，但其他原因亦可引起四肢厥冷，如阳郁、热厥等，因此临床对"四肢厥冷"的出现，要全面观察，入细辨证，不可仅以此为准。

②少阴寒化证是少阴病的严重阶段，它常出现在心肾衰竭类疾病，阳气的存亡是疾病转化的关键，因此要积极抢救，不可有丝毫延误。

③少阴病转化到一定阶段，会出现阴盛格阳现象，即阴盛于下，格阳于上，但其"阴盛"为本，"格阳"为标，切不可被假象所迷惑。

（2）Key points for syndrome differentiation

a. Cold limbs is one symptom of shaoyin cold-transformation syndrome. But there are other factors that may contribute to cold limbs，such as yang stagnation，heat syncope，etc. Therefore，for the occurrence of "cold limbs"，doctors must examine comprehensively and differentiate carefully，and this syndrome can not be taken as the only one for "cold limbs".

b. Shaoyin cold-transformation syndrome is the critical stage of shaoyin disease，which usually occurs in cardiorenal failure. Existence of yang qi is crucial for transformation of diseases. Consequently，much weight should be attached to emergent salvation，and delayed treatment must be avoided.

c. Phenomenon of predominant yin rejecting yang may arise at some stage of shaoyin cold-transformation syndrome，that is，the internal excessive yin refuses yang to transmit inside and force it to stay outside，"yin predominance" is the root cause，while "rejecting yang" is the superficial manifestations. Doctors should not get confused by false manifestations.

（六）厥阴病证
2.2.6 Jueyin syndrome

厥阴病为病变的末期阶段，这时正气与邪气将做胜败的相争，病变的表现极为错综复杂。但其主要证候不外乎寒热错杂和厥热胜复两种。病变多表现在肝胆二经并夹胃，阳气的恢复与否决定着本病的转归。

Jueyin syndrome appears at the last stage of syndrome transformation when healthy qi and pathogenic factors struggle against each other to win. Therefore, the syndrome is marked by complex pathological changes of two types, complex changes and mixture of cold and heat as well as alternation of cold and heat. Syndrome transformation usually occurs in liver meridian and gallbladder meridian together with the area of the stomach, and sequela of jueyin syndrome depends on whether yang qi could be recovered or not.

（1）主要脉证

消渴，气上冲心，心中疼热，饥而不欲食，食则吐蛔。

①寒热错杂：是指主要见症而言。口渴不止，气上冲心，心中疼热，是上热；饥而不欲食，食则吐蛔，是下寒。治以寒温并用，和胃安蛔，用乌梅丸之类。

②厥热胜复：四肢厥冷时间短，而发热时间长，是阴消阳长，其病向愈；四肢厥冷时间长，发热时间短，为阳消阴长，其病为进；先发冷后发热为病轻，先发热后厥冷为病重。

（1）Main clinical manifestations

Consumptive thirst, qi rushing up into the heart, painful and feverish sensation in the heart, hunger but with no appetite, postcibal vomiting of ascaris.

a. Syndrome of complex changes and mixture of cold and heat: This is the main syndrome. Continuous thirst, qi attacking the heart and painful and feverish sensation of the heart are symptoms of upper-heat syndrome; hunger without appetite and postcibal vomiting of ascaris belong to lower-cold syndrome.

Prescription: Use cooling and warming methods simultaneously, regulate the stomach and relieve colic pain caused by ascaris.

Formulas: Wumei Wan (Pill).

b. Syndrome of alternation of cold and heat: Short duration of cold limbs with lingering fever indicates declination of yin and yang growing and a favorable prognosis; lingering cold limbs with short duration of fever suggests declination of yang while yin growing, serious advancement of the disease; cold sensation followed by fever indicates unserious condition of it, feverish sensation followed by cold suggests seriousness of it.

（2）辨证要点

①形成厥冷的原因很多，如寒厥、热厥、痰厥、蛔厥、脏厥、饮厥等，虽然有些不属于厥阴病，而属杂病范畴，但在临床上仍须认真辨证，分清厥证的形成原因，然后才能对症下药。

②厥阴病发生厥逆的机制只有一个，那就是"阴阳气不相顺接"，"阴阳气"就是手足三阴三阳之气。关键就是里边的阳气不能外达，寒厥是寒盛而阳虚于里，热厥是热盛而阳郁于里，同样都是"阴阳气不相顺接"所致。热多于厥为病退，厥多于热为病进，厥热相等为病愈。

（2）Key points for syndrome differentiation

a. Cold limbs may occur in many cases such as cold syncope, heat syncope, syncope due to phlegm or ascaris, visceral syncope as well as that of fluid retention. Though some of them only fall into miscellaneous diseases rather than jueyin syndrome, the factors that cause jueyin diseases must be distinguished carefully so as to apply suitable therapeutical methods to some specific syndrome.

b. Pathogenesis for cold limbs in jueyin syndrome is that yin qi and yang qi（qi in three yin meridians of hand and foot, as well as three yang meridians of hand and foot）fail to supplement each other. To be exact, yang qi trapped internally fail to reach outward to the four limbs. Cold syncope is caused by predominance of yin which brings about yang asthenia in the interior, while heat syncope is due to superabundance of yang which gives rise to internal stagnation of yang. Though both of them are caused by the same pathogenesis, failure of yin qi and yang qi to supplement each other, syndrome of exuberant heat with insufficient cold indicates decline of the disease, while that of exuberance of cold with insufficient heat suggests advancement of the disease; and equal degree of cold and heat is indicative of healing.

三、病因辨证
2.3　Syndrome differentiation of pathogenic factors

导致疾病的因素有多种多样，但归纳起来不外乎六淫、七情、饮食劳倦、外伤等。病因辨证，是通过临床上病人所表现出来的症状、体征，再结合各种病因的致病特点，从而推断出致病的因素，为治疗提供有针对性的证候依据。

Pathogenic factors that cause a disease are various, in general, they include six climate factors, intemperance of seven emotions, improper diet, overstrain and fatigue, traumatic injury and so on. To differentiate pathogenic factors is to distinguish syndromes by combining physical signs, clinical manifestation as well as case history of a patient, and then to infer the pathogenic factors that cause a disease and to provide corresponding information for the treatment of a disease.

（一）六淫辨证
2.3.1　Syndrome differentiation of six climate pathogenic factors

六淫包括风、寒、暑、湿、燥、火，以及传染性极强的疫疠之气。

Six climate pathogenic factors include wind, cold, summer-heat, dampness, dryness, fire, as well as epidemic pathogens.

1. 风淫证候

2.3.1.1　Pathogenic wind syndrome

风为百病之长，其性轻扬，善行数变，具有发病迅速，游走不定，消退也快等特点。

①外风特点：恶寒发热，头痛汗出，鼻塞流涕，咳嗽痰多，舌苔薄白，脉浮。治以祛风解表为主，用桂枝汤、杏苏散之类。

②内风特点：轻则头晕，目眩，肢体麻木，重则四肢抽搐，半身不遂，语言謇涩，神志昏迷，兼有六经形证者。治以平肝熄风，用天麻钩藤饮或牛黄至宝丹之类。

Pathogenic wind is known as the leading pathogen of all diseases, or origin of all diseases, characterized by light and drifting movement, skilled at frequent changes, causing rapid outbreak of diseases as well as quick disappearance.

a. Exogenous wind pathogen：Aversion to cold, fever, headache and sweating, stuffy and runny nose, cough with profuse sputum, thin whitish tongue fur as well as floating pulse.

Prescription：Dispel pathogenic wind to relieve external syndrome.

Formulas：Guizhi Tang（Decoction）, as well as Xing Su San（Powder）.

b. Endogenous wind pathogen：Dizziness, vertigo, numb limbs in unsevere cases; spasm, hemiplegia, slurred speech, coma as well as symptoms combined with six meridian syndromes of wind stroke in severe cases.

Prescription：Suppress hyperactive liver to calm endogenous wind.

Formulas：Tianma Gouteng Yin（Decoction）, or Niuhuang Zhibao Dan（Pill）.

2. 寒淫证候

2.3.1.2　Pathogenic cold syndrome

寒为阴邪，其性寒凉，凝滞、收引，易伤及人的阳气，阻碍气血的运行。

①外寒特点：感受寒邪较轻，症见恶寒发热，无汗头痛，身痛，腰痛，骨节疼痛，咳嗽，舌苔薄白，脉象浮紧。治以祛风散寒，用麻黄汤或大青龙汤之类。

②中寒特点：感受寒邪较重，症见全身恶寒战栗，四肢冰凉，手足挛痛，倦卧不动，昏迷不语，脉象沉伏。治以温脾益气，用附子理中汤之类。

③内寒特点：素体阳气虚弱，寒从内生，症见面色苍白，畏寒喜热，腹痛腹泻，手足不温，舌质淡白，舌苔薄白。治以温阳健脾益肾，用参附汤或芪附汤之类。

Cold belongs to yin pathogen and it is characterized by cold and cool nature, stagnancy and contraction with the susceptibility to impairing yang qi and obstructing qi and blood circulation.

a. External cold syndrome：Human body has been slightly invaded by external cold pathogens, with manifestations such as aversion to cold, fever, headache without sweating, aching sensation of the body and loins, pain in bones and knuckles, cough, thin whitish tongue fur as well as floating and tense pulse.

Prescription: Dispel wind and cold.

Formulas: Mahuang Tang (Decoction), or Large Qinglong Tang (Decoction).

b. Syndrome of cold in the middle: Human body has been seriously invaded by external cold pathogens, with clinical manifestations as sudden aversion to cold and shudder, cold limbs, spasm and painful sensation of hands and feet, fatigue with unwillingness to move, coma with aphasia as well as sunken and deep-sited pulse.

Prescription: Warm the spleen and benefit qi.

Formulas: Fuzi Lizhong Tang (Decoction).

c. Internal cold syndrome: Constitutional asthenia of yang qi and endogenous cold generated from the interior with clinical manifestations as pale complexion, aversion to cold but preference for heat, abdominal pain with diarrhea, cold limbs, pale whitish tongue as well as thin whitish fur.

Prescription: Warm yang and invigorate the spleen and kidney.

Formulas: Shen Fu Tang (Decoction), or Qi Fu Tang (Decoction).

3. 暑淫证候
2.3.1.3　Pathogenic summer-heat syndrome

暑为阳邪，其性炎热升散，其病多热象，最易耗气伤阴，且常夹湿，与湿混合，难以分解。

①伤暑：寒热头痛，恶热，汗出，烦躁，呕吐，腹泻，唇干，口渴，气促，四肢乏力，小便短赤，舌质红，苔白腻或黄腻。多发生在静卧或贪饮纳凉之时。治以温散寒湿，辛凉涤暑，用新加香薷饮、黄连香薷饮、藿香正气散之类。

②中暑：突然晕倒，神志不清，发热烦躁，气促，口渴，出冷汗或无汗，舌绛干燥，脉象洪大无力。多发生在高温环境下的人。治以清暑益气，用人参白虎汤之类。

Summer-heat is yang pathogen with a sign of heat syndrome, characterized by scorching sensation with ascending and dispersing tendency, susceptibility to consuming qi and impairing yin. Furthermore, it is usually complicated or mixed with dampness. Therefore, it is hard to differentiate summer-heat from dampness.

a. Sunstroke syndrome: Headache with alternation of cold and fever, aversion to hot, sweating, restlessness, vomiting, diarrhea, dry lips with thirst, short breath, lassitude, short brownish urination as well as reddish tongue with greasy whitish fur or with greasy yellowish fur. Sunstroke usually occurs when lying in quietness or drinking profuse cold water as well as intake of cold food.

Prescription: Warm cold, dispel dampness and eliminate summer-heat with cool-natured medicinal herbs.

Formulas: Xinjia Xiangru Yin (Decoction), Huanglian Xiangru Yin (Decoction), as well as Huoxiang Zhengqi San (Powder).

b. Heat stroke: Sudden faint, obnubilation, fever with irritancy, short breath, thirst, cold sweating or no sweating, dry deep-reddish tongue with weak full large pulse. It usually occurs when patients are in high temperature.

Prescription：Clear summer-heat and benefit qi.

Formulas：Renshen Baihu Tang（Decoction）.

4. 湿淫证候
2.3.1.4　Pathogenic dampness syndrome

湿是一种黏滞的阴邪，一般多见于久居湿地，或外感雾露，涉水雨淋而致。湿邪的特点是重浊、黏滞、缠绵，病程较久，难以速愈。临床有内湿、外湿之不同。

1）外湿：身重难以转侧，肢体疼痛，关节屈伸不利，皮肤潮湿，头汗出，口不渴，脉象濡缓，舌苔白腻。治以芳香透表，渗湿泄热，用三仁汤或藿朴夏苓汤之类。

2）内湿：内湿有湿浊中于上、中、下三焦之别。

①中于上焦：头涨头重，胸脘痞闷，口淡乏味，不思饮食，或饮而不多，舌苔白腻。治以宣通肺气，健脾化湿，用三仁汤之类。

②中于中焦：脘腹胀满，饮食不化，嗳气，大便溏薄，自汗出，肢体无力，舌苔白腻而厚。治以辛开苦降，用半夏泻心汤之类。

③中于下焦：下肢肿胀，小便淋浊，大便反溏，痢疾，妇女白带，舌苔白腻，脉象沉细。治以温健脾肾，用双补丸或术附汤方之类。

Dampness is a sticky and stagnant yin pathogen, usually seen in those who live in wetland for a long time, or in those invaded by fog and dew or water as well as in those drenched by rain. Pathogenic dampness factor is marked by heaviness, turbidity, stickiness, stagnancy, long duration as well as difficulty to be healed. Clinically, dampness is classified into external and internal dampness.

1）Exogenous（external）dampness syndrome：Heavy sensation over the body with difficulty to turn sideward, aching sensation over limbs and body, inflexible arthral flexion and extension, damp and wet skin, sweating over the head without thirst, soft and moderate pulse as well as greasy whitish fur.

Prescription：Eliminate external syndrome and promote eruption with aromatic-natured herbs, resolve dampness and purge heat.

Formulas：Sanren Tang（Decoction）, or Huo Pu Xia Ling Tang（Decoction）.

2）Endogenous（internal）dampness syndrome is divided into 3 types：

a. Stagnation of dampness and turbidity in upper energizer：Heavy and distending sensation of the head, fullness and oppression in the chest, bland taste of the mouth, anorexia, or oligodipsia as well as greasy whitish tongue fur.

Prescription：Disperse lung qi, invigorate the spleen and resolve dampness.

Formulas：Sanren Tang（Decoction）.

b. Stagnation of dampness and turbidity in middle energizer：Distention and fullness in the epigastrium and abdomen, indigested food, eructation, thin loose stool, spontaneous sweating, weak limbs and thick greasy whitish tongue fur.

Prescription：Disperse with pungent herbs and descend with bitter herbs.

Formulas：Banxia Xiexin Tang（Decoction）.

c. Stagnation of dampness and turbidity in lower energizer：Swollen legs, turbid urine with stranguria, loose stool with diarrhea, leucorrhea in women, greasy whitish tongue fur and sunken and thin pulse.

Prescription：Warm and invigorate the spleen and the kidney.

Formulas：Shuangbu Wan（Pill）, or Zhu Fu Tang（Decoction）.

5. 燥淫证候
2.3.1.5 Pathogenic dryness syndrome

燥性干燥，易伤津液。燥又为秋天之主令，有温燥与凉燥之分。此外，还有内燥，多因出汗、呕吐、泄下伤其津液而致。

1）外燥：秋季初期，久晴无雨，阳光暴烈，人感之多为温燥；日过中秋，西风肃杀，凉气袭来，人感之多为凉燥。

①温燥：身热有汗，口渴，咽痛，咳嗽，胸痛，或痰中带血，气促鼻干，舌尖边红赤，苔薄白少津，脉象浮数或弦涩。治以宣肺润燥，用桑杏汤之类。

②凉燥：恶寒重发热轻，头痛鼻塞，无汗唇燥，咽干，咳嗽，气喘，舌苔白而少津，脉象浮弦而涩。治以调和营卫，苦温肃肺，用杏苏散之类。

2）内燥：内热时起，皮肤干燥，口咽干燥，指甲干，毛发干枯易折，干咳，舌面干燥无津液，脉象弦涩。治以清燥救肺，用清燥救肺汤之类。

Pathogenic dryness is dry in nature, regarded as the leading characteristic of autumn, with a tendency to impair body fluids. It can be classified into warm and cool dryness. Besides, there also exists endogenous dryness due to sweating, vomiting as well as diarrhea which leads to impairment of body fluids.

1）Exogenous Dryness：In early autumn, it is always sunny with intensely hot sunshine and scarce rain, so usually people can be attacked by warm dryness. However, the weather turns windy and cool after mid-autumn, as a result, people may be affected by cool dryness.

a. Warm dryness：Fever with sweating, thirst, pain in throat, cough, painful sensation over the chest, sputum mingled with blood, short breath, dry sensation in the nose, reddish tongue tip and margins, thin dry whitish tongue fur as well as floating and fast pulse or taut and astringent pulse.

Prescription：Disperse lung qi and moisten dryness.

Formulas：Sang Xing Tang（Decoction）.

b. Cool dryness：Severe aversion to cold, light fever, headache, stuffy nose, dry lips without sweating, dry throat, cough, panting, dry whitish fur as well as floating, taut and astringent pulse.

Prescription：Regulate nutrient qi and defensive qi and depurate the lung heat with warm-

and-bitter natured herbs.

Formulas：Xing Su San（Powder）.

2）Endogenous dryness：Frequent onset of endogenous heat，dry and rough skin，dry mouth and throat，dry lusterless fingernail，dry lusterless and easily broken hair，dry cough，dry tongue without fluids as well as taut and astringent pulse.

Prescription：Moisten dryness to salvage the lung.

Formulas：Qingzao Jiufei Tang（Decoction）.

6. 火淫证候
2.3.1.6 Pathogenic fire syndrome

火虽属外感之一，但此火非外感之火，而是在体内产生的。各种精神活动过度都能生火，此即"七情化火"。外感之邪到了人体内也可转化为火，此即"六淫皆可化火"。

火的表现多种多样，大致可分实火与虚火两大类。临床上多以火淫所发作的部位进行分类。

①实火：实火以胃肠经为多，如壮热、口渴、腹满便秘；或温病热入营血，症见谵语，烦躁，吐血，衄血，或狂越而走，舌质红绛，脉象洪数等。治以清热泻火，凉血解毒，用白虎汤、清营汤、犀角地黄汤、安宫牛黄丸之类。

②虚火：虚火多为五脏阴伤所致，如见低热、干咳、口咽干燥，遗精，盗汗，五心烦热，口舌糜烂，或骨弱尿浊，或小便涩赤，舌质红赤，苔干，脉象细数等。治以养血、滋阴、清热，用六味地黄汤、知柏地黄汤、大补阴丸、当归六黄汤之类。

Although fire belongs to one of exogenous pathogens，here，it refers to the endogenous fire generated from human body. Any intemperate emotional activities can give rise to it，namely，"seven emotions transforming into fire". Furthermore，when transmiting into human body，the six exogenous climatic pathogens，wind，cold，summer-heat，dampness，dryness and fire，can transform into fire，which is the so-called "six pathogenic factors can transform into fire".

Generally，fire can be divided into sthenic and asthenic fire. However，clinically，it is classified according to the region where it breaks out.

a. Sthenic fire：It usually occurs in the meridians of the stomach and intestines，such as high fever，thirst，abdominal fullness as well as constipation；or it is caused by invasion of pathogenic febrile factors into nutrient as well as blood phase，with manifestations as delirium，restlessness，hematemesis，epistaxis，or running wildly，deep-reddish tongue，full and fast pulse.

Prescription：Clear away heat，purge fire，cool blood and relieve internal toxin.

Formulas：Baihu Tang（Decoction），or Qingying Tang（Decoction），or Xijiao Dihuang Tang（Decoction），or Angong Niuhuang Wan（Pill）.

b. Asthenic fire：It is caused by impairment of yin in viscera，and its clinical manifestations are low fever, dry cough, dry mouth and throat, seminal emission, night sweating, dysphoria and feverish sensation over five centres (the chest, palms and soles), erosion of mucous membrane of the oral cavity, or weakness of bones and turbid urine, or brownish and obstructive urination, reddish tongue with dry fur as well as thin and fast pulse.

Prescription：Nourish blood and yin and clear away heat.

Formulas：Liuwei Dihuang Tang (Decoction), Zhi Bo Dihuang Tang (Decoction), or Large Buyin Wan (Pill), Danggui Liuhuang Tang (Decoction).

7. 疫疠证候
2.3.1.7 Epidemic pathogenic syndrome

疫疠乃指具有传染性的不正常之气，如特殊的气候变化，恶劣的自然环境，空气中弥漫的腐败秽浊之气，尤其是大灾之后自然条件的破坏，都会导致疫疠之气弥漫，诱发传染病的发生。疫疠是一种严重的具有传染性的流行病，其发病急骤，蔓延迅速，传染之广与传播之快常出乎人们的预料。现将几种常见证候叙述如下。

①瘟疫证候：因感受疫疠之气而得，发病急剧，病情险恶，并有传染性，变化多端。初起憎寒而后发热，日后但热而不寒；初得之二三日，脉象不浮不沉而数，头痛身疼，昼夜发热，日晡益甚，舌苔白如积粉。治以开达膜原，避秽化浊，用达原饮之类。

②疫疹病候：因感染燥热疫毒而引起的发疹性疫毒。初期身体发热，头痛如劈，斑疹透露，或红或赤，或紫或黑，脉象滑数。如果初起脉象细数沉伏，昏愦如迷，四肢逆冷，头汗如雨，其痛如劈，腹内搅肠欲吐不吐，欲泄不泄，摇头鼓颔，此为"闷疫"。治以清热解毒，凉血泻火，用清瘟败毒散之类。

③瘟黄病候：因感受瘟毒夹有湿热而引起的猝然发黄的病候。初起发热恶寒，随即出现黄疸，全身、齿垢、白眼珠黄色深，名为急黄。严重者四肢厥冷，神昏谵语，直视，甚至舌卷而囊缩，寻衣摸床。治以清热祛湿，利疸退黄，用加味茵陈蒿汤之类。

④疫痢病候：因肠道感染疫毒所引起。发病急速，发热恶寒，身痛口渴，腹痛如绞，痢下赤白，一日数十行，大便腐臭，肛门灼热，毒邪剧则神昏谵语，抽搐痉挛，或兼夹斑疹，舌苔厚腻，脉象不定。治以清热解毒凉血，用白头翁汤加金银花、生地黄、赤芍、牡丹皮、秦皮等。

⑤疫毒发颐证候：耳下两颐肿硬且痛，连面皆肿，喉赤肿痛，壮热口渴，时有睾丸肿痛，甚至神昏嗜睡，或惊厥，舌苔黄厚，脉象浮沉俱大。治以疏风消肿，清热解毒，用普济消毒饮之类。

Epidemic pathogen refers to infective abnormal qi, caused by such factors as special weather condition, terrible natural environment, air mingled with putrid foul odor, in particular, air permeated with epidemic pathogens after disasters, accompanied with the damage of natural environment, which could induce onset of infectious diseases. Epidemic pathogenic syndrome signifies epidemic diseases with severe infectivity, characterized by sudden outbreak and fast spread. The wide range and fast speed of spreading is usually out of what people could expect. The following are the commonly seen syndromes of it.

a. Epidemic infectious syndrome: A patient can contract the disease after being infected with pestilent pathogens. Pestilence is featured by sudden outbreak, severe conditions of the illness, infectivity as well as different variations, with clinical manifestations like aversion to cold followed by fever at the initial stage, fever sensation without aversion to cold the following day, neither floating nor sunken but fast pulse during the next days, headache as well as painful sensation of the body, persistent fever during the day and the night, even high fever particularly in the afternoon (15~17 o'clock), as well as whitish tongue fur like wearing with powder.

Prescription: Eliminate pathogenic factors retained in Moyuan (the region between thorax and diaphragm), and resolve internal turbid and foul substance.

Formulas: Dayuan Yin (Decoction).

b. Epidemic syndrome with eruption of rashes: Epidemic syndrome with eruption of rashes is caused by being infected with dry and heat pestilence. At the initial stage, feverish sensation of the body, headache like head being chopped, reddish or purplish or blackish macule or eruption of rashes as well as fast and slippery pulse. At the beginning of the appearance of macule and eruptions, "oppressed pestilence syndrome" will arise with manifestations like thin fast sunken and deep-sited pulse, coma, cold limbs, sweating over the head like rain, headache with chopping painful sensation, abdominal discomfort due to failure to vomit and diarrhea, head shaking as well as swollen jaw.

Prescription: Clear away heat, resolve internal toxin and cool blood to purge fire.

Formulas: Qingwen Baidu San (Powder).

c. Syndrome of fulminant jaundice: Syndrome of fulminant jaundice refers to sudden onset of jaundice due to infection of pestilent pathogens complicated with damp-heat. At the initial stage, fever with aversion to cold followed by sudden onset of jaundice, with signs such as yellowish coloration over the whole body, odontia incrustans, as well as dark yellow coloration of the white part of the eyeball, known as "fulminant jaundice". In serious cases, symptoms such as cold limbs, coma, delirium, euthyphoria even with shrunk tongue and abnormal manners as looking for clothes and touching bed can arise.

Prescription: Clear away heat, eliminate dampness, purge fire from the gallbladder and remove jaundice.

Formulas: Jiawei Yinchenhao Tang (Decoction).

d. Syndrome of fulminant dysentery: Syndrome of fulminant dysentery is due to intestinal tract being infected with pestilent pathogens. It is characterized by sudden onset, fever with aversion to cold, painful sensation over the body, thirst, colic pain in the abdomen, frequent red-white dysentery, feces with putrid and foul odor, scorching sensation of the anus, coma and delirium, twitching and spasm in case of serious pestilent pathogens, or complicated with eruption of maculae and thick greasy fur and unfixed pulse condition.

Prescription: Clear away heat and relieve internal toxin to cool blood.

Formulas：Baitouweng Tang （Decoction） combined with Jinyinhua （*Flos Lonicerae*），Shengdihuang （*Radix Rehmanniae Recens*），Chishao （*Radix Paeoniae Rubra*），Mudanpi （*Cortex Moutan Radicis*） and Qinpi （*Cortex Fraxini*）.

e. Syndrome of acute suppurative parotitis due to pestilence：It is characterized by swollen，hard and painful sensation over the region of the entire parotid gland under the ears as well as swollen face，reddish painful swollen throat，high fever with thirst，accompanied with frequent painful swollen spermary，even coma and somnolence，or convulsion，thick yellowish tongue fur as well as large，floating and sunken pulse.

Prescription：Expel wind，resolve swellings and relieve heat and internal toxicity.

Formulas：Puji Xiaodu Yin （Decoction）.

8. 辨证要点
2.3.1.8 Key points for syndrome differentiation

六淫与疫疬之气乃指自然界的异常气候。随着科学技术的发展，人类对自然界气候的变化预测越来越提前，使得人们对六淫与疫疬致病有了预防与适度对抗的时间和空间。对此人们应当注意以下几个问题。

①重视对气候和空气质量的预测，以便预防某些传染病的发生与传播。

②注意自身防护措施，如生活环境的卫生，个人的衣着与饮食卫生等。

③六淫致病以"风"为首，风可携带湿邪、寒邪、热邪、火邪、燥邪等，因此在辨证的时候，要注意兼夹证候，不可一味地祛风。

④疫疬之气，伤人最速，害人最厉，如"非典"病毒、甲型 H1N1 病毒等，对于此类疫疬的辨证，要分秒必争地做出判断，要有严格的防范措施。

⑤对于病因的辨证，既要吸收前人的经验，更要注重当前的实际和现代科技的有效成果，以便及时控制病情的发展。

Six climate and epidemic pathogenic factors refer to abnormal natural climate. With the development of science and technology，change of climate has been predicted in advance increasingly，which provides time and room for human to prevent themselves from six climate pathogenic factors as well as epidemic pathogenic diseases. However，much weight should be attached to the following：

a. Attention should be paid to the prediction to climate and air quality so as to guard against onset and spread of some infectious diseases.

b. Some self-defensive measures should be taken，for instance，to keep a clean living environment，to wear tidy personal clothes as well as to keep a healthy diet.

c. Pathogenic wind is the leading pathogen that causes diseases，it can combine with pathogen of dampness，cold，summer-heat，fire，as well as dryness. Therefore，in syndrome differentiation，dispelling wind pathogen simply regardless of other complicated syndromes of pathogenic wind should be avoided.

d. Epidemic pestilent pathogens do the severest harm to people at the fastest speed，for instance, SARS and influenza virus H1N1. In differentiating those syndromes, diagnosis must be made immediately and serious prevention measures must be taken.

e. As for differentiating etiology of a syndrome, on the basis of absorbing experience handed down, much weight should be attached to current situation as well as advanced technological achievements so as to control the advancing process of diseases in time.

（二）七情辨证
2.3.2 Syndrome differentiation of seven emotion

七情，即喜、怒、忧、思、悲、恐、惊。七情致病主要见于内伤杂病。七情致病常见于气血阴阳的变化，如暴喜伤阳，暴怒伤阴，气郁化火，气逆血乱，并能伤及五脏六腑。

Seven emotions refer to different emotional responses of a person to environmental stimulation, namely, over-joy, fury, anxiety, excessive thinking, grief, fear and fright. Intemperate activities of the seven emotions may bring about miscellaneous diseases with abnormal change of qi, blood, yin and yang due to internal impairment of these emotions to zang-fu organs. For instance, sudden over-joy can impair yang, fury could impair yin, stagnancy of qi can transform into fire, and adverse qi can cause disorder of blood circulation, which, in turn, may give rise to dysfunction of zang-fu organs.

（1）主要脉证

①过喜：过喜伤心，症见心神不安，甚则语无伦次，举止失常；喜则气缓，还可见心气缓散不收。

②过怒：过怒伤肝，症见面色青暗，两目怒视，怒极则血菀于上，可致神昏暴厥；若怒气不得发越，则会导致精神病。

③过忧：过忧伤肺，症见情志抑郁，闷闷不乐，神疲乏力，食欲欠佳，甚则失眠，精神失常，日渐消瘦。

④过思：过思伤脾，症见饮食不馨，睡眠欠安，健忘，思维紊乱，肌肉消瘦，精神不振，四肢困顿。

⑤过悲：过悲亦伤肺，症见面色惨淡，神气不足，垂头丧气，叹息连声，偶有所触，即泪涌欲哭。

⑥过恐：过恐伤肾，症见神气不足，易恐，时时怵惕不安，如人将捕之之状。

⑦过惊：过惊伤肝，症见暴受惊吓，即目瞪口呆，彷徨失措，情绪不宁，甚至思维错乱，语言颠倒，举止失常。

（1）Main clinical manifestations

a. Syndrome of over-joy: Over-joy may impair the heart, for instance, unease of mind, even incoherent speech, and abnormal manners. Over-joy may also bring about slow flow of qi, even failure to receive the heart qi.

b. Syndrome of fury: Fury can impair the liver, with such clinical manifestations as dark cyanotic complexion, bloodshot eyes, extreme fury may cause coma as well as sudden syncope due to upper flow of blood. Failure to give out fury may lead to abnormal mental disease.

c. Syndrome of anxiety: Excessive anxiety may impair the lung, with the following clinical manifestations: emotional depression, bad mood, dispiritedness, lassitude, reduced appetite, even insomnia, abnormal mental activity and emaciation.

d. Syndrome of excessive thinking: Excessive thinking can impair the spleen, with clinical manifestations such as poor appetite, disturbed sleep, amnesia, disordered thinking, emaciation, dispiritedness as well as exhausted limbs.

e. Syndrome of grief: Grief may induce impairment to the lung, with clinical manifestations such as pale complexion, insufficient energy and qi, dispiritedness, frequent sighs and susceptibility to cry at stimulus.

f. Syndrome of fear: Excessive fear may bring about impairment to the kidney, with clinical manifestations such as insufficient energy and qi, susceptibility to fear, frequent uneasy mood and feeling of being captured.

g. Syndrome of fright: Fright may hurt the liver, with the clinical manifestations such as sudden shock, fixed position of mouth and eyes, feeling like being attacked by panic, uneasy mood, even confused thinking, incoherent speech as well as abnormal manners.

（2）辨证要点

①七情辨证，要注意病人的心理变化，详细询问病人的发病原因和变化过程，以便正确地捕捉致病因素，为治疗提供可靠的依据。

②七情致病的因素，也不是一成不变的。如前人所说"喜极而泣""乐极生悲"等，都是常见的。因此要细致观察，注意病人微小的心理变化。

③七情郁结常常导致气滞，进而不思饮食；由气滞又可使血分郁结，出现气滞血瘀的证候。

④七情证候与脏腑内伤有密切关系，临床辨证要结合脏腑、气血进行辨证。

（2）Key points for syndrome differentiation

a. Attention should be paid to psychological changes of a patient. Doctors should inquire about the cause of the outbreak as well as the development of a disease in order to obtain correct information about factors that causing the disease and to provide reliable data for treatment.

b. The factors of seven emotions causing diseases are not fixed but changeable. For instance, "excessive joy can give rise to crying" and "too much great pleasure would bring about grief". As a result, careful examination must be involved in syndrome differentiation, and attention must be given to any psychological change of a patient.

c. Qi stagnation is caused by depression of seven emotions, which could affect appetite. Qi stagnation could cause blood stasis, thus, giving rise to syndrome of qi stagnation and blood stasis.

d. Syndromes caused by seven emotions are closely related to internal impairment of zang-fu organs, therefore, clinically, syndrome differentiation should be combined with syndromes of zang-fu organs as well as those of qi and blood.

四、卫气营血辨证
2.4 Syndrome differentiation of defensive qi, qi, nutrient qi, and blood

卫气营血辨证是对外感温热病的一种辨证方法。它是从不同层面、不同阶段、不同轻重程度去辨别证候性质的一种方法。

卫气营血辨证，即辨别卫分证、气分证、营分证、血分证四种证候。病在表者，为卫分证；病入里者，为气分证；气之后为营分证，再深一层为血分证。病在卫分与气分者，病变会涉及肺、胃、肠、胆等几个脏器；病在营分、血分者，病变多涉及肝、肾、心与心包等脏器。

Syndrome differentiation of defensive qi, qi, nutrient qi, and blood is a method to differentiate the syndrome of exogenous epidemic febrile disease from different level, stage as well as degrees of seriousness of a disease.

Syndrome differentiation of defensive qi, qi, nutrient qi, and blood is to differentiate the syndromes of defensive phase, qi phase, nutrient phase as well as blood phase. Syndrome of defensive phase refers to epidemic exogenous febrile pathogens are in the superficies, qi phase syndrome suggesting pathogenic factors invading the interior, nutrient phase syndrome indicating pathogenic factors invading into nutrient phase, and the last one, blood phase syndrome, signifying that pathogenic factors go beyond the above three and invade into blood phase. If pathogenic factors invade the area between defensive phase and qi phase, the disease will spread to the lung, stomach, intestines, gallbladder, etc; if pathogenic factors invade the area between nutrient and blood phase, the disease will transmit to the liver, kidney, heart as well as pericardium.

（一）卫分证候
2.4.1 Syndrome of defensive phase

卫分证候，是温热病的表证，常见于外感温热病的初期。温热病的卫分证候与肺关系密切，因肺合皮毛，主一身之表，"肺位最高，邪必先伤"，故卫分证候常伴有肺经病变。

Syndrome of defensive phase refers to external syndrome of epidemic febrile disease, usually seen at the initial stage of epidemic febrile disease. It is closely related to the lung, for the lung associates the skin and body hair, and dominates the surface of whole body. Thus, "among visceral organs, the lung holds the highest position, so it must be the first region attacked by pathogenic factors." Consequently, the syndrome is always accompanied with diseases in lung meridian.

（1）主要脉证

发热，微恶风寒，舌边尖红，脉象浮数。常伴有头痛、咳嗽，口干微渴，咽喉肿痛等。治以辛凉解表，用银翘散或桑菊饮之类。

（1）Main clinical manifestations

Fever with slight aversion to wind and cold, reddish tongue tip and reddish margin, fast floating pulse, usually accompanied with headache, cough, dry mouth with mild thirst as well as swollen and painful throat.

Prescription：Relieve the superficies with pungent-cool natured medicinal herbs.

Formulas：Yinqiao San（Powder）, or Sang Ju Yin（Decoction）.

（2）辨证要点

卫分证候为温热病的表证，即初期证候。它的特点是发热、咳嗽、脉浮、舌质红赤等。这是由于温热之邪侵犯卫分，卫分受束，肺失宣降，热伤津液所致。如果出现口渴引饮，则是温热之邪侵入气分，已非卫分证候了。

（2）Key points for syndrome differentiation

Defensive phase syndrome is an external one of epidemic febrile disease, usually seen at the initial stage of this disease. The syndrome is characterized by fever, cough, floating pulse, reddish tongue, etc, due to invasion of pathogenic febrile factors into defensive phase, defensive phase being encumbered, failure of the lung to disperse as well as heat impairing body fluid. Thirst with desire to drink indicates that pathogenic febrile factors have invaded qi phase. At this time, it is no longer a syndrome of defensive phase.

（二）气分证候
2.4.2　Syndrome of qi phase

气分证候，属于温热病的里证，即病邪由表入里，与正气抗争的阳热实证。常见的证候主要是热壅于肺、热扰胸膈、热迫大肠和热在肺胃等。

Qi phase syndrome is an internal one of epidemic febrile disease, indicating pathogenic factors invading from the exterior into the interior, a syndrome of yang, heat and sthenia due to the struggle between pathogenic factors and healthy qi, with common symptoms such as accumulation of heat in the lung, disturbance of heat in the chest and diaphragm, attack of heat in the large intestine as well as heat accumulation in the lung and stomach.

（1）主要脉证

发热，不恶寒反恶热，汗出，口渴，舌红苔黄，脉象洪数。治以清热泻火，用白虎汤之类。

①热壅于肺：兼见咳喘，胸痛，咳吐黄稠痰。治以清热宣肺，利窍逐饮，用千金苇茎汤加杏仁、石膏之类。

②热扰胸膈：兼见心烦懊恼，坐卧不安。治以清心除烦，用栀子豉汤之类。

③热迫大肠：兼见胸痞，烦渴，下利赤白，甚则谵语。清热解毒凉血，用白头翁汤之类。

④热在肺胃：兼见自汗，喘急，烦闷，渴甚，苔黄燥，脉数。治以两清肺胃，用麻杏石甘汤之类。

（1）Main clinical manifestations

Fever, aversion not to cold but to heat, sweating with thirst, reddish tongue with yellowish fur as well as full and fast pulse.

Prescription：Clear away heat and purge fire.

Formulas：Baihu Tang（Decoction）.

a. Accumulation of heat in the lung：fever, aversion not to cold but to heat, reddish tongue with yellowish fur as well as fast pulse, combined with cough, asthma, pain in the chest and expectoration of thick yellowish sputum.

Prescription：Clear heat to disperse the lung, relieve constipation and promote defecation and urination by purging retention of water and fluid.

Formulas：Qianjin Weijing Tang（Decoction）combined with Xingren（*Semen Armeniacae Amarum*）and Shigao（*Gypsum Fibrosum*）.

b. Disturbance of heat in the chest and diaphragm：Fever, aversion not to cold but to heat, reddish tongue with yellowish fur as well as fast pulse, combined with vexation and restlessness.

Prescription：Clear away fire from the heart and relieve restlessness.

Formulas：Zhizi Chi Tang（Decoction）.

c. Attack of heat in the large intestine：Fever, aversion not to cold but to heat, reddish tongue with yellowish fur as well as fast pulse, combined with fullness and distention in the chest, polydipsia, red and white dysentery, and even delirium.

Prescription：Clear away heat, eliminate toxin and cool blood.

Formulas：Baitouweng Tang（Decoction）.

d. Heat accumulation in the lung and stomach：Fever, aversion not to cold but to heat, reddish tongue, combined with spontaneous sweating, dyspnea with rapid respiration, irritancy, severe thirst, dry and yellowish fur as well as fast pulse.

Prescription：Clear away heat from the lung and the stomach.

Formulas：Mahuang Xingren Shigao Gancao Tang（Decoction）.

（2）辨证要点

气分证候是温热之邪入里，病邪呈现亢盛阶段。它的特点是发热、汗出、口渴、脉洪数，表现出明显的热盛伤津的病性。如果热壅于肺（这是很常见的），会兼见咳嗽、气喘、胸痛、咳吐黄痰的症状，还可以出现热迫大肠、热扰胸膈等证候，临床必须细致鉴别，明确病位，正确治疗。

（2）Key points for syndrome differentiation

Qi phase syndrome is the stage of hyperactivity of pathogenic factors due to invasion of pathogenic febrile factors into the interior. The syndrome is characterized by fever, sweating, thirst, full and fast pulse, and the obvious manifestation of exuberant heat impairing fluid. Exuberance of heat in the lung (which is quite common) can be complicated with symptoms as cough, short breath, chest pain, expectoration of yellowish sputum, even heat attacking the large intestine, and heat disturbing the chest and diaphragm and so on. Thus, the location of diseases must be differentiated carefully and clearly to ensure correct treatment for patients.

（三）营分证候
2.4.3　Syndrome of nutrient phase

营分证候，是温热病邪内陷的严重阶段。营行脉中，内舍于心。故营分证候以营阴受损和心神被扰为其特点。营分介于气分与血分之间，若病邪由营分转入气分，为病情好转；若病邪由营分转入血分，则表示病情加重，应当积极治疗。

Nutrient phase syndrome occurs at the serious stage when pathogenic febrile factors invade internally. The heart is located in the thorax, governing the blood and vessels and housing the mind, while the nutrient qi flows in the vessels. When the pathogenic febrile factors invade nutrient phase, some of them could retain in the heart. Therefore, the syndrome is characterized by consumption of nutrient yin and disturbance of the mind. Because nutrient phase is located between qi phase and blood phase, transmission of pathogenic factors from nutrient phase into qi phase is a favorable prognosis of the disease; if pathogenic factors transmit from nutrient phase into blood phase, it is a sign of aggravation of a disease. Therefore, an effective treatment should be taken.

（1）主要脉证

身热夜甚，口渴不甚，心烦不眠，甚或神昏谵语，斑疹隐现，舌质红绛，脉象细数。治以清热凉营，用清营汤之类。

（1）Main clinical manifestations

Severe fever at night, mild thirst, vexation with insomnia, or even coma and delirium, indistinct eruption of maculae, deep-reddish tongue and thin and fast pulse.

Prescription：Clear away heat and cool nutrient qi.

Formulas：Qingying Tang (Decoction).

（2）辨证要点

营分证候与阳明病的证候有些类同，如身热、口渴与阳明经证类同，神昏谵语与阳明腑证类同。其区别点在于,营分之热,夜热尤甚,口反不甚渴,脉象细数;而阳明经的热象是大热,大渴,脉象洪数。再者,营分之谵语,伴见舌质红绛、无垢苔,而无阳明腑证的腹痛腹胀、大便秘结、舌苔有厚苔垢,以此为别。

(2) Key points for syndrome differentiation

Syndrome of nutrient phase is similar to that of yangming in some aspects. For instance, symptoms such as feverish sensation over the body and thirst are the same to those in yangming meridian syndrome, and coma and delirium are the same to those in yangming fu syndrome. The first difference lies in that syndrome of nutrient phase has severe fever at night, mild thirst and thin fast pulse while yangming meridian syndrome has high fever, severe thirst as well as full fast pulse. And the second difference is that symptoms such as delirium, deep-reddish tongue without greasy fur in the syndrome of nutrient phase are not accompanied with abdominal pain and fullness, constipation as well as thick tongue fur, existing in yangming fu syndrome.

(四) 血分证候
2.4.4 Syndrome of blood phase

血分证候,是卫气营血证候的最后阶段,也是温热病发作过程中最为严重的阶段。心主血而肝藏血,故热入血分,首先影响到心、肝两脏;另外,热邪久羁,势必伤及肾中真阴,故血分证候以心、肝、肾三脏病变为主。临床除热势严重外,以耗血、动血、阴伤、动风为其特征。

Syndrome of blood phase is the last among those of defensive qi, qi, nutrient qi and blood, and it occurs at the critical stage of the development of epidemic febrile disease. The heart dominates blood and the liver stores blood, if pathogenic febrile factor invades blood phase, it will immediately affect the heart and the liver. Furthermore, prolonged retention of pathogenic febrile factors must impair kidney yin, as a result, differentiation of blood phase syndrome should focus on the heart, liver and kidney. Clinically, in addition to severe fever, consumption of blood, disturbance of blood, impairment of yin and generation of wind are regarded as the main feature of this syndrome.

(1) 主要脉证

具有发热、神志不清症状。

①血分实热证:在营分证候基础上,更见烦热躁扰,神昏谵语,斑疹透露,色紫或黑,吐血,衄血,便血,尿血,或有抽搐,颈项强直,角弓反张,牙关紧闭,窜视,舌质深绛或紫,脉象细数,或弦数。治以清热凉血,用犀角地黄汤(以水牛角代犀角)之类。

②血分虚热证:多由实热演变而来,症见持续低热,夜热早凉,五心烦热,热退无汗,口干咽燥,神疲耳鸣,肢体干瘦,或见手足蠕动,瘛疭,舌上少津,脉象虚细。

治以滋阴清热，用青蒿鳖甲汤之类。

（1）Main clinical manifestations

Fever, confused state of mind and so on.

a. Sthenic heat syndrome of blood phase：More serious symptoms than those manifesting in the syndrome of nutrient phase such as dysphoria with disturbance of dryness and heat, delirium, eruption of purplish and blackish maculae, haematemesis, epistaxis, hematochezia, hematuria, or convulsion, stiffness of neck, opisthotonos, lockjaw, upward staring of eyes, deep-reddish or purplish tongue, thin fast pulse or taut fast pulse.

Prescription：Clear away heat and cool blood.

Formulas：Xijiao Dihuang Tang（Decoction）〔Xijiao（*Cornu Rhinoceri*）can be replaced with Shuiniujiao（*Cornu Bubali*）〕.

b. Asthenic heat syndrome of blood phase：It usually evolves from sthenic heat syndrome, with manifestations such as continuous dull fever, aggravation of fever at night but alleviation in the next morning, feverish sensation over five centre（palms, soles, and the chest）, alleviation of fever with no sweating, dry mouth and throat, dispiritedness and tinnitus, emaciation, or tremor of hands and feet, flaccidity, dry tongue with less fluid as well as weak thin pulse.

Prescription：Nourish yin and clear away heat.

Formulas：Qinghao Biejia Tang（Decoction）.

（2）辨证要点

温热之邪进入血分，证候呈现阴虚与血热并存的特点。实热者多有出血症状，虚热者以夜热早凉、久羁不愈为特点。不论虚热与实热，肝肾之阴必被耗竭之极，甚则出现阴虚风动症状。热邪进入血分，是疾病发展的危重阶段，医者不可有丝毫懈怠。

（2）Key points for syndrome differentiation

Blood phase syndrome refers to invasion of pathogenic and febrile factors into blood phase, characterized by coexistence of yin asthenia with blood heat. Sthenic heat is featured by bleeding, while asthenic heat is manifested by prolonged retention of evening fever and alleviation of it the following morning. Both syndromes can severely consume liver and kidney yin, even bringing about asthenic yin and endogenous wind. Invasion of pathogenic and febrile factors into the blood phase indicates the serious stage of epidemic febrile disease, which, therefore, must not be neglected.

五、三焦辨证

2.5 Syndrome differentiation of triple energizer

三焦辨证是温热病辨证方法之一。清代吴鞠通在所著的《温病条辨》中，依据《黄帝内经》关于三焦所属部位的概念，结合温热病传变规律的特点，将温热病分为三个所属部位来叙述，即上焦证候、中焦证候、下焦证候，依次来说明温热病初期、中期、末期三个不同阶段的演变过程。就其证候的特点来看，上焦包括手太阴肺经和手厥阴心包经的证候，中焦包括足阳明胃经和足太阴脾经的证候，下焦包括足少阴肾经和足厥阴肝经的证候。

Syndrome differentiation of triple energizer is one of the methods of differentiating epidemic febrile disease. Based on the concept that triple energizer is located in the viscera of human body of *Huangdi Neijing* (*Huangdi's Internal Classic*), Wu Jutong from the Qing Dynasty puts forward in his *Wenbing Tiaobian* (*Analysis of Epidemic Febrile Disease*) that epidemic febrile disease can be divided into three syndromes, syndromes of upper energizer, of middle energizer and of lower energizer by combining the law of transmission of epidemic febrile disease and explains in turn the developing process of the disease at three different stages according to the region where the disease occurs. As far as the characteristics of epidemic febrile disease is concerned, syndromes of upper energizer include syndrome of lung meridian of hand taiyin and that of pericardium meridian of hand jueyin; syndromes of middle energizer involve syndrome of stomach meridian of foot yangming and that of spleen meridian of foot taiyin; syndromes of lower energizer include syndrome of kidney meridian of foot shaoyin and that of liver meridian of foot jueyin.

（一）上焦证候

2.5.1 Syndrome differentiation of upper energizer

上焦者，膈肌以上之属。"温邪上受，首先犯肺，逆传心包。"温邪进犯，自口鼻而入，鼻通于肺，肺主皮毛，所以温病初期，即现肺卫受邪的症状。温邪犯肺有两种转归：一是顺传，即由上焦传入中焦，肺经传入阳明胃经；二是逆传，即由肺经传入心包经，出现温邪内陷心包的证候。

Upper energizer refers to the area above the diaphragm. "Up-attack of pathogenic febrile factors starts from the lung and then transmits adversely into the pericardium." Invasion of pathogenic febrile factors begins from the mouth and nose. The nose is connected with the lung, which is associated with the skin and body hair. Therefore, at the initial stage of epidemic febrile disease, signs of invasion of pathogenic factors into the lung are manifested. About the invasion of pathogenic factors into the lung, there are two ways, one is "due transmission", that is, pathogenic febrile factors transmit from upper energizer and into middle energizer, and from lung meridian to yangming stomach meridian; while the other is "adverse transmission", indicating pathogenic febrile factors invade from lung meridian and transmit into pericardium meridian, thus, manifestation of pathogenic febrile factors sinking into the pericardium arises.

（1）主要脉证

身热自汗，微恶风寒或不恶风寒，口渴，或不渴而咳，午后热甚；脉象浮数或两寸独大；若邪入心包，则神昏谵语，舌謇肢厥。治以辛凉解表，用银翘散、桑菊饮；若邪入心包，用清宫汤或安宫牛黄丸之类。

（1）Main clinical manifestations

Fever with spontaneous sweating, slight aversion to wind and cold, or no aversion to wind and cold, thirst, or cough with no thirst, severe fever in the afternoon; fast and floating pulse or large pulse on the cun portion of both hands; invasion of pathogenic febrile factors into the pericardium meridian may bring about coma and delirium, unsmooth tongue movement and cold limbs.

Prescription：Relieve the external syndrome with pungent-cool natured Chinese medicinal herbs.

Formulas：Yinqiao San (Powder), Sang Ju Yin (Decoction); for invasion of pathogenic factors into the pericardium meridian, Qinggong Tang (Decoction), or Angong Niuhuang Wan (Pill) can be used.

（2）辨证要点

上焦辨证的要点是，要辨明温热病初起的顺传与逆传。初起的证候即感冒的初期症状，可由表入里，由上焦传入中焦，呈现脾胃证候，此为顺传；也可能由顺传转变为逆传，即由上焦证候传入心包。而顺传与逆传则有两种不同的结果，顺传者易愈，逆传者危重。因此，不可忽视上焦证候的调治，不使逆传是治疗的关键。

（2）Key points for syndrome differentiation

Differentiation of syndromes of upper energizer should be focused on the difference between due transmission and adverse transmission at the initial stage of epidemic febrile disease. The symptoms at the initial stage are those of the primary stage of cold. Pathogenic febrile factors can be transmitted from the external into the internal, or from the upper energizer into the middle energizer, manifesting the syndromes of the spleen and stomach, which is called due transmission. However, due transmission can turn into adverse transmission, namely, diseases in the upper energizer could transmit into the pericardium. Due transmission and adverse transmission can bring about different outcomes. Diseases caused by the former can be easily cured, while those caused by the latter are usually severe and critical. Thus, treatment for syndromes in the upper energizer should not be neglected, and it is essential to avoid the occurrence of adverse transmission, treating the disease at stage of due transmission.

（二）中焦证候
2.5.2　Syndrome differentiation of middle energizer

中焦者，膈肌以下，神阙以上之位。温病自上焦始，顺传至中焦，呈现脾胃证候。脾主静，喜燥而恶湿，喜静而恶动；胃主动，喜润而恶燥，喜动而恶止。中焦有疾从湿化，则出现太阴脾经湿遏证候；如果从热化，则出现阳明胃经燥热证候。

Middle energizer refers to the region below the diaphragm and above Shenque（CV 8）. Invasion of pathogenic febrile factors starts from upper energizer and transmits into middle energizer by due transmission, manifesting syndromes of the stomach and spleen. The spleen pertain to yin, which controls cooling with preference for dryness and immobility and aversion to dampness and motions; while the stomach pertains to yang, with preference for moistening and motions with aversion to dryness and motionlessness. If pathogenic factors in middle energizer transform into dampness, then syndrome of obstruction of dampness in taiyin spleen meridian may arise; if they transform into heat, syndrome of dryness and heat in yangming stomach may appear.

（1）主要脉证

分太阴湿化证和阳明燥化证。

①太阴湿化证：身热不扬，午后较甚，胸闷身重，腹满呕逆，大便溏薄，舌苔滑腻，脉象较缓。治以理气化湿，用三仁汤之类。

②阳明燥化证：面目俱赤，呼吸气粗，大便秘结，腹满腹痛，口干咽燥，唇裂舌焦，苔黄或焦黑，脉象沉涩。治以通腑泻实，用大承气汤、小承气汤之类。

（1）Main clinical manifestations

Main clinical manifestations can be divided into two syndromes, dampness transformation in taiyin meridian and dryness transformation in yangming meridian.

a. Syndrome of transformation of dampness in taiyin meridian：

Manifestations：Dull fever, aggravation of fever in the afternoon, chest oppression and heavy sensation over the body, abdominal fullness, vomiting, loose and thin stool, slippery and greasy tongue fur as well as moderate pulse.

Prescription：Regulate qi and resolve dampness.

Formulas：Sanren Tang（Decoction）.

b. Syndrome of transformation of dryness in yangming meridian：

Manifestations：Flushed complexion and eyes, hoarse breath, constipation, fullness and painful sensation over the abdomen, dry mouth and throat, dry and fissured lips, dry scorching tongue with yellowish tongue fur or scorching blackish fur as well as sunken and astringent pulse.

Prescription：Dredge fu organs and purge stagnation of sthenic heat.

Formulas：Large Chengqi Tang（Decoction）, as well as Small Chengqi Tang

（Decoction）.

（2）辨证要点

中焦证候的辨证要点，是区别湿化与燥化。病从燥化，热势明显，如发热、面赤、便秘、舌干等；而病从湿化，湿遏显露，如身热不扬、身重、胸闷、苔腻、脉缓等。抓住重点，不难区别。

（2）Key points for syndrome differentiation

Differentiation of syndromes of middle energizer should be focused on the difference between transformation of dryness and that of dampness. Diseases due to transformation of dryness are marked by obvious fever, presenting such symptoms as fever, flushed cheeks, constipation and dryness of tongue, while diseases caused by transformation of dampness are characterized by appearance of dampness obstruction with symptoms as dull fever, heavy sensation of the body, chest oppression, greasy fur as well as moderate pulse. If the tips could be kept in mind, it would be easy to distinguish them.

（三）下焦证候
2.5.3　Syndrome differentiation of lower energizer

下焦者，神阙以下，小腹之部位。温病传至下焦，必然耗及肝肾之阴，乙癸同源，肝肾受灼，肝之阴血与肾之阴精，就会日渐耗灼，呈现肝肾阴虚或阴虚风动之证候。

Lower energizer refers to the region below Shenque （CV 8） and above the lower abdomen. Transmission of pathogenic febrile factors into lower energizer must consume liver yin as well as kidney yin. "乙" （the liver） and "癸" （the kidney） are derived from the same source, lower energizer. （Zang-fu organs are attributed to "five phase theory" and to "heavenly stems and earthly branches" of ancient Chinese calendar, in which, "乙" pertaining to wood, the liver; "癸" pertaining to water, the kidney. Therefore, "乙" "癸" are derived from the same origin, both of them belong to lower energizer.） The liver and the kidney being scorched, could give rise to gradual consumption of yin-blood of the liver and yin-essence of the kidney. Therefore, syndrome of asthenic yin of the liver and kidney as well as that of endogenous liver wind due to yin asthenia will appear.

（1）主要脉证

分肝肾阴虚证和阴虚风动证。

①肝肾阴虚证：身热面赤，手足心热甚于手背，口干，舌燥，耳鸣，神倦，舌苔薄干，脉象虚大。治以滋养肝肾，用杞菊地黄丸之类。

②阴虚风动证：身热缠绵，手足蠕动，或瘛疭，心中憺憺大动，精神疲倦，甚或时时欲脱，舌绛苔少，脉象虚弱。治以滋阴熄风，用大定风珠之类。

（1）Main clinical manifestations

Syndromes of lower energizer include asthenic yin of the liver and kidney and endogenous liver wind due to yin asthenia.

a. Syndrome of asthenic yin of the liver and kidney：

Manifestations：Fever and flushed cheeks, feverish sensation over the palms and soles even over the back of hands, dry mouth and tongue, tinnitus, dispiritedness, thin dry fur as well as weak and large pulse.

Prescription：Moisten and nourish the liver and kidney.

Formulas：Qi Ju Dihuang Wan（Pill）.

b. Syndrome of endogenous liver wind due to yin asthenia：

Manifestations：Lingering fever of the body, tremor or flaccidity of the hands and feet, severe palpitation and empty sensation in the heart, lassitude, even with susceptibility to syncope with convulsions, deep-reddish tongue with scanty fur as well as weak pulse.

Prescription：Nourish yin and suppress wind.

Formulas：Large Dingfeng Zhu Large Wind-expelling Decoction（Pill）.

（2）辨证要点

温热之邪传入下焦，引起肾阴亏虚与肝风内动的病变。肾为水脏，主藏阴精，邪热伤及肾阴，会出现手足心热于手背、口燥、咽干、神疲、心烦不眠等症状；而邪热伤及肝阴，肝为风木之脏，阴虚风动，则会见到手足蠕动，甚则瘛疭，脉虚舌绛等虚多邪少症状。两者不难鉴别。

（2）Key points for syndrome differentiation

Invasion and transmission of pathogenic febrile factors into lower energizer causes deficiency of kidney yin and endogenous liver wind. The kidney is the viscus of water, dominating the storage of yin and essence. If pathogenic febrile factors impair kidney yin, symptoms such as feverish sensation over the palms and soles even over the back of hands, dry mouth and throat, dispiritedness and vexation can appear. The liver is the viscus attributed to wind and wood, if pathogenic febrile factors impair liver yin, yin asthenia will result in endogenous liver wind, thus, symptoms such as tremor or flaccidity of the hands and feet, deep-reddish tongue as well as weak pulse may occur. It is not hard to distinguish the above syndromes.

六、脏腑辨证

2.6　Syndrome differentiation of zang-fu organs

脏腑辨证是以脏腑证候分类的辨证方法。

脏腑辨证是以脏腑的生理功能与病理反应为依据，以虚、实、寒、热不同性质为纲目而归纳的一种内伤杂病辨证方法。脏腑辨证包括脏病辨证、腑病辨证，以及脏腑兼病辨证，还有相关脏腑的经脉辨证。

Syndrome differentiation of zang-fu organs deals with different syndromes of zang-fu organs.

On basis of physiological function as well as pathological reaction of zang-fu organs, differentiation of zang-fu organs involves syndrome differentiating methods summed up about internal impairment diseases with distinct features of asthenia, sthenia, cold and heat as the outline. It includes syndromes of zang organs, fu organs, complicated syndromes of zang and fu organs as well as meridian syndromes related to zang-fu organs.

（一）肝病证候
2.6.1　Syndrome of liver diseases

1. 肝气郁结证
2.6.1.1　Syndrome of liver qi depression

胸胁或少腹闷胀窜痛，善太息，或咽部梅核气，或颈部瘿瘤，或癥瘕，情志抑郁易怒；妇女可见乳房胀痛，月经不调，痛经，甚则闭经，舌质暗红，苔白腻，脉象弦紧。治以疏肝理气，或破积散结，用柴胡疏肝散或鳖甲煎丸之类。

Main clinical manifestations: Distention, fullness and migratory pain in the chest, hypochondrium or lower abdomen, frequent sigh, or sensation of imagined bolus like foreign body in throat, or goiter and scrofula in the neck, or abdominal mass, emotional depression with susceptibility to anger, distending pain over the breast, irregular menstruation, dysmenorrhea and even amenorrhea in women, deep-reddish tongue with greasy whitish tongue fur as well as taut and tense pulse.

Prescription: Soothe the liver to regulate qi, or relieve stagnation and resolve masses.

Formulas: Chaihu Shugan San (Powder), or Biejia Jian Wan (Pill).

2. 肝火上炎证
2.6.1.2　Syndrome of liver fire hyperactivity

头晕脑涨，面红目赤，口苦口干，急躁易怒，失眠，或做噩梦，大便秘结，耳鸣如潮，舌红苔黄，脉象弦数。治以泻肝清热，用龙胆泻肝汤之类。

Main clinical manifestations: Dizziness and distending sensation over the head, flushed cheeks and eyes, bitter taste and dryness of the mouth, restlessness with susceptibility to rage, insomnia, or nightmare, constipation, tidal tinnitus, reddish tongue with yellowish fur as well as fast and taut pulse.

Prescription: Purge the liver to clear away heat.

Formulas: Longdan Xiegan Tang (Decoction).

3. 肝阳上亢证

2.6.1.3 Syndrome of liver yang hyperactivity

眩晕耳鸣，头目涨痛，面红目赤，急躁易怒，失眠多梦，头重脚轻，舌质红赤，脉象弦而有力，或弦细数。治以平肝潜阳，用羚角钩藤汤之类。

Main clinical manifestations：Vertigo and tinnitus, distending pain over the head and eyes, flushed cheeks and eyes, irritancy with susceptibility to rage, insomnia and dreaminess, heavy sensation of the head and light sensation of the feet, reddish tongue as well as taut, powerful pulse or taut, thin and fast pulse.

Prescription：Calm the liver and suppress yang.

Formulas：Lingjiao Gouteng Tang（Decoction）.

4. 肝风内动证

2.6.1.4 Syndrome of endogenous liver wind

肝风内动有肝阳化风、热极生风、阴虚风动和血虚生风四种证候。

According to the causes, the syndromes can be divided into liver yang transforming into wind, extreme heat generating wind, yin asthenia stirring wind, and blood asthenia generating wind.

（1）肝阳化风

眩晕欲仆，头痛而摇，颈项强硬不舒，语言謇涩，手足麻木，步履不正，或猝然昏倒，不省人事，口眼㖞斜，半身不遂，舌强不语，喉中痰鸣，舌质暗红，苔腻，脉象弦有力。治以滋阴平肝熄风，用镇肝熄风汤之类。

（1）Syndrome of liver yang transforming into wind

Main clinical manifestations：Vertigo, head shaking with headache, neck stiffness and discomfort, slurred speech, numbness of hands and feet, abnormal gait, or even sudden collapse with coma, facial distortion, hemiplegia, aphasia with stiffness of the tongue, sputum rale in the throat, deep-reddish tongue with greasy fur and taut and powerful pulse.

Prescription：Nourish yin and calm the liver to suppress wind.

Formulas：Zhengan Xifeng Tang（Decoction）.

（2）热极生风

高热神昏，躁扰如狂，手足抽搐，颈项强直，甚则角弓反张，两目上视，牙关紧闭，舌质绛，脉象弦数。治以清热凉肝熄风，用羚角钩藤汤、安宫牛黄丸之类。

（2）Syndrome of extreme heat generating wind

Main clinical manifestations：High fever with unconsciousness, mania with disturbance of dryness, spasm and twitching of hands and feet, stiff neck, even episthotonos, up-staring eyes, lockjaw, deep-reddish tongue as well as taut and fast pulse.

Prescription：Suppress wind by clearing away heat and cooling the liver.

Formulas：Lingjiao Gouteng Tang (Decoction), as well as Angong Niuhuang Wan (Pill).

（3）阴虚风动

多见于热病后期。症见手足蠕动，午后潮热，五心烦热，口咽干燥，形体消瘦，舌红少津，脉象细数。治以滋阴熄风，用青蒿鳖甲汤之类。

（3）Syndrome of yin asthenia stirring wind (usually seen at the advanced stage of epidemic febrile disease)

Main clinical manifestations：Tremor of hands and feet, tidal fever in the afternoon, feverish sensation over five centre (palms, soles, and the chest), dry mouth and throat, emaciation, reddish tongue with scanty fluid as well as thin and fast pulse.

Prescription：Nourish yin to suppress wind.

Formulas：Qinghao Biejia Tang (Decoction).

（4）血虚生风

多有出血先兆。症见手足蠕动，肌肉瞤动，关节拘急不利，肢体麻木，头晕耳鸣，面黄无华，爪甲不荣，舌质淡红，脉象弦细。治以养血熄风，用定振丸之类。

（4）Syndrome of blood asthenia generating wind (usually combined with sign of bleeding)

Main clinical manifestations：Tremor of hands and feet, muscular twitching, spasm and unsmooth movement of joints, numbness of limbs and body, dizziness and tinnitus, sallow complexion, lusterless nails, pale reddish tongue as well as taut and thin pulse.

Prescription：Nourish blood to suppress wind.

Formulas：Dingzhen Wan (Pill).

5. 肝经湿热证
2.6.1.5　Dampness and heat in liver meridian

胁肋胀痛灼热，厌食，口苦泛呕，小便短赤，大便不调，或胁下有痞块，舌质红赤，脉象弦数。或寒热往来，身目发黄，或阴囊湿疹，瘙痒难忍，或睾丸肿胀热痛，或妇女带下黄而臭，外阴瘙痒等。治以清利湿热，用茵陈蒿汤或茵陈五苓散。

Main clinical manifestations：Distending pain as well as scorching sensation in the chest and hypochondrium, anorexia, bitter taste with vomiting, scanty and brownish urine, irregular defecation, lumps under the hypochondrium, reddish tongue as well as taut and fast pulse. Or alternation of cold and fever, yellow coloration of body as well as eyes, or eczema in the scrotum with unbearable itchy sensation, or swollen and distending pain and fever over the spermary, or yellowish leucorrhea with foul discharge as well as pruritus vulvae in women.

Prescription：Clear away heat and eliminate dampness.

Formulas：Yinchenhao Tang (Decoction), or Yinchen Wuling San (Powder).

6. 寒滞肝脉证
2.6.1.6 Syndrome of cold stagnation in liver meridian

少腹牵引睾丸坠胀冷痛，或阴囊收缩引痛，受寒更甚，得热则缓，舌苔白滑，脉象沉弦，或弦迟。治以温经暖肝，用暖肝煎之类。

Main clinical manifestations：Lower abdominal cold pain, sagging distending pain of the spermary, or contraction and pain of scrotum, aggravation with cold and alleviation with warmth, slippery whitish tongue fur as well as sunken and taut pulse or taut and slow pulse.

Prescription：Warm the meridian and liver.

Formulas：Nuangan Jian (Decoction).

7. 肝经经脉证
2.6.1.7 Syndrome of liver meridian

颠顶头痛，两胁胀痛，目赤，面青，耳聋，颊肿，噫干，筋挛，睾丸抽缩，颓疝，遗尿，小便癃闭，女子前阴胀痛。

Main clinical manifestations：Headache, distending pain in the chest and hypochondrium, flushed eyes, cyanotic complexion, deafness, swollen cheeks, eructation with fetid odor, twitching tendons, contraction of hard and swollen spermary, sagging and distending pain or numbness of spermary without itching sensation, enuresis, blocked urination, distending pain in external genitalia in women.

8. 肝病兼证
2.6.1.8 Complicated syndromes of liver diseases

（1）肝火犯肺证

咳呛气逆，胸胁疼痛或不舒，性急易怒，痰少而黏或带血，目赤口苦，咽干声哑，或见头痛头晕，小便短赤，大便秘结，舌质红，苔黄而干，脉象弦数或弦细数。治以清肝泻肺，用黛蛤散之类。

（1）Syndrome of liver fire invading the lung

Main clinical manifestations：Choked cough with adverse flow of qi, pain in the chest and hypochondrium or discomfort sensation, irritancy and susceptibility to rage, sparse sticky sputum or mingled with blood, flushed eyes and bitter taste of the mouth, dry throat with hoarse voice, or accompanied with headache as well as dizziness, scanty and brownish urine, constipation, reddish tongue with dry and yellowish fur as well as taut and fast pulse or taut, thin and fast pulse.

Prescription：Clear away liver fire and purge lung heat.

Formulas：Dai Ge San（Powder）.

（2）肝气犯胃证

胃脘痞满时痛，引及两胁胀痛或窜痛，嗳气吞腐，善太息，舌苔薄白或薄黄，脉弦。治以泻肝和胃，用四逆散合左金丸之类。

（2）Syndrome of liver qi invading the stomach

Main clinical manifestations：Epigastric distention and fullness with occasional pain involving distending pain or wandering pain in the hypochondrium，belching with acid regurgitation，frequent sigh，thin，whitish or thin，yellowish tongue fur as well as taut pulse.

Prescription：Purge liver fire and harmonize the stomach.

Formulas：Sini San（Powder）combined with Zuojin Wan（Pill）.

（3）肝脾不和证

两胁胀满或疼痛，脘腹痞满，食欲减退，烦躁易怒，善太息，腹痛欲泻，月经不调，舌苔白腻，脉象弦缓。治以调理肝脾，用逍遥散之类。

（3）Syndrome of imbalance between the liver and the spleen

Main clinical manifestations：Distention，fullness or pain in the hypochondrium，epigastric and abdominal distention and fullness，reduced appetite，restlessness with susceptibility to rage，frequent sigh，abdominal pain with desire to diarrhea，irregular menstruation，greasy whitish tongue fur as well as taut and moderate pulse.

Prescription：Regulate qi in the liver as well as in the spleen.

Formulas：Xiaoyao San（Powder）.

（4）肝胆不宁证

虚烦不眠，或噩梦惊恐，触事易惊，或善恐如人将捕之状，短气乏力，目视无力，口苦，呕吐苦水，舌苔薄白，脉象弦细。治以养肝清胆宁神，用酸枣仁汤之类。

（4）Syndrome of discomfort of the liver and gallbladder

Main clinical manifestations：Dysphoria with insomnia，or fright with nightmare，susceptibility to panic，or frightened feeling like being captured，short breath with lassitude，weakness of vision，bitter taste with vomiting，thin and whitish tongue fur as well as taut and thin pulse.

Prescription：Nourish the liver，clear the gallbladder and tranquilize the mind.

Formulas：Suanzaoren Tang（Decoction）.

（5）肝肾阴虚证

两颧嫩红，面色憔悴，头眩目干，腰膝酸软，耳鸣耳聋，夜半咽喉干痛，骨蒸盗汗，手足心热，男子遗精，女子少腹痛，月经不调，舌红无苔，脉象弦细。治以滋阴降火，用一贯煎之类。

（5）Yin asthenia syndrome of the liver and the kidney

Main clinical manifestations：Tender pale-reddish cheeks, emaciated complexion, dizziness with dry eyes, aching and weakness of the loins and knees, tinnitus and deafness, dry and painful throat at midnight, steaming bone with night sweating, feverish sensation over palms and soles, seminal emission in male, abdominal pain and irregular menstruation in women, reddish tongue without fur as well as taut and thin pulse.

Prescription：Nourish yin and descend fire.

Formulas：Yiguan Jian（Decoction）.

（6）肝肾阴虚阳亢证

头昏目眩，少寐多梦，烦热颧红，心悸易怒，头重脚轻，四肢无力，腰酸遗精，舌质光红，脉象弦细数。治以滋阴潜降，用知柏地黄汤合建瓴汤之类。

（6）Syndrome of yin asthenia and yang hyperactivity in the liver and the kidney

Main clinical manifestations：Vertigo and dizziness, sleeplessness or dreaminess, dysphoria with flushed cheeks, palpitation with susceptibility to rage, heavy sensation of the head, weakness and fatigued limbs, aching loins and seminal emission, reddish mirror-like tongue as well as taut, thin and fast pulse.

Prescription：Nourish yin and suppress hyperactive yang.

Formulas：Zhi Bo Dihuang Tang（Decoction）combined with Jianling Tang（Decoction）.

9. 辨证要点
2.6.1.9 Key points for syndrome differentiation

①肝脏"体阴而用阳"。体阴者，包括肝血、肝精与水分等。用阳者，指肝气的疏通与条达。肝脏之疾，常常是体不足而用有余，肝体不足即肝血不足、肝精亏虚等，而肝气有余，如肝气郁结、肝气横逆、肝阳上亢、肝火上炎、肝风内动等。

②肝寒证，仅仅限于感受寒邪，凝于前阴所致的寒疝，或少腹的寒性疼痛，其他部位极少有肝寒症状。

③肝脏病常常呈现本虚标实证候，即阴不足而阳有余的证候，临证须仔细辨证。

④肝虚证，多与肾阴不足、精不化血有关，这是由于"乙癸同源"的缘故。乙者肝也，癸者肾也。由于肾阴不足而导致肝阴不足的病证屡见不鲜，辨证时，不可忽视这个问题。

a. The liver pertains to yin in nature but it functions as yang. "The liver pertains to yin in nature" refers to that blood, essence and body fluid in the liver are characterized by yin, but "it functions as yang" signifying that the liver qi acts freely and disperses normally. Diseases in the liver are usually due to deficiency of liver blood or deficiency of liver essence and surplus liver qi, bringing about qi stagnation, up-flow of liver qi, hyperactivity of liver yang, up-flaming of liver fire as well as endogenous wind in the liver.

b. Cold syndrome of the liver is only confined to cold hernia caused by stagnation of exogenous cold pathogen in the external genitalia, or pain in the lower abdomen due to cold. The syndrome hardly occurs in other region of the body.

c. Liver diseases usually display syndromes with asthenia as the root cause, and sthenia as the superficial manifestations, that is, syndrome of deficiency of yin with sufficient yang. Therefore, clinically, such syndromes must be differentiated carefully.

d. Syndrome of asthenic liver is related to kidney-yin deficiency and failure of essence to transform into blood, which is due to the fact that "乙" and "癸" have the same source. "乙" indicates the liver, and "癸" refers to the kidney. (Zang-fu organs are attributed to "five phase theory" and "heavenly stems and earthly branches" of ancient Chinese calendar, in which, "乙" pertaining to wood, the liver; "癸" pertaining to water, the kidney. Therefore, "乙" "癸" are derived from the same source, both of them belong to lower energizer.) There are quite a lot of syndromes caused by deficiency of kidney-yin, leading to insufficiency of liver-yin, which can not be neglected in syndrome differentiation.

（二）心病证候
2.6.2 **Syndrome of heart diseases**

1. 心虚证
2.6.2.1 Asthenia syndrome of the heart

（1）心血虚证

心悸，怔忡，健忘，失眠，面色萎黄无华，舌质淡红，脉象细弱。治以补血养心安神，用四物汤之类。

（1）Syndrome of asthenic heart blood

Main clinical manifestations：Palpitation, amnesia, insomnia, sallow complexion, pale reddish tongue as well as thin and weak pulse.

Prescription：Replenish blood and nourish the heart to tranquilize the mind.

Formulas：Siwu Tang (Decoction).

（2）心气虚证

心悸，怔忡，胸闷气短，乏力，畏寒，自汗，面色淡白或㿠白，舌质淡红，脉象虚弱。治以补益心气，用养心汤之类。

（2）Syndrome of asthenic heart qi

Main clinical manifestations：Palpitation, chest oppression with short breath, lassitude, aversion to cold, spontaneous sweating, pale complexion, pale reddish tongue as well as weak pulse.

Prescription：Supplement heart and benefit qi.

Formulas：Yangxin Tang (Decoction).

（3）心阴虚证

心悸，怔忡，心烦，虚惊，失眠，手足心热，盗汗，舌质红绛，舌面偏干，脉象细数。治以滋阴养心安神，用补心汤、朱砂安神丸之类。

（3）Syndrome of asthenic heart yin

Main clinical manifestations：Palpitation, vexation, feeling alarmed about nothing, insomnia, feverish sensation over palms and soles, night sweating, deep-reddish tongue with slight dryness as well as thin and fast pulse.

Prescription：Nourish yin and the heart to tranquilize the mind.

Formulas：Buxin Tang (Decoction), as well as Zhusha Anshen Wan (Pill).

（4）心阳虚证

心悸，怔忡，形寒肢冷，倦怠乏力，动则汗出，面色㿠白，或晦暗，舌质淡暗胖大，脉象迟缓或细弱。治以温心阳，益心气，用养心汤或四逆汤之类。

（4）Syndrome of asthenic heart yang

Main clinical manifestations：Palpitation, cold limbs and body, lassitude and fatigue, sweating after movement, pale or tarnished complexion, dull darkish and enlarged tongue as well as slow and moderate pulse or thin and weak pulse.

Prescription：Warm heart yang and benefit heart qi.

Formulas：Yangxin Tang (Decoction), or Sini Tang (Decoction).

2. 心实证

2.6.2.2 Sthenia syndrome of the heart

（1）心火旺证

烦躁不宁，喜笑不休，躁动不安，发狂怒骂，其则神昏谵语，或见吐血、衄血，口舌生疮，或见肌肤疮疡，溃烂疼痛，舌质红赤，脉象实大。治以清心泻火，用清心化痰丸或礞石滚痰丸之类。

（1）Syndrome of superabundant heart fire

Main clinical manifestations：Fidget, non-stop joy and laughing, restlessness, mania with rage, even delirium or unconsciousness, or usually accompanied with hematemesis, rhinorrhagia, ulceration and pain of the mouth and tongue as well as the superficial skin, reddish tongue as well as powerful and large pulse.

Prescription：Clear away heat from the heart and purge fire.

Formulas：Qingxin Huatan Wan (Pill), or Mengshi Guntan Wan (Pill).

（2）心脉痹阻证

心胸闷痛，或如针刺，彻及肩背，时发时止，舌质暗红，或有瘀斑，脉象沉涩，或沉缓。若形体肥胖，胸闷憋痛，舌苔白腻者，为痰阻心脉证。治以活血化瘀，用血府逐瘀汤；或宽胸化痰，用瓜蒌薤白半夏汤之类。

（2）Syndrome of obstruction of heart vessels

Main clinical manifestations：Oppression and pain in the chest and heart, or occasional piercing pain over the back and shoulders, deep-reddish tongue or coupled with petechiae as well as sunken and astringent pulse, or sunken and moderate pulse. Symptoms such as obese figure of body with oppression and pain in the chest as well as greasy and whitish tongue fur indicate of phlegm obstruction of heart vessels.

Prescription：Activate blood and dissolve stasis with formula of Xuefu Zhuyu Tang (Decoction)；or ease the chest and resolve phlegm with formula of Gualou Xiebai Banxia Tang (Decoction).

3. 心寒证
2.6.2.3　Cold syndrome of the heart

症见心悸，恍惚不安，肢冷恶寒，唇甲青紫，舌质暗红，脉象沉迟。治以温阳散寒，用参附汤之类。

Main clinical manifestations：Palpitation, unease and absent-mindedness, cold limbs and aversion to cold, cyanotic lips and nails, deep-reddish tongue as well as sunken and slow pulse.

Prescription：Warm yang and dispel cold.

Formulas：Shen Fu Tang (Decoction).

4. 心经经脉证
2.6.2.4　Syndrome of heart meridian

症见目黄，咽干，心痛，胁痛，口渴引饮，臑臂内侧后缘疼痛，或厥冷，掌中热痛。

Main clinical manifestations：Yellow coloration of eyes, dry throat, pain in the heart as well as in the hypochondrium, thirst with desire for drink, pain in posterior border of inner part of arms, or cold limbs, pain and feverish sensation over the palms.

5. 心病兼证
2.6.2.5　Complicated syndromes of heart diseases

（1）心脾两虚证

面色萎黄，食欲减退，气短神怯，健忘，怔忡，少寐，盗汗，腹胀便溏，妇女月经不调，舌质淡红，脉象细弱无力。治以补益心脾，用归脾丸之类。

（1）Asthenia syndrome of the heart and the spleen

Main clinical manifestations：Sallow complexion, reduced appetite, short breath and timidity due to qi deficiency, amnesia, palpitation, sleeplessness, night sweating, abdominal distention with loose stool, irregular menstruation in women, pale reddish tongue as well as thin and weak pulse.

Prescription：Supplement the heart and benefit the spleen.

Formulas：Guipi Wan (Pill).

（2）心胆俱虚证

触事易惊，虚烦不眠，噩梦多，心烦喜呕，口干口苦，舌质淡红，脉象弦细无力。治以补益心胆，宁神安魂，用十味温胆汤之类。

（2）Asthenia of the heart and the gallbladder

Main clinical manifestations：Susceptibility to fright, dysphoria with insomnia, nightmare, vexation with preference for vomiting, dry mouth with bitter taste, pale reddish tongue as well as taut and thin pulse.

Prescription：Supplement the heart, benefit the gallbladder and tranquilize the mind and spirit.

Formulas：Shiwei Wendan Tang (Decoction).

（3）心肾不交证

虚烦不眠，怔忡健忘，夜梦遗精，潮热盗汗，目眩，耳鸣，耳聋，腰酸腿软，舌红苔少，脉象细数。治以交通心肾，用黄连阿胶汤或交泰丸之类。

（3）Syndrome of disharmony between the heart and the kidney

Main clinical manifestations：Dysphoria with insomnia, palpitation with amnesia, seminal emission in dreams, tidal fever and night sweating, dizziness, tinnitus, deafness, aching and weakness of loins and legs, reddish tongue with scanty fur as well as thin and fast pulse.

Prescription：Restore normal coordination between the heart and kidney.

Formulas：Huanglian Ejiao Tang (Decoction) or, Jiaotai Wan (Pill).

6. 辨证要点
2.6.2.6 Key points for syndrome differentiation

①心病证候的虚证，从八纲上分大体可以分为阴虚证与阳虚证。阴虚证包括阴虚与血虚，心悸、怔忡、失眠是其共有症，区别在于有无虚热征兆，阴虚证有热象，如手足心热、盗汗、舌质红绛、脉象细数等。阳虚证包括气虚与阳虚，心悸、怔忡、胸闷、自汗是其共有症，区别点是有无寒象，阳虚证寒象明显，如形寒肢冷、脉象迟缓无力等。

②心病证候的实证，主要是指心火旺证与心脉痹阻证。心火旺证往往夹有痰火扰心，其指征为舌质红绛、舌苔黄腻、脉象滑数、大便秘结等。心脉痹阻证，要注意血瘀证与痰浊证的区别，血瘀证以心痛为主，而痰浊证以胸闷为主，前者舌质紫暗，后

者舌苔厚腻，可相鉴别。

③心病兼证还有心肺气阴两虚证，这在心脏病中也是常见的证候，其共有症状为气短、动则汗出、畏风、脉象细弱等，兼有心脏病的心悸、怔忡，或有结代脉，以及肺脏病的咳嗽、时时虚热、吐痰等。

④心胃同病，这是以经脉为联系的常见病证，《素问·平人气象论》曰："胃之大络，名曰虚里，贯膈络肺，出于左乳下，其动应衣，脉宗气也。"其临床症状除心前区闷痛外，必然伴有胃脘痞硬、恶心、干呕等，或因饮食不慎发作心绞痛。

a. Asthenia syndrome of heart diseases can be classified into yin and yang asthenia according to eight principles of syndrome differentiation. Asthenic yin syndrome includes yin and blood asthenia, with palpitation and insomnia as their common symptoms. The difference lies in that existence of asthenic heat in yin asthenia syndrome, such as feverish sensation over palms and soles, night sweating, deep-reddish tongue as well as thin and fast pulse. While yang asthenia syndrome involves qi asthenia and yang asthenia, with their common symptoms being palpitation, chest oppression as well as spontaneous sweating. The difference of yang asthenia from yin asthenia lies in that manifestation of obvious cold exists in yang asthenia syndrome such as cold limbs and body as well as weak, slow and moderate pulse.

b. Sthenia in syndromes of heart diseases mainly includes exuberance of heart fire and obstruction of heart vessels. Exuberance of heart fire syndrome is usually complicated with phlegmatic fire disturbing the heart, presenting symptoms such as deep-reddish tongue, greasy yellowish fur, fast and slippery pulse as well as constipation. Syndrome differentiation of obstruction of heart vessels should focus on the difference between blood stasis and phlegm turbidity. Pain in the heart is the main symptom of the former, while the leading manifestation of the latter is chest oppression, on the other hand, dark purplish tongue of the former is in sharp contrast with thick greasy fur of the latter.

c. Qi asthenia and yin asthenia of the heart and lung, as the common syndromes of heart diseases, belong to complicated syndromes of the diseases, too. Both of them have the following symptoms in common, such as short breath, sweating with movement, aversion to wind, thin weak pulse, and they are usually accompanied with symptom of palpitation of heart disease, or with slow and intermittent or slow-intermittent-regular pulse as well as symptoms of cough, occasional asthenic fever and sputum of lung disease.

d. "Heart and stomach diseases can have the same symptoms", the common one associated with meridians. Just as what is stated in the chapter "*On the pulse conditions of healthy people*" of *Suwen* (*Plain Questions*), "The major collaterals of the stomach is Xuli (apex of the heart), which runs through the diaphragm and connects with the lung from below the left breast. Its pulsation can be felt because of the propelling of Zongqi (Pectoral qi)." In addition to oppression and pain in the precordial region, clinical manifestations of the syndrome must be accompanied with hard lumps in the epigastrium, nausea, retching, etc, or angina pectoris caused by unsuitable diet.

（三）脾病证候
2.6.3 Syndrome of spleen diseases

1. 脾虚证
2.6.3.1 Asthenia syndrome of the spleen

（1）脾气虚证

食后胃脘不适，腹胀肠鸣，大便溏薄，语言气怯，四肢乏力，或见脱肛，或见胃下垂，舌质淡红，苔薄白，脉象濡缓。治以补气升阳，用补中益气汤之类。

（1）Syndrome of qi asthenia of the spleen

Main clinical manifestations：Epigastric discomfort after meals, abdominal distention with borborygmus, thin and loose stool, timidity in speaking due to qi deficiency, weak limbs with lassitude, or prolapse of the rectum, or gastroptosis, pale reddish tongue with thin whitish fur as well as soft and moderate pulse.

Prescription：Replenish qi and lift yang.

Formulas：Buzhong Yiqi Tang（Decoction）.

（2）脾阳虚证

胃脘冷痛，时泛清水，腹胀，便溏，喜热饮，小便清利，少气懒言，舌质淡红，苔白滑，脉象濡弱，或缓迟。治以温运脾阳，用理中汤之类。

（2）Syndrome of yang asthenia of the spleen

Main clinical manifestations：Epigastric cold and pain, occasional regurgitation of clear saliva, abdominal distention, loose stool, preference for hot drink, smooth urination, no desire to speak due to lack of qi, pale reddish tongue with slippery whitish fur as well as soft and feeble pulse, or slow and moderate pulse.

Prescription：Warm splenic yang to promote transportation as well as transformation of the spleen.

Formulas：Lizhong Tang（Decoction）.

2. 脾实证
2.6.3.2 Sthenia syndrome of the spleen

（1）寒湿困脾证

饮食不香，胃脘痞满，口甜而黏，头重身困，大便不实或溏泻，舌苔白腻，脉象濡细。治以健脾化湿，用胃苓汤之类。

（1）Syndrome of cold and dampness encumbering the spleen

Main clinical manifestations：Poor appetite, epigastric distention and fullness, sweet and sticky taste of the mouth, heavy sensation of the head and body, loose stool or diarrhea, greasy whitish tongue fur as well as soft and thin pulse.

Prescription：Tonify the spleen and resolve dampness.

Formulas：Weiling Tang（Decoction）.

（2）湿热内蕴证

胃脘及两胁痞胀，不思饮食，身重体困，面、目、身黄，皮肤发痒，小便色赤不利，舌苔黄腻，脉象濡数。治以清热利湿，用茵陈蒿汤、四苓散之类。

（2）Syndrome of damp heat encumbering the spleen

Main clinical manifestations：Distention and fullness in the epigastrium and hypochondrium, poor appetite, heavy sensation over the head and body, yellow coloration of the body, eyes and complexion, itching skin, unsmooth brownish urine, greasy yellowish tongue fur as well as soft and fast pulse.

Prescription：Clear away heat and induce diuresis by removing dampness.

Formulas：Yinchenhao Tang（Decoction）, as well as Siling San（Powder）.

3. 脾经经脉证
2.6.3.3　Syndrome of spleen meridian

症见舌根疼痛，身体不能动摇，食物不下，心内烦扰，心下掣痛，大便稀薄，或痢疾，或水闭于内不能排泄，或面、目、一身尽黄，不能安睡，勉强站立则股膝内侧发肿而厥冷，足大趾不能运动。

Main clinical manifestations：Pain in the root of tongue, failure of the body to move or shake, indigested food in the stomach, vexation and disturbance of the mind, dragging pain in the epigastrium, thin and loose stool, or dysentery, or failure of internal blocked fluid to be discharged, or yellow coloration of the body, eyes and complexion, inability to sleep, cold sensation due to swelling inside the thighs and knees when standing up with efforts, and failure of the hallux to move.

4. 脾病兼证
2.6.3.4　Complicated syndromes of spleen diseases

（1）脾胃不和证

胃脘痞满，绵绵作痛，食入不化，嗳气呃逆，甚则呕吐，舌苔薄白，脉象沉细。治以调和脾胃，用香砂六君子汤之类。

（1）Syndrome of incoordination between the spleen and the stomach

Main clinical manifestations：Distention, fullness and lingering pain in the epigastrium, indigested food in the stomach, belching and hiccup, even vomiting, thin whitish tongue fur as well as sunken and thin pulse.

Prescription：Harmonize the spleen and the stomach.

Formulas：Xiang Sha Liujunzi Tang（Decoction）.

（2）脾肾阳虚证

畏寒肢冷，少气懒言，大便溏薄，或五更泄泻，舌苔薄白，脉象沉细。治以健脾温肾，用理中汤合四神丸之类。

（2）Syndrome of yang asthenia of the spleen and kidney

Main clinical manifestations：Aversion to cold and cold limbs，no desire to speak due to lack of energy，thin and loose stool，or diarrhea at dawn，thin whitish fur as well as sunken and thin pulse.

Prescription：Invigorate the spleen and warm the kidney.

Formulas：Lizhong Tang（Decoction）combined with Sishen Wan（Pill）.

（3）脾湿犯肺证

咳嗽，咯吐痰涎，胸闷气短，胃纳不佳，舌苔微腻，脉象滑而缓。治以燥湿化痰，用二陈汤或平胃散之类。

（3）Syndrome of splenic dampness attacking the lung

Main clinical manifestations：Cough，expectoration with sputum and saliva，chest oppression with short breath，poor appetite，slight greasy tongue fur as well as slippery and moderate pulse.

Prescription：Dry dampness and resolve phlegm.

Formulas：Erchen Tang（Decoction），or Pingwei San（Powder）.

（4）心脾两虚证

见心病兼证。

（4）Asthenia syndrome of the heart and spleen（the detailed description can be seen in the complicated syndromes of heart diseases）.

5. 辨证要点

2.6.3.5 Key points for syndrome differentiation

①脾病的虚证与实证是相对的，即脾虚证常常夹有实证。脾虚失运，水湿内停，即为本虚标实证。在治疗上，视虚证与实证的轻重和缓急，一般轻证，先当健脾，化其水湿；标实证突出时，可以标本兼治。

②脾病与湿浊有着密切关系。如虚证的湿浊不化，实证的寒湿困脾，热证的湿热内蕴等。因此在治疗时，要参以燥湿、化湿、利湿、逐水等方药，以利于湿去脾运自复。

③中医学认为，脾与胃以膜相连，但脾病多虚证、寒证，胃病多实证、热证，古人有"实则阳明（胃），虚则太阴（脾）"之说，即是此意。另外，还要注意脾病与其他脏腑的关系，因为脾为中央土，主运四旁，治疗脾病对其他脏腑疾病的恢复非常重要。

a. Splenic asthenia and sthenia are a pair of relative syndromes, that is, splenic asthenia is usually complicated by sthenia. Failure of the spleen to transport and internal retention of dampness is a syndrome with asthenia as the root cause and sthenia as the superficial symptoms. Clinically, attention should be paid to the serious and urgent degree of a syndrome. For an unserious disease, the first place should be given to invigorating the spleen and resolving dampness. If sthenic symptoms in the superficies manifest strikingly, both the root cause and the superficial symptoms should be taken into consideration and treated simultaneously.

b. Spleen diseases are closely related to turbid dampness, such as unresolved turbid dampness in an asthenia syndrome, obstruction of cold dampness in the spleen in a sthenia syndrome as well as internal accumulation of damp heat in a heat syndrome. Therefore, in treating, the following prescriptions such as drying dampness, resolving dampness, removing dampness through diuresis or purging edema would be adopted to eliminate dampness, thus, transporting function of the spleen could be restored spontaneously.

c. In TCM, it is held that the spleen is connected with the stomach by a piece of membrane. Spleen diseases are usually manifested as asthenia and cold syndromes, while stomach diseases have manifestations of sthenia as well as heat syndrome. This is in accordance with the ancient statement "all sthenia syndromes belong to yangming diseases (stomach diseases), while all asthenia syndromes are taiyin diseases (spleen diseases)". In addition, much weight should be attached to the relationship between spleen diseases and other zang-fu organ diseases, for the spleen pertains to earth and it is located in the center, dominating and nourishing the other four zang-fu organs, so treatment of spleen disease is of great significance to restore normal function of other organs.

（四）肺病证候
2.6.4　**Syndrome of lung diseases**

1. 肺虚证
2.6.4.1　Asthenia syndrome of the lung

（1）肺阴虚证

咳呛气逆，痰少质黏，咯吐不利；咳嗽痰中带血，或为血丝，或为血块；潮热盗汗，午后颧红，少寐失眠；口干咽燥，或声音嘶哑，舌质红赤，苔少，脉象细数。治以滋阴润肺，用百合固金汤之类。

（1）Yin asthenia of the lung

Main clinical manifestations：Choked cough with adverse qi flow, sparse sticky sputum with difficulty to expectorate；sputum mingled with blood or mingled with clot of blood when coughing；tidal fever and night sweating, flushed cheeks in the afternoon, sleeplessness or even insomnia；dry mouth and throat, or hoarse voice, reddish tongue with scanty fur as well as thin and fast pulse.

Prescription：Nourish yin and moisten the lung.

Formulas：Baihe Gujin Tang（Decoction）.

（2）肺气虚证

咳而短气，痰液清稀；倦怠懒言，声音低怯；面色㿠白，形寒畏风，或时有自汗，舌质淡红，苔薄白，脉象虚弱。治以补益肺气，用补肺汤之类。

（2）Qi asthenia of the lung

Main clinical manifestations：Short breath due to cough, sparse clear sputum；fatigue and no desire to speak, low and feeble voice；pale complexion, cold limbs and aversion to wind, or occasional spontaneous sweating, pale reddish tongue with thin whitish fur as well as weak pulse.

Prescription：Supplement and benefit lung qi.

Formulas：Bufei Tang（Decoction）.

2. 肺实证
2.6.4.2 Sthenia syndrome of the lung

（1）风寒束肺证

恶寒发热，头痛身困，无汗，鼻塞流涕，咳嗽，痰液稀薄，舌苔薄白，脉象浮紧。治以发散风寒，用麻黄汤之类。

（1）Syndrome of wind cold encumbering the lung

Main clinical manifestations：Aversion to cold and fever, headache and heaviness sensation over the body, no sweating, stuffy nose with clear snivel, cough, thin clear sputum, thin and whitish tongue fur as well as floating and tense pulse.

Prescription：Dispel wind and cold.

Formulas：Mahuang Tang（Decoction）.

（2）寒饮内阻证

咳嗽频频，气急而喘，痰黏白且量多，舌苔白滑，脉象浮紧。治以温化寒饮，用小青龙汤之类。

（2）Syndrome of internal obstruction of cold and fluid

Main clinical manifestations：Frequent cough, asthma with rapid respiration, profuse sticky whitish sputum, slippery whitish tongue fur as well as floating and tense pulse.

Prescription：Resolve cold and fluid retention by warming.

Formulas：Small Qinglong Tang（Decoction）.

（3）痰浊阻肺证

咳嗽气喘，喉中痰鸣，痰黏稠不易咳出，胸胁支满，倚息不得卧，苔黄而腻，脉象滑或滑数。治以泻肺降气，用葶苈大枣泻肺汤之类。

（3） Syndrome of turbid phlegm obstructing the lung

Main clinical manifestations：Cough and asthma，sputum rale in the throat，thick sticky sputum with difficulty to expectorate，distention and fullness in the chest and hypochondrium，failure to sleep due to panting in sleeping position，greasy yellowish tongue fur as well as slippery pulse or slippery and fast pulse.

Prescription：Purge lung heat and send down adverse qi flow.

Formulas：Tingli Dazao Xiefei Tang （Decoction）.

（4） 邪热乘肺证

咳嗽之声洪亮，气喘息粗，痰稠色黄，或咳出腥臭脓血，咳则胸痛引背，鼻干鼻煽，烦渴引饮，咽喉肿痛，大便干结，小便短赤，舌质干红，苔黄燥或黄干腻，脉象滑数。治以清泻肺热，用千金苇茎汤或泻肺汤之类。

（4） Syndrome of pathogenic heat attacking the lung

Main clinical manifestations：Sonorous cough，asthma with rapid respiration，thick yellowish sputum，or expectoration of stinking foul pus and blood，cough coupled with chest pain as well as pain in the back，dry sensation in the nose and flapping of nasal wings，polydipsia with desire to drink，painful and swollen throat，dry feces，scanty brownish urine，dry reddish tongue with dry yellowish fur or greasy dry yellowish fur as well as slippery and fast pulse.

Prescription：Purge heat in the lung.

Formulas：Qianjin Weijing Tang （Decoction） or Xiefei Tang （Decoction）.

3. 肺经经脉证
2.6.4.3　Syndrome of lung meridian

症见胸部胀满，气喘作咳，缺盆中疼痛，口渴，心中烦躁，臑臂部的内侧前缘作痛，或厥冷，或掌心发热。

Main clinical manifestations：Distention and fullness in the chest，cough with asthma，pain in the supraclavicular fossa，thirst，restlessness，pain in anterior border of inner upper limbs，or cold limbs，or feverish sensation over the palms.

4. 肺病兼证
2.6.4.4　Complicated syndromes of lung diseases

（1） 心肺气虚证

心悸咳喘，气短乏力，动则尤甚，胸部憋闷，痰液清稀，面色㿠白，精神疲倦，舌淡苔白，脉象沉弱或结代。治以补益心肺，用保元汤之类。

（1） Syndrome of qi asthenia in the heart and the lung

Main clinical manifestations: Palpitation, cough, asthma, short breath and lassitude, aggravation of the above symptoms after movement, chest oppression, thin and clear sputum, pale complexion, dispiritedness, pale tongue with whitish fur as well as weak and sunken pulse or slow-intermittent pulse or slow-intermittent-regular pulse.

Prescription: Replenish and benefit the heart and lung.

Formulas: Baoyuan Tang (Decoction).

（2）脾肺气虚证

久咳不止，气短而喘，痰多稀白，食欲不振，腹胀便溏，声怯懒言，倦怠乏力，面色㿠白，甚则面浮足肿，舌淡苔白，脉象细弱。治以补脾益肺，用六君子汤之类。

（2）Syndrome of qi asthenia in the spleen and the lung

Main clinical manifestations: Continuous cough without stop, asthma with short breath, profuse clear whitish sputum, poor appetite, abdominal distention and loose stool, weak voice and no desire to speak, fatigue and lassitude, pale complexion, even facial edema and swollen feet, pale tongue with whitish fur as well as thin and weak pulse.

Prescription: Supplement the spleen and benefit the lung.

Formulas: Liujunzi Tang (Decoction).

（3）肺肾阴虚证

咳嗽痰少，口燥咽干，或声音嘶哑，或痰中带血，形体消瘦，骨蒸潮热，颧红盗汗，男子遗精，女子月经不调，舌红苔少，脉象细数。治以滋阴养肺，用生脉散之类。

（3）Syndrome of yin asthenia in the lung and the kidney

Main clinical manifestations: Cough and sparse sputum, dry mouth and throat, or hoarse voice, or sputum mingled with blood, emaciation, bone steaming with tidal fever, flushed cheeks with night sweating, seminal emission in male, irregular menstruation in women, reddish tongue with scanty fur as well as thin and fast pulse.

Prescription: Moisten yin and nourish the lung.

Formulas: Shengmai San (Powder).

5. 辨证要点
2.6.4.5 Key points for syndrome differentiation

①肺为清虚之脏，主皮肤，主鼻窍，主宗气的储藏与运行。"风寒入，外撞鸣；虚劳损，内撞鸣"。肺为娇脏，易伤不易愈。不管是外感六淫，或是七情内伤，或是饥饱劳逸，都可以伤及肺的气阴，使其发生虚损劳伤。由此可知，肺病是非常多见的。

②肺与大肠相表里，大肠的实热常常使肺气不得宣降；而肺气壅塞，也使大肠不得正常传导。所以，在对肺病辨证的时候，要注意大肠的宣通情况，以便使腑通而脏安。

③肺病证候的主要见症是恶寒、发热、咳嗽、咳痰、气喘、胸闷、胸痛、咯血、

咽干、自汗、声哑等，这些症状涉及肺的气阴和阻塞肺络的痰液等，辨证时虚实是大纲，其次是肺热或肺寒。

a. The lung is a clean, weak, tender and delicate viscus. It dominates the skin, connecting with the nose, governing storage and circulation of thoracic qi. In TCM, it is held that "Invasion of pathogenic wind and cold factors can give rise to tracheitis and asthma, excessive inner consumption like speaking too much could also result in impairment of lung yin and lung qi, thus, symptoms such as hoarse voice and throat pain may appear". The lung is a delicate viscus with susceptibility to being injured and difficulty to be healed. Lung qi and lung yin could get impaired by invasion of exogenous six climatic factors or inner impairment by intemperance of seven emotions, or improper diet as well as overstrain and fatigue, thus, giving rise to asthenic disease due to internal impairment. Consequently, lung diseases are commonly seen in clinical practice.

b. The lung is connected with the large intestine internally and externally. Sthenic heat in the large intestine results in failure of lung qi to disperse and descend, leading to qi blockage in the lung, which, in turn, causes dysfunction of the large intestine in transportation. Therefore, in differentiating syndromes of lung diseases, attention should be paid to conditions of the large intestine in transportation to ensure the normal function of zang-fu organs.

c. The main symptoms of syndrome of lung diseases are aversion to cold, fever, cough, expectoration of sputum, asthma, chest oppression and pain, hemoptoe, dry throat, spontaneous sweating as well as hoarse voice, etc, which are involved with lung qi and lung yin as well as phlegm that obstructs lung collaterals. Therefore, asthenia and sthenia should be referred to as the focus in syndrome differentiation, and lung heat or lung cold is the secondary to take into account.

（五）肾病证候
2.6.5 Syndrome of kidney diseases

1. 肾阳虚证
2.6.5.1 Syndrome of kidney yang asthenia

（1）肾气不固证

面色淡白，腰膝酸软，听力减退，小便频数，甚则不禁，早泄滑精，舌苔淡白，脉象细弱。治以固摄肾气，用大补元煎之类。

（1）Syndrome of failure to store kidney qi

Main clinical manifestations：Pale complexion, aching and weakness of the loins and knees, auditory hypofunction, frequent urination, even incontinence of urine, premature ejaculation and involuntary emission, pale tongue fur as well as thin and weak pulse.

Prescription：Reinforce kidney qi.

Formulas：Large Buyuan Jian（Decoction）.

（2）肾气不纳证

短气喘逆，动则尤甚，喘逆时汗出，且小便失禁，甚则痰鸣，面色浮白，舌质淡红，苔薄白，脉象虚弱。治以补肾纳气，用人参胡桃汤之类。

（2）Syndrome of failure of the kidney to receive qi

Main clinical manifestations：Short breath and dyspnea，aggravation of dyspnea after movement，sweating accompanied with dyspnea，incontinent urine，even sputum rale，weak and pale complexion，pale reddish tongue with thin whitish fur as well as weak pulse.

Prescription：Supplement the kidney to receive qi.

Formulas：Renshen Hutao Tang（Decoction）.

（3）肾阳不振证

面色淡白无华，形寒肢冷，腰膝酸软，阳痿，头昏耳鸣，舌苔淡白，脉象沉弱或迟缓。治以温补肾阳，用桂附地黄丸或右归丸之类。

（3）Syndrome of kidney yang asthenia

Main clinical manifestations：Pale and lusterless complexion，cold limbs and body，aching and weakness of the loins and knees，impotence，dizziness and tinnitus，pale tongue fur as well as sunken and weak pulse or slow and moderate pulse.

Prescription：Warm and replenish kidney yang.

Formulas：Gui Fu Dihuang Wan（Pill），or You Gui Wan（Pill）.

（4）肾虚水泛证

水泛肌肤，则见周身浮肿，下肢尤甚，按之如泥，腰膝酸软，尿少；水泛为痰，则咳逆上气，痰多稀薄，动则喘息，舌苔淡白，脉象沉滑。治以温阳化水，用真武汤或济生肾气丸之类。

（4）Syndrome of edema due to asthenic kidney

Main clinical manifestations：Anasarca due to retention of fluid in the muscles and superficial skin，especially the region below the waist，pressing the finger onto the area is like pressing into the mud，aching and weakness of the loins and knees，oliguria；retention of fluid resulting in phlegm，cough and adverse flow of qi，profuse clear sputum，dyspnea after movement，pale tongue fur as well as sunken and slippery pulse.

Prescription：Warm yang and resolve edema.

Formulas：Zhenwu Tang（Decoction），or Jisheng Shenqi Wan（Pill）.

2. 肾阴虚证

2.6.5.2 Syndrome of kidney yin asthenia

（1）肾阴亏虚证

形态虚弱，头晕耳鸣，健忘少寐，腰膝酸软，或有遗精，口咽干燥，舌红苔少，脉象细弱。治以滋养肾阴，用六味地黄丸之类。

（1）Syndrome of kidney yin asthenia

Main clinical manifestations：Weakness of the body and emaciation, dizziness and tinnitus, amnesia and insomnia, aching and weakness of the loins and knees, or seminal emission, dry mouth and throat, reddish tongue with scanty fur as well as thin and weak pulse.

Prescription：Nourish the kidney and moisten yin.

Formulas：Liuwei Dihuang Wan（Pill）.

（2）阴虚火旺证

颧唇红赤，潮热盗汗，腰脊酸痛，虚烦不眠，阳举遗精，口咽干燥，小便黄赤，大便秘结，舌质红赤，苔少，脉象细数。治以滋阴降火，用知柏地黄丸之类。

（2）Syndrome of yin asthenia due to exuberant fire

Main clinical manifestations：Flushed cheeks and lips, tidal fever and night sweating, aching sensation of the loins and back, dysphoria and insomnia, frequent seminal emission due to yang sufficiency, dry mouth and throat, yellow or brownish urine, constipation, reddish tongue with scanty fur as well as thin and fast pulse.

Prescription：Moisten yin and send down the fire.

Formulas：Zhi Bo Dihuang Wan（Pill）.

3. 肾经经脉证

2.6.5.3 Syndrome of kidney meridian

症见心如饥饿状，心跳善恐，口热舌干，咽肿，心内烦扰，脊股部后缘疼痛，痿废厥冷，嗜睡，足下热而痛。

Main clinical manifestations：Hungery sensation, heart throb with susceptibility to fright, feverish sensation of the mouth and dry tongue, swelling throat, vexation and disturbance of the mind, pain in posterior border of the spine, buttocks and thighs, flaccid and cold limbs, somnolence, feverish and painful sensation over the soles of the feet.

4. 肾病兼证
2.6.5.4 Complicated syndromes of kidney diseases

（1）肾虚脾弱证

大便溏泻，完谷不化，滑泻难禁，神疲肢冷，腹胀少食，肢软无力，舌淡苔薄，脉象沉迟。治以补火生土，用四神丸之类。

（1）Asthenia of the kidney and spleen

Main clinical manifestations: Loose stool, indigested food, incontinent diarrhea, dispiritedness and cold limbs, abdominal distention with reduced appetite, flaccid and weak limbs, pale tongue with thin fur as well as sunken and slow pulse.

Prescription: Benefit fire and generate earth (Reinforce kidney yang to warm and supplement splenic qi).

Formulas: Sishen Wan (Pill).

（2）水气凌心证

心悸不宁，水肿，胸腹胀满，咳喘短气，不能平卧，四肢厥冷，指唇青紫，舌质淡暗，脉象虚弱。治以温化水气，用真武汤之类。

（2）Syndrome of fluid attacking the heart

Main clinical manifestations: Palpitation and disturbance of the heart, edema, distention and fullness in the chest and abdomen, cough and dyspnea with short breath, inability to lie on the back, cold limbs, cyanotic fingernail and lips, dull darkish tongue as well as weak pulse.

Prescription: Warm and resolve edema.

Formulas: Zhenwu Tang (Decoction).

5. 辨证要点
2.6.5.5 Key points for syndrome differentiation

①一般而言，肾病无表证与实证，肾之热属阴虚之变，肾之寒属阳虚之变，对此应明辨清楚。

②肾阴虚者，往往导致阴虚火旺之证，呈现阴虚内热之变；肾阳虚者，常常犯及脾经，呈现脾肾阳虚证候。常需知此，以明辨证。

③肾与膀胱相表里，膀胱病变属虚寒者，多由肾阳虚所致；而肾阳的气化不及，也会使水湿停留于下焦形成膀胱湿热证，这在临床上也是常见的。

④肾病的兼症与五脏都有关系，如水不涵木的肾虚肝旺证、水不上乘的心肾不交证、水泛高原的肺咳喘证，以及肾阳不振的火不生土证等。认识这些病证，对解决疑难病非常重要。

a. Generally speaking, kidney disease does not include external syndrome and sthenia syndrome. Heat in the kidney is transformed from kidney yin asthenia, while cold in the kidney is transformed from kidney yang asthenia, which should be differentiated clearly.

b. Kidney yin asthenia tends to give rise to syndrome of exuberant fire due to yin asthenia, presenting manifestations of endogenous heat due to yin asthenia. Kidney yang asthenia usually causes invasion of pathogenic factors into spleen meridian, giving rise to manifestations of yang asthenia of the spleen and kidney, which should be kept in mind to differentiate syndromes carefully.

c. The kidney and bladder are related to each other internally and externally. Bladder disease due to asthenia, and cold is usually caused by kidney yang asthenia. However, failure of kidney yang to transform qi may give rise to syndrome of dampness and heat in the bladder due to dampness retention in lower energizer, which is a usual clinical manifestation.

d. Complicated syndromes of kidney disease are related to five-zang organs, for instance, kidney asthenia and liver hyperactivity due to failure of water (the kidney) to nourish wood (the liver), disharmony between the heart and kidney due to failure of kidney yin to flow upward, cough and dyspnea in the lung caused by edema and fluid retention in upper energizer, as well as deficiency of kidney yang due to failure of fire (the heart) to generate earth (the spleen). Recognition of these syndromes is of great significance to deal with stubborn diseases.

（六）胆病证候
2.6.6　Syndrome of gallbladder diseases

1. 胆虚证
2.6.6.1　Asthenia syndrome of the gallbladder

头晕欲呕，易惊少寐，视物模糊，舌苔薄滑，脉象弦细。治以养心神，和肝胆，用酸枣仁汤之类。

Main clinical manifestations：Vertigo with desire to vomit, susceptibility to fright and insomnia, blurred vision, thin slippery fur as well taut and thin pulse.

Prescription：Nourish the heart and mind and harmonize the liver and gallbladder.

Formulas：Suanzaoren Tang (Decoction).

2. 胆实证
2.6.6.2　Sthenia syndrome of the gallbladder

目眩耳聋，头晕，胸胁苦满，呕吐苦水，易怒，寐少梦多，或寒热往来，舌质红赤，苔黄，脉象弦数有力。治以泻胆清热，用龙胆泻肝汤之类。

Main clinical manifestations：Dizziness and deafness, vertigo, distention and fullness in the chest and hypochondrium, vomiting of bitter saliva, susceptibility to rage, insomnia and dreaminess, or alternate attack of cold and heat, reddish tongue with yellowish fur as well as powerful, taut and fast pulse.

Prescription：Purge heat in the gallbladder.

Formulas：Longdan Xiegan Tang（Decoction）.

（七）小肠病证候
2.6.7 Syndrome of small intestine diseases

1. 小肠虚寒证
2.6.7.1 Syndrome of asthenic cold in the small intestine

小腹隐痛，喜温喜按，肠鸣溏泻，小便频数不爽，舌质淡红，苔薄白，脉象细缓。治以温通小肠，用吴茱萸散之类。

Main clinical manifestations：Dull pain in the lower abdomen, preference for warmth and pressing, loose stool or diarrhea with borborygmus, frequent unsmooth urination, pale reddish tongue with thin whitish fur as well as thin and moderate pulse.

Prescription：Warm and dredge the small intestine.

Formulas：Wuzhuyu San（Powder）.

2. 小肠实热证
2.6.7.2 Syndrome of sthenic heat in the small intestine

心烦口疮，咽痛耳聋，小便短涩，或茎中痛，脐腹作胀，矢气后稍快，舌质红赤，苔黄，脉象滑数。治以清利实热，用导赤散或凉膈散之类。

Main clinical manifestations：Dysphoria and ulcer in the mouth, pain in the throat and deafness, scanty urine and inhibited urination, or pains in the penis, distention in the navel and abdomen, alleviation of distention with flatus, reddish tongue with yellowish fur as well as slippery and fast pulse.

Prescription：Clear away sthenic heat.

Formulas：Daochi San（Powder）or Liangge San（Powder）.

3. 小肠气痛证
2.6.7.3 Syndrome of pain in the small intestine due to qi stagnation

小腹急痛，连及腰背，下控睾丸，舌苔白滑，脉象沉弦或弦滑。治以行气散结，用天台乌药散之类。

Main clinical manifestations：Colic pain in the lower abdomen involving the loins, the back as well as the spermary, slippery whitish fur as well as sunken and taut pulse or taut and slippery pulse.

Prescription：Promote qi circulation and disperse lumps.

Formulas：Tiantai Wuyao San（Powder）.

（八）胃病证候
2.6.8　Syndrome of stomach diseases

1. 胃寒证
2.6.8.1　Stomach cold syndrome

胃脘痞满作痛，隐隐不止，喜热喜按，泛吐清水，呕吐呃逆，舌苔白滑，脉象沉迟。治以温胃散寒，用高良姜汤之类。

Main clinical manifestations：Lingering distention and pain in the epigastrium, preference for warmth and pressing, regurgitation of clear saliva, vomiting and hiccup, greasy whitish fur as well as sunken and slow pulse.

Prescription：Warm the stomach and dispel cold.

Formulas：Gaoliangjiang Tang（Decoction）.

2. 胃热证
2.6.8.2　Stomach heat syndrome

口渴喜冷饮，消谷善饥，呕吐嘈杂，或食入即吐，口臭，牙龈肿痛、腐烂或出血，舌质红，苔黄，脉象滑数。治以清胃泻火，用清胃散之类。

Main clinical manifestations：Thirst with preference for cold drink, polyphagia and frequent eating, vomiting with gastric upset, or vomiting right after eating, halitosis, swelling, pain, ulceration or bleeding of the gum, reddish tongue with yellowish fur as well as slippery and fast pulse.

Prescription：Clear away heat in the stomach and purge fire.

Formulas：Qingwei San（Powder）.

3. 胃虚证
2.6.8.3　Asthenia syndrome of the stomach

胃脘痞满，饮食不化，时时嗳气，大便不实，说话气怯，舌质淡红，脉象虚弱。治以益气建中，用黄芪建中汤之类。

Main clinical manifestations：Distention and fullness in the epigastrium, indigested food, frequent eructation, loose stool, timidity and fright in speaking due to qi deficiency, pale reddish tongue as well as weak pulse.

Prescription：Benefit qi and invigorate middle energizer.

Formulas：Huangqi Jianzhong Tang（Decoction）.

4. 胃实证
2.6.8.4 Sthenia syndrome of the stomach

食滞胃脘，脘腹胀满，大便不爽，口中秽浊，嗳腐吞酸，或呕吐，舌苔薄黄，脉象滑而数。治以消导化滞，用保和丸之类。

Main clinical manifestations: Food retention in the epigastrium, gastric and abdominal distention and fullness, unsmooth defecation, foul and turbid odor of the mouth, eructation with fetid odor and acid regurgitation, or vomiting, thin yellowish tongue fur as well as slippery and fast pulse.

Prescription: Remove indigested food and resolve retention.

Formulas: Baohe Wan (Pill).

（九）大肠病证候
2.6.9 Syndrome of large intestine diseases

1. 大肠寒证
2.6.9.1 Large intestine cold syndrome

腹痛肠鸣，大便溏薄，小便清长，舌苔白滑，脉缓。治以散寒止泻，用胃苓汤之类。

Main clinical manifestations: Abdominal pain with borborygmus, thin loose stool, thin clear urine, slippery whitish tongue fur as well as moderate pulse.

Prescription: Dispel cold and stop diarrhea.

Formulas: Weiling Tang (Decoction).

2. 大肠热证
2.6.9.2 Large intestine heat syndrome

①口燥唇焦，大便秘结，或大便腐臭，肛门灼热肿痛，小便短赤，舌苔黄燥，脉数。治以清热泻结，用凉膈散之类。

②若见赤白下痢，里急后重，发热，腹痛，舌苔黄腻，脉象滑数，为湿热痢疾。治以清利湿热，用芍药汤或白头翁汤之类。

a. Main clinical manifestations: Dry mouth and scorching lips, constipation, or stool with putrid foul odor, scorching sensation, swelling and pain over the anus, scanty and brownish urine, dry yellowish fur as well as fast pulse.

Prescription: Clear away heat and purge constipation.

Formulas: Liangge San (Powder).

b. Manifestation of the following symptoms such as red-white dysentery, tenesmus, fever, abdominal pain, greasy yellowish tongue fur as well as slippery and fast pulse indicates damp-heat dysentery.

Prescription：Eliminate dampness and heat.

Formulas：Shaoyao Tang（Decoction）or Baitouweng Tang（Decoction）.

3. 大肠虚证
2.6.9.3 Asthenia syndrome of the large intestine

泄泻日久，肛门下脱，四肢不温，舌苔薄白，脉象细微。治以厚肠固摄，用真人养脏汤之类。

Main clinical manifestations：Chronic diarrhea, prolapse of the anus, cold limbs, thin whitish tongue fur as well as thin and indistinct pulse.

Prescription：Consolidate the intestine by astringing method.

Formulas：Zhenren Yangzang Tang（Decoction）.

4. 大肠实证
2.6.9.4 Sthenia syndrome of the large intestine

腹痛拒按，或发热呕逆，便秘，或排便不爽，苔黄，脉象沉实。治以清热导滞，用承气汤之类。

Main clinical manifestations：Unpressable pain in the abdomen, or fever with vomiting, constipation, or unsmooth defecation, yellowish tongue fur as well as sunken and powerful pulse.

Prescription：Clear away heat and relieve stagnation by purgation.

Formulas：Chengqi Tang（Decoction）.

（十）膀胱病证候
2.6.10 Syndrome of bladder diseases

1. 膀胱虚寒证
2.6.10.1 Asthenic cold syndrome of the bladder

小便频数，淋漓不禁，或遗尿，舌质淡红，苔白润，脉象沉细。治以固摄肾气，用桑螵蛸散之类。

Main clinical manifestations：Frequent urination with incontinent and dripping urine, or spontaneous urination, pale reddish tongue with moist whitish fur as well as sunken and thin pulse.

Prescription：Consolidate and store kidney qi.

Formulas：Sangpiaoxiao San（Powder）.

2. 膀胱实热证

2.6.10.2　Sthenic heat syndrome of the bladder

小便短赤不利，尿色黄赤，或混浊不清，尿时茎中热痛，甚则淋漓不畅，或见脓血砂石，舌红苔黄，脉数。治以清利湿热，用八正散之类。

Main clinical manifestations：Unsmooth urination with scanty brownish urine, or yellow brownish urine, or turbid unclear urine, fever and pain sensation of the penis, even dripping or obstructive urination, or accompanied with pus, blood as well as urinary calculi, reddish tongue with yellowish fur as well as fast pulse.

Prescription：Eliminate dampness and heat by inducing diuresis.

Formulas：Bazheng San（Powder）.

下篇　常见病治疗

Section B　Treatment for some common diseases

古代中医学对疾病的命名，多是以症状、病因或病变部位而拟定的，如以症状命名的咳嗽、喘证、水肿、眩晕，以病因命名的中风、郁证、虫积，以病变部位命名的肺痨、胃痞、胸痹等。但在现代中医学著作里，以西医学立名的亦不少见。为了方便国外热爱中医学的朋友学习，本书采用西医学病名立篇，并与中医学病名对照，以便读者能深入地学习与应用。

In TCM, terminology of diseases is based on their specific symptoms and etiology, or regions where pathological changes occur. For instance, diseases such as cough, dyspnea, edema and vertigo are named after their symptoms, while stroke, depression and parasitic malnutrition are named after their causes. There are still other diseases named after the regions where pathological changes occur, such as lung-lao (namely, pulmonary tuberculosis, a disease in the lung), stomach-pi (stomach distention and fullness, a disease in the stomach), as well chest-bi (namely, ischemic heart disease, a disease in the chest). However, in modern Chinese medicinal books, there are quite a few diseases which are named after their corresponding terminology in Western medicine. In this book, terminology of the diseases in Western medicine has been adopted and their TCM corresponding terms are also listed so as to provide convenience for TCM lovers abroad.

一、感冒

1　Common cold

[概说] Summary

感冒，作为一个病名，最早见于中国北宋《仁斋直指方》一书，并指出可用参苏饮治疗。但现代医学所说的感冒不仅与中医学所指的感冒相同，而且还包括中医学所说的"伤风"等病证。

感冒发生的病变部位仅限于肺卫，极少传变。一般病程为 3~7 天，身体强壮的人，通过适当休息，适量饮水，多可痊愈。但若反复发作，导致肺气不足，抗病能力下降，就会出现内伤证候，如气短、汗出、形寒、肢冷，变生其他疾病。因此，感冒虽非大病，也要从预防入手，积极治疗，防患于未然。

The term of "common cold", as a disease, appears in the Northern Song Dynasty for the first time in the book *Renzhai Zhi Zhi Fang* (*Effective Recipes from Renzhai House*), which holds that Shen Su Yin (Decoction) can be applied to treat it. However, "common cold" not only has the same meaning as in modern medicine, it also includes the syndromes such as "cold due to invasion of exogenous wind" in TCM.

Common cold can only bring about pathological change to the lung, and it scarcely transmits to other parts of body. The general course of the disease is about 3 ~ 7 days. Many healthy people can get recovered through proper rest and drinking water. Frequent catching cold could cause insufficient lung qi, as a result, patients' resistance against diseases would decline, from which other symptoms due to internal impairment, for instance, shortness of breath, sweating, cold limbs and body could arise and they could, in turn, lead to other diseases. Therefore, though it is not a serious disease, treatment for it should start from prevention, and patients should take precautions as early as possible.

〔辨证论治〕 Syndrome differentiation and treatment

（一）实证
1.1 Sthenia syndrome

1. 风寒感冒
1.1.1 Wind-cold common cold

【症状】恶风恶寒，或发热或未发热，鼻塞声重，鼻流清涕，咳嗽，喉痒，痰稀薄，头痛，肢体酸痛，无汗，舌苔薄白，脉象浮紧，发热时浮数。

【分析】风寒感冒主要是风寒外袭，肺卫受邪所致。风寒外袭，卫气被遏，卫气不能卫外，故见恶风恶寒；若卫气可以抵抗外邪，则见发热，卫气弱而不能抵御外邪，则不见发热。肺主呼吸，开窍于鼻，鼻被风寒所遏，窍道不利，故见鼻塞声重、鼻流清涕、咳嗽、喉痒、痰稀薄等症状；风寒客于皮毛，寒为阴邪，郁遏卫阳，故见头痛、无汗、肢体酸痛。邪客于表，则舌苔薄白；浮紧为风寒客表之脉，浮数为发热之脉象。

【治法】辛温解表，宣肺散寒。

【方药】荆防败毒散或葱豉汤。荆防败毒散为辛温发表之剂，方中荆芥、防风、羌活、独活等为驱散风寒之要药，对于恶寒无汗、肢体酸痛等风寒表证，最为适宜；前胡、桔梗、茯苓、甘草等有宣肺止咳祛痰之功效。葱豉汤为辛温散寒之轻剂，也为食疗之方，用于风寒感冒之轻证。若鼻塞重者，加苍耳子；痰多白黏者，加橘红、杏仁等。

Clinical manifestations：Aversion to wind and cold, fever or no fever, stuffy nose with low voice, clear snivel, cough, throat itching, thin sputum, or accompanied with headache, aching sensation of limbs and body, no sweating, whitish and thin tongue fur, floating and tense pulse or floating and fast pulse with fever.

Analysis：Cold syndrome due to wind cold is caused by pathogenic cold and wind attacking the surface of body. Aversion to wind and cold is due to wind cold attacking the superficies, resulting in failure of stagnated defensive qi to defend the superficies. Fever is caused when defensive qi could prevent the attack of pathogenic wind and cold. If defensive qi is too weak to resist attack of exogenous pathogens, fever will not arise. The lung governs respiration and opens into the nose. Stuffy nose with low voice, clear snivel, cough, throat itching and clear sputum are due to obstruction of wind cold as well as unsmooth air passage. Headache, anhidrosis and aching sensation of limbs and body are caused by attack of pathogenic wind cold in the skin and hair, and stagnation of defensive yang by cold pathogen. Whitish and thin tongue fur is due to invasion of pathogens on the surface of the body. Floating and tense pulse indicates attack of wind cold on the superficies, while floating and fast pulse is a sign of fever.

Prescription: Relieve superficial syndrome with pungent-warm herbs and disperse the lung and wind cold.

Formulas: Jing Fang Baidu San (Powder), or Congchi Tang (Decoction of Chinese green onion stalk and fermented soybean). The former formula, Jing Fang Baidu San, is pungent in flavor and warm in nature, has an action of inducing sweating to relieve exterior syndrome, in which, Jingjie (*Herba Schizonepeta*), Fangfeng (*Radix Saposhnikoviae*), Qianghuo (*Rhizoma et Radix Notopterygii*), and Duhuo (*Radix Angelicae Pubescentis*) can expel wind cold, so it is very suitable to treat the superficial syndrome of wind and cold with symptoms such as aversion to cold, anhidrosis and aching sensation of the limbs and body. The other herbs in the formula have the function of dispersing the lung, arresting cough and resolving phlegm, such as Qianhu (*Radix Peucedani*), Jiegeng (*Radix Platycodi*), Fuling (*Poriae Cocos*) and Gancao (*Radix Glycyrrhizae*). The latter one, Congchi Tang, pungent in flavor and warm in nature, belongs to a light diaphoretic prescription, with the action of dispersing cold. It can also be used as a dietetic therapy for wind-cold type common cold. Cang'erzi (*Fructus Xanthii*) can be added for severe stuffy nose, Juhong (*Exocarpium Citri Rubrum*) and Xingren (*Semen Armeniacae Amarum*) can be added for profuse, whitish and sticky sputum.

附：风寒夹湿感冒

Complicated syndrome of common cold: Wind-cold common cold complicated with dampness

【症状】恶寒发热，但热势不扬，头重如裹，骨节疼痛，舌苔白腻，脉象浮濡。

【分析】感受雾露之湿，或冒受雨淋，湿邪着表，则恶寒发热，但湿邪重浊，故热势不扬；湿邪蒙蔽清阳，故头重如裹；湿伤骨节，骨节失养，故疼痛明显；其舌苔、脉象均为湿邪之象。

【治法】疏风散湿。

【方药】羌活胜湿汤。方中取羌活、独活、川芎、防风散风祛湿；藁本辛温，入膀胱经，上至头项，发散风寒，尤擅祛湿；蔓荆子为辛苦之品，性善上行，性不太燥，较为平和，可以升发人体的阳气，以便把湿邪祛除掉。

Clinical manifestations: Aversion to cold and dull fever, distending headache like being wrapped, pain in the bones and knuckles, whitish and greasy tongue fur, floating and soft pulse.

Analysis: Aversion to cold and fever are caused by exogenous dampness of fog or dew, or by being drenched in rain, resulting in stagnation of damp pathogen in the superficial skin. Dull fever is due to heaviness and turbidity of dampness. Distending headache like being wrapped is caused by invasion of pathogenic damp factors in the head which prevents lucid yang from rising. Obvious pain sensation is due to pathogenic damp impairing bones and knuckles, which results in malnutrition of bones and knuckles; greasy whitish tongue fur and floating soft pulse are manifestations of pathogenic dampness.

Prescription: Expel wind and disperse dampness.

Formulas: Qianghuo Shengshi Tang (Decoction). In this formula, Qianghuo (*Rhizoma et Radix Notopterygii*), Duhuo (*Radix Angelicae Pubescentis*), Chuanxiong (*Rhizoma Ligustici Chuanxiong*) and Fangfeng (*Radix Saposhnikoviae*) are used for expelling wind and dispersing dampness. Gaoben (*Rhizoma Ligustici*), pungent in flavor and warm in nature, attributive to bladder meridian, can travel to top of the head to dispel wind cold, and it is especially good at dispelling dampness; Manjingzi (*Fructus Viticis*), pungent and bitter in flavor, neutral in nature, bears a tendency to lift upward. Therefore, it can improve generation of yang qi to eliminate pathogenic dampness factor with its mild action.

2. 风热感冒
1.1.2 Wind-heat common cold

【症状】发热，微恶风寒，头痛，鼻塞，流浊涕，咳痰黄稠，口干欲饮，有汗出，咽喉焮红疼痛，舌苔薄黄，脉象浮数。

【分析】风为阳邪，与热相合，必然发热，虽有汗出，但邪不从汗解；风热上受，肺失清肃，则头痛、鼻塞、流浊涕、咳痰黄稠；风热熏蒸于清窍，并灼伤肺阴，故见口干欲饮，咽喉焮红疼痛；苔薄黄、脉浮数，为风热客于肌表之象。

【治法】辛凉解表，祛风清热。

【方药】银翘散或桑菊饮。两方均为辛凉解表之常用方剂，前者取金银花、连翘、薄荷之辛凉，配荆芥、淡豆豉之辛温，退热作用较强；佐以牛蒡子、桔梗、甘草清肺利咽，并辅以竹叶、鲜芦根清上焦之热，对风热感冒之发热、咽喉疼痛者，效果尤佳。后者作用较弱，对上呼吸道感染者效果满意。

Clinical manifestations: Fever, slight aversion to wind and cold, headache, stuffy nose with turbid snivel, cough with yellowish thick sputum, thirst with desire for drink, sweating, swollen sore throat, yellowish and thin tongue fur as well as floating and fast pulse.

Analysis: Wind, as a pathogenic factor of yang nature, coupled with pathogenic heat, gives rise to fever. Though accompanied with sweating, pathogenic factor cannot be relieved through sweating. Headache, stuffy nose with turbid snivel, cough and yellowish thick sputum are due to upper invasion of wind heat and loss of depuration of the lung; thirst with desire for drink and swollen sore throat are caused by wind heat fumigating the upper orifice and scorching lung yin; thin yellowish tongue fur and floating and fast pulse are signs of wind heat invading the superficies of the skin.

Prescription: Relieve the superficial syndrome with pungent-cool natured herbs and disperse wind heat.

Formulas: Yin Qiao San (Powder), or Sang Ju Yin (Decoction). Both of the formulas are common recipes with pungent-cool nature. In the former, Jinyinhua (*Flos Lonicerae*), Lianqiao (*Fructus Forsythiae*) and Bohe (*Herba Menthae*) are pungent in flavor and cool in nature, combined with pungent-warm natured Jingjie (*Herba Schizonepetae*) and Dandouchi (*Semen Sojae Preperatum*), have the strong action of expelling heat; Niubangzi (*Fructus Arctii*), Jiegeng (*Radix Platycodonis*) and Gancao (*Radix Glycyrrhizae*) can be combined to clear away heat in the lung and ease the throat; Zhuye (*Herba Lophatheri*) and Fresh Lugen (*Rhizoma Phragmitis*) can be added to clear away heat from upper energizer, which is particularly effective for symptoms of fever and sore throat in common cold due to wind heat. The latter one, with a weak action, can have a very satisfactory curative effect to upper respiratory tract infection.

3. 表寒里热感冒
1.1.3 Common cold of exogenous cold with endogenous heat

【症状】发热恶寒，头痛无汗，肢体酸痛，鼻塞声重，咽喉肿痛，咳嗽，痰黏稠，舌边尖红赤，苔薄白或薄黄，脉象浮数。

【分析】素体热盛，或素有痰火，感受风寒，则热郁于里，寒居于表，形成表寒里热，即所谓"寒包火"之候。寒袭于表，故见发热恶寒、头痛无汗、肢体酸痛；其他咽喉肿痛、咳嗽、脉舌之象，均为里热所致。

【治法】疏风宣肺，散寒清热。

【方药】麻杏石甘汤加羌活、独活、鱼腥草。麻杏石甘汤为清热解表之剂，麻黄配羌活、独活解表散寒，杏仁、石膏、甘草配鱼腥草清肺解热。若表寒较重，肢节酸痛明显，可加桂枝、苏叶；肺热较重，咳嗽、咽燥，可加沙参、黄芩；大便秘结者，可加生大黄沸水泡饮。

Clinical manifestations: Fever, aversion to cold, headache, anhidrosis, aching sensation of the limbs and body, stuffy nose with low voice, swollen sore-throat, cough with sticky and thick sputum, reddish margins and tip of tongue, thin whitish tongue fur or thin yellowish fur as well as floating and fast pulse.

Analysis: Persistent exuberance of endogenous heat, or prolonged phlegmatic fire, complicated by invasion of wind and cold, gives rise to stagnation of heat on the interior, but accumulation of cold on the exterior, resulting in the syndrome of exogenous cold and endogenous heat, namely, "fire enveloped by cold". Fever and aversion to cold, headache, anhidrosis and aching sensation of the limbs and body are caused by attack of pathogenic cold on the superficies; other manifestations such as swollen sore throat, cough, reddish margins and tip of tongue, thin whitish tongue fur or thin yellowish fur and floating and fast pulse are caused by internal heat.

Prescription：Expel wind, disperse the lung, dissipate cold and clear away heat.

Formulas：Mahuang Xingren Shigao Gancao Tang (Decoction) coupled with Qianghuo (*Rhizoma et Radix Notopterygii*), Duhuo (*Radix Angelicae Pubescentis*) and Yuxingcao (*Herba Houttuyniae*). Mahuang Xingren Shigao Gancao Tang is used to clear away heat and relieve superficies. Mahuang (*Herba Ephedrae*), in combination with Qianghuo and Duhuo, has an effect of relieving superficies and dispersing cold, Xingren (*Semen Armeniacae Amarum*), Shigao (*Gypsum Fibrosum*), Gancao (*Radix Glycyrrhizae*), together with Yuxingcao (*Herba Houttuyniae*), can clear away lung heat and relieve fever. Guizhi (*Ramulus Cinnamomi*) and Suye (*Folium Perillae*) can be added for severe exogenous cold and arthrodynia of the extremities. Shashen (*Radix Glehniae*) and Huangqin (*Radix Scutellariae*) can be added for severe lung heat, cough and dry throat. Shengdahuang (*Radix et Rhizoma Rhei*), soaked in boiling water for oral use, can be added for constipation.

4. 暑湿感冒
1.1.4 Common cold due to summer-heat and dampness

【症状】发热恶风，身热有汗，头痛身困，心烦口渴，小便短赤，舌苔黄腻，脉象濡数。

【分析】暑湿感冒，发于夏季，暑为阳邪，湿为阴邪，暑湿之邪袭于肌表，则发热恶风、身热有汗；湿邪重浊，外蒙清窍，则头痛身困；小便短赤，为暑湿之邪下注之象；舌苔黄腻与脉象濡数，为夏季暑湿感冒之特点。

【治法】解表清暑，芳香化湿。

【方药】新加香薷饮。方用金银花、连翘清热解毒，香薷、厚朴、白扁豆芳香化湿。若口淡无味，可加藿香、佩兰、荷叶之类芳香醒脾；若湿重于暑，头涨胸闷、身楚不适，可用薷藿汤解表化湿。

Clinical manifestations：Fever, aversion to wind, sweating, headache, lassitude, dysphoria, thirst, scanty and brownish urine, greasy yellowish tongue fur and soft and fast pulse.

Analysis：Common cold due to summer-heat and dampness breaks out in summer. Summer-heat is a pathogenic yang factor, while dampness is a pathogenic yin factor, attack of pathogenic summer-heat and dampness on the superficies gives rise to fever, aversion to wind and sweating; headache and lassitude are due to heaviness and turbidity of pathogenic dampness which blocks the orifices. Scanty and brownish urine is caused by downward discharge of pathogenic summer-heat and dampness. Yellowish and greasy tongue fur and soft and fast pulse are manifestations of common cold due to summer-heat and dampness.

Prescription：Relieve superficial symptoms with aromatic natured drug, clear away summer-heat and eliminate dampness.

Formulas：Xinjia Xiangru Yin (Decoction). In this formula, Jinyinhua (*Flos Lonicerae*) and Lianqiao (*Fructus Forsythiae*) have the action of clearing away heat, Xiangru

(*Herba Moslae*), Houpo (*Cortex Magnoliae Officinalis*) and Baibiandou (*Semen Dolichoris Album*), aromatic in flavor, can eliminate dampness. For bland taste of the mouth, Huoxiang (*Herba Agastachis*), Peilan (*Herba Eupatorii*) and Heye (*Folium Nelumbinis*), can be used to invigorate the spleen. For summer-heat and dampness syndrome with predominant dampness, distending headache and chest oppression, and discomfort over the whole body, Ru Huo Tang (Decoction) can be used to relieve superficies and resolve dampness.

(二) 虚证
1. 2 Asthenia syndrome

1. 气虚感冒
1.2.1 Common cold due to qi asthenia

【症状】恶寒发热，但热势不高，时感形寒，自汗，头痛鼻塞，咳嗽，痰液稀薄，语声低怯，气短，乏力，舌苔薄白，脉象浮而无力。

【分析】素体气虚者，最易感冒，气虚则卫外之力减弱，易受风寒之袭，恶寒发热、头痛鼻塞、咳嗽、痰液稀薄、苔白，为风寒表证；气短、乏力、语声低怯、脉浮而无力，为气虚之征。

【治法】益气解表，调和营卫。

【方药】参苏饮或黄芪桂枝五物汤。前者为气虚感冒而设，方中有人参、茯苓、甘草等益气扶正，苏叶、葛根、前胡疏风祛邪，桔梗、半夏、枳壳宣肺化痰，陈皮、木香理气和中，生姜、大枣调和营卫，适用于气虚感冒热势不高、咳嗽、气短、形寒恶风者。后者以黄芪益气固表，桂枝汤调和营卫，疏散风寒，适用于气虚感冒，凛凛恶寒，肢体酸困不适者。

Clinical manifestations: Aversion to cold, dull fever, occasional sensation of cold limbs, spontaneous sweating, headache and stuffy nose, cough, thin sputum, timidity and low voice, short breath, lassitude, thin and whitish tongue fur, floating and weak pulse.

Analysis: A patient with qi asthenic constitution is liable to catch a cold. Qi asthenia leads to weakness or failure of defensive qi to protect the superficies from attack of exogenous wind and cold pathogens. Aversion to cold, fever, headache with stuffy nose, cough, thin sputum, and whitish tongue fur are signs of external syndrome of wind and cold; short breath, lassitude, timidity and low voice and floating and weak pulse are manifestations of qi asthenia.

Prescription: Invigorate qi, relieve the superficies and harmonize nutrient qi and defensive qi.

Formulas: Shen Su Yin (Decoction), or Huangqi Guizhi Wuwu Tang (Decoction). The former is applicable to common cold due to qi asthenia, in which, Renshen (*Radix Ginseng*), Fuling (*Poriae Cocos*) and Gancao (*Radix Glycyrrhizae*) have an action of benefiting healthy qi; Suye (*Folium Perillae*), Gegen (*Radix Puerariae*) and Qianhu

（*Radix Peucedani*）can dispel wind pathogen；Jiegeng（*Radix Platycodonis*）, Banxia（*Rhizoma Pinelliae*）and Zhiqiao（*Fructus Aurantii*）can disperse the lung and resolve phlegm；Chenpi（*Pericarpium Citri Reticulatae*）and Muxiang（*Radix Aucklandiae*）have an effect of regulating qi and harmonizing the spleen and stomach；Shengjiang（*Rhizoma Zingiberis Recens*）and Dazao（*Fructus Jujubae*）, with the effect of harmonizing nutrient qi and defensive qi, can be used for symptoms such as dull fever, cough, short breath, cold limbs and aversion to wind of the syndrome of common cold due to qi asthenia. In the latter, Huangqi（*Radix Astragali seu Hedysari*）has the action of invigorating qi to strengthen superficies；Guizhi Tang（Decoction）, with the action of harmonizing nutrient qi and defensive qi and expelling wind and cold, is applicable to the syndrome of common cold due to qi asthenia with manifestations as aversion to cold, huddled posture with cold, and aching and discomfort of limbs and body.

2. 阳虚感冒
1.2.2　Common cold due to yang asthenia

【症状】恶寒重，发热轻，甚则蜷缩、寒战，或稍有发热，头痛，骨节疼痛，面色㿠白，四肢不温，舌质淡胖，苔白，脉象沉细无力。

【分析】阳虚之人，卫外能力最差，所以感受风寒时以恶寒明显，发热次之；四肢不温，面色㿠白，是阳虚者形体表现；寒邪凝遏阳脉经络，则头痛、骨节疼痛；舌质淡胖、苔白、脉沉细，均为阳虚之兆。

【治法】温阳解表。

【方药】桂枝加附子汤。阳虚之体，感受恶寒，首先要温阳散寒，而桂枝加附子汤即是温阳散寒之主剂。方中桂枝汤辛温散寒，温经达表；附子大辛大热，温通经脉，是辅助阳气的最佳选择。

Clinical manifestations：Severe aversion to cold, dull fever, even huddled posture in severe cases, or mild fever, headache, painful sensation of bones and knuckles, pale complexion, cold limbs, bulgy pale tongue, whitish fur as well as thin, sunken and weak pulse.

Analysis：Constitutional yang asthenia results in weakness of defensive qi to guard against exogenous pathogens, leading to obvious aversion to cold and dull fever. Cold limbs and pale complexion are manifestations of yang asthenic physique. Headache and painful sensation of bones and knuckles are due to obstruction of stagnant pathogenic cold in yang meridians and collaterals；bulgy pale tongue with whitish fur and thin, sunken and weak pulse are signs of yang asthenia.

Prescription：Warm yang and relieve the superficies.

Formulas：Guizhi Fuzi Tang（Decoction）. The prescription of warming yang and expelling cold should be adopted for constitutional yang asthenia complicated by exogenous pathogenic cold factor. Guizhi Fuzi Tang is a main recipe for warming yang and expelling cold, of which, Guizhi (*Ramulus Cinnamomi*), pungent in flavor, warm in nature, has the effect of dispersing cold and warming the meridians, Fuzi (*Radix Aconiti Lateralis Preparata*), severe pungent and hot in nature, is the best choice for warming meridians and activating yang qi.

3. 血虚感冒
1.2.3 Common cold due to blood asthenia

【症状】发热，但热势不高，头痛，有汗，面色无华，唇舌淡红，心悸，头晕，舌苔淡红，脉象浮而无力，或有结代脉。

【分析】素体血虚，或于产后，或因失血，感受外邪，既有外感症状，又有血虚症状。外感症状如发热、头痛、脉浮等，血虚症状如头晕、心悸、唇舌淡红、汗出等。有的会出现结代脉，这是阴血不足，不能充盈脉道所致。

【治法】养血解表。

【方药】葱白七味饮。方以葱白、淡豆豉、葛根、生姜发汗解表，又有生地黄、麦冬养血滋阴，更有味甘体轻之劳水（甘澜水）以养脾胃，使汗出表解而不伤正。如恶寒较重，可加苏叶、荆芥；身热甚者，可加金银花、连翘；出血未止，可加芦根、藕节、白及等。

Clinical manifestations: Dull fever, headache, sweating, pale or sallow complexion, pale lips and tongue, palpitation and dizziness, pale reddish tongue fur, floating and weak pulse or slow and intermittent pulse, or slow-intermittent-regular pulse.

Analysis: This syndrome is caused by constitutional blood asthenia because of delivery, or due to loss of blood complicated by invasion of exogenous pathogenic factors. Therefore, it involves symptoms of exogenous syndrome as well as those of blood asthenia. Symptoms of exogenous pathogens syndrome include fever, headache and floating pulse, while dizziness, palpitation, pale reddish lips and tongue and sweating belong to syndrome of blood asthenia. In some cases, slow and intermittent pulse, or slow-intermittent-regular pulse may appear because of failure of insufficient yin blood to fill up blood vessels.

Prescription: Nourish blood and relieve the superficies.

Formulas: Congbai Qiwei Yin (Decoction). In this formula, Congbai (*Allium Fislulosum*), Dandouchi (*Semen Sojae Preperatum*), Gegen (*Radix Puerariae*) and Shengjiang (*Rhizoma Zingiberis Recens*) are used to induce sweating so as to relieve superficies. Shengdihuang (*Radix Rehmanniae Recens*) and Maidong (*Radix Ophiopogonis*) are used to nourish blood and moisten yin, Laoshui [or Ganlan water (in terms of TCM, the water for our daily use is heavy and salty, but if it is raised up with a gourd ladle for thousands of times, it will become light and sweet. Therefore, the water produced in this way is called Laoshui or Ganlan water)] can invigorate the spleen and stomach so as to achieve the effect of inducing sweating and relieving the exogenous syndrome without impairing healthy qi of the body. For severe aversion of cold, Suye (*Folium Perillae*), and Jingjie (*Herba Schizonepetae*) can be combined; for fever, Jinyinhua (*Flos Lonicerae*) and Lianqiao (*Fructus Forsythiae*) can be added；for high non-stop bleeding, Lugen (*Rhizoma Phragmitis*), Oujie (*Nodus Nelumbinis Rhizomatis*) and Baiji (*Hyacinth Bletilla*) can be combined.

4. 阴虚感冒
1.2.4　Common cold due to yin asthenia

【症状】发热，微恶风寒，或自汗，或盗汗，或无汗，头痛，口干咽燥，干咳，或痰中带血丝，手足心热，舌质红赤，苔少津，脉象细数。

【分析】阴虚之体，感受外邪，易从热化，多出现肺燥伤阴之候，如发热、汗出、干咳、头痛、痰中带血丝等。手足心热、舌质红赤、脉象细数，是阴虚内热证候。形体消瘦、口干咽燥是其体质特点。

【治法】滋阴解表。

【方药】加减葳蕤汤。方中以甘平柔润之葳蕤（玉竹）滋阴增液、润肺生津为主药，葱白、淡豆豉、薄荷、桔梗解表宣肺、止咳利咽为臣药，白薇凉血清热除烦为佐药，甘草、大枣甘润滋脾为使药。全方滋阴清热而不碍解表，发汗解表而不伤阴津，用于阴虚外感最为适宜。

Clinical manifestations：Fever, slight aversion to wind and cold, spontaneous sweating, or night sweating, or no sweating, headache, dry mouth and throat, dry cough, sputum mingled with blood, feverish sensation over the palms and soles, reddish tongue, dry tongue fur and thin and fast pulse.

Analysis：Fever, sweating, dry cough, headache, sputum mingled with blood are due to dryness of the lung impairing yin because patients with asthenic constitution are prone to being attacked by invasion of exogenous pathogenic factors, which can transform into heat. Feverish sensation over the palms and soles, reddish tongue, thin and fast pulse are signs of endogenous heat due to yin asthenia. Emaciation and dry mouth and throat are signs of yin asthenic constitution.

Prescription：Nourish yin and relieve superficial symptoms.

Formulas：Jiajian Weirui Tang (Decoction). In the formula, Weirui (*Rhizom a Polygonati Odorati*), sweet in flavor, plain, soft and moist in nature, has the effect of nourishing yin, moistening the lung and promoting the production of body fluid, so it used as sovereign drug；Congbai (*Allium fislulosum*), Dandouchi (*Semen Sojae Preperatum*), Bohe (*Herba Menthae*), and Jiegeng (*Radix Platycodi*) are used as ministerial drug to relieve the superficies, disperse the lung and relieve cough and sore throat；Baiwei (*Radix Cynanchi Atrati*), with the action of cooling blood and clearing away heat and restlessness serves as assistant drug；Gancao (*Radix Glycyrrhizae*) and Dazao (*Fructus Jujubae*), sweet in flavor, is used as courier drug to moisten the spleen. Combined together, the formula has the action of nourishing yin and clearing heat, meanwhile, it does not hinder relieving the superficies. Furthermore, this formula is the best choice for common cold due to yin asthenia, for it can induce sweating and relieve the superficies without impairing yin fluid.

二、流行性感冒

2 Influenza

〔**概说**〕 Summary

流行性感冒（简称流感）为常见的传染病，一年四季均可发生，但以春季发生较多。一般 2~3 年发生小流行，10~15 年发生大流行。流感的潜伏期为 1~3 天，起病急，始见恶寒、发热，体温迅速上升至 39 ℃ 或以上，伴有头痛、全身酸痛、软弱无力、咽干喉痛，有的出现鼻塞、流涕、打喷嚏等。一般 3~4 天退热，其他症状亦随之消失。

流行性感冒属于中医学"温病"范畴，多由外界风热火燥毒邪所引起，俗称"风温""热感冒"。与普通感冒的区别在于，本病起病急、恶寒发热重，属阳证、热证、实证者居多，因此治疗上多用辛凉、苦寒、甘寒药物。但亦有风寒表证者，依据感受外邪性质与个人体质不同而决定证候性质。

Influenza is a common infectious disease occurring in all the seasons of a year, and spring is its high-incidence season in particular. In general, influenza occurs in a small scale every 2~3 years, however, it can be a popular epidemic every 10~15 years in a large scale. The latent period of influenza may be 1~3 days. Influenza is characterized by sudden onset, aversion to cold, fever, and temperature may rise to 39 ℃ or above 39℃. Usually, influenza is complicated with headache, aching and weakness sensation over the whole body, dry and sore throat. Sometimes symptoms such as stuffy nose, runny nose and sneeze may appear. Generally, fever can be relieved after 3~4 days, and other symptoms will disappear with it.

Influenza pertains to the category of "epidemic febrile disease" in TCM. It is usually caused by exogenous pathogenic factors such as wind, heat, fire as well as dryness, therefore, influenza is known as "wind epidemic febrile disease", or "wind-heat cold syndrome". In contrast with common cold, influenza is marked by rapid onset, severe aversion to cold, high fever, and it belongs to yang syndrome, heat syndrome and sthenia syndrome. Consequently, pungent-cool, or bitter-cold, or sweet-cold natured Chinese medicinal herbs are mostly adopted for treating it. However, the disease may manifest a wind-cold external syndrome, diagnosis of the syndromes of the disease should be based on characteristics of various pathogenic factors as well as constitution of a patient.

〔**辨证论治**〕 Syndrome differentiation and treatment

1. 邪在肺卫

2.1 Invasion of pathogenic factors into the lung

【症状】发热，微恶风寒，头痛，咳嗽，口渴，无汗或微有汗出，舌边尖红，苔薄白，脉象浮数。

【分析】风温之邪伤及肺卫，卫气被遏，开合失司，故见发热、微恶风寒、无汗或微有汗。风热上扰则头痛，肺气失宣则咳嗽；脉浮、苔薄是表证之象；口渴、脉数、舌边尖红，为热之征象。

【治法】辛凉解表，疏风泄热。

【方药】银翘散。本方为辛凉平剂，为治疗风热感冒之主方。方中金银花、连翘、竹叶、薄荷清热宣透表邪，淡豆豉、荆芥以助发汗解表之力，牛蒡子、桔梗、甘草宣肺止咳，芦根生津止渴。用于风温初起，发热恶风无汗者，若出现高热，可加黄芩、知母、生石膏，以清解卫气之热毒；若咽干痛者，可加射干、山豆根，以解毒利咽。

Clinical manifestations: Fever, slight aversion to wind and cold, headache, cough, thirst, no sweating or slight sweating, reddish tongue tip and margin, thin whitish fur as well as floating and fast pulse.

Analysis: Fever, slight aversion to wind and cold, no sweating or slight sweating are caused by invasion of pathogenic wind and warm factors into the lung, which results in impairment of the lung, obstruction of defensive qi, as well as failure of disordered qi in dominating the opening and closing of yang. Headache is due to wind heat attacking upward and disturbing the head; cough is due to failure of lung qi to disperse; floating pulse and thin fur are signs of external syndrome; thirst, fast pulse and reddish tongue tip are manifestations of heat syndrome.

Prescription: Relieve external pathogens with pungent-cool natured drug, expel wind and purge heat.

Formulas: Yinqiao San (Powder). This is a major formula for treating wind-heat cold, marked by pungent, cold and neutral nature. In this formula, Jinyinhua (*Flos Lonicerae*), Lianqiao (*Fructus Forsythiae*), Zhuye (*Herba Lophatheri*) and Bohe (*Herba Menthae*) have an effect of clearing away heat and dispelling external pathogens; Dandouchi (*Semen Sojae Preperatum*) and Jingjie (*Herba Schizonepeta*) can induce sweating to relieve exterior syndrome; Niubangzi (*Fructus Arctii*), Jiegeng (*Radix Platycodi*) and Gancao (*Radix Glycyrrhizae*) can disperse lung heat to stop cough; Lugen (*Rhizoma Phragmitis*) can promote production of body fluid to stop thirst. This formula can be used for treating such symptoms as fever, aversion to wind and no sweating at the initial stage of wind-warm syndrome. For high fever, Huangqin (*Radix Scutellariae*), Zhimu (*Rhizoma Anemarrhenae*) and Shengshigao (*Gypsum Fibrosum*) can be added to resolve toxic heat of defensive qi; for dry and sore throat, Shegan (*Rhizoma Belamcandae*) and Shandougen (*Radix Sophorae Tonkinensis*) can be combined to resolve toxic heat and ease throat.

2. 邪热壅肺

2.2 Accumulation of pathogenic heat in the lung

【症状】高热，口渴，咳嗽，气喘，大汗出，大便秘结，小便短赤，舌质红，苔黄，脉象滑数。

【分析】邪热壅肺多是在卫分症状之后出现，为卫分之邪传里的证候。热势弛张，病位在肺，故见高热、咳嗽、气喘、大汗出；热伤津液，则上见口渴，下见便秘和小便短赤；舌红、苔黄、脉数均为热盛之象。

【治法】清热宣肺。

【方药】麻杏石甘汤加味。方中麻黄、杏仁开宣肺气，石膏清泻肺经之热，甘草调和胃气。只是此方清肺止咳之力略显单薄，故加黄芩、鱼腥草、金银花以清泻肺热。痰多黄稠，可加知母、瓜蒌皮、芦根清肺化痰；腑气不通，可加大黄清热通腑；口渴不解，可加北沙参、麦冬、石斛滋阴清肺。

Clinical manifestations：High fever, thirst, cough, dyspnea, profuse sweating, dry feces and scanty brownish urine, reddish tongue with yellowish fur as well as slippery and fast pulse.

Analysis：This syndrome usually occurs after the syndrome of defensive phase, suggesting internal transmission of pathogenic factors into the interior. High fever, cough, dyspnea and profuse sweating are due to rapid outbreak and development of exuberant heat and the lung being the location of the disease; thirst, dry feces and scanty brownish urine are caused by impairment of fluid by heat; reddish tongue with yellowish fur and slippery and fast pulse are signs of hyperactive heat.

Prescription：Clear away heat and disperse the lung.

Formulas：Mahuang Xingren Shigao Gancao Tang Jiawei (Modified Mahuang Xingren Shigao Gancao Decoction). In this formula, Mahuang (*Herba Ephedrae*) and Xingren (*Semen Armeniacae Amarum*) can disperse lung qi, Shigao (*Gypsum Fibrosum*) can purge heat from the lung meridian, and Gancao (*Radix Glycyrrhizae*) can regulate stomach qi. Because the effect of this formula is not strong enough in clearing away lung heat and stopping cough, so Huangqin (*Radix Scutellariae*), Jinyinhua (*Flos Lonicerae*) and Yuxingcao (*Herba Houttuyniae*) can be combined to purge lung heat. For profuse and thick yellowish sputum, Zhimu (*Rhizoma Anemarrhenae*), Gualoupi (*Pericapium Trichosanthis*) and Lugen (*Rhizoma Phragmitis*) can be added to clear away lung heat and resolve phlegm. For stagnant qi in fu organs, Dahuang (*Radix et Rhizoma Rhei*) can be added to clear away heat and promote qi circulation in fu organs, Beishashen (*Radix Glehniae*), Maidong (*Radix Ophiopogonis*) and Shihu (*Herba Dendrobii*) can be combined to nourish yin and clear away lung heat.

3. 热在气分

2.3　Invasion of pathogenic heat into qi phase

【症状】高热，烦渴，喜冷饮，面赤，大汗出，舌质红，苔黄燥，脉象洪数。

【分析】热在气分，即邪热进入阳明经气分。热势外扬，故见高热、面赤、大汗出；热耗津液，则烦渴、喜冷饮；舌红苔燥、脉洪数，为热势炽盛之象。

【治法】清热生津。

【方药】白虎汤加味。方中生石膏清泻气分之热；知母寒润，助生石膏以清热；甘草、粳米养胃生津。若热势不退，可加金银花、芦根、石斛、竹叶以加强清热生津之效；若高热病人突然出现汗出肢冷，四肢不温，脉转微细，为阳气衰败之象，急宜扶阳救逆，用人参、附子等辛温之品，或可救逆。

Clinical manifestations：High fever, polydipsia with preference for cold drink, flushed cheeks, profuse sweating, reddish tongue with dry yellowish fur as well as full and fast pulse.

Analysis：Heat in qi phase refers to pathogenic heat factor invading into qi phase of the yangming meridian. High fever, flushed cheeks and profuse sweating are due to heat spreading outward；polydipsia with preference for cold drink is caused by heat consuming body fluid；reddish tongue with dry fur and full and fast pulse are signs of superabundant heat.

Prescription：Clear away heat and promote production of body fluid.

Formulas：Baihu Tang Jiawei (Modified Baihu Decoction). In this formula, Shengshigao (*Gypsum Fibrosum*) has the action of purging heat of qi phase；Zhimu (*Rhizoma Anemarrhenae*), cold and moist in nature, can clear away heat with Shengshigao；Gancao (*Radix Glycyrrhizae*) and Jingmi (*Semen Oryzae Sativae*) can nourish the stomach and promote production of fluid. Jinyinhua (*Flos Lonicerae*), Lugen (*Rhizoma Phragmitis*), Shihu (*Herba Dendrobii*) and Zhuye (*Herba Lophatheri*) can be added to reinforce the effect of heat-clearing and promoting production of fluid；for declination of yang qi with such symptoms as high fever, sweating, cold limbs, indistinct thin pulse, Renshen (*Radix Ginseng*) and Fuzi (*Radix Aconiti Lateralis Preparata*), pungent and warm in nature, can be added to strengthen yang to rescue from collapse.

4. 热结胃肠
2.4 Accumulation of heat in the stomach and intestines

【症状】午后高热，腹部胀满或痛而拒按，大便秘结，泻下黄臭稀水，时有谵语，神志不清，舌苔黄燥，脉象数大有力。

【分析】实热结于胃肠，胃肠运行障碍，故腹部胀满；若燥粪内结不通，则腹部痛而拒按；大肠失于传导，则大便秘结，或纯利稀水；阳明实热，上攻心神，则神志不清，时有谵语；舌苔黄燥、脉象数大，为有形实邪结聚之征。

【治法】攻下清热。

【方药】偏于燥结的，用调胃承气汤；偏于腹满胀痛的，用小承气汤；病势较重，舌苔焦黄或有芒刺，用大承气汤。三方内药物功效为：大黄苦寒泻热，芒硝咸寒泻下，厚朴、枳实行气破坚，推动大黄、芒硝的泻下作用。若舌苔焦黄或有芒刺，可于方中加入增液汤，即生地黄、玄参、麦冬养阴生津，有利于泻热润燥。

Clinical manifestations：High fever in the afternoon, unpressable distention and fullness or pain in the abdomen, dry feces, or diarrhea with discharge of yellowish thin and foul undigested food, occasional delirious speech, unconsciousness, yellowish dry tongue fur as well as fast, large and powerful pulse.

Analysis: Distention and fullness or pain in the abdomen are due to dysfunction of the stomach and intestines because of sthenic heat accumulation in the stomach and intestines; abdominal unpressable pain is due to retention of dry feces and difficulty in defecation; constipation or diarrhea with watery dysentery is due to failure of the large intestine in transportation; unconsciousness with occasional delirious speech is caused by sthenic heat in yangming meridian attacking upward into the heart and mind; yellowish dry fur and fast, large and powerful pulse are signs of accumulation of tangible sthenic pathogens.

Prescription: Remove stagnation by purgation and clear away heat.

Formulas: Tiaowei Chengqi Tang (Decoction) for dry accumulation; Small Chengqi Tang (Decoction) for abdominal distention, fullness and pain; Large Chengqi Tang (Decoction) for serious syndrome with scorching yellow fur or prickly tongue.

The actions of the herbs in the above formulas are as follows: Dahuang (*Radix et Rhizoma Rhei*), bitter and cold in nature, can purge heat; Mangxiao (*Natrii Sulfas*), salty and cold in nature, can cause diarrhea; Houpo (*Cortex Magnoliae Officinalis*) and Zhishi (*Fructus Aurantii Immaturus*) can activate qi and soften dry feces to promote purging action of Dahuang and Mangxiao. For scorching yellow fur or prickly tongue, Zengye Tang (Decoction), consisting of Shengdihuang (*Radix Rehmanniae Recens*), Xuanshen (*Radix Scrophulariae*) and Maidong (*Radix Ophiopogonis*), can be added to nourish yin and promote production of fluid, for it is very helpful to purge heat and moisten dryness.

5. 热入营血
2.5 Invasion of pathogenic heat into nutrient phase and blood phase

【症状】发热夜甚，烦躁不安或谵语神昏，或发斑疹，或见衄血，口燥而不甚渴，舌红绛而干，脉象细数。

【分析】若气分热毒不解，内传营血，则发热夜甚；热入心包，心神被扰，则谵语神昏；热毒迫血妄行，则发斑疹或衄血；邪热内伤营血，虽口燥而不渴饮；舌红绛而干，脉象细数，为邪热内伤营血，伤阴耗津之象。

【治法】清营透热，清心开窍。

【方药】清营汤加味。方中犀角（现多用水牛角代替）、黄连凉营清热；生地黄、玄参、麦冬、丹参滋阴凉血；金银花、连翘、竹叶清热解毒，并能透邪。若出现斑疹或衄血者，可加牡丹皮、紫草、大青叶、赤芍以凉血解毒；若神昏谵语，可选安宫牛黄丸、至宝丹等清心开窍。

Clinical manifestations: Severe fever especially at night, restlessness, delirious speech and unconsciousness, or eruption of maculae, or accompanied with rhinorrhagia, dry mouth with no thirst for drink, dry deep-reddish tongue as well as thin and fast pulse.

Analysis: Severe fever at night is due to transmission of unrelieved toxic heat pathogen from qi phase into nutrient phase as well as blood phase; coma and delirious speech are due to invasion of pathogenic heat into the pericardium disturbing the mind. Eruption of maculae, or rhinorrhagia is due to toxic heat pathogen causing extravasation of blood; dry mouth with no thirst for drink is caused by pathogenic heat impairing nutrient qi as well as blood; dry deep-reddish tongue and thin and fast pulse are signs of pathogenic heat impairing nutrient qi as well as blood and consuming yin and body fluid.

Prescription: Clear away heat in nutrient phase and regain consciousness by purging heart fire.

Formulas: Qingying Tang Jiawei (Modified Qingying Decoction). In this formula, Xijiao (*Cornu Rhinoceri*), which can be replaced with Shuiniujiao (*Cornu Bubali*) and Huanglian (*Rhizoma Coptidis*) can cool nutrient qi and blood and clear away heat; Shengdihuang (*Radix Rehmanniae Recens*), Xuanshen (*Radix Scrophulariae*), Maidong (*Radix Ophiopogonis*) and Danshen (*Radix Salviae Miltiorrhizae*) have an action of nourishing yin and cooling blood; Jinyinhua (*Flos Lonicerae*), Lianqiao (*Fructus Forsythiae*) and Zhuye (*Herba Lophatheri*) have an effect of clearing away heat to relieve toxic pathogens as well as letting out pathogenic factors. For eruption of macula or rhinorrhagia, Mudanpi (*Cortex Moutan Radicis*), Zicao (*Radix Arnebiae*), Daqingye (*Folium Isatidis*) and Chishao (*Radix Paeoniae Rubra*) can be added to cool blood and relieve toxic factors. For delirious speech and unconsciousness, Angong Niuhuang Wan (Pill) as well as Zhibao Dan (Pill) can be used to regain consciousness by purging heart fire.

6. 阴伤风动
2.6 Endogenous wind due to impairment of yin

【症状】身热不甚，手足心热，面色潮红，精神疲倦，心悸，手足蠕动，甚则瘛疭，或耳聋失聪，口燥，舌干绛，脉象虚数或结代。

【分析】温热病后期，由于热邪久羁，耗伤肝肾之阴，形成热邪内伏，久而不退，但热势不甚之状态。阴虚内热，则手足心热、面色潮红；阴血不足，神失所养，则精神疲倦、心悸；阴不敛阳，虚风内动，故手足蠕动，甚则瘛疭；肾精不能上承，则见耳聋失聪；口燥、舌干绛，是阴液枯耗之征；脉象虚数或结代，为正虚热恋、血脉瘀阻之象。

【治法】滋阴清热，养血熄风。

【方药】青蒿鳖甲汤合大定风珠加减。青蒿鳖甲汤中的青蒿与鳖甲相配，以滋阴清热、入络搜风为主药；辅以牡丹皮、生地黄、知母凉血养阴，生津润燥，对夜热早凉，热势不退较宜。大定风珠以地黄、麦冬、阿胶、鸡子黄滋阴补血；五味子、甘草酸甘化阴，龟板、鳖甲、生牡蛎潜阳熄风。本方以治虚风内动为主要功效，但此方偏于滋腻，适用于热势已除，唯虚风内动者。

Clinical manifestations: Mild fever, feverish sensation over palms and soles, flushed complexion, dispiritedness and lassitude, palpitation, tremor of hands and feet, even flaccidity of hands and feet, or deafness, dry mouth, dry deep-reddish tongue as well as weak and fast pulse, or slow and intermittent pulse, or slow-intermittent-regular pulse.

Analysis: At the advanced stage of epidemic febrile disease, prolonged accumulation of pathogenic heat factors consumes and impairs yin of the liver and kidney, which cause prolonged internal accumulation of pathogenic heat and mild fever; feverish sensation over palms and soles and flushed complexion are caused by endogenous heat generated from yin asthenia; dispiritedness, lassitude and palpitation are due to failure of insufficient yin blood to nourish the heart and mind; tremor or even flaccidity of hands and feet is due to endogenous asthenic wind because of failure of yin to constrain yang; deafness is due to failure of asthenic kidney essence to transport upwards; dry mouth and dry, dark reddish tongue are manifestations of yin fluid consumption; weak and fast pulse, or slow and intermittent pulse, or slow-intermittent-regular pulse is a sign of obstruction in vessels due to asthenia of healthy qi and accumulation of superabundant heat.

Prescription: Nourish yin to clear away heat and tonify blood to stop endogenous wind.

Formulas: Qinghao Biejia Tang (Decoction) combined with Large Dingfeng Zhu (Modified Large Wind-expelling Pill) Jiajian.

In Qinghao Biejia Tang, Qinghao (*Herba Artemisiae Annuae*) combined with Biejia (*Carapax Trionycis*), as the principal drug, can nourish yin, clear away heat, and remove wind from collaterals; Mudanpi (*Cortex Moutan Radicis*), Shengdihuang (*Radix Rehmanniae Recens*) and Zhimu (*Rhizoma Anemarrhenae*) can be used as adjuvant drug to cool blood, nourish yin and promote production of fluid to moisten dryness, and they are suitable for treating evening fever which can be alleviated in the next morning. In Large Dingfeng Zhu, Dihuang (*Radix Rehmanniae Recens*), Maidong (*Radix Ophiopogonis*), Ejiao (*Colla Corii Asini*) and Jizihuang (hen egg yolk) can nourish yin and supplement blood; Wuweizi (*Fructus Schisandrae Chinensis*) and Gancao (*Radix Glycyrrhizae*), sour and sweet in flavor, have an action of nourishing yin; Guiban (*Plastrum Testudinis*), Biejia (*Carapax Trionycis*) and Shengmuli (*Concha Ostreae*), can be used to treat the syndrome of asthenic endogenous wind with the action of suppressing hyperactive yang to stop wind. Because it could cause stagnant dampness and dysfunction of the spleen and stomach, this formula is clinically used for the syndrome of asthenic endogenous wind with pathogenic heat eliminated.

三、急性支气管炎

3 Acute bronchitis

〔概说〕 Summary

急性支气管炎属于中医学"伤风咳嗽""痰饮"等病证范畴。其病的发生与肺、脾功能失调有关。发生的原因不但与四季不正的邪气有关,而且与饮食不节亦有关联。

中医治疗急性支气管炎分证明确，药效显著，并有扶助正气、祛邪外出的作用，受到病人的青睐。

Acute bronchitis pertains to "cough due to common cold" "retention of phlegm and fluid" in TCM. The onset of the disease is related to dysfunction of the lung and spleen, and its occurrence is mainly caused by pathogenic factors generated from abnormal climate of the four seasons as well as improper diet. With clear syndrome-differentiation and its special function of strengthening healthy qi and expelling pathogens, treatment for the disease by means of TCM can surely achieve a remarkable curative effect.

〔辨证论治〕 Syndrome differentiation and treatment

1. 风寒外束，肺失宣降
3.1　Failure to disperse lung qi due to exogenous wind cold

【症状】咳嗽，痰液稀薄，发热恶寒，鼻塞流涕，喉痒声重，或兼头痛，无汗出，舌苔薄白，脉象浮紧。

【分析】外感风寒，内舍于肺，肺气不得宣发，则见咳嗽、发热恶寒；寒邪郁闭，可见鼻塞流涕；风痰内扰，则喉痒声重；头部阳气被郁，则头痛；卫阳被遏，无汗出；舌苔与脉象均为风寒郁遏之象。

【治法】疏风散寒，宣肺化痰。

【方药】三拗汤、小青龙汤。三拗汤，仅三味药，即麻黄、甘草、杏仁，具有宣肺解表、止咳化痰的作用。小青龙汤为发散风寒、解表蠲饮、止咳平喘之药剂。方取麻黄、桂枝发汗解表，除外寒而宣肺气；干姜、细辛温肺化痰，并助麻黄、桂枝解表；半夏祛痰和胃；五味子、芍药养血敛气，同时不使麻、桂发散太过；炙甘草益气和中，调和辛散、酸收之度。此方对外感风寒，肺气不宣导致咳嗽频频、痰多稀薄、不得平卧者，非常有效。

Clinical manifestations: Cough, clear thin sputum, fever and aversion to cold, stuffy and runny nose, itching throat and low voice, or complicated by headache, no sweating, thin whitish fur as well as floating and tense pulse.

Analysis: Cough and fever with aversion to cold are due to failure of lung qi to disperse because of exogenous wind cold encumbering the lung; stuffy and runny nose is due to internal obstruction of pathogenic cold factors; itching throat and low voice are due to internal disturbance of phlegmatic wind; headache is due to obstruction of yang qi in the head; no sweating is due to stagnation of defensive yang; thin whitish fur and floating and tense pulse are signs of stagnation of wind cold.

Prescription: Dispel wind cold, disperse lung qi and resolve phlegm.

Formulas: San'ao Tang (Decoction), as well as Small Qinglong Tang (Decoction). San'ao Tang, made up of Mahuang (*Herba Ephedrae*), Gancao (*Radix Glycyrrhizae*) and

Xingren (*Semen Armeniacae Amarum*), have the action of dispersing lung qi, relieving exterior syndrome, stopping cough and resolving phlegm. Small Qinglong Tang is a recipe for dispelling wind cold, relieving exterior syndrome, eliminating fluid retention as well as arresting cough and asthma, in which, Mahuang (*Herba Ephedrae*) and Guizhi (*Ramulus Cinnamomi*) have an action of inducing sweating to relieve exterior syndrome, dispelling external cold and dispersing lung qi; Ganjiang (*Rhizoma Zingiberis*) and Xixin (*Herba Asari*) can warm the lung and resolve phlegm, assisting Mahuang and Guizhi to relieve exterior syndrome; Banxia (*Rhizoma Pinelliae*) can reduce phlegm and harmonize the stomach; Wuweizi (*Fructus Schisandrae Chinensis*) and Shaoyao (*Radix Paeoniae*) have the function of nourishing blood and astringing qi, meanwhile, they can prevent Mahuang and Guizhi from inducing excessive sweating; Zhigancao (*Radix Glycyrrhizae Preparata*) can benefit qi, harmonize middle energizer and regulate the degree of pungent-flavored herbs in dispersing and that of sour-flavor drug in astringing. The recipe is of great effect to such symptoms as frequent cough, profuse thin clear sputum and inability to lie on the back because of exogenous wind cold and failure to disperse lung qi.

2. 风热犯表，肺失宣畅
3.2 Failure to disperse the lung due to wind heat attacking the superficies

【症状】咳嗽痰稠，咳而不爽，身热，口渴，咽痛，或见头痛恶风，汗出，舌苔白而燥，脉象浮数。

【分析】风热犯肺，肺气不得宣畅，故见咳嗽；热灼津液，则痰黏稠，且咳而不爽；肺热耗津，口渴咽痛；风热客于肌表，则有头痛恶风、汗出之症；舌苔白燥，脉象浮数，表明风热在肺在表。

【治法】疏风清热，宣肺止咳。

【方药】桑菊饮。方中桑叶、菊花、薄荷疏风清热，宣透肌表；杏仁、桔梗、甘草利咽止咳；连翘、芦根清热生津，使肺热得解，咳嗽自止。咽痒者，加蝉蜕除风，山豆根清热利咽；胸闷痰黄者，加黄芩清肺，瓜蒌皮宽胸化痰。

Clinical manifestations: Cough with thick sputum, unsmooth coughing, fever, thirst, sore throat, or headache with aversion to wind, sweating, dry whitish fur as well as floating and fast pulse.

Analysis: Cough is due to invasion of wind heat into the lung and failure of the lung to disperse and descend qi; cough with thick sputum and unsmooth process of coughing are due to pathogenic heat scorching fluid; thirst and sore throat are due to pulmonary heat consuming fluid; headache with aversion to wind and sweating are due to invasion of pathogenic wind heat into the superficies of the skin; dry whitish fur and floating and fast pulse indicate wind heat retaining in the lung and muscular superficies.

Prescription: Dispel wind to clear away heat, disperse the lung qi and stop cough.

Formulas: Sang Ju Yin (Decoction). In the recipe, Sangye (*Folium Mori*), Juhua

(*Florist's chrysanthemum*) and Bohe (*Herba Menthae*) can dispel wind, clear away heat and expel pathogenic factors from superficial muscles; Xingren (*Semen Armeniacae Amarum*), Jiegeng (*Radix Platycodonis*) and Gancao (*Radix Glycyrrhizae*) have the action of relieving sore throat and stopping cough; Lianqiao (*Fructus Forsythiae*) and Lugen (*Rhizoma Phragmitis*) can clear away heat and promote production of fluid so as to relieve lung heat and arrest cough. For itching throat, Chantui (*Periostracum Cicadae*) can be added to dispel wind; Shandougen (*Radix Sophorae Tonkinensis*) can be added to clear away heat and ease the throat. For chest oppression and yellowish sputum, Huangqin (*Radix Scutellariae*) could be combined to eliminate lung heat, and Gualoupi (*Pericarpium Trichosanthis*) may be used to ease chest oppression and resolve phlegm.

3. 燥热伤津,肺失清润

3.3 Loss of depuration and moisture of the lung due to pathogenic dry and heat factors impairing fluid

【症状】 干咳无痰,或痰少不易咳出,或痰中带血丝,咽干鼻燥,咳甚则胸痛,大便干燥,小便短赤,舌质红赤,苔薄黄而干,脉象浮数。

【分析】 风燥外伤,或体质阴虚内燥,表邪入里化热,灼伤肺津而干咳无痰;"燥胜则干",故见咽干鼻燥,若伤及络脉,则会痰中带血丝;若频频作咳,肺气不能宣通,又不能肃降,所以气不通,故见胸痛;肺与大肠相表里,肺津缺少,也会引起大肠燥结,热耗则小便短赤;舌脉均为燥热之象。

【治法】 清热生津,润燥救肺。

【方药】 清燥救肺汤加减。方中桑叶、石膏清肺中燥热,阿胶、麦冬养阴润燥,黑芝麻既补阴又能补气,人参、甘草补肺气,杏仁、枇杷叶清肺下气、止咳祛痰。痰不易咳喘者,加瓜蒌、贝母清化热痰;痰中带血者,加生地黄、白茅根滋阴清热止血;咽干者,加玄参滋阴清热;胸痛者,加赤芍、藕节化瘀清热。

Clinical manifestations: Dry cough without sputum, or sparse sputum with difficulty to expectorate, or sputum mingled with blood, dry throat and nose, chest pain with aggravation of cough, dry feces, scanty brownish urine, reddish tongue with dry thin yellowish fur as well as floating and fast pulse.

Analysis: Dry cough without sputum is due to heat transformed from exogenous pathogens, which scorches and impairs fluid of the lung because of impairment of exogenous pathogenic dryness and wind together with endogenous dryness resulting from constitutional yin asthenia; dry throat and nose are due to "exuberance of dryness"; sputum mingled with blood is caused by impairment of collaterals by heat; chest pain is caused by qi stagnation due to frequent cough as well as failure of the lung to disperse and depurate. The lung and the large intestine are interior-exteriorly related. Reduced pulmonary fluid could cause dryness accumulation, giving rise to dry feces; scanty brownish urine is due to pathogenic heat consuming the lung fluid; reddish tongue with dry thin yellowish fur and floating and fast pulse indicate dryness and heat.

Prescription：Clear away heat, promote production of fluid and moisten dryness to rescue the lung.

Formulas：Qingzao Jiufei Tang Jiajian（Modified Decoction of Qingzao Jiufei）. In this formula, Sangye（*Folium Mori*）and Shigao（*Gypsum Fibrosum*）can clear away dryness and heat of the lung, Ejiao（*Colla Corii Asini*）and Maidong（*Radix Ophiopogonis*）have the action of nourishing yin and moistening dryness, Heizhima（*Semen sesami nigrum*）can replenish yin and qi, Renshen（*Radix Ginseng*）and Gancao（*Radix Glycyrrhizae*）can supplement qi of the lung, Xingren（*Semen Armeniacae Amarum*）and Pipaye（*Folium Eriobotryae*）have the effect of clearing away lung heat, descending qi, stopping cough as well as eliminating phlegm. For difficulty to expectorate sputum, Gualou（*Fructus Trichosanthis*）and Beimu（*Bulbus Fritillaria*）can be added to clear away heat and resolve phlegm；for sputum mingled with blood, Shengdihuang（*Radix Rehmanniae Recens*）and Baimaogen（*Rhizoma Imperatae*）can be added to nourish yin and purge heat and stop bleeding；for dry throat, Xuanshen（*Radix Scrophulariae*）can be combined to nourish yin and purge heat；for chest pain, Chishao（*Radix Paeoniae Rubra*）and Oujie（*Nodus Nelumbinis Rhizomatis*）could be added to resolve stasis and clear away heat.

四、慢性支气管炎
4 Chronic bronchitis

〔概说〕 Summary

慢性支气管炎属于中医学"咳嗽""痰饮""喘息"等范畴。它以咳嗽、咯痰为主要症状，但在炎症后期，气喘成为经常性，变成咳嗽、咯痰、气喘症状组合。如果重视预防措施，及早防治，就可以阻止慢性支气管炎的发展。

In terms of TCM, chronic bronchitis belongs to the scope of "cough" "retention of phlegmatic fluid" "asthma", etc. Its main clinical symptoms include cough and expectoration. However, at the advanced stage of the disease, asthmatic breath is the frequent symptom, which turns into the combination of cough, expectoration and asthma. Precautious measures should be taken timely so as to prevent the development of this disease.

〔辨证论治〕 Syndrome differentiation and treatment

1. 痰湿咳嗽
4.1 Cough due to phlegmatic dampness

【症状】咳嗽痰多，痰白而黏，胸脘闷满，食纳不佳，四肢无力，舌苔白腻，脉象濡滑。

【分析】脾虚健运失调，以致痰湿内生，上渍于肺，阻遏气机，故咳嗽、痰白而黏，此即"脾为生痰之源，肺为贮痰之器"之意。痰阻胸膈，气机不利，所以胸脘作闷；湿浊困于脾胃，则不欲饮食，四肢无力；舌苔白腻、脉象濡滑，为痰湿内聚，气失宣畅之征。

【治法】健脾燥湿，理气化痰。

【方药】二陈汤加味。方中半夏燥湿化痰，陈皮理气化痰，气顺则痰降，气行则痰化；茯苓健脾利湿，甘草健脾和中。诸药合用，脾得健运，湿去痰消，脾运健则湿自化，湿得去则痰自消。若痰多湿重，胸闷明显，加苍术、厚朴、薏苡仁、杏仁，以增强燥湿化痰之力；证属寒痰者，加干姜、细辛以温化之；属风痰者，加胆南星、白附子以祛风化痰；痰滞胸膈，食欲不振，苔腻脉滑者，加三子养亲汤顺气降逆，化痰消食。

Clinical manifestations: Cough with profuse, whitish and sticky sputum, oppression and fullness of the chest and epigastrium, poor appetite, weak limbs, whitish greasy tongue fur as well as soft and slippery pulse.

Analysis: Cough with whitish and sticky sputum is due to dysfunction of asthenic spleen in transformation and transportation and internal accumulation of phlegmatic dampness in the lung, which causes inhibited flow of lung qi. It is in accord with the saying "The spleen is the source of generation of phlegm, and the lung is the utensil for storing phlegm". Oppression and fullness of the chest and epigastrium are due to retention of phlegm in the chest and diaphragm which hinder qi movement. Poor appetite and weak limbs are caused by obstruction of phlegmatic turbidity and dampness in the spleen and stomach. Whitish greasy tongue fur and slippery and soft pulse are signs of internal accumulation of phlegmatic dampness which prevents lung qi from dispersing and descending.

Prescription: Invigorate the spleen, dry dampness, regulate qi and resolve phlegm.

Formulas: Erchen Tang Jiawei (Modified Erchen Decoction). In the formula, Banxia (*Rhizoma Pinelliae*) can dry dampness to resolve phlegm, Chenpi (*Pericarpium Citri Reticulatae*) has an effect of resolving phlegm by regulating qi, therefore, smooth qi circulation can reduce phlegm, while activation of qi could resolve phlegm. Fuling (*Poriae Cocos*) has an action of invigorating the spleen and resolving dampness; Gancao (*Radix Glycyrrhizae*) can invigorate the spleen and harmonize middle energizer (the spleen and stomach). Combined together, these Chinese medicinal herbs can relieve dysfunction of the spleen in transportation and eliminate dampness and phlegm. For profuse damp phlegm and obvious chest oppression, Cangzhu (*Rhizoma Atractylodis*), Houpo (*Cortex Magnoliae Officinals*), Yiyiren (*Semen Coicis*) and Xingren (*Semen Armeniacae Amarum*) can be added to strengthen the ability of drying dampness and resolving phlegm. For cold phlegm, Ganjiang (*Rhizoma Zingiberis*) and Xixin (*Herba Asari*) can be combined to warm and resolve phlegm. For wind phlegm, Dannanxing (*Rhizoma Arisaematis Cum Bile*) and Baifuzi (*Rhizoma Typhonii*) can be combined to expel wind and resolve phlegm. For phlegm retention in the chest and diaphragm, poor appetite, greasy tongue fur and slippery pulse, Sanzi Yangqin Tang, the decoction of combination of Zisuzi (*Fructus Perillae*), Baijiezi (*Semen Sinapis*) and Laifuzi (*Semen Raphani*), can be added to lower the adverse rise of qi, resolve phlegm and relieve food retention.

2. 痰热咳嗽
4.2　Cough due to phlegmatic heat

【症状】咳嗽，痰黄稠而不易咯出，甚则痰中带血，胸闷，口干口苦，咽干痛，舌苔黄腻或黄白相兼，脉象滑数。

【分析】痰热蕴肺，肺失宣降，故咳嗽、痰黄稠而不易咯出；痰热化火，灼肺伤络，则见痰中带血、咽痛；肺气不利，故胸闷；苔黄、脉滑数，均为痰热之象。

【治法】清热肃肺，豁痰止咳。

【方药】清金化痰汤。方用黄芩、栀子、知母、桑白皮清热肃肺；陈皮、桔梗、瓜蒌仁理气化痰；麦冬、贝母、甘草润肺止咳；茯苓健脾渗湿。全方共奏清热肃肺、豁痰止咳的功效。若肺热壅盛，咳而喘满，壮热口渴，去桔梗、陈皮，加金银花、鱼腥草、石膏、葶苈子等清热泻肺。

Clinical manifestations: Cough with yellowish and thick sputum with difficulty to expectorate, even sputum mingled with blood, chest oppression, dryness of mouth and bitter taste, dry and sore throat, yellowish greasy tongue fur, or yellowish and whitish fur mingled together and slippery and fast pulse.

Analysis: Cough with yellowish and thick sputum with difficulty to expectorate is due to failure of the lung to disperse resulting from accumulation of phlegmatic heat in the lung; sputum mingled with blood and sore throat are caused by transformation of fire from phlegmatic heat, which scorches the lung and impairs the collaterals; chest oppression is due to inhibited flow of lung qi; yellowish tongue fur with slippery and fast pulse is the sign of phlegmatic heat.

Prescription: Clear away heat to depurate the lung and resolve phlegm to arrest cough.

Formulas: Qingjin Huatan Tang (Decoction). In this formula, Huangqin (*Radix Scutellariae*), Zhizi (*Fructus Gardeniae*), Zhimu (*Rhizoma Anemarrhenae*) and Sangbaipi (*Cortex Mori Radicis*) have the action of clearing away heat and dispersing the lung; Chenpi (*Pericarpium Citri Reticulatae*), Jiegeng (*Radix Platycodonis*) and Gualouren (*Semen Trichosanthis*) can regulate qi and resolve phlegm; Maidong (*Radix Ophiopogonis*), Beimu (*Bulbus Fritillaria*) and Gancao (*Radix Glycyrrhizae*) can moisten the lung and relieve cough; Fuling (*Poriae Cocos*) has the action of invigorating the spleen and eliminating dampness. Combined together, all the medicinal herbs in the formula have the function of clearing away heat to depurate the lung and resolving phlegm to arrest cough. For exuberance of lung heat, cough with dyspneal fullness, high fever and thirst, Jinyinhua (*Flos Lonicerae*), Yuxingcao (*Herba Houttuyniae*), Shigao (*Gypsum Fibrosum*) and Tinglizi (*Semen Descurainiae*) could be added to clear away heat and purge fire of the lung, in the meantime, Jiegeng (*Radix Platycodonis*) and Chenpi (*Pericarpium Citri Reticulatae*) should be removed from this formula.

3. 肝火犯肺咳嗽
4.3 Cough due to liver fire attacking the lung

【症状】咳嗽气逆，咳则连声，甚则咳吐鲜血，或痰带血丝，胸胁窜痛，性急易怒，烦热口苦，咽喉干燥，面红目赤，舌苔薄黄少津，脉象弦数。

【分析】肝火犯肺咳嗽，乃由情志不遂，肝气郁结，久而化火所致。肝火犯肺，肺失清肃，则咳嗽气逆；木火刑金，肺络损伤，则咳吐鲜血，或痰带血丝；胁为肝之分野，肝火肆逆，则胁痛；其他如性急易怒、烦热口苦、咽喉干燥、面红目赤等，均为肝火炽盛之象；苔黄、脉弦数，为肝郁化火、肺热伤津之征。

【治法】清肝泻肺。

【方药】黛蛤散合泻白散加味。黛蛤散（青黛、海蛤壳）清肝豁痰，泻白散（地骨皮、桑白皮）清泻肺热、止咳平喘。火热较盛，咳嗽连声，可加栀子、牡丹皮、浙贝母、枇杷叶，以增强清热止咳之功效。

Clinical manifestations: Persistent cough with adverse flow of lung qi, even hematemesis with fresh blood, or sputum mingled with blood, wandering pain in the chest and hypochondrium, irritability and susceptibility to rage, dysphoria and bitter taste, dryness of the throat, flushed cheeks and eyes, thin yellowish tongue fur with scanty saliva as well as taut and fast pulse.

Analysis: Cough due to liver fire attacking the lung results from emotional upset, transformation of fire from liver depression; cough with adverse flow of lung qi is due to liver fire attacking the lung, which loses deputation; hematemesis with fresh blood, or sputum mingled with blood is due to impairment of lung collaterals resulting from wood fire impairing metal (the liver pertains to wood, and the lung pertains to metal); the hypochondrium is the dividing line of the liver, pain in chest and hypochondrium is caused by adverse flow of hyperactive liver fire; other symptoms such as irritability, susceptibility to rage, bitter taste, dryness of throat as well as flushed cheeks and eyes, are the manifestations of hyperactivity of liver fire; yellowish fur and taut and fast pulse are due to transformation of fire from liver depression and lung heat impairing fluid.

Prescription: Clear away heat from the liver and purge the lung.

Formulas: Dai Ge San (Powder) combined with Xie Bai San (Powder) Jiawei. Dai Ge San includes two medicinal herbs, Qingdai (*Indigo Naturalis*) and Haigeke (*Concha Meretricis seu Cyclinae*), both of them have the action of clearing away liver fire and phlegmatic heat. In the formula of Xie Bai San, Digupi (*Cortex Lycii*) and Sangbaipi (*Cortex Mori*) can be effective to purge lung heat and arrest cough and asthma; for hyperactive fire and lingering cough, Zhizi (*Fructus Gardeniae*), Mudanpi (*Cortex Moutan Radicis*), Zhebeimu (*Bulbus Fritillariae Thunbergii*) and Pipaye (*Folium Eriobotryae*) can be added to strengthen the effect of clearing away heat and arresting cough.

4. 气虚咳嗽
4.4 Cough due to qi asthenia

【症状】咳嗽声低无力，气短，痰涎清稀，精神疲倦，畏风，自汗，易于感冒，舌苔薄白，脉象虚弱。

【分析】素体虚弱，肺气不足，或脾虚运化不健，不能生化水谷给养于肺，则肺气日虚。肺气虚弱，则咳嗽无力、气短声怯、痰液稀薄；肺气虚弱，卫外能力降低，则畏风、自汗、易于感冒；舌苔薄白、脉象虚弱，均为气虚之象。

【治法】补益肺气，化痰宁嗽。

【方药】补肺汤加味。方中用人参、黄芪补益肺气；熟地黄、五味子滋肾敛肺，共同起到肺肾双补的作用；配以紫菀、桑白皮止咳平喘。若痰多清稀者，可加炒白术、茯苓，以增强补益脾肺、益气固表的功效；若有喘息者，可加款冬花，以助止咳化痰之力。

Clinical manifestations：Cough with weak and low voice, shortness of breath, thin and clear saliva and sputum, spiritual lassitude, aversion to wind, spontaneous sweating, susceptibility to catching cold, thin and whitish tongue fur as well as weak pulse.

Analysis：Constitutional asthenia, insufficiency of lung qi or dysfunction of asthenic spleen in transporting and transforming leads to failure of the spleen to transform food and provide nourishment for the lung, which results in gradual asthenia of lung qi, thus, bringing about cough with weak and low voice, shortness of breath as well as thin and clear saliva and sputum；aversion to wind, spontaneous sweating, and susceptibility to catching cold are due to insufficiency of lung qi, which gives rise to weakness of it to protect the superficies；thin and whitish tongue fur and weak pulse are signs of qi asthenia.

Prescription：Replenish lung qi and resolve phlegm to stop cough.

Formulas：Bufei Tang Jiawei (Modified Bufei Decoction). In the formula, Renshen (*Radix Ginseng*) and Huangqi (*Radix Astragali seu Hedysari*) can replenish lung qi；Shudihuang (*Radix Rehmanniae Praeparata*) and Wuweizi (*Fructus Schisandrae Chinensis*), with the action of nourishing the kidney and astringing the lung to arrest persistent cough, can supplement both the lung and the kidney. The formula can be used together with Ziwan (*Radix Asteris*) and Sangbaipi (*Cortex Mori*) to arrest cough and asthma. For profuse thin sputum, stir-baked Baizhu (*Rhizoma Atractylodis Macrocephalae*) and Fuling (*Poriae Cocos*) can be added to strengthen the effect of replenishing the spleen and lung, benefiting qi and strengthening the exterior；for dyspnea, Kuandonghua (*Flos Farfarae*) can be added to help relieve cough and resolve phlegm.

5. 阴虚咳嗽

4.5　Cough due to yin asthenia

【症状】干咳无痰，或痰少咯出不爽，口干咽燥，或见咯血，舌质红赤，苔少，脉象细数。

【分析】阴虚内燥，肺失滋润，以致肃降无权，肺气上逆，肺阴耗伤，故出现一派肺气失宣的症状；若肺络受伤，则见咯血；舌红苔少、脉象细数，为阴虚内燥之征。

【治法】养阴润肺，宁嗽止咳。

【方药】二冬二母汤。方中用麦冬、天冬滋阴润燥；知母、贝母清润止咳。口干舌燥者，加北沙参、生地黄、百合养阴润燥；咳嗽甚者，加百部、黄芩、桑白皮、瓜蒌皮清肺润燥止咳；咯血者，加白及、仙鹤草、藕节止血。

Clinical manifestations：Dry cough with no sputum, or scanty sputum with difficulty to expectorate, dry mouth and throat, or hematemesis, reddish tongue with thin fur and thin and fast pulse.

Analysis：Endogenous dryness due to yin asthenia deprives the lung of moisture and of the function of depuration, leading to adverse flow of qi, consumption and impairment of lung yin, which brings about failure to disperse lung qi; hematemesis is due to impairment of the lung collaterals; reddish tongue with thin fur and thin and fast pulse are signs of endogenous dryness due to yin asthenia.

Prescription：Nourish yin, moisturize the lung and arrest cough.

Formulas：Erdong Ermu Tang (Decoction). In the formula, Maidong (*Radix Ophiopogonis*) and Tiandong (*Radix Asparagi*) have the effect of nourishing yin and moistening dryness, Zhimu (*Rhizoma Anemarrhenae*) and Beimu (*Bulbus Fritillaria*) can clear away heat and moisten lung so as to arrest cough. For dryness of the mouth and throat, Beishashen (*Radix Glehniae*), Shengdihuang (*Radix Rehmanniae Recens*) and Baihe (*Bulbus Lilii*) can be added to nourish yin and moisten dryness; for severe cough, Baibu (*Radix Stemonae*), Huangqin (*Radix Scutellariae*), Sangbaipi (*Cortex Mori*) and Gualoupi (*Pericapium Trichosanthis*) can be combined with the formula to clear away heat from the lung and moisten dryness so as to arrest cough; for hematemesis, Baiji (*Rhizoma Bletillae*), Xianhecao (*Herba Agrimoniae*) and Oujie (*Nodus Nelumbinis Rhizomatis*) can be added to stop bleeding.

6. 阳虚咳嗽

4.6　Cough due to yang asthenia

【症状】咳嗽反复发作，痰涎清稀，头晕目眩，面色㿠白，形寒肢冷，易感冒，大便溏薄，小便不利，舌质淡暗，苔薄白滑，脉象沉迟或沉缓。

【分析】脾肾阳虚，水气上泛，是本证发作的主要病机。阳虚失运，水气停滞，则上干于肺，故咳嗽、痰涎清稀；阳虚失于温养作用，故头晕目眩、形寒肢冷、易于感冒；脾阳虚则大便溏薄，肾阳虚则小便不利；苔白滑、脉沉迟或沉缓，为阳虚水停之征。

【治法】温养脾肾，化气行水。

【方药】真武汤加味。方中以附子温阳补肾，以祛寒水；茯苓、白术健脾利水，导水下行；生姜温散水气；白芍收敛正气，不使正气随水气下泄。此方重在温肾行水。若咳甚者，加干姜、五味子、细辛散寒化饮，敛肺止咳；胸胁满闷者，加白芥子、旋覆花祛痰降气；气短乏力者，加党参益气；大便稀薄、次数多者，加干姜、肉豆蔻温中止泻。

Clinical manifestations: Frequent cough, thin and clear sputum and saliva, dizziness, pale complexion, cold body and limbs, susceptibility to catching cold, loose stool, dysuria, dull color of tongue with thin slippery whitish fur, as well as slow and sunken pulse or moderate and sunken pulse.

Analysis: Pathogenesis for the onset of the syndrome is yang asthenia of the spleen and kidney, which gives rise to retention of fluid in the muscles. Cough with thin and clear sputum and saliva is due to failure of asthenia of splenic yang to transport and retained fluid and edema, which invades adversely to the lung; dizziness, cold body and limbs, and susceptibility to catching cold are caused by failure of asthenic yang to warm and nourish; loose stool is due to asthenic spleen yang; dysuria is caused by yang asthenia of the kidney; whitish slippery fur and slow and sunken pulse or moderate and sunken pulse are manifestations of yang asthenia and fluid retention.

Prescription: Warm and nourish the spleen and kidney, and transform qi to promote diuresis.

Formulas: Zhenwu Tang Jiawei (Modified Zhenwu Decoction). In the formula, Fuzi (*Radix Aconiti Lateralis Preparata*) has the action of warming yang and tonifying the kidney; Fuling (*Poriae Cocos*) and Baizhu (*Rhizoma Atractylodis Macrocephalae*) can invigorate the spleen and alleviate fluid retention by guiding it to flow downward; Shengjiang (*Rhizoma Zingiberis Recens*) can warm and resolve dampness, Baishao (*Radix Paeoniae Alba*) has an effect of astringing healthy qi in order that it could not flow downward with fluid. The main effect of the formula is to warm the kidney and promote diuresis; for severe cough, Ganjiang (*Rhizoma Zingiberis*), Wuweizi (*Fructus Schisandrae Chinensis*), and Xixin (*Herba Asari*) can be added to disperse cold, resolve fluid retention and astringe lung qi to arrest cough; for oppression and fullness of the chest and hypochondrium, Baijiezi (*Semen Brassicae*) and Xuanfuhua (*Flos Inulae*) can be used to eliminate phlegm and depress adverse flow of qi; for short breath and lack of energy, Dangshen (*Radix Codonopsis*) can be combined to replenish qi; for loose stool, Ganjiang (*Rhizoma Zingiberis*) and Roudoukou (*Semen Myristicae*) can be added to warm middle energizer and relieve diarrhea.

五、支气管哮喘

5 Bronchial asthma

〔**概说**〕 Summary

支气管哮喘简称哮喘，又称过敏性哮喘，是一种常见的呼吸道慢性炎症性疾病。这种炎症与普通因细菌、病毒感染引起的炎症有着本质的不同。病人的气道对外界的刺激存在高反应性，这种高反应性可因接触环境中的过敏原、冷空气等诱因而触发。本病属于中医学"哮喘"病范畴，多发于秋冬季节，春季次之，夏季则缓解。

中医学认为，本病的发生和进展与肺、脾、肾三脏功能失调有关。肺主呼吸，脾主运化，肾主纳气；肺肾气虚，则浊气不出，清气失纳，引起呼吸困难；脾失健运，则生痰，痰阻气道，亦会引起呼吸不畅。病发时以实喘为主，以外邪犯肺，肺失宣降，脾湿生痰为主要病机；缓解时，以虚喘为主，以脾肺两虚，肾不纳气为主要病机。两者治疗有本质上的区别。

Bronchial asthma, known as "asthma" or "allergic asthma", is a common chronic inflammation of the respiratory tract. It differs in nature from other common inflammatory diseases caused by infection of bacteria or virus. Respiratory airway has hyperresponsiveness to external stimulation, which can be triggered by contact with allergens of the surroundings, cold air and so on. In terms of TCM, this disease falls into the scope of "asthma". Autumn and winter are highest-incidence seasons of this disease, spring being the second. While in summer, syndrome of asthma may be relieved.

In TCM, it is held that the onset and development of bronchial asthma are related to dysfunction of the lung, spleen and kidney. The lung governs respiration, the spleen dominates transportation and transformation, and the kidney controls receiving of qi. Dyspnea is caused by adverse flow of turbid qi and failure to receive lucid qi because of qi asthenia of the lung and kidney. Failure of the spleen to transport and transform food generates phlegm, which inhibits respiratory tract, thus, leading to unsmooth breath. At the stage of the outbreak of the disease, dyspnea is of sthenic nature, mainly caused by invasion of exogenous pathogenic factors into the lung, failure of the lung to disperse and descend, as well as phlegm generated from splenic dampness. When the symptoms get relieved, dyspnea displays asthenic nature, with its main pathogenesis being asthenic spleen and lung and failure of the kidney to receive qi. Therefore, treatment for both types of asthma should be different in nature.

〔辨证论治〕 Syndrome differentiation and treatment

（一）实喘（发作期）
5.1　Sthenic asthma （the stage of onset）

1. 风寒束肺
5.1.1　Asthma due to wind cold encumbering the lung

【症状】咳嗽，气喘，胸闷，痰白清稀，口不渴，初期多兼有恶寒发热、无汗头痛、鼻喉发痒等症，舌质不红，舌苔薄白，脉象浮紧。

【分析】初期发作多呈现风寒表证，如恶寒发热，无汗头痛，苔薄白，脉浮等；因肺合皮毛，主呼吸，为气之主，风寒袭表，引起肺气不得宣降，津液凝聚为痰，堵塞气道，故咳嗽气喘；风邪干于清窍，则鼻喉发痒。如此症状反复发作，则风寒之邪遗患于肺，"寒入肺俞"，成为病根，每遇风寒，就会发为哮喘。

【治法】辛温解表，宣肺平喘。

【方药】麻黄汤加减。方中麻黄、桂枝辛温发汗，杏仁降气平喘，甘草调和诸药。如表证不重，可去桂枝，即为宣肺平喘的三拗汤；喘甚，加苏子、前胡降气平喘；痰多，加半夏、橘红；痰白黏稠，加胆南星、白芥子燥湿化痰；胸闷憋气，加枳壳、紫苏梗、桔梗。

Clinical manifestations：Cough, shortness of breath, chest oppression, whitish and thin and clear sputum, no thirst, complicated with such symptoms as aversion to cold, fever, no sweating, headache, itching nose and throat, non-reddish tongue, whitish thin fur as well as floating and tense pulse at the initial stage of the disease.

Analysis：The symptoms at the initial stage of the disease are manifested as an external syndrome of wind cold, such as aversion to cold and fever, headache without sweating, whitish thin tongue fur as well as floating pulse. The lung is closely connected with the skin and body hair, dominating qi and respiration. Cough with asthma is due to pathogenic wind and cold factors attacking the superficies and coagulation of phlegm from fluid, which obstructs the airway because of failure of lung qi to disperse and descend. Itching nose and throat are caused by pathogenic wind factor attacking the upper orifices. Frequent occurrence of the above symptoms leads to pathogenic wind cold impairing the lung, "cold invading Feishu （BL13）", which becomes the root cause for asthma. Each time when wind and cold pathogens attack the superficies, patients can contract asthma.

Prescription：Relieve the superficies with pungent-warm herbs and disperse the lung to arrest asthma.

Formulas：Mahuang Tang Jiajian （Modified Mahuang Decoction）. In the formula, Mahuang （*Herba Ephedrae*） and Guizhi （*Ramulus Cinnamomi*）, pungent and warm in nature, have an action of inducing sweating; Xingren （*Semen Armeniacae Amarum*） can depress adverse flow of qi, Gancao (*Radix Glycyrrhizae*) can regulate the above herbs. If the exterior syndrome is not serious, Guizhi can be removed, and the modified formula is the so-called San'ao Tang (Decoction), which has the action of dispersing lung heat and arresting asthma; for severe asthma, Suzi (*Fructus Perillae*) and Qianhu (*Radix Peucedani*) can be added to descend adverse flow of qi and arrest asthma; for profuse sputum, Banxia (*Rhizoma Pinelliae*) and Juhong (*Exocarpium Citri Rubrum*) could be added; for whitish, sticky and thick sputum, Dannanxing (*Rhizoma Arisaematis Cum Bile*) and Baijiezi (*Semen Sinapis*) can be combined to dry dampness and resolve phlegm; for chest oppression, Zhiqiao (*Fructus Aurantii*), Zisugeng (*Caulis Perllae*) and Jiegeng (*Radix Platycodonis*) can be added.

2. 外寒内饮
5.1.2 Asthma due to external cold and internal retention of fluid

【症状】喘息，咳嗽，痰多稀薄如水状，恶寒发热，形寒肢冷，背冷，口不渴或渴喜热饮，舌苔白滑，脉象弦紧。

【分析】寒饮内伏，心肺之阳气无以振作，故形寒肢冷并背寒；寒饮堵塞气道，则咳嗽喘息；稀薄之痰如水状，乃寒饮内伏之明证；无热邪之扰，故口不渴或喜热饮；苔白脉弦，为寒饮内伏之征。

【治法】温肺散寒，解表化饮。

【方药】小青龙汤。方中麻黄、桂枝解表散寒；细辛、干姜辛散水饮；五味子收敛肺气，芍药养血敛气；半夏降逆化痰；炙甘草益气和中。八味配伍，可使风寒解，水饮去，宣降有权，肺气清肃，诸症自平。若咳呛内热者，可加生石膏、芦根；痰鸣、喘息不得卧者，可加葶苈子、射干；痰多闷气，可加紫菀、款冬花。

Clinical manifestations: Asthma with cough, watery and thin sputum, aversion to cold and fever, cold body and limbs, cold sensation of the back, no thirst, or thirst with desire for hot drink, whitish slippery tongue fur and taut and tense pulse.

Analysis: Cold body and limbs and cold sensation of back are due to internal retention of cold and fluid and failure to vitalize yang and qi in the heart and lung; dyspnea with cough is caused by cold and fluid obstructing the respiration tract; thin sputum like water is the obvious manifestation of internal retention of cold and fluid; no thirst, or thirst with desire for hot drink results from no disturbance of pathogenic heat factor; whitish fur and taut pulse are signs of internal retention of cold and fluid.

Prescription: Warm the lung and expel cold, relieve exterior pathogens and resolve retention of fluid.

Formulas: Small Qinglong Tang (Decoction). In the formula, Mahuang (*Herba Ephedrae*) and Guizhi (*Ramulus Cinnamomi*) have the action of relieving exterior syndrome and expelling cold; Xixin (*Herba Asari*) and Ganjiang (*Rhizoma Zingiberis*), pungent in flavor, can disperse retention of fluid; Wuweizi (*Fructus Schisandrae Chinensis*) has the effect of astringing lung qi, Shaoyao (*Radix Paeoniae*) can nourish blood and astringe qi;

Banxia (*Rhizoma Pinelliae*) can descend adverse qi and resolve phlegm, Zhigancao (*Radix Glycyrrhizae Preparata*) has an effect of replenishing qi and harmonizing the spleen and stomach. Combined together, the eight herbs can expel wind cold, eliminate fluid retention and improve the function of the lung in dispersing and descending so as to remove the above symptoms. For cough and stagnation of endogenous heat, Shengshigao (*Gypsum Fibrosum*) and Lugen (*Rhizoma Phragmitis*) can be combined; for sputum rale, asthma and inbility to rest, Tinglizi (*Semen Lepidii seu Descurainiae*) and Shegan (*Rhizoma Belamcandae*) could be added; for profuse sputum and chest oppression, Ziwan (*Radix Asteris*) and Kuandonghua (*Flos Farfarae*) can be added.

3. 风热犯肺
5.1.3 Asthma due to wind heat invading the lung

【症状】发热恶风，有汗，口渴欲饮，咳喘气粗，甚则鼻张息肩，痰黄而黏稠，舌质红赤，舌苔黄腻，或薄白而干，脉象浮数。

【分析】风热外袭，肺卫不得宣发，肺气郁闭，发为咳喘；邪热迫肺，灼津为痰，故痰黄而黏稠；热灼津液，故口渴欲饮；舌质红赤，苔黄腻，脉象浮数，均为风热犯肺、灼津为痰之象。

【治法】祛风清热，宣肺平喘。

【方药】桑菊饮加味。桑菊饮为治疗风热感冒的主方，是祛风清热的代表方剂之一。若发热口渴较甚者，加生石膏、知母清热泻火；实热便秘者，加生大黄、决明子等；痰黄难以咯出者，加瓜蒌皮、桑白皮。

Clinical manifestations: Fever and aversion to wind, sweating, thirst with desire for drink, cough and dyspnea with deep breath, even with flaring of nares and elevated shoulders, thick and sticky and yellowish sputum, reddish tongue, yellowish greasy tongue fur or thin whitish dry fur as well as floating and fast pulse.

Analysis: Cough with dyspnea is due to wind heat invading the lung, failure of the lung to disperse results in stagnation of lung qi; yellowish and thick and sticky sputum results from pathogenic heat invading the lung and scorching fluid; thirst with desire to drink is due to heat scorching fluid; reddish tongue with yellowish greasy tongue fur and floating and fast pulse are signs of wind heat invading the lung and pathogenic heat scorching fluid.

Prescription: Expel wind, clear away heat and disperse the lung to relieve asthma.

Formulas: Sang Ju Yin Jiawei (Modified Sang Ju Decoction). Sang Ju Yin is an essential formula for the syndrome of cold due to wind heat, and it is also one of the typical recipe for expelling wind and clearing away heat. For severe thirst, the recipe is often combined with Shengshigao (*Gypsum Fibrosum*) and Zhimu (*Rhizoma Anemarrhenae*) to clear away heat and purge fire; for sthenic heat and constipation, Shengdahuang (*Radix et Rhizoma Rhei*) and Juemingzi (*Semen Cassiae Torae*) can be added to the recipe; for yellowish sputum with difficulty to expectorate, Gualoupi (*Pericapium Trichosanthis*) and Sangbaipi (*Cortex Mori*) can be added to th recipe.

4. 痰湿壅肺

5.1.4 Asthma due to phlegmatic dampness in the lung

【症状】气喘，咳嗽，痰多而黏腻，咯吐不利，胸中满闷，喉中如有黏痰黏着，时时恶心，舌苔白腻，脉象弦滑。

【分析】湿痰上着于肺，肺气不得宣畅，故为喘、咳、闷、恶心等；其他均为痰湿之象。湿痰留着于体内，是喘证的主要证候之一，一有风寒外袭，或饮食过于甘肥，就会使痰喘加重。若痰湿久蕴，亦可化热转为痰热证候，不可不辨。

【治法】祛痰降逆，宣肺平喘。

【方药】三子养亲汤合二陈汤。三子养亲汤（紫苏子、白芥子、莱菔子）降逆、祛痰、平喘；二陈汤（陈皮、半夏、茯苓、甘草）健脾、降逆、化痰。若有化热之象者，可加黄芩、瓜蒌皮、桑白皮等清肺宣化之品。

Clinical manifestations：Asthma with cough, profuse and thick and sticky sputum with difficulty to expectorate, chest oppression and fullness, frequent nausea with a sensation of the throat being stuck with sputum, whitish and greasy tongue fur and taut and slippery pulse.

Analysis：Asthma with cough, chest oppression and nausea are due to retention of phlegmatic dampness in the lung and failure of lung qi to disperse and descend. Other symptoms are manifestations of phlegmatic dampness. Internal retention of damp phlegm is one major syndrome of asthma, which can be aggravated with invasion of wind cold or excessive intake of sweet or greasy food. Prolonged retention of phlegmatic dampness can be transformed into the syndrome of phlegmatic heat. Therefore, treatment for asthma must be based on syndromes differentiation.

Prescription：Eliminate phlegm, descend adverse flow of qi, and disperse the lung to subdue asthma.

Formulas：Sanzi Yangqin Tang (Decoction) combined with Erchen Tang (Decoction). Sanzi Yangqin Tang, made up of Zisuzi (*Fructus Perillae*), Baijiezi (*Semen Sinapis*) and Laifuzi (*Semen Raphani*), is used to descend adverse flow of qi, eliminate phlegm and subdue asthma. Erchen Tang, consisting of Chenpi (*Pericarpium Citri Reticulatae*), Banxia (*Rhizoma Pinelliae*), Fuling (*Poriae Cocos*) and Gancao (*Radix Glycyrrhizae*), has an effect of invigorating the spleen, descending adverse flow of qi, and resolving phlegm. For symptoms of transformation of heat, Huangqin (*Radix Scutellariae*), Gualoupi (*Pericapium Trichosanthis*), and Sangbaipi (*Cortex Mori*) may be added to disperse lung qi and resolve phlegm.

5. 痰热壅肺

5.1.5 Asthma due to accumulation of phlegmatic heat in the lung

【症状】喘急面红，咳嗽，胸闷烦热，口干口苦，痰黄而稠，或虽是白痰，但黏稠难以咯出，舌质红赤，苔黄腻而干，脉象滑数。

【分析】风寒入里可以化热，或肺胃素有蕴热，或嗜食辛辣厚味食物，或湿痰蕴积化热，皆可形成痰热壅肺证候。痰热阻塞气道，使得肺气不得宣降，而为咳嗽、喘息、胸闷。

【治法】清热化痰，宣肺平喘。

【方药】麻杏石甘汤加味。麻黄配杏仁，宣肺平喘；麻黄配石膏，发散郁热；生甘草清热止咳。如里热重者，可加黄芩、板蓝根、鱼腥草清热解毒祛痰；若痰多喘急，可加桑白皮、瓜蒌皮、葶苈子祛痰平喘；便秘、腹胀，可加大黄、决明子、瓜蒌仁通腑泄浊，以利肺气的肃降。

Clinical manifestations：Asthma with rapid respiration, flushed cheek, cough, chest oppression with dysphoria, dry mouth and bitter taste, yellowish and sticky sputum, or whitish and sticky sputum with difficulty to expectorate, reddish tongue with yellowish and greasy and dry fur as well as slippery and fast pulse.

Analysis：This syndrome is caused by heat transformed from invasion of pathogenic wind cold in the interior, or prolonged accumulation of heat in the lung and the stomach, or excessive intake of pungent and savory food, or heat transformed from accumulation of phlegmatic dampness. Cough, dyspnea, rapid respiration and chest oppression are caused by failure of the lung to disperse because of accumulation of phlegmatic heat obstructing the respiration tract.

Prescription：Clear away heat, resolve phlegm and disperse the lung to subdue asthma.

Formulas：Mahuang Xingren Shigao Gancao Tang Jiawei (Modified Mahuang Xingren Shigao Gancao Decoction). In the formula, Mahuang (*Herba Ephedrae*), in combination with Xingren (*Semen Armeniacae Amarum*), can disperse the lung and subdue asthma; Mahuang, in combination with Shigao (*Gypsum Fibrosum*), can disperse stagnated heat; Gancao (*Radix Glycyrrhizae*) has an effect of clearing away heat to stop cough. For severe internal heat, Huangqin (*Radix Scutellariae*), Banlangen (*Radix Isatidis*) and Yuxingcao (*Herba Houttuyniae*) can be added to relieve heat, toxin and dispel phlegm; for profuse phlegm and rapid respiration, Sangbaipi (*Cortex Mori*), Gualoupi (*Pericapium Trichosanthis*) and Tinglizi (*Semen Lepidii seu Descurainiae*) can be added to eliminate phlegm and suppress asthma; for constipation and abdominal distention, Dahuang (*Radix et Rhizoma Rhei*), Juemingzi (*Semen Cassiae Torae*) and Gualouren (*Semen Trichosanthis*) could be added to remove stagnated qi in fu-organ and purge turbid qi so as to help depurate and depress lung qi.

6. 外寒里热

5.1.6 Asthma due to external cold and endogenous heat

【症状】恶寒发热，有汗或无汗，喘急烦闷，痰黄而稠，咳吐不利，口渴，咽干，舌尖红赤，苔薄白微黄，脉象浮数。

【分析】风寒之邪，在表不解，入里化热，或里有郁热，外受风寒，寒束于外，热郁于内，使得肺气不得宣降，发为喘急、烦闷等症。若里热郁甚，侵犯肺络，"肺主气"失职，进一步侵犯心脏，发为高热、神昏、痉厥等，则为危重之候。

【治法】解表清里，化痰平喘。

【方药】定喘汤。方中麻黄、杏仁宣肺平喘；黄芩、桑白皮清泻伏热；苏子、半夏降气化痰；白果、款冬花敛肺气之耗散；甘草调和诸药。全方清中有散，发中有收，收散结合，有利于肺气的宣发与肃降。

Clinical manifestations：Aversion to cold and fever，sweating or no sweating，asthma with rapid respiration and irritancy，yellowish and thick sputum with difficulty to expectorate，thirst and dry throat，reddish tongue tip with whitish or pale yellowish thin fur as well as floating and fast pulse.

Analysis：Unrelieved pathogenic wind and cold factors invade into the interior and transform into heat，or internal stagnation of heat，combined with invasion of exogenous wind cold，gives rise to pathogenic cold encumbering the superficies with heat stagnating in the interior，which leads to failure to disperse and descend lung qi. The above factors result in asthma with rapid respiration and irritancy. Invasion of internal stagnation of heat into the lung collaterals gives rise to failure of the lung to govern qi，which，in turn，attacks the heart and results in critical symptoms such as high fever，coma as well as syncope with convulsion.

Prescription：Relieve the external pathogens，eliminate internal heat and resolve phlegm to subdue asthma.

Formulas：Dingchuan Tang（Decoction for arresting asthma）. In the formula，Mahuang（*Herba Ephedrae*）and Xingren（*Semen Armeniacae Amarum*）have the action of dispersing the lung and arresting dyspnea；Huangqin（*Radix Scutellariae*）and Sangbaipi（*Cortex Mori*）can purge latent heat；Suzi（*Fructus Perillae*）and Banxia（*Rhizoma Pinelliae*）can descend adverse flow of qi and resolve phlegm；Baiguo（*Semen Ginkgo*）and Kuandonghua（*Flos Farfarae*）have an effect of astringing consumption of lung qi；Gancao（*Radix Glycyrrhizae*）is used to harmonize the above herbs. The whole formula combines the function of eliminating，dispersing，relieving as well as astringing，which are very helpful to promote dispersing and descending lung qi.

（二）虚喘（缓解期）
5.2 Asthenic asthma（the stage of alleviation）

1. 脾肺两虚
5.2.1 Asthma due to asthenia of the spleen and lung

【症状】喘促短气，咳痰稀薄，乏力，自汗畏风，饮食减少，面色苍白，舌质淡红，苔薄白，脉象细弱；或面红，口干，盗汗，咽喉干痒不利，舌质红赤，苔少，脉象细数。

【分析】肺主气，肺气不足，则喘促短气；肺合皮毛，肺卫不固，则自汗畏风；脾不健运，故饮食减少；若肺阴不足，则虚火上炎，故见面红、口干、盗汗、咽喉干痒等；其脉舌之象，反映了肺脾虚弱的本质。

【治法】健脾益气，补土生金。

【方药】补中益气汤合生脉散。补中益气汤（由黄芪、人参、白术、炙甘草、当归、陈皮、升麻、柴胡、生姜、大枣组成）为健脾益气的主方，具有补益脾肺之气、升举阳气的作用；生脉散（由人参、麦冬、五味子组成）为益气养阴的主方，是养心肺气阴的主剂。两方合用，以补益脾肺之气为主，兼以养肺阴，可谓脾肺并调、阴阳兼理之方。如痰液稀薄，形寒、口不渴，为肺虚寒证，可于上方去麦冬，加干姜温养阳气；如肺阴虚明显者，应以生脉散为基础方，酌加百合、南沙参、北沙参、玉竹、石斛等，或用百合固金汤加味。脾虚湿盛者，可改用六君子汤加干姜、细辛、五味子，平时可用香砂六君子丸平调之。

Clinical manifestations: Asthma with rapid respiration and short breath, cough with thin sputum, lack of energy, spontaneous sweating, aversion to wind, reduced appetite, pale complexion, pale reddish tongue with whitish thin fur, as well as thin and feeble pulse; or flushed cheek, dry mouth, night sweating, dry and itching throat, reddish tongue with scanty fur as well as thin and fast pulse.

Analysis: Asthma with rapid respiration and short breath are due to qi deficiency resulting from hypofunction of the lung in governing qi; the lung dominates the skin and hair, spontaneous sweating and aversion to wind are caused by weakness of the lung to protect the superficies; reduced appetite is due to failure of the spleen in transportation and transformation of food; flushed cheek, dry mouth, night sweating, and dry itching throat are due to deficiency of lung yin which gives rise to up-flaming of asthenic fire; reddish tongue with scanty fur as well as thin and fast pulse is the reflection of asthenic lung and spleen.

Prescription: Invigorate the spleen, tonify qi and generate metal by supplementing earth (the spleen pertains to earth, and the lung to metal).

Formulas: Buzhong Yiqi Tang (Decoction) combined with Shengmai San (Powder). Buzhong Yiqi Tang, consisting of Huangqi (*Radix Astragali seu Hedysari*), Renshen (*Radix Ginseng*), Baizhu (*Rhizoma Atractylodis Macrocephalae*), Zhigancao (*Radix Glycyrrhizae Preparata*), Danggui (*Radix Angelicae Sinensis*), Chenpi (*Pericarpium Citri Reticulatae*), Shengma (*Rhizoma Cimicifugae*), Chaihu (*Radix Bupleuri*), Shengjiang (*Rhizoma Zingiberis Recens*) and Dazao (*Fructus Jujubae*), has an action of nourishing qi in the lung and spleen and strengthening yang qi, and it is an essential formula for invigorating the spleen and tonifying qi. Shengmai San, made up of Renshen (*Radix Ginseng*), Maidong (*Radix Ophiopogonis*) and Wuweizi (*Fructus Schisandrae Chinensis*), is the main formula for nourishing yin and qi, and it is also used to strengthen qi and yin in the heart and lung. Combined together, both formulas can have the function of nourishing yin and qi as well as strengthening lung yin. Therefore, the formula can regulate not only the spleen and lung, but also yin and yang. For asthenic cold in the lung with symptoms such as thin and clear sputum, cold limbs and no thirst, Maidong (*Radix Ophiopogonis*) should be removed from the formula, Ganjiang (*Rhizoma Zingiberis*) can be added to warm and nourish yang qi; for obvious asthenic yin of the lung, Baihe (*Bulbus Lilii*), Nanshashen (*Radix Adenophorae*), Beishashen (*Radix Glehniae*), Yuzhu (*Rhizoma Polygonati Odorati*) and Shihu (*Herba Dendrobii*) can be combined with Shengmai San, or Baihe Gujin Tang Jiawei (Modified Baihe Gujin Decoction) can be applied to replace the above formula; for exuberant dampness due to splenic asthenia, Liujunzi Tang, combined with Ganjiang (*Rhizoma Zingiberis*), Xixin (*Herba Asari*) and Wuweizi (*Fructus Schisandrae Chinensis*), can take the place of the above formula, or Xiang Sha Liujunzi Wan (Pill) can be used to regulate the syndrome.

2. 肾阳虚衰
5.2.2　Asthma due to yang asthenia of the kidney

【症状】喘促日久，呼多吸少，活动则喘促更甚，痰多而稀薄，汗出，形寒肢冷，神怯，面目虚浮，精神困倦，乏力，足胫浮肿，舌质淡暗，苔薄白，脉象沉细无力或浮大而空。

【分析】本证多由房劳伤肾，或大病久病之后，肾精亏虚，或肺病日久，金不生水所致。肾为元气之根，肾虚则元气不纳，故喘促而气不接续；阳虚阴盛，故形寒肢冷；水气不化，则面目虚浮并足胫浮肿；肾为"作强之官"，肾虚则精神困倦，乏力神怯；肾阳虚极，还可见暴然喘促、大汗淋漓、肢冷神脱、烦躁不安、脉大无根、唇舌青紫等危证。故对此证候，不可掉以轻心。

【治法】温肾纳气。

【方药】金匮肾气丸。本方为温肾之祖方，但丸者，缓也，不宜救急，当改为汤剂为宜。是方取熟地黄、山茱萸、山药补益肾精，并有纳气平喘作用；取茯苓、牡丹皮、泽泻泄浊化瘀，并有健脾缓急作用；主药附子、桂枝温肾扶阳，为恢复肾阳之主剂。若在方中加入人参、蛤蚧，以补肾纳气，其平喘作用更好。若汗出如油，大口喘气，脉大无根，可急用参附龙骨牡蛎汤（由人参、附子、生姜、大枣、龙骨、牡蛎组成），加麦冬、五味子、蛤蚧、桂心等，扶元救脱，固摄肾气。

Clinical manifestations: Prolonged asthma with rapid respiration, more exhalation but less inhalation, aggravation of asthma with movement, profuse and thin sputum, sweating, cold body and limbs, timidity, asthenic facial edema, lassitude, lack of energy, edema of legs and feet, pale and darkish tongue with thin and whitish fur as well as thin, sunken and weak pulse or floating large and hollow pulse.

Analysis: This syndrome is usually caused by impairment of the kidney due to intemperance of sexual life, or by deficiency of kidney essence from severe or prolonged disease, or by failure of metal (the lung) to generate water (the kidney) resulting from prolonged lung disease. The kidney is the root of primordial qi, asthenia of the kidney results in failure of the kidney to receive primordial qi, thus, giving rise to asthma with rapid respiration and more exhalation but less inhalation; cold body and limbs is due to asthenia of yang and excess of yin; asthenic edema of the face, legs and feet is caused by failure to activate qi to promote diuresis; the kidney is similar to an official with great power or strength, lassitude and timidity are due to asthenic kidney; abrupt dyspnea with rapid respiration, profuse sweat, cold limbs, depletion of spirit, restlessness, cyanotic or purplish tongue and lips as well as rootless large pulse are signs of critical diseases, caused by extreme deficiency of kidney yang. Therefore, the syndrome must be treated carefully.

Prescription: Warm the kidney to receive qi.

Formulas: Jingui Shenqi Wan (Pill). This is a recipe handed down from ancestors for warming the kidney. However, the action of pills is moderate, it cannot be used to cope with critical cases. Therefore, pills should be replaced by decoction with the same herbs. In the formula, Shudihuang (*Radix Rehmanniae Preparata*), Shanzhuyu (*Fructus Corni*) and Shanyao (*Rhizoma Dioscoreae*) have the effect of tonifying kidney essence as well as receiving qi to arrest dyspnea. Fuling (*Poriae Cocos*), Mudanpi (*Cortex Moutan Radicis*) and Zexie (*Rhizoma Alismatis*) can purge turbidity, resolve blood stasis, invigorate the spleen and alleviate critical diseaseas. Fuzi (*Radix Aconiti Lateralis Preparata*) and Guizhi (*Ramulus Cinnamomi*), as the leading herbs here, are essential for restoring kidney yang. Renshen (*Radix Ginseng*) and Gejie (*Gecko*) can be added to tonify kidney essence and receive qi in order to improve the action of arresting dyspnea. For dyspnea with rapid respiration, profuse sweat as well as large and rootless pulse, Shen Fu Longgu Muli Tang (Decoction) including Renshen (*Radix Ginseng*), Fuzi (*Radix Aconiti Lateralis Preparata*), Shengjiang (*Rhizoma Zingiberis Recens*), Dazao (*Fructus Jujubae*), Longgu (*Os Draconis*) and Muli (*Concha Ostreae*), is used with Maidong (*Radix Ophiopogonis*), Wuweizi (*Fructus Schisandrae Chinensis*), Gejie (*Gecko*) and Guixin (*Cortex Cinnamomi*) to rescue collapse of qi so as to strengthen kidney qi.

3. 肾阴不足
5.2.3　Asthma due to insufficiency of kidney yin

【症状】喘促气短，耳鸣，腰酸，口干，心烦，手足心热，潮热盗汗，烦劳则喘甚，小便黄赤，舌质红赤，脉象细数。

【分析】肾阴不足，精与气不能互生，气虚不纳，故喘促气短；"阴虚生内热"，故有手足心热、潮热盗汗等症状；阴虚一样不能作劳，心烦、形劳都会使喘促加重；其他舌脉之象，均为阴虚内热之征。

【治法】滋阴补肾，纳气平喘。

【方药】七味都气丸、河车大造丸等。七味都气丸为六味地黄丸加五味子而成。六味地黄丸为滋阴之主剂，具有滋阴降火的作用，加用五味子，意在加强肾的纳气作用，五味子虽有五味之称，但以酸甘二味为主，其气温、酸甘可以养阴纳气，气温有利于抑制六味地黄丸的过寒之性，又有利于元气的温养。河车大造丸为明代张景岳所拟定的名方，药物由紫河车、龟板、黄柏、牛膝、天冬、麦冬、熟地黄组成。具有滋阴补肾、清热平喘的功效。凡阴虚之支气管哮喘、老年性肺气肿、肺结核、慢性肾炎、男女不育不孕症等，均可选用。

Clinical manifestations：Asthma with rapid respiration，short breath，tinnitus，aching sensation of the loins，dry mouth，irritancy，feverish sensation over the palms and soles，tidal fever and night sweating，aggravation of asthma with overstrain，yellowish and brownish urine，reddish tongue as well as thin and fast pulse.

Analysis：Asthma with rapid respiration and shortness of breath is due to failure to receive qi because of insufficiency of kidney yin，which brings about failure of the interdependence of essence and kidney qi；feverish sensation over the palms and soles with tidal fever and night sweating is due to "endogenous heat generated from yin asthenia"；aggravation of dyspnea is caused by yin asthenia，irritancy and overstrain；reddish tongue as well as thin and fast pulse is manifestation of yin asthenia and endogenous heat.

Prescription：Nourish yin，tonify the kidney and receive qi to subdue dyspnea.

Formulas：Qiwei Duqi Wan（Pill），Heche Dazao Wan（Pill），etc. Qiwei Duqi Wan is made up of Liuwei Dihuang Wan and Wuweizi（*Fructus Schisandrae Chinensis*）. Liuwei Dihuang Wan，with the effect of nourishing yin as well as reducing fire pathogen，is an essential formula to nourish yin. Together with Wuweizi，the newly combined "Qiwei Duqi Wan" is to reinforce the function of the kidney in receiving qi. Wuweizi，although named after "Wuwei" —the five flavors in Chinese language，is mainly characterized by sour and sweet flavor with the action of nourishing yin and receiving qi. With its warm nature，Wuweizi can restrain excessive cold nature of Liuwei Dihuang Wan，and promote the function of warming and nourishing primordial qi. Heche Dazao Wan，designed by Zhang Jingyue from the Ming Dynasty，consists of Ziheche（*Placenta Hominis*），Guiban（*Plastrum Testudinis*），Huangbo（*Cortex Phellodendri*），Niuxi（*Radix Achyranthis Bidentatae*），Tiandong（*Radix Asparagi*），Maidong（*Radix Ophiopogonis*）and Shudihuang（*Radix Rehmanniae Preparata*），having an action of nourishing yin，tonifying the kidney，clearing away heat as well as subduing dyspnea. And it can also be used to treat diseases due to yin asthenia such as bronchial asthma，senile pulmonary emphysema，tuberculosis，chronic nephritis，sterility in male and infertility in female，and so on.

六、肺气肿

6 Emphysema

〔概说〕 Summary

肺气肿是指终末细支气管的远端部分，包括呼吸性细支气管、肺泡壁、肺泡囊和肺泡的持久性扩大，并伴有肺泡壁破坏的病理状态。肺气肿包括代偿性肺气肿和阻塞性肺气肿，本节重点叙述阻塞性肺气肿。

阻塞性肺气肿，是由慢性支气管炎或其他原因逐渐引起的细支气管不完全阻塞或狭窄，使得终末细支气管远端气腔过度充气，并伴有气腔壁膨胀、破裂而产生，临床上常继发于慢性支气管炎、支气管哮喘和肺纤维化，尤以慢性支气管炎为多见。

Emphysema refers to the persistent expansion of the far-ends of bronchiole involving respiratory bronchus, alveolar walls, sacs and pulmonary alveoli, and accompanied by pathological state of the damage of alveolar walls. It is classified into compensatory and obstructive emphysema, the latter being the focus of this chapter.

Obstructive emphysema is caused by partial obstruction or stenosis of bronchiole because of chronic bronchitis and other factors, resulting in excessive inflation of the far-ends of bronchiole and abnormal increase of the size and rupture of the air cavity. It occurs after the onset of chronic bronchitis, bronchial asthma as well as pulmonary fibrosis, and the first is commonly seen in clinical practice.

〔辨证论治〕 Syndrome differentiation and treatment

1. 肺肾阳虚

6.1 Emphysema due to yang asthenia of the lung and kidney

【症状】喘促日久，呼长吸短，咳声低微，气不接续，动则喘息更甚，痰多而清稀，腰膝酸软，汗出肢冷，夜尿多，严重者面青唇紫，面浮肢肿，舌质淡白，苔薄白，脉象沉细无力。

【分析】喘促日久，必然肺虚及肾，或劳伤肾气，肾虚则摄纳无力，吸不归根，气不归原，故呼长吸短；肺气虚，则咳声低微，时时汗出；肺气不足，气不化津，水液停聚于肺，并随气上逆，所以出现痰液清稀；肾阳不能温养其府，故腰膝酸软，肢体不温；阳虚失于温化，则夜尿多，并会出现面浮肢肿；严重者，阳气欲脱，面青唇紫；脉舌均为阳虚之候。

【治法】益气补肺，温肾纳气。

【方药】玉屏风散合金匮肾气丸。玉屏风散中的黄芪为补气之首，外可固表止汗，内则大补脾肺之气；白术益气健脾，脾健则肺气可生；防风走表祛风散邪。三药合用，如屏风所至。现代医学研究认为，黄芪是珍贵的草药，它可恢复和强化机体的免疫能力，增加干扰素和白细胞的活性，促进体内有毒物质的排出，使人的精力旺盛，加大对疾病的抵抗能力，对慢性病毒感染、慢性免疫功能低下、职业性过劳综合征等"亚健康"人群，具有良好的治疗作用。

金匮肾气丸为温阳补肾之要药，其具体药效参见"支气管哮喘"一节。它与玉屏风散合用，使肺肾兼顾，金水相生，方中的山药、茯苓等，加强了益气健脾的作用，脾健则土可生金，又有利于肺气的恢复。这样上焦得固，中焦得健，下焦得纳，气归于根，其喘促自然有望平复。

Clinical manifestations: Prolonged dyspnea with rapid respiration, long exhalation but short inhalation with incontinuous breath, aggravated dyspnea with movements, low and weak cough, profuse and thin and clear sputum, aching sensation of the loins and knees, cold body and limbs with sweating, frequent urination at night, edema of the face and limbs even with cyanotic and purplish face and lips, pale whitish tongue with thin and whitish fur as well as thin, sunken and weak pulse.

Analysis: Long exhalation but short inhalation is caused by prolonged dyspnea with rapid respiration, which gives rise to deficiency of the lung involving the kidney and insufficient reception of qi, thus, failing to supplement kidney qi, or it is caused by consumption of kidney qi due to overstrain; low and weak cough and frequent sweating are due to deficiency of lung qi; thin and clear sputum is caused by deficiency of lung qi which results in failure of qi to transform fluid, retention of fluid in the lung and upper invasion of fluid with qi; aching sensation of the loins and limbs and cold body are caused by failure of asthenic kidney yang to warm and nourish the body; frequent urination at night and edema of the face and limbs are due to insufficiency of kidney yang and its failure in warming and transforming fluid; cyanotic and purplish face and lips in severe cases are caused by depletion of yang qi; pale whitish tongue with thin and whitish fur as well as thin, sunken and weak pulse are signs of yang asthenia.

Prescription: Replenish qi, tonify the lung and warm the kidney to receive qi.

Formulas: Yupingfeng San (Powder) combined with Jingui Shenqi Wan (Pill). In Yupingfeng San, Huangqi (*Radix Astragali seu Hedysari*) is the best Chinese medicinal herb to replenish qi, with the action of strengthening exterior and reducing sweat as well as supplementing qi of the spleen and lung; Baizhu (*Rhizoma Atractylodis Macrocephalae*) is used to benefit qi and invigorate the spleen, promoting generation of lung qi; Fangfeng (*Radix Saposhnikoviae*) is applied for exterior syndrome by dispelling pathogenic wind factor. Combined together, the three herbs can serve as "a folding screen" to prevent invasion of diseases. In modern medicine, it is held that Huangqi is a very precious herb with an action of restoring immune competency of human body and strengthening the activity of interferon and leucocyte so as to promote elimination of poisonous substance and restore vitality of patients, as a result, immune system could resist invasion of pathogens. Consequently, Huangqi is effective for treating chronic infection of virus, hypofunction of chronic immune system as well as syndrome of professional fatigue and overstrain in "subhealthy" people.

Jingui Shenqi Wan (Pill) is a principal recipe for warming yang and invigorating the kidney, and it has been discussed in the section of *Bronchial Asthma*. The combination of it with Yupingfeng San can supplement the lung and kidney, promote the inter-generation of metal (the lung) and water (the kidney). Shanyao (*Rhizoma Dioscoreae*) and Fuling (*Poriae Cocos*) in the formula could improve the effect of benefiting qi and invigorating the spleen (earth), which, in turn, can promote the function of metal (the lung) and help restore lung qi. In this way, upper energizer could be strengthened, middle energizer get invigorated, and qi could be directed into its source, the lower energizer. Thus, the symptom of asthma with rapid respiration could be removed.

2. 肺肾阴虚

6.2   Emphysema due to yin asthenia of the lung and kidney

【症状】喘促气短，动则喘甚，咳嗽少痰，或痰黏难以咳出，手足心热，潮热盗汗，口干欲饮，男子或有遗精，女子或有闭经，舌质红赤，苔少，脉象细数。

【分析】肺为水上之源，肾为元气之主，肺肾之间，母子相连，以少阳三焦为其通道，两者在生理上，相互资生；在病理上，相互影响。肺主清肃，性喜柔润，肺阴不足，虚热内生，肺被热蒸，气逆而上，则生咳嗽；久咳伤肺，则会引起宗气不足，宗气虚则肺的呼吸功能下降，因而喘促气短；热灼津液，故痰少而黏；肺肾阴虚，则见手足心热、潮热盗汗、口干欲饮；阴虚火动，男子会有遗精，女子会有闭经；舌红苔少，脉象细数，为阴虚火动之象。

【治法】滋补肺肾。

【方药】七味都气丸合生脉散。方解见"支气管哮喘"。七味都气丸与生脉散合用，前者补肾扶元，后者益肺生脉，使得金水相生，阴复热散，心肺兼顾，血脉通畅，其喘促自然平息。

Clinical manifestations：Asthma with rapid respiration and short breath, aggravation of dyspnea with movements, cough and scanty sputum or sticky sputum and difficulty to expectorate, feverish sensation over the palms and soles, tidal fever and night sweating, dry mouth with desire to drink, seminal emission in male, amenorrhoea in female, reddish tongue with scanty fur as well as thin and fast pulse.

Analysis：According to the theory of five phases, the lung pertains to metal, and the kidney pertains to water. Metal can generate water, therefore, the lung is regarded as the source or the mother of water (the kidney). The lung being the source of water, the kidney being the root of primordial qi, the relationship between the lung and kidney is just like that of mother and child. With shaoyang meridian and triple-energizer being their passage, the lung is associated with the kidney. Therefore, physiologically they form a relationship of intergeneration. However, from the perspective of pathology, they are mutually affected. The lung governs depuration, with preference for soft and moist substance. Insufficiency of lung yin gives rise to endogenous asthenic heat, which fumigates the lung, resulting in adverse flow of qi and cough; persistent cough impairs the lung and leads to deficiency of thoracic qi, which results in hypofunction of the lung in governing respiration, thus, giving rise to dyspnea with rapid respiration and shortness of breath; scanty and sticky sputum is due to heat scorching body fluid; feverish sensation over the palms and soles, tidal fever and night sweating and dry mouth with desire to drink are due to yin asthenia of the lung and kidney; seminal emission in male or amenorrhoea in female is caused by hyperactivity of fire because of yin asthenia; reddish tongue with scanty fur and thin and fast pulse are manifestations of fire hyperactivity because of yin asthenia.

Prescription：Moisten the lung and nourish the kidney.

Formulas：Qiwei Duqi Wan（Pill）combined with Shengmai San（Powder）. It has been discussed in the section of *Bronchial Asthma*. The former, Qiwei Duqi Wan, has the action of tonifying the kidney and restoring kidney qi, while the latter, Shengmai San, can benefit the lung and promote circulation of blood in the vessels. Combined together, they could achieve the effect of mutual generation of metal and water, restoring yin and dispelling heat, which could promote smooth circulation of blood in the vessels and subdue dyspnea with rapid respiration.

七、慢性胃炎

7　Chronic gastritis

〔**概说**〕 Summary

慢性胃炎是一种以胃黏膜炎症为主要病理变化的慢性疾病。临床表现多种多样，但以胃痛，或上腹部痞满、闷胀为主要症状，常伴有食欲不振、嗳气、恶心、呕吐、泛酸等症。本病属于中医学中的"胃脘痛""呕吐"等范畴。

中医学对慢性胃炎的治疗，有着独特的疗效优势，常以补泻兼施、寒热并用、升降有序、收散结合的治疗方法而取效。若配合饮食疗法，效果更为明显。临床上分为虚证与实证两大类。

Chronic gastritis refers to a chronic disease marked by pathological changes of gastric mucous membranes. Though it has got various clinical manifestations, the disease is mainly characterized by symptoms of stomachache, distention, fullness and oppression over the upper abdomen. It is usually accompanied with poor appetite, belching, nausea, vomiting as well as acid regurgitation. In terms of TCM, chronic gastritis pertains to "epigastric pain" "vomiting", and so on.

Treatment for chronic gastritis by means of TCM therapeutic methods is unique and of great curative effect, including combining supplementation with purgation, cold-natured drugs with hot-natured drugs, integrating uplifting with descending as well as astringing with dispersing. If combined with dietary therapy, the curative effect of the disease would be more obvious. In clinical practice, the disease is divided into sthenia syndrome and asthenia syndrome.

〔辨证论治〕 Syndrome differentiation and treatment

（一）实证
7.1 Sthenia syndrome

1. 寒凝气滞

7.1.1 Retention of pathogenic cold and qi stagnation

【症状】胃痛突然发作，疼痛剧烈，畏寒喜热，得温痛减，口不渴，喜热饮，口流清涎，舌苔薄白而滑，脉象弦紧或弦迟。

【分析】由于胃脘部受寒，或饮食生冷，而致寒积胃中。寒为阴邪，其性凝滞，阳气被寒邪所遏，胃失通降，故发疼痛；寒邪主事，欲散寒邪，故喜热畏寒，并喜热饮；口流清涎，为胃寒之象；苔白而滑，为寒凝所致；弦脉主痛，紧脉与迟脉主寒，脉证互参，为寒凝气滞之征。

【治法】温胃散寒，行气止痛。

【方药】良附丸加味。良附丸由高良姜、香附二味组成。高良姜温胃散寒，香附行气止痛。若寒重者，加干姜、吴茱萸；气滞甚者，加木香、陈皮；呕恶甚者，加苏叶、生姜；不思饮食者，加麦芽、鸡内金；大便稀薄，一日数次者，加肉豆蔻、炒山药；若胃脘疼痛，舌苔腻而润者，可改用半夏泻心汤，辛开苦降、燥湿清热。

Clinical manifestations: Acute pain in the epigastrium, aversion to cold and preference for warmth, alleviation of pain with warmth, no thirst, preference for hot drink, regurgitation of clear saliva and fluid, thin and whitish and slippery fur as well as taut and tense pulse or taut and slow pulse.

Analysis: Accumulation of cold in the stomach is due to exogenous pathogenic cold factors attacking the stomach, or intake of raw and cold food. Cold is a pathogenic factor of yin with the nature of stagnancy, cold pathogen obstructing yang qi and failure of stomach qi to transport and descend cause epigastric pain; aversion to cold and preference for warmth and hot drink are due to tendency to dispel hyperactive pathogenic cold; regurgitation of clear saliva and fluid indicates cold in the stomach; whitish slippery fur is caused by stagnation of cold; taut pulse indicates pain, tense pulse and slow pulse suggest cold syndrome. The above pulse conditions as well as manifestations signify the syndrome of cold retention and qi stagnation.

Prescription: Warm the stomach to dispel cold and activate qi to stop pain.

Formulas: Liangfu Wan Jiawei (Modified Liangfu Pill). Liangfu Wan is made up of Gaoliangjiang (*Rhizoma Alpiniae Officinarum*) and Xiangfu (*Rhizoma Cyperi*). Gaoliangjian has an action of warming the stomach and dispelling cold, Xiangfu can activate qi to stop pain. For severe cold, Ganjiang (*Rhizoma Zingiberis*) and Wuzhuyu (*Fructus Evodiae*) can be added; for heavy qi stagnation, Muxiang (*Radix Aucklandiae*) and Chenpi (*Pericarpium*

Citri Reticulatae）can be added；for severe vomiting，Suye（*Folium Perillae*）and Shengjiang（*Rhizoma Zingiberis Recens*）can be combined；for poor appetite，Maiya（*Fructus Hordei Germinatus*）and Jineijin（*Endothelium Corneum Gigeriae Galli*）can be combined；for frequent defecation with loose and thin stool each day，Roudoukou（*Semen Myristicae*）and stir-baked Shanyao（*Rhizoma Dioscoreae*）can be added；for epigastric pain and greasy and moist fur，Banxia Xiexin Tang（Decoction），pungent and bitter in flavor，can be used to replace Liangfu Wan with its action of dispersing，descending qi，drying dampness and clearing heat.

2. 饮食积滞
7.1.2　Food retention

【症状】胃脘胀满，疼痛拒按，嗳腐吞酸，或呕吐不消化食物，吐后胃脘较舒，不思饮食，大便不爽，舌苔厚腻，脉象弦滑。

【分析】饮食不洁或不节，食滞中焦，脾胃纳运失常，胃失和降，故胃脘胀满而疼痛，或呕吐不消化食物；胃气上逆，则嗳腐吞酸；脾胃被食物所遏制，故不思饮食；腑气不通，故大便不爽；苔厚腻、脉弦滑，均为食滞之象。

【治法】消食和胃。

【方药】保和丸。方中山楂消油腻腥膻之食，神曲消酒食陈腐之积，麦芽消五谷之积，莱菔子下气消胀；伤食必有湿，故用茯苓健脾而渗湿；积久必生热，故用连翘散结而清热；半夏和胃而健脾；陈皮能升能降，和胃理气。人以胃气为本，本方正是为消除胃中食积而设，食积消除，胃气恢复，所以名为"保和丸"。

Clinical manifestations：Distention and fullness in the epigastrium，unpressable pain，eructation with fetid odor and acid regurgitation，or vomiting undigested food，restored comfortable sensation in the stomach after vomiting，poor appetite，unsmooth defecation，thick greasy fur as well as taut and slippery pulse.

Analysis：Distention，fullness and pain in the epigastrium or vomiting undigested food are caused by failure of stomach qi to descend due to food retention in middle energizer and dysfunction of the spleen and stomach in transportation and transformation because of improper diet or excessive intake of food；eructation with fetid odor and acid regurgitation are due to adverse flow of stomach qi；poor appetite is caused by obstruction of food in the spleen and stomach；unsmooth defecation is due to qi stagnation in fu organs；thick and greasy fur and taut and slippery pulse are signs of food retention.

Prescription：Eliminate indigested food and harmonize the stomach.

Formulas：Baohe Wan（Pill）. In this formula，Shanzha（*Fructus Crataegi*）can help digest greasy food as well as food with smell of fish and mutton，Shenqu（*Massa Medicata Fermentata*）has an action of helping eliminate retention of alcoholic drink and stale and decayed food，Maiya（*Fructus Hordei Germinatus*）can eliminate retention of food of refined and coarse grains，Laifuzi（*Semen Raphani*）can send down qi and get rid of epigastric distention；dyspepsia due to improper diet or intemperance of eating must result in retention of dampness, so Fuling (*Poriae Cocos*) can be used to invigorate the spleen and resolve dampness; prolonged food retention must generate endogenous heat, so Lianqiao (*Fructus Forsythiae*) can be combined to disperse stagnation and clear away heat; Banxia (*Rhizoma Pinelliae*) can harmonize the stomach and invigorate the spleen; Chenpi (*Pericarpium Citri Reticulatae*) has an action of lifting, descending as well as regulating stomach qi. Stomach qi is the source of life of human being. The formula is designed to eliminate food retention in the stomach. With food retention eliminated, stomach qi could be restored, thus, it is named as "Baohe wan (Pill)".

3. 肝郁气滞
7.1.3　Stagnation of qi and liver depression

【症状】胃脘胀痛，攻痛两胁，按之较舒，善太息，每遇烦恼、郁闷而痛作，苔多薄白，脉象沉弦。

【分析】情志不舒，肝气不得疏泄，横逆犯胃，则引起胃脘胀痛；两胁为肝经之分野，气郁于本经，故两胁攻痛；善太息者，肝气欲舒展也；苔薄白、脉沉弦，为肝郁湿阻之象；如夹食，苔必厚腻；欲化火，则舌质转红，脉亦带数象。

【治法】疏肝理气。

【方药】柴胡疏肝汤。方中以柴胡、赤芍、川芎、香附疏肝解郁为主药；陈皮、甘草顺气和中为佐药，共收理气止痛之效。若泛酸者，加黄连、吴茱萸；痛甚者，加川楝子、延胡索；不思食者，加生麦芽、鸡内金。

Clinical manifestations: Distending pain in the epigastrium involves the hypochondrium, alleviation of pain with pressing, frequent sigh, occurrence of pain accompanied with vexation and emotional depression, thin whitish tongue fur as well as sunken and taut pulse.

Analysis: Epigastric distending pain is caused by emotional depression, which fails to disperse liver qi, thus, giving rise to adverse flow of stagnated liver qi attacking the stomach; the hypochondrium are the line by which liver meridians are divided, qi stagnation in liver meridian gives rise to pain in the hypochondrium; frequent sigh indicates susceptibility of liver qi to being dispersed; thin whitish tongue fur and sunken and taut pulse are signs of obstruction of dampness due to liver qi stagnation; thick and greasy fur indicates food retention, tongue turning into reddish and fast pulse suggest transformation of fire from qi stagnation.

Prescription: Soothe the liver and regulate qi.

Formulas: Chaihu Shugan Tang (Decoction). In the recipe, Chaihu (*Radix Bupleuri*), Chishao (*Radix Paeoniae Rubra*), Chuanxiong (*Rhizoma Ligustici Chuanxiong*) and Xiangfu (*Rhizoma Cyperi*), with the action of soothing the liver and dispelling qi oppression, are used as principal drug; Chenpi (*Pericarpium Citri reticulatae*) and Gancao (*Radix Glycyrrhizae*), with the action of guiding qi downward and harmonizing middle energizer, are used as assistant drug to achieve the effect of regulating qi and stopping pain. For acid regurgitation, Huanglian (*Rhizoma Coptidis*) and Wuzhuyu (*Fructus Evodiae*) can be added; for worsening pain, Chuanlianzi (*Fructus Meliae Toosendan*) and Yanhusuo (*Rhizoma Corydalis*) could be added; for poor appetite, Shengmaiya (*Fructus Hordei Germinatus*) and Jineijin (*Endothelium Corneum Gigeriae Galli*) can be combined.

（二）虚证
7.2 Asthenia syndrome

1. 脾胃虚寒
7.2.1 Asthenic cold of the spleen and stomach

【症状】胃痛隐隐，泛吐清水，喜按喜暖，得食则减，神疲乏力，手足不温，饮食减少，大便溏薄，舌质淡红，脉象细弱。

【分析】脾寒胃弱，纳食不多，健运迟缓，故胃痛隐隐，喜按喜暖；泛吐清水，为胃寒之象；大便溏薄，为脾失健运所致；脾主四肢，脾阳虚弱，不能温阳四肢，故手足不温；舌质淡红、脉象细弱，为中焦虚寒，阳气不足的表现。

【治法】温阳益气健中。

【方药】黄芪建中汤加味。方用黄芪补益中气，饴糖补虚健中；合用桂枝温阳散寒，白芍、甘草和中止痛；生姜、大枣健脾胃而和营卫。如泛吐清水，加陈皮、半夏；吐酸水者，去饴糖，加黄连、吴茱萸；胃寒痛甚者，加良附丸。

Clinical manifestations: Dull pain in the stomach, regurgitation of clear fluid and saliva, preference for pressing and warmth, alleviation of pain with intake of food, dispiritedness and lack of energy, cold limbs, reduced appetite, loose stool, pale reddish tongue as well as thin and weak pulse.

Analysis: Dull pain in the stomach and preference for pressing and warmth are due to anorexia and slow transportation and transformation of the spleen because of cold in the spleen and asthenia of the stomach; regurgitation of clear fluid and saliva is a sign of cold in the stomach; loose stool is caused by dysfunction of the spleen; the spleen dominates the limbs, failure of asthenic yang of the spleen to warm the limbs gives rise to cold limbs; pale reddish tongue and thin and weak pulse are signs of asthenic cold in middle energizer and insufficiency of yang qi.

Prescription: Warm yang, benefit qi and invigorate middle energizer.

Formulas: Huangqi Jianzhong Tang Jiawei (Modified Huangqi Jianzhong Decoction). In the recipe, Huangqi (*Radix Astragali seu Hedysari*) has an effect of supplementing qi in middle energizer, Yitang (*Saccharum Granorum*) can replenish asthenia and strengthen middle energizer; Guizhi (*Ramulus Cinnamomi*) has an action of warming yang and expelling cold, Baishao (*Radix Paeoniae Alba*) and Gancao (*Radix Glycyrrhizae*) can regulate middle energizer and stop pain, Shengjiang (*Rhizoma Zingiberis Recens*) and Dazao (*Fructus Jujubae*) can invigorate the spleen and the stomach and reconcile nutrient qi and defensive qi. For regurgitation of clear fluid and saliva, Chenpi (*Pericarpium Citri reticulatae*) and Banxia

(*Rhizoma Pinelliae*) can be added; for acid regurgitation, Yitang should be removed from this fomula, and Huanglian (*Rhizoma Coptidis*) and Wuzhuyu (*Fructus Evodiae*) can be added; for worsening pain and cold in the stomach, Liangfu Wan (Pill) can be combined.

2. 脾胃阴虚

7.2.2 Yin asthenia of the spleen and stomach

【症状】胃脘隐隐作痛，有灼热感，烦渴欲饮，口燥咽干，饮食减少，大便干结，舌质红赤，苔少，脉象细数或弦细。

【分析】阴虚作痛，常因肝郁化火，灼伤脾胃之阴，或因胃热素盛，或因寒邪入里化热，或长期服用辛燥之药，使脾胃之阴暗伤日久，所以呈现一派阴虚内燥之症，如隐痛灼热、烦渴欲饮、口燥咽干等。最为明证的是：舌质红赤、苔少、脉象细数，这是与其他慢性胃炎中的胃脘痛所不同的，这也是本证的辨证要点。

【治法】养阴益胃。

【方药】益胃汤合竹叶石膏汤。方用沙参、麦冬、玉竹、生地黄甘润养阴益胃；竹叶、石膏甘寒清胃泻热；半夏降逆；甘草、大枣甘润和中。如是肝火犯胃，当养肝清胃，方用一贯煎，方用生地黄、枸杞子滋阴；沙参、麦冬益胃；当归养血活血；川楝子疏肝理气。吞酸者，加瓦楞子、川贝母；食少者，加生麦芽、山楂、神曲等。

Clinical manifestations: Dull pain in the epigastrium, scorching sensation, polydypsia with desire for drink, dry mouth and throat, reduced appetite, constipation, reddish tongue with scanty fur as well as thin and fast pulse or taut and thin pulse.

Analysis: Pain due to yin asthenia is usually caused by fire transformed from liver qi stagnation scording yin in the spleen and stomach, or by persistent hyperactive heat in the stomach, or by heat transformed from invasion of pathogenic cold factors into the interior, or by taking pungent-dry flavored drugs for a long time. Prolonged impairment of yin in the spleen and stomach by these factors brings about the syndrome of yin asthenia and endogenous dryness with the following manifestations such as dull pain, scorching sensation, polydypsia with desire for drink as well as dry mouth and throat. The most obvious sign of this syndrome is reddish tongue with scanty fur as well as thin and fast pulse, which is different from epigastric pain in other syndromes of chronic gastritis. Therefore, it is the key point for syndrome differentiation.

Prescription: Nourish yin and benefit the stomach.

Formulas: Yiwei Tang (Decoction) combined with Zhuye Shigao Tang (Decoction). In the formula, Shashen (*Adenophora stricta*), Maidong (*Radix Ophiopogonis*), Yuzhu (*Rhizoma Polygonati Odorati*) and Shengdihuang (*Radix Rehmanniae Recens*), sweet and moist in nature, can nourish yin and tonify the stomach; Zhuye (*Herba Lophatheri*) and Shigao (*Gypsum Fibrosum*) may clear away heat in the stomach with their sweet and cold nature; Banxia (*Rhizoma Pinelliae*) has an action of descending adverse flow of qi; Gancao (*Radix Glycyrrhizae*) and Dazao (*Fructus Jujubae*), sweat and moist in nature, can harmonize middle energizer. For liver fire attacking the stomach, Yiguan Jian (Decoction) should be applied to nourish the liver and clear away stomach fire, of which, Shengdihuang and Gouqizi (*Fructus Lycii*) have an action of nourishing yin; Shashen and Maidong can benefit stomach qi; Danggui (*Radix Angelicae Sinensis*) has an effect of nourishing blood and promoting circulation of blood; and Chuanlianzi (*Fructus Meliae Toosendan*) can soothe the liver and regulate qi. For acid regurgitation, Walengzi (*Concha Arcae*) and Chuanbeimu (*Bulbus Fritillariae Cirrhosae*) should be combined; for reduced appetite, Shengmaiya (*Fructus Hordei Germinatus*), Shanzha (*Fructus Crataegi*) as well as Shenqu (*Massa Medicata Fermentata*) should be added.

八、慢性腹泻

8　Chronic Diarrhea

〔**概说**〕　Summary

慢性腹泻是指排便次数多于平日，粪便稀薄，水分增多，或含未消化食物，或含脓血。其病程应在 2 个月以上，或间歇期在 2~4 周内的复发性腹泻。

慢性腹泻属于中医学"泄泻"范畴，中医学对该病早有认识，指出"泄泻之本，无不由乎脾胃"。说明脾胃是发生腹泻的主要环节。对其治疗，中医学积累有丰富的经验，许多治疗方药已被西医所接受并在临床使用。

Chronic diarrhea refers to the pathological condition marked by frequent discharge of loose and watery stool, or indigested food, or stool mingled with pus, blood and mucus. Generally speaking, the course of chronic diarrhea can last over two months. However, recurrent diarrhea can have its intermission about 2~4 weeks.

In terms of TCM, chronic diarrhea is classified into "diarrhea" and the recognition of the disease starts from the early time. It is thought that "Diarrhea is usually caused by the stomach or spleen", which indicates that the stomach and the spleen are the key organs that cause diarrhea. As to the treatment for the disease, lots of useful experience has been accumulated, and many formulas have been accepted and applied to clinical practice even by doctors of Western medicine nowadays.

〔**辨证论治**〕　Syndrome differentiation and treatment

1. 肝郁脾虚

8.1　Syndrome of asthenic spleen and stagnation of liver qi

【**症状**】平时有胸胁闷胀，嗳气食少，每因抑郁、恼怒或精神紧张时，发生腹痛泄泻，伴有小腹胀气，舌质淡红，苔薄白，脉象弦细。

【分析】病由肝气郁结，横逆脾土，脾土受伤，失于健运所致。每因肝气不舒时发作，脾不健运，水谷之湿不能运化，故发作腹痛泄泻；胸胁闷胀、嗳气食少，是肝气郁结之征；舌质淡红、苔薄白，脾虚使也；脉象弦细，为肝郁之象。

【治法】抑肝扶脾。

【方药】痛泻要方加味。方用白术健脾，白芍柔肝益阴，陈皮理气醒脾，防风辛散疏肝。四药合用，具有疏肝补脾、调和胃肠之功。若舌边红赤者，加左金丸（黄连、吴茱萸）以收清泻肝火、健脾和胃之效。

Clinical manifestations: Frequent distention and fullness in the chest and hypochondrium, belching and poor appetite. Outbreak of diarrhea due to abdominal pain at the time of emotional depression, rage or nervousness is accompanied with distention and fullness of the lower abdomen, reddish tongue, thin and whitish fur as well as thin and taut pulse.

Analysis: This syndrome is caused by stagnation of liver qi and invasion of adverse flow of liver qi into the spleen, which give rise to impairment of the spleen and dysfunction of the spleen in transportation. Outbreak of diarrhea and pain over the lower abdomen accompanied with stagnation of liver qi are due to failure to disperse liver qi and dysfunction of the spleen in transporting and transforming food; distention and fullness in the chest and hypochondrium, belching and little repast are manifestations of stagnation of liver qi; reddish tongue with thin whitish fur is due to splenic asthenia; taut and thin pulse is a sign of liver qi stagnation.

Prescription: Restrain stagnation of liver qi and strengthen the spleen.

Formulas: Tongxie Yaofang Jiawei (Modified essential formula for severe diarrhea). In the formula, Baizhu (*Rhizoma Atractylodis Macrocephalae*) can invigorate the spleen; Baishao (*Radix Paeoniae Alba*) has an action of softening the liver and benefiting yin; Chenpi (*Pericarpium Citri Reticulatae*) can regulate qi and reinforce the spleen; Fangfeng (*Radix Sapos nikoviae*), pungent in flavor, has an effect of dispersing and dispelling stagnation of liver qi, Combined together, the above herbs can dispel stagnation of liver qi, invigorate the spleen and harmonize the stomach and intestines. For reddish tongue tip and margin, Zuojin Wan (Pill), including Huanglian (*Rhizoma Coptidi*s) and Wuzhuyu (*Fructus Evodiae*), can be added to purge liver fire, invigorate the spleen and harmonize the stomach.

2. 食滞中焦

8.2　Food retention in middle energizer

【症状】腹痛肠鸣，泻下粪便臭如败卵，泻后痛减，伴有不消化食物，嗳腐吞酸，食欲减退，食后胃脘痞满，舌苔厚腻，脉滑。

【分析】本证由饮食不节，宿食内停，伤及胃肠所致。宿食内停，使脾胃升降的功能失常，故腹痛肠鸣；饮食不化，浊气上逆，则嗳腐吞酸；食积不化而腐败，则泻下粪便如败卵；浊物得以泻下，故泻后痛减；胃肠为饮食所伤，则食欲减退，食后胃脘痞满；舌苔厚腻、脉滑，为食滞内困之象。

【治法】消食导滞。

【方药】保和丸（组成与方义见"慢性胃炎"）。若腹痛明显者，可加木香、槟榔；食滞化热，大便黏滞不爽，加黄连、黄芩、大黄；如果食滞较重，脘腹胀满，可因势利导，依据"通因通用"的原则，改用枳实导滞丸，本方以大黄、枳实为主药，推荡积滞，使邪有出路，从而达到邪去正安的效果。

Clinical manifestations：Abdominal pain with borborygmus, stool with putrid and foul odor like that of decayed egg, alleviation of pain after diarrhea with indigested food, eructation with fetid odor and acid regurgitation, reduced appetite, gastric fullness after meals, thick and greasy tongue fur as well as slippery pulse.

Analysis：Abdominal pain with borborygmus is caused by excessive intake of food and internal retention of food in the stomach as well as dysfunction of the stomach and spleen in receiving and transporting food; eructation with fetid odor and acid regurgitation are due to retention of indigested food leading to adverse flow of turbid qi; stool with putrid and foul odor like that of decayed egg is due to decaying of indigested food; alleviation of pain after diarrhea is due to discharge of putrid stool; reduced appetite and gastric fullness after meals are due to excessive intake of food which impairs the stomach and intestines; thick and greasy tongue fur as well as slippery pulse is a sign of internal food stagnation.

Prescription：Promote digestion of food and discharge dyspeptic retention.

Formulas：Baohe Wan（Pill）（It has been discussed in the section of *Chronic Gastritis*）. For obvious abdominal pain, Muxiang（*Radix Aucklandiae*）and Binlang（*Semen Arecae*）can be added; for transformation of heat from food retention and sticky unsmooth defecation, Huanglian（*Rhizoma Coptidis*）, Huangqin（*Radix Scutellariae*）and Dahuang（*Radix et Rhizoma Rhei*）should be combined with the formula; for severe food stagnation and distending fullness in the stomach and abdomen, Zhishi Daozhi Wan（Pill）can be used to replace Baohe Wan according to the principle of "treating diarrhea with purgative" to discharge stool. Dahuang and Zhishi（*Fructus Aurantii Immaturus*）, with the action of discharging food stagnation, are used as the essential drug of the formula to achieve the effect of expelling pathogens and reinforcing healthy qi.

3. 脾胃虚弱
8.3 Asthenia of the spleen and stomach

【症状】大便时溏时泻，迁延反复，水谷不化，稍进油腻食物，则大便次数明显增多，饮食减少，食后脘腹不舒，面色萎黄，精神疲倦，舌苔淡白，脉象细弱。

【分析】劳力过度，伤及脾胃之气，使脾胃虚弱，清阳之气不能升发，运化失常，清浊不分，故大便时溏时泻，水谷不化；脾虚运化无权，则饮食减少，或食后脘腹胀满；久泻伤及气血，故面色萎黄、精神疲倦；舌苔淡白、脉象细弱，均为脾虚胃弱之象。

【治法】健脾益胃。

【方药】参苓白术散。方中人参、白术、茯苓、甘草为补气之祖方——四君子汤，具有健脾益气和胃的作用；砂仁、陈皮、桔梗、白扁豆、怀山药、莲子、薏苡仁，理气健脾化湿，是治疗脾虚泄泻的常用药物。若脾阳不振，阴寒内盛，可改用附子理中汤温中散寒；若久泻不止，中气下陷，兼有脱肛者，可用补中益气汤健脾止泻，益气升阳。

Clinical manifestations: Persistent alternation of loose stool and diarrhea with indigested food, abnormal frequency of defecation due to intake of greasy food, reduced appetite, gastric and abdominal discomfort after meals, sallow complexion, lassitude, pale tongue fur as well as thin and weak pulse.

Analysis: Overstrain impairs gastrosplenic qi and asthenia of the spleen and stomach, giving rise to failure of lucid yang qi to rise, dysfunction of the spleen to transport and transform as well as failure to separate lucidity from turbidity, which causes occasional loose stool and diarrhea with indigested food; reduced appetite or gastric and abdominal discomfort after meals is caused by failure of the spleen to transport and transform; sallow complexion and lassitude are due to chronic diarrhea impairing qi and blood; pale tongue fur and thin and weak pulse are signs of asthenia of the spleen and stomach.

Prescription: Invigorate the spleen and benefit the stomach.

Formulas: Shen Ling Baizhu San (Powder). In the formula, Renshen (*Radix Ginseng*), Baizhu (*Rhizoma Atractylodis Macrocephalae*), Fuling (*Poriae Cocos*) and Gancao (*Radix Glycyrrhizae*) constitute Sijunzi Tang, a secret recipe handed down from ancestors for supplementing qi, which possesses the action of invigorating the spleen, benefiting qi as well as harmonizing the stomach; Sharen (*Fructus Amomi Villosi*), Chenpi (*Pericarpium Citri Reticulatae*), Jiegeng (*Radix Platycodonis*), Baibiandou (*Semen Dolichoris Album*), Huaishanyao (*Rhizoma Dioscoreae*), Lianzi (*Semen Nelumbinis*) and Yiyiren (*Semen Coicis*) can regulate qi, invigorate the spleen and resolve dampness, and they are also commonly used for diarrhea due to spleen asthenia. For hypoactivity of spleen yang and hyperactivity of yin cold, Fuzi Lizhong Tang (Decoction) can replace the above recipe to warm middle energizer and dispel cold. For prolonged diarrhea, sinking of gastrosplenic qi coupled with prolapse of the anus, Buzhong Yiqi Tang (Decoction) could be used to invigorate the spleen and stop diarrhea by benefiting qi and lifting yang.

4. 寒湿内停

8.4 Internal retention of cold and dampness

【症状】泄泻清稀，甚则大便如水样，腹痛肠鸣，胃脘痞闷，饮食减少，苔白腻，脉象濡缓。若兼外感风寒，则恶寒发热，头痛，肢体酸痛，苔薄白，脉象浮紧。

【分析】本证由于寒湿之邪侵袭肠胃，使脾胃升降功能失调，清浊不分，传导失司，故见泄泻清稀。寒湿内停，使气机阻塞不通，故腹痛肠鸣；寒湿蒙蔽清阳，则胃脘痞闷，饮食减少。若外感风寒，则会出现恶寒发热、肢体酸痛等风寒外束症状。

【治法】温化寒湿，芳香化浊。

【方药】轻者用平胃散，重者用胃苓汤；兼风寒表证，用藿香正气散。

平胃散由苍术、厚朴、橘皮、甘草、生姜、大枣组成，具有健脾、燥湿散寒的作用。胃苓汤乃平胃散与五苓散组合而成，五苓散由茯苓、猪苓、泽泻、白术、桂枝组成，功能行气利水。藿香正气散中的紫苏叶、白芷解表散寒；藿香辛温散寒，芳香化浊；陈皮、半夏理气化浊，和中止呕；厚朴、大腹皮理气除满；茯苓、白术健脾化湿。本方既能疏风散寒、解表祛湿，又能健脾和中、调理肠胃。不管是外湿或内湿侵袭胃肠，该方均可使胃肠功能得到恢复，泄泻自止。

Clinical manifestations: Diarrhea with thin and clear stool even with watery stool, abdominal pain with borborygmus, gastric fullness and oppression, reduced appetite, greasy and whitish tongue fur as well as soft and moderate pulse. If the syndrome is complicated with exogenous wind cold, the disease can present the following signs such as aversion to cold, fever, headache, aching sensation of body and limbs, thin and whitish tongue fur as well as floating and tense pulse.

Analysis: Diarrhea with thin and clear stool is due to pathogenic cold and dampness factors attacking the stomach and intestines, which gives rise to hypofunction of the spleen and stomach in descending and ascending, failure to separate lucidity from turbidity as well as dysfunction of the spleen and stomach in transportation of food. Abdominal pain with borborygmus is caused by obstruction of qi due to retention of cold and dampness; gastric fullness, oppression and reduced appetite are due to cold and dampness blocking lucid yang; syndrome of wind cold encumbering the superficies with such symptoms as aversion to cold, fever and aching sensation of the body and limbs will arise if the syndrome is complicated with exogenous wind cold.

Prescription: Resolve cold and dampness by warming and dissolve turbidity by applying aromatic natured herbs.

Formulas: Pingwei San (Powder) for common or unserious cases, Weiling Tang (Decoction) for severe cases, as well as Huoxiang Zhengqi San (Powder) if the syndrome is complicated with syndrome of exogenous wind and cold.

Pingwei San consists of Cangzhu (*Rhizoma Atractylodis*), Houpo (*Cortex Magnoliae Officinals*), Jupi (*Exocarpium Citri Grandis*), Gancao (*Radix Glycyrrhizae*), Shengjiang (*Rhizoma Zingiberis Recens*) and Dazao (*Fructus Jujubae*), and it possesses an effect of invigorating the spleen, drying dampness as well as expelling cold. Weiling Tang is the combination of Pingwei San and Wuling San. Wuling San, made up of Fuling (*Poriae Cocos*), Zhuling (*Polyporus Umbellatus*), Zexie (*Rhizoma Alismatis*), Baizhu (*Rhizoma Atractylodis Macrocephalae*) and Guizhi (*Ramulus Cinnamomi*), has an action of promoting qi circulation and inducing diuresis. In Huoxiang Zhengqi San, Zisuye (*Folium Perillae*) and Baizhi (*Radix Angelicae Dahuricae*) can relieve superficies and expel cold; Huoxiang (*Herba Agastachis*), pungent in flavor, warm in nature, has a function of expelling cold and dissolving turbidity; Chenpi (*Pericarpium Citri reticulatae*) and Banxia (*Rhizoma Pinelliae*) can regulate qi, dissolve turbidity, harmonize the stomach and spleen and stop vomiting;

Houpo (*Cortex Magnoliae Officinals*) and Dafupi (*Pericarpium Arecae*) are used to promote qi circulation and remove distention and fullness; Fuling (*Poriae Cocos*) and Baizhu (*Rhizoma Atractylodis Macrocephalae*) can invigorate the spleen and resolve dampness. This recipe has not only the action of dispelling wind, expelling cold, relieving superficies as well as resolving dampness, but it could also invigorate the spleen, harmonize the stomach and regulate the stomach and intestines. Whether dampness comes from the exterior or it is generated from the interior, the above formulas can restore normal function of the stomach and intestines, which, in turn, can relieve diarrhea naturally.

5. 湿热壅滞
8.5　Stagnation of dampness and heat

【症状】泄泻腹痛，泻下急迫，或泻而不爽，大便黄褐色，气味秽臭，肛门灼热，烦热口渴，小便短赤，舌苔黄腻，脉象滑数或濡数。

【分析】湿热壅滞大肠，则泻下急迫；湿热互结，故泻而不爽；湿热下注，壅滞不化，则呈现肛门灼热、粪便气味秽臭、小便短赤等症状；舌苔黄腻、脉象滑数等，为湿热内盛之象。

【治法】清热利湿。

【方药】葛根芩连汤加味。葛根芩连汤为治疗湿热泄泻的首选方药，方中葛根解肌清热，煨用能升清止泻；黄芩、黄连苦寒清热燥湿；甘草甘缓和中。偏湿重者，加薏苡仁、赤小豆；夹食积者，加神曲、山楂、麦芽；发热、头痛者，加金银花、连翘、薄荷；小便短赤者，加六一散（冲服）。

Clinical manifestations: Fulmination of diarrhea with abdominal pain, or diarrhea with unsmooth sensation, dark yellowish stool with putrid and foul odor, scorching sensation of the anus, dysphoria and thirst, scanty and brownish urine, yellowish and greasy tongue fur as well as floating and fast pulse or soft and fast pulse.

Analysis: Fulmination of diarrhea is due to stagnation of heat in the large intestine; diarrhea with unsmooth sensation is caused by accumulation of dampness and heat; scorching sensation of the anus, stool with putrid and foul odor and scanty brownish urine are due to stagnation and downward migration of unresolved damp heat; greasy and yellowish tongue fur and floating and fast pulse are signs of exuberance of internal dampness and heat.

Prescription: Clear away heat and resolve dampness.

Formulas: Gegen Huangqin Huanglian Tang Jiawei (Modified Gegen Huangqin Huanglian Decoction). It is the best choice for damp-heat diarrhea. In the recipe, Gegen (*Radix Puerariae*) is used to clear away heat by expelling pathogenic factors from the muscles, and Gegen roasted in hot ashes can lift lucid yang and stop diarrhea; Huangqin (*Radix Scutellariae*) and Huanglian (*Rhizoma Coptidis*), bitter and cold in nature, can clear away heat and dry dampness; Gancao (*Radix Glycyrrhizae*), sweet in flavor, can harmonize the stomach and spleen to a moderate degree. For severe dampness, Yiyiren (*Semen Coicis*) and

Chixiaodou (*Semen Phaseoli*) could be added; for food retention, Shenqu (*Massa Medicata Fermentata*), Shanzha (*Fructus Crataegi*) and Maiya (*Fructus Hordei Germinatus*) should be added; for fever and headache, Jinyinhua (*Flos Lonicerae*), Lianqiao (*Fructus Forsythiae*) and Bohe (*Herba Menthae*) can be combined; for scanty and brownish urine, Liuyi San (Powder), taken for oral use, can be combined with the above recipe.

6. 肾阳虚衰
8.6 Asthenia and declination of kidney yang

【症状】黎明之前脐腹作痛，肠鸣即泻，泻后即安，平时形寒肢冷，腰膝酸软，舌淡苔白，脉象沉细。

【分析】肾阳虚馁，不能温煦脾土，黎明之前，阳气未振，阴寒未退，寒邪作祟，故脐腹作痛；肠鸣者，寒邪主事也；泻后寒邪去也，故泻后即安；其他均为脾肾阳虚之象。

【治法】温补脾肾，固涩止泻。

【方药】理中汤合四神丸。理中汤温中健脾；四神丸中，补骨脂温补肾阳，吴茱萸、肉豆蔻温中散寒，五味子收敛止泻。两个方子，一个偏于温补脾阳，一个偏于温补肾阳，两方配伍，相得益彰，用于脾肾阳虚之泄泻，疗效突出。若泄泻日久，中气下陷，适当加入升阳固涩之品，如黄芪、升麻、柴胡、诃子、赤石脂等，有固本扶正之效。

Clinical manifestations: Abdominal pain in the peri-navel region before the dawn, diarrhea with borborygmus, alleviation after diarrhea, cold body and limbs, aching and weakness of the loins and knees, pale tongue with whitish fur as well as thin and sunken pulse.

Analysis: Asthenic kidney yang fails to warm the spleen. Hypofunction of yang qi and retaining of yin and cold before the dawn result in hyperactivity of pathogenic cold factors, which gives rise to abdominal pain in the peri-navel region; borborygmus indicates the domination of cold pathogen; alleviation after diarrhea is due to elimination of cold pathogen; other symptoms are signs of yang asthenia of the spleen and kidney.

Prescription: Warm and supplement the spleen and kidney, induce astringency and relieve diarrhea.

Formulas: Lizhong Tang (Decoction) combined with Sishen Wan (Pill). Lizhong Tang has an action of warming middle energizer (the spleen and stomach) and invigorating the spleen. In Sishen Wan, Buguzhi (*Fructus Psoraleae*) can warm and supplement kidney yang, Wuzhuyu (*Fructus Evodiae*) and Roudoukou (*Semen Myristicae*) can warm middle energizer and expel cold, Wuweizi (*Fructus Schisandrae Chinensis*) has an effect of inducing astringency and stopping diarrhea. The former recipe is prone to warming splenic yang, while the latter is prone to warming kidney yang, combined together, both of them could achieve an remarkable effect for treating diarrhea due to yang asthenia of the spleen and kidney. For prolonged chronic diarrhea and qi sinking in middle energizer, Huangqi (*Radix Astragali seu*

Hedysari）, Shengma（*Rhizoma Cimicifugae*）, Chaihu（*Radix Bupleuri*）, Hezi（*Fructus Chebulae*）and Chishizhi（*Halloysitum Rubrum*）can be added to lift yang and induce astringency so as to strengthen healthy qi, however, the amount of these herbs should be based on various cases.

九、胃及十二指肠溃疡

9　Gastroduodenal ulcer

〔**概说**〕 Summary

　　胃及十二肠溃疡是一种具有反复发作倾向的慢性胃肠道疾病，因溃疡的形成和发展与胃液中的胃酸及胃蛋白酶的消化有关，故又称消化性溃疡。

　　本病以胃痛、嗳气、泛酸、恶心、呕吐、食欲不振为主要表现。根据临床症状与病因病机，可将本病归属于中医学中的"胃脘痛""嘈杂""吞酸""痞满"等范畴。从汉代张仲景，到元代李东垣，迨至清代叶天士等医学家，对本病的辨证论治都积有丰富的临床经验，他们的经验用方至今仍被中西医所喜用。

Gastroduodenal ulcer refers to chronic pathological change in the stomach and intestines with a tendency to frequent outbreak. It is also known as digestive ulcer, since its formation and development are related to gastric acid and pepsin.

Clinically, the disease is marked by stomachache, belching, nausea, vomiting, poor appetite, etc. According to its clinical manifestations, etiology and pathogenesis, the disease can pertain to"epigastric pain""epigastric discomfort""acid regurgitation"or"distending fullness" in TCM. Lots of useful clinical experience has been collected by TCM experts such as Zhang Zhongjing from the Han Dynasty, Li Dongyuan from the Yuan Dynasty, as well as Ye Tianshi from the Qing Dynasty, and has been applied in TCM as well as Western medicine up to now.

〔**辨证论治**〕 Syndrome differentiation and treatment

1. 肝胃气滞

9.1　Syndrome of qi stagnation in the liver and stomach

　　【症状】胃脘胀痛，攻撑两胁，嗳气或呃逆频繁，得矢气而痛减，大便不爽，胃脘痛每因情绪变化而发作，舌苔薄白，脉象弦略紧。

　　【分析】本证由肝气犯胃而作。肝气犯胃，使中焦气机升降失常，气滞中焦，并攻撑两胁，故胃脘及胁痛；胃失和降，则会嗳气或呃逆；得矢气则胃气暂缓，故痛减；胃气通降无力，故大便不爽；情绪变化则肝气失和，故胃痛随之发作；其脉象与舌苔为肝胃不和之象。

【治法】疏肝理气，和胃止痛。

【方药】柴胡疏肝散加味。方用柴胡、陈皮、川芎、香附、枳壳疏肝和胃，白芍、甘草缓急止痛，服后肝气舒达，血脉通畅，胃气和降，营卫自和，疼痛自除。嗳气较重者，加旋覆花、沉香，以顺气降逆；有化热征象者，加黄连、栀子，以清肝泻火；舌质有瘀点者，加丹参、赤芍，以活血化瘀。

Clinical manifestations： Distending pain in the epigastrium which attacks bilateral hypochondrium, frequent belching or hiccup, alleviation of pain with flatus, unsmooth defecation, outbreak of epigastric pain with emotional upset, thin and whitish tongue fur as well as taut and slightly tense pulse.

Analysis： The syndrome is caused by liver qi attacking the stomach. Distending pain in epigastrium involving the hypochondrium is due to liver qi attacking the stomach and failure of qi in middle energizer to descend and ascend, which gives rise to stagnated qi in middle energizer attacking bilateral hypochondrium； belching or hiccup is caused by failure of the stomach to descend； alleviation of epigastric pain is due to discharge of flatus alleviating qi stagnation in the stomach； unsmooth defecation is due to weakness of stomach qi to descend； occurrence of epigastric pain with emotional depression is due to disorder of liver qi； thin and whitish tongue fur and slightly tense pulse are manifestations of disharmony of the liver and stomach.

Prescription： Soothe the liver to regulate qi circulation and harmonize the stomach to stop pain.

Formulas： Chaihu Shugan San Jiawei （Modified Chaihu Shugan Powder）. In the recipe, Chaihu （*Radix Bupleuri*）, Chenpi （*Pericarpium Citri reticulatae*）, Chuanxiong （*Rhizoma Ligustici Chuanxiong*）, Xiangfu （*Rhizoma Cyperi*） and Zhiqiao （*Fructus Aurantii*） can soothe the liver and harmonize the stomach, Baishao （*Radix Paeoniae Alba*） and Gancao （*Radix Glycyrrhizae*） can relax spasm and relieve pain. The formula can achieve the effect of soothing liver qi, activating blood circulation, descending stomach qi and harmonizing nutrient qi and defensive qi after being taken. As a result, pain could be relieved automatically. For the symptom of severe belching, Xuanfuhua （*Flos Inulae*） and Chenxiang （*Lignum Aquilariae Resinatum*） should be added to regulate qi and descend adverse flow of qi； for internal heat transformation, Huanglian （*Rhizoma Coptidis*） and Zhizi （*Fructus Gardeniae*） should be added to remove heat from the liver and to purge fire； for tongue with petechiae, Danshen （*Radix Salviae Miltiorrhizae*） and Chishao （*Radix Paeoniae Rubra*） can be combined to activate blood and dissolve stasis of blood.

2. 脾胃虚寒

9.2　Asthenic cold in the spleen and stomach

【症状】胃脘隐痛，喜按喜暖，遇冷或劳累时加重，空腹痛甚，食后痛减，泛吐清水，不欲饮食，四肢倦怠，手足不温，大便溏薄，舌质淡嫩，苔薄白，脉象沉细弱。

【分析】本证由脾阳不足，胃失温养所致。寒滞中焦，故胃脘隐痛；寒得暖而散，气得按而行，故喜按喜暖；寒冷或劳累都可加重胃痛；食后痛减，为胃气得养所致；脾胃虚寒，水不运化而入上泛，则吐清水；脾胃所主者，四肢也，脾胃失养，故四肢倦怠，手足不温；脾虚生湿，下注于肠，故大便溏薄；脉舌为脾胃虚弱之象。

【治法】温中健脾，暖胃止痛。

【方药】黄芪建中汤合良附丸。方中黄芪为主药，有补气健脾、祛寒温中之效；桂枝、高良姜、香附，均为温阳理气止痛之药，共为辅药；另有白芍、甘草，有缓急止痛功效；生姜散寒健脾。泛酸者，加瓦楞子、浙贝母、吴茱萸，温中抑酸；肠鸣者，加防风、荜茇；大便溏薄者，可加肉豆蔻、补骨脂。

Clinical manifestations: Dull pain in epigastrium, aggravation of pain with cold or overstrain, or with emptiness of the stomach, alleviation of pain after meals, preference for pressure and warmth, regurgitation of clear fluid and saliva, no appetite, lassitude and cold limbs, loose stool, pale and tender tongue with whitish and thin fur as well as sunken, thin and weak pulse.

Analysis: This syndrome is caused by asthenia of spleen yang and loss of warmth and nourishment of the stomach. Dull pain in epigastrium is caused by retention of pathogenic cold in middle energizer; preference for pressure and warmth is due to the fact that cold could be dispelled with warmth and qi could be activated with pressure; aggravation of pain in epigastrium is due to cold or overstrain; alleviation of pain after meals is due to the fact that stomach qi has obtained nutrition; regurgitation of clear fluid and saliva results from adverse attack of body fluid because of failure of asthenic cold of spleen and stomach to transport; the spleen and stomach govern the limbs, lassitude and cold limbs are due to loss of nourishment of the spleen and stomach; loose stool is due to dampness generated from splenic asthenia, which migrates downward into the intestines; pale and tender tongue with thin and whitish fur as well as thin, weak and sunken pulse is a sign of asthenia of the spleen and stomach.

Prescription: Invigorate the spleen by warming middle energizer, and stop pain by warming the stomach.

Formulas: Huangqi Jianzhong Tang (Decoction) combined with Liangfu Wan (Pill). In the recipe, Huangqi (*Radix Astragali seu Hedysari*), used as principal drug, has an effect of supplementing qi, invigorating the spleen, expelling cold and warming middle energizer; Guizhi (*Ramulus Cinnamomi*), Gaoliangjiang (*Rhizoma Alpiniae Officinarum*) and Xiangfu (*Rhizoma Cyperi*) are used as assistant drug to warm yang and regulate qi so as to stop pain; Baishao (*Radix Paeoniae Alba*) and Gancao (*Radix Glycyrrhizae*) can relax spasm and relieve pain; Shengjiang (*Rhizoma Zingiberis Recens*) has an action of dispelling cold and invigorating the spleen. For acid regurgitation, Walengzi (*Concha Arcae*), Zhebeimu (*Bulbus Fritillariae Thunbergii*) and Wuzhuyu (*Fructus Evodiae*) can be added to warm middle energizer and restrain acid regurgitation; for borborygmus, Fangfeng (*Radix Saposhnikoviae*) and Biba (*Fructus Piperis Longi*) should be added; for loose stool,

Roudoukou (*Semen Myristicae*) and Buguzhi (*Fructus Psoraleae*) should be combined with the recipe.

3. 肝胃郁热
9.3 Stagnation of heat in the liver and stomach

【症状】胃脘灼痛、嘈杂，痛势急迫，情绪易怒，泛酸烧心，口干口苦，大便干结，小便短赤，舌苔黄腻，脉象弦数。

【分析】肝胃郁热是由于肝气郁结，久而不解，郁而化热，并伤及胃阴所引起。气郁不解，故胃脘灼痛、嘈杂；郁热上攻，则泛酸烧心、口干口苦；郁热伤津，故便干溺赤；脉象与舌苔为肝胃郁热之象。

【治法】疏肝泻热，和胃止痛。

【方药】化肝煎（《景岳全书》）加减。方中以白芍酸寒柔肝养阴、缓急止痛；青皮、陈皮疏肝理气；牡丹皮、栀子清泻肝火；泽泻、贝母泻热散结。胁痛甚者，加川楝子、郁金清肝泻火；口干苦甚者，加麦冬、石斛滋养胃阴；大便干结，可加决明子、火麻仁润燥通便。

Clinical manifestations：Acute and rapid scorching pain in the epigastrium, epigastric discomfort, susceptibility to rage, acid regurgitation with heart-burning sensation, dry mouth with bitter taste, constipation, scanty and brownish urine, yellowish and greasy tongue fur as well as taut and fast pulse.

Analysis：The syndrome is caused by prolonged stagnation of unrelieved liver qi, which transforms into heat and impairs stomach yin. Scorching pain in the epigastrium and epigastric upset are due to unrelieved liver qi transforming heat; acid regurgitation with heart-burning sensation and dry mouth with bitter taste are caused by heat transformed from qi stagnation which attacks upwards; constipation as well as scanty and brownish urine is due to stagnated heat impairing body fluid; yellowish and greasy tongue fur and taut and fast pulse are signs of heat stagnation in the liver and stomach.

Prescription：Soothe the liver to purge heat, regulate the stomach and stop pain.

Formulas：Huagan Jian Jiajian (Modified Huagan Decoction). The recipe is quoted from *Jingyue Quanshu (Complete Works of Jingyue)*. In the recipe, Baishao (*Radix Paeoniae Alba*), sour in flavor and cold in nature, can moisten the liver, nourish yin, and relax spasm and pain; Qingpi (*Pericarpium Citri Reticulatae Viride*) and Chenpi (*Pericarpium Citri reticulatae*) can soothe the liver and regulate qi; Mudanpi (*Cortex Moutan Radicis*) and Zhizi (*Fructus Gardeniae*) have an action of clearing away heat and purging fire; Zexie (*Rhizoma Alismatis*) and Beimu (*Bulbus Fritillaria*) can purge heat and disperse stagnation. For pain in the hypochondrium, Chuanlianzi (*Fructus Meliae Toosendan*) and Yujin (*Radix Curcumae*) should be added to clear away heat from the liver and purge fire; for dry mouth with bitter taste, Maidong (*Radix Ophiopogonis*) and Shihu (*Herba Dendrobii*) should be combined to nourish stomach yin; for constipation, Juemingzi (*Semen Cassiae Torae*) and

Huomaren (*Fructus Cannabis*) can be added to moisten dryness so as to relax the bowels.

4. 胃阴亏虚
9.4 Asthenia of stomach yin

【症状】胃脘隐隐灼痛，午后尤甚，口燥咽干，心烦易躁，大便干结，舌质红赤，苔薄干，脉象细数。

【分析】本证多见于阴虚之体，或过食辛辣食品，伤及胃阴，使胃失濡养所致。胃阴不足，胃失濡养，胃络不和，故隐隐灼痛；阴虚则口燥咽干；阴虚内热，故心烦易躁；大肠失去濡养，则大便干结；舌质与脉象均为阴虚内热之象。

【治法】濡养胃阴，和胃止痛。

【方药】益胃汤加味。益胃汤由沙参、麦冬、玉竹、生地黄四味药与冰糖组成。重在濡养胃阴，使胃阴充足，络脉柔润，更无肠燥，则胃脘隐隐灼痛自然消失。若口干甚，可加石斛、芦根甘寒养阴润燥；大便干结甚者，可用生大黄沸水冲泡，取液缓缓饮之。

Clinical manifestations: Dull scorching pain in the epigastrium, aggravation of pain in the afternoon, dry mouth and throat, irritancy with susceptibility to restlessness, constipation, reddish tongue with thin and dry fur as well as thin and fast pulse.

Analysis: The syndrome is usually caused by constitutional asthenia of yin, or by excessive intake of pungent food which impairs stomach yin, giving rise to loss of moisture and nutrition of the stomach. Dull scorching pain in the epigastrium is due to insufficiency of stomach yin, which brings about loss of moisture and nutrition of the stomach as well as disharmony of stomach collaterals; dry mouth and throat is due to yin asthenia; irritancy with susceptibility to restlessness is due to endogenous heat generated from yin asthenia; constipation is caused by loss of proper moisture and nutrition of the intestines; reddish tongue with thin and dry fur and thin and fast pulse are signs of yin asthenia generating endogenous heat.

Prescription: Nourish stomach yin and harmonize the stomach to stop pain.

Formulas: Yiwei Tang Jiawei (Modified Yiwei Decoction). Yiwei Tang, made up of Shashen (*Radix Adenophorae*), Maidong (*Radix Ophiopogonis*), Yuzhu (*Rhizoma Polygonati Odorati*), Shengdihuang (*Radix Rehmanniae Recens*) as well as Bingtang (*Saccharum sinensis Roxb*), has a main function of nourishing stomach yin, aiming at supplementing stomach yin so as to enrich yin, soften and moisten the collaterals, and eliminate dryness in the intestines. As a result, dull scorching pain of the epigastrium could disappear spontaneously. For severe dry mouth, Shihu (*Herba Dendrobii*) and Lugen (*Rhizoma Phragmitis*) can be added to nourish yin and moisten dryness with the sweet and cold nature; for serious constipation, Shengdahuang (*Radix et Rhizoma Rhei*) can be made into drink by processing it in boiling water, and patients shouldn't drink it profusely and rapidly.

5. 瘀血停滞

9.5　Retention of blood stasis

【症状】胃脘疼痛日久，如刀割，如针刺，痛有定处，且痛处拒按，食后痛剧，或见呕血、便血，舌质暗红，苔白腻，脉象弦涩。

【分析】本证由胃痛日久，由气分入于血分，血分瘀阻所致。瘀血之重者，痛如刀割，瘀血之轻者，如针刺；瘀血为有形之物，故拒按；进食则扰动瘀血，故疼痛加重；瘀血处如有破裂，则会呕血、便血；舌质暗红与脉象弦涩，均为瘀阻之象。

【治法】化瘀通络，理气止痛。

【方药】失笑散合丹参饮。失笑散由蒲黄与五灵脂组成，两味药均为活血化瘀止痛药，只是蒲黄偏于气分，五灵脂偏于血分，方名取"失笑"者，是形容见效快也。丹参饮由丹参、檀香、砂仁三味药组成，丹参为活血化瘀药，檀香、砂仁为宽胸理气药，三味配伍，具有理气活血止痛之效。以上两方组合，共奏理气活血止痛的效果。如果食后痛甚者，可加神曲、麦芽、鸡内金，以促消食化瘀止痛；便血、呕血者，可酌加仙鹤草、白及、阿胶等，以加快止血作用。

Clinical manifestations: Prolonged pain with sensation of being cut with a knife or stabbing pain with fixed position in the epigastrium, unpalpable pain with aggravation after meals, or complicated with vomiting of blood or hematochezia, dark reddish tongue with whitish greasy fur as well as taut and astringent pulse.

Analysis: The syndrome is caused by prolonged pain in the epigastrium, transmission of pathogenic factors from qi phase into blood phase, as well as obstruction of blood in blood phase. Pain with sensation of being cut with a knife is due to severe blood stasis, while stabbing pain is due to slight blood stasis; unpalpable pain is due to the fact that blood stasis is tangible; aggravation of pain after meals is due to disturbance of blood stasis because of intake of food; vomiting of blood or hematochezia is caused by stasis of blood having been broken into pieces; dark reddish tongue and taut and astringent pulse are signs of obstruction of blood.

Prescription: Dissolve stasis of blood to promote blood circulation in collaterals and regulate qi to stop pain.

Formulas: Shixiao San (Powder) combined with Danshen Yin (Decoction). Shixiao San consists of Puhuang (*Pollen Typhae*) and Wulingzhi (*Faeces Togopteri*). Both herbs can activate blood circulation and stop pain, Puhuang is prone to treating diseases in qi phase, while Wulingzhi is prone to curing diseases in blood phase. The name of the formula, "Shixiao San" is derived from its sudden curable effect. Danshen Yin is made up of Danshen (*Radix Salviae Miltiorrhizae*), Tanxiang (*Lignum Santali Albi*) and Sharen (*Fructus Amomi Villosi*). Of them, Danshen has an action of activating blood and dissolving stasis, Tanxiang and Sharen can relieve chest oppression and regulate qi. Used together, ingredients of the recipe can regulate qi, activate blood and stop pain. The combination of both formulas could achieve the effect of regulating qi, activating blood as well as stopping pain. For aggravation of pain after meals, Shenqu (*Massa Medicata Fermentata*), Maiya (*Fructus Hordei Germinatus*) and Jineijin (*Endothelium Corneum Gigeriae Galli*) can be added to promote digestion of food, resolve blood stasis and arrest pain; for vomiting of blood or hematochezia, appropriate amount of Xianhecao (*Herba Agrimoniae*), Baiji (*Rhizoma Bletillae*) and Ejiao (*Colla Corii Asini*) can be added to promote the effect of arresting bleeding.

十、胃下垂

10 Gastroptosis

〔概说〕 Summary

胃下垂是指人体站立时胃的下缘达骨盆，胃小弯弧线的最低点降到髂嵴连线以下的病变。本病多见于女性（尤以经产妇生育较多者）、瘦长体型者、消化性疾病进行性消瘦者，以及卧床少动者。本病发生的机理为固定胃的韧带张力减弱，内脏平滑肌张力低下，腹壁脂肪减少，腹肌迟缓。但坚持治疗，预后较好。

胃下垂以上腹部不适，多在餐后、站立时及劳累后加重，易饱胀、厌食、嗳气、恶心及便秘等为主要症状。属于中医学"胃缓"范畴。中医学对此病的认识与治疗积有丰富的经验。早在元代，李东垣在《脾胃论》一书中创拟补中益气汤，以治疗脾胃虚弱、中气下陷为其专长，此方补气升陷作用明显，至今已成为治疗胃下垂的首选方剂。

Gastroptosis refers to the pathological condition that the lower margin of the stomach reaches the pelvis, and the lowest curvature notch of the stomach is lower than the iliac crest level in standing position. This disease is usually seen in women (particularly those after multiple deliveries) or slim figure and gradual emaciation because of digestive disease, as well as those lying in bed with few movements. Pathogenesis of the disease is due to decline of the strain of ligament in supporting the stomach, which causes hypotonia of plain muscles of viscera, reduced fat of abdominal wall as well as slow movements of abdominal muscles. Favorable prognosis could be achieved by means of persistent treatment.

The main clinical manifestations of gastroptosis are marked by discomfort of the upper abdomen, aggravation of discomfort after meals, in standing position and overstrain, susceptibility to feeling full of the stomach, anorexia, belching, nausea, as well as constipation, etc. Gastroptosis pertains to "slow movement of the stomach" in terms of TCM. And ancient TCM practitioners have accumulated plenty of experience about treatment for the disease. As early as in the Yuan Dynasty, in *Treatise on the Spleen and Stomach*, Li Dongyuan talked about his creative formula of Buzhong Yiqi Tang (Decoction) for treating syndromes of asthenia of the spleen and stomach as well as sinking of qi in middle energizer. With its obvious action in tonifying qi and lifting sunken qi, the formula has become the best choice among formulas of treating gastroptosis up to now.

〔**辨证论治**〕 Syndrome differentiation and treatment

1. 脾虚下陷
10.1 Syndrome of splenic qi sinking

【症状】脘腹胀满，食后、站立或劳累时加重，食欲减退，形体消瘦，面色萎黄，少气无力，大便稀薄而少，舌质淡红、边有齿痕，舌苔薄白，脉象濡细虚弱。

【分析】脾胃虚弱，运化无力，所以脘腹胀满，而凡中气下陷者，食后、站立、劳累等，都会使中气下陷加重，所以这类病人以半卧位比较舒服；脾的运化能力减退，故食欲自然不振，气血生化不及，日久便会形体消瘦、面色萎黄；"气不足便为寒"，湿气不化，下注于肠，则大便稀薄而少；舌质、舌苔与脉象，均呈现脾胃气虚之象。

【治疗】健脾益胃，升阳举陷。

【方药】补中益气汤加味。此方以黄芪、人参、白术三味健脾益气为主药；气虚则血虚，故取当归补血，陈皮理气，不使气机紊乱，共为辅药；气虚下陷，方用柴胡、升麻升发阳气，为佐药；甘草甘温和中，为使药。根据经验，用补中益气汤治疗胃下垂，一般要加枳壳或枳实；若是用来治疗子宫下垂，加入车前子效果更好。大便稀薄，可加炒山药、炒薏苡仁；腹胀甚者，可加厚朴花、代代花；食欲不振者，可加砂仁、麦芽。

Clinical manifestations: Distention and fullness of the epigastrium and the abdomen, aggravation after meals, in standing position as well as with overstrain, reduced appetite, emaciation, sallow complexion, weakness and lack of energy, thin loose and scanty stool, pale reddish tooth-marked tongue, thin whitish fur as well as soft, thin and weak pulse.

Analysis: Distention and fullness in the epigastrium and the abdomen are due to weakness and asthenia of the spleen and stomach as well as failure of the spleen and stomach in transportation and transformation; for symptom of qi sinking, feeling comfortable in semi-lying position is due to aggravation of qi sinking after meals, in standing position as well as with overstrain; reduced appetite is caused by dysfunction of the spleen; emaciation and sallow complexion are due to prolonged insufficient production of qi and blood; "insufficiency of qi can result in cold", thin loose and scanty stool is caused by downward migration of unresolved stagnation of damp qi; pale reddish tooth-marked tongue with thin whitish fur and soft, thin and weak pulse are signs of qi asthenia in the spleen and stomach.

Prescription: Invigorate the spleen, strengthen the stomach and rise yang to lift sunken qi.

Formulas: Buzhong Yiqi Tang Jiawei (Modified Decoction of Buzhong Yiqi). In this formula，Huangqi （*Radix Astragali seu Hedysari*），Renshen （*Radix Ginseng*） and Baizhu （*Rhizoma Atractylodis Macrocephalae*） are used as sovereign drug to invigorate the spleen and benefit qi；qi asthenia gives rise to blood deficiency，so Danggui （*Radix Angelicae Sinensis*），with the action of tonifying blood，and Chenpi （*Pericarpium Citri Reticulatae*），having the effect of regulating qi and eliminating qi disorder，are combined as ministerial drug；qi asthenia will bring about qi sinking，therefore，Chaihu （*Radix Bupleuri*） and Shengma （*Rhizoma Zingiberis Recens*） are used as assistant drug to lift yang qi；Gancao （*Radix Glycyrrhizae*），sweet and warm in nature，is used as courier drug to regulate middle energizer. Generally speaking，according to clinical experience，in treating gastroptosis with Buzhong Yiqi Tang，Zhiqiao （*Fructus Aurantii*） or Zhishi （*Fructus Aurantii Immaturus*） should be combined；for prolapse of the uterus，Cheqianzi （*Semen Plantaginis*） can be added to achieve a better curative effect. For thin loose stool，stir-baked Shanyao （*Rhizoma Dioscoreae*） and stir-baked Yiyiren （*Semen Coicis*） could be used；for worsening abdominal distention，Houpohua （*Flos Magnoliae Officinalis*） and Daidaihua （*Cirus aurantium anara Engl*） may be added；for poor appetite，Sharen （*Fructus Amomi Villosi*） and Maiya （*Fructus Hordei Germinatus*） could be combined.

2. 脾虚食滞
10.2　Syndrome of food retention due to spleen asthenia

【症状】脘腹胀坠，食后加重，厌食呕吐，嗳腐吞酸，形体消瘦，大便溏薄，舌苔白腻，脉象沉细不滑利。

【分析】本证由体质虚弱，脾胃气馁，饮食停滞所致。由于食滞不化，故脘腹胀坠，食后加重；胃纳力弱，脾运不及，则厌食呕吐；食滞生腐，气逆而上，故嗳腐吞酸；此证日久，形体消瘦；气不化食，传导失司，故大便稀薄；食滞日久，则舌苔厚腻；脉象沉细不滑利，为食滞不化之象。

【治疗】健脾和胃，消食导滞。

【方药】四君子汤合保和丸。四君子汤为健脾益气之主方，保和丸为消食导滞之主方。两方组合，补气而不壅滞，消食而不伤气。只是在应用时，不要随意去掉保和丸中的连翘。从表面上看，连翘似乎与食积无关，但食滞在内是会生湿热的，湿热一生，就会使气分郁滞，郁滞久了，也会生热。因此，用连翘清热散结，会使食滞快一些消退。

Clinical manifestations：Aggravation of prolapsing sensation and distention of the epigastrium and abdomen after meals, anorexia and vomiting, eructation with fetid odor and acid regurgitation, emaciation, thin loose stool, greasy whitish fur as well as sunken, thin and unsmooth pulse.

Analysis：This syndrome is caused by asthenic constitution, qi asthenia of the spleen and stomach as well as food retention. Prolapsing sensation and distention of the epigastrium and abdomen with aggravation after eating are due to retention of indigested food；anorexia and vomiting are due to weakness of the stomach to receive food and dysfunction of the spleen in transportation；eructation with fetid odor and acid regurgitation are caused by up-attacking of adverse flow of qi because of food retention producing decayed and putrid odor and qi；emaciation is due to prolonged condition of this syndrome；thin loose stool is due to failure of food to transform into qi and dysfunction of the spleen in transportation；thick greasy fur is due to prolonged retention of food；sunken，thin and unsmooth pulse is a sign of indigested food retention.

Prescription：Invigorate the spleen and regulate the stomach，promote digestion of food and discharge food retention.

Formulas：Sijunzi Tang（Decoction）combined with Baohe Wan（Pill）. Sijunzi Tang is an essential recipe for invigorating the spleen and benefiting qi，and Baohe Wan is a principal formula used to eliminate indigested food and guide stagnation of qi. Combined together，both formulas can tonify qi without causing stagnation，and eliminate indigestion of food without impairing qi. In clinical practice，Lianqiao（*Fructus Forsythiae*）can not be removed from the recipe of Baohe Wan，although it appears to be irrelevant to food retention. Dampness and heat generated from food retention can bring about stagnation in qi phase，and prolonged stagnation could result in heat. Therefore，clearing away heat and dispersing stagnation by means of Lianqiao could eliminate food retention quickly.

3. 肝胃不和
10.3　Syndrome of disharmony between the liver and the stomach

【症状】胃脘胀满连及两胁，每遇情绪激动则加重，平时有失眠、多梦，心急烦躁，或善太息，嗳气，大便不调，舌苔白腻，脉象弦细。

【分析】本证由肝郁不和，横逆犯胃所引起。胃居中焦，肝布两胁，情志不遂，肝失条达，则胃脘胀痛并及两胁，情绪激动则肝郁更甚，故必疼痛加重；"肝主魂"，肝失条达，魂不守舍，则失眠、多梦；善太息、嗳气，均为肝胃之气失序所引起；其他如大便不调，以及脉舌之象，显示气机不顺、运化不及之病机。

【治疗】疏肝和胃，理气消胀。

【方药】柴胡疏肝散加味。方取柴胡疏肝，配香附、枳壳理气；川芎活血；白芍、甘草缓急止痛。胃脘胀满者，加厚朴花、代代花理气消胀；失眠多梦者，加酸枣仁、合欢皮理气宁心安神；大便不调者，加山药、炒白术健脾整肠。

Clinical manifestations：Epigastric distention and fullness involving the hypochondrium，aggravation with emotional activity，occasional insomnia and dreaminess，irritancy and restlessness in daily life，or frequent sigh，belching，irregular defecation，greasy whitish fur as well as taut and thin pulse.

Analysis：This syndrome is caused by stagnated qi in the liver attacking adversely upward into the stomach. The stomach is located in middle energizer，and the liver is in the region of the hypochondrium，epigastric distention and fullness involving the hypochondrium is caused by failure of the liver in dispersion because of emotional upset，and aggravation of epigastric pain is due to worsening stagnation of the liver because of agitated emotion; "the liver dominates the spirit", insomnia and dreaminess are caused by mental derangement because of failure of the liver in dispersion; frequent sigh and belching are caused by qi disorder of the liver and stomach; other symptoms such as irregular defecation and whitish greasy fur as well as taut and thin pulse indicate disorder of qi movement and dysfunction of the spleen in transportation and transformation.

Prescription: Soothe the liver, harmonize the stomach and regulate qi to eliminate distention.

Formulas: Chaihu Shugan San Jiawei (Modified Chaihu Shugan Powder). In the recipe, Chaihu (*Radix Bupleuri*) is used to soothe the liver, Xiangfu (*Rhizoma Cyperi*) and Zhiqiao (*Fructus Aurantii*) are combined to regulate qi; Chuanxiong (*Rhizoma Ligustici Chuanxiong*) can promote blood circulation; Baishao (*Radix Paeoniae Alba*) and Gancao (*Radix Glycyrrhizae*) can relax spasm and relieve pain. For epigastric distention and fullness, Houpohua (*Flos Magnoliae Officinalis*) and Daidaihua (*Cirus aurantium anara Engl*) may be added to regulate qi and eliminate distention; for insomnia and dreaminess, Suanzaoren (*Semen Ziziphi Spinosae*) and Hehuanpi (*Cortex Albiziae*) could be combined to regulate qi and tranquilize the mind and heart; for irregular defecation, Shanyao (*Rhizoma Dioscoreae*) and stir-baked Baizhu (*Rhizoma Atractylodes Macrocephaia*) may be used together with the above recipe to invigorate the spleen and regulate the bowels.

4. 胃阴不足
10.4　Syndrome of yin deficiency of the stomach

【症状】脘腹胀满，并隐隐坠痛，口干口燥，烦渴喜饮，嗳气呃逆，嘈杂不饥，胃中灼热，舌质红赤，少津少苔，脉象沉细数。

【分析】本证由胃阴不足，胃失濡养，虚热内生所致。与体质、饮食习惯有密切关系。胃阴不足，胃失濡养，气机乖逆，故胀满坠痛、嗳气呃逆；阴虚内热，津液缺乏，则口干口燥、烦渴喜饮；热蕴于内，不得发散，故胃中灼热；其脉舌之象，为阴虚之明证。

【治法】滋养胃阴，润燥和胃。

【方药】益胃汤加味。方中沙参、麦冬、玉竹、生地黄、冰糖，皆属甘润养阴益胃之品，为滋养胃阴之主方。若烦渴喜饮，可加天花粉、石斛养阴止渴；嗳气呃逆，可加竹茹、生姜降气和胃；嘈杂不饥，可加生山楂、乌梅增加食欲。

Clinical manifestations: Epigastric and abdominal distention and fullness, dull pain with prolapsing sensation, dry mouth and throat, polydipsia with preference for drink, belching and hiccups, epigastric upset without sense of hunger, scorching sensation of the stomach, reddish tongue with scanty fluid, scanty fur as well as sunken and thin and fast pulse.

Analysis: This syndrome is caused by loss of proper nourishing and moistening of the stomach as well as generation of endogenous asthenic heat. It is closely related to constitution and dietary habit. Distention, fullness and prolapsing sensation as well as belching and hiccups are due to insufficient stomach-yin and loss of proper nourishing and moistening of the stomach, which gives rise to attack of adverse flow of qi; dry mouth and throat and polydipsia with preference for drink are due to lack of body fluid because of endogenous heat and asthenic yin; scorching sensation of the stomach is due to failure to disperse accumulation of endogenous heat; reddish tongue with scanty fluid, scanty fur as well as sunken and thin and fast pulse are obvious manifestations of yin asthenia.

Prescription: Nourish stomach yin and moisten dryness to harmonize the stomach.

Formulas: Yiwei Tang Jiawei (Modified Yiwei Decoction). In the formula, Shashen (*Adenophora stricta*), Maidong (*Radix Ophiopogonis*), Yuzhu (*Rhizoma Polygonati Odorati*), Shengdihuang (*Radix Rehmanniae Recens*) and Bingtang (*crystal sugar*), sweat and moist in nature, have an action of nourishing yin and benefiting stomach, so it is used as the major formula for nourishing stomach yin. For polydipsia with preference for drink, Tianhuafen (*Radix Trichosanthis*) and Shihu (*Herba Dendrobii*) can be added to nourish yin and stop thirst; for belching and hiccups, Zhuru (*Caulis Bambusae in Taenia*) and Shengjiang (*Rhizoma Zingiberis Recens*) can be added to descend qi and harmonize the stomach; for epigastric upset without sense of hunger, Shengshanzha (*Fructus Crataegi*) and Wumei (*Fructus Mume*) should be combined to promote appetite.

十一、胆囊炎
11　Cholecystitis

〔概说〕 Summary

胆囊炎有急性与慢性之分，本文主要叙述慢性胆囊炎。

慢性胆囊炎可由急性胆囊炎反复迁延发作而来，也可由胆囊慢性炎症而发作。其主要致病因素为细菌感染、病毒感染、结石刺激、寄生虫感染、胆固醇代谢障碍等。

慢性胆囊炎的主要症状为反复发作性上腹痛，疼痛多发作于右上腹或中上腹，少数可发生于胸骨后或左上腹，并向右肩胛下区放射，常于晚上或饱餐后发作。当胆囊管或胆总管发生胆石嵌顿时，可发生胆绞痛。缓解期可无症状，间或有上腹部不适、嗳气、泛酸、厌油腻等。

胆囊炎属于中医学"腹胀""胆胀""胁痛"等范畴。多由于七情内伤、肝失疏泄，饮食不节、湿热内生，或饮食不洁、浊气郁结等发生。其病位在肝胆，但多涉及脾胃。

Cholecystitis includes acute cholecystitis and chronic cholecystitis. This chapter is focused on chronic cholecystitis.

The outbreak of chronic cholecystitis is due to delayed treatment for acute cholecystitis, or frequent occurrence of acute cholecystitis. Chronic inflammation of gallbladder may also develop into chronic cholecystitis. Pathogenesis of the disease includes bacterial or viral infection, stimulation of gallstones of the gallbladder, infection of parasites as well as cholesterol dysbolism.

The main clinical manifestation of chronic cholecystitis is marked by frequent occurrence of upper abdominal pain, usually in right upper abdomen or in middle upper abdomen, and in a few cases, pain can appear from behind the chest bone or in left upper abdomen with a tendency to spreading to the region below the right shoulder blade. The onset of chronic cholecystitis usually occurs in the evening or after a full meal. When gallstones block the cystic duct, symptoms of biliary colic may arise. With the alleviation of colic pain, biliary colic may disappear, or it is accompanied with occasional discomfort over the upper abdomen, belching, acid regurgitation as well as aversion to greasy food.

In terms of TCM, cholecystitis belongs to "abdominal distention" "gallbladder distention" or "hypochondriac pain", and so on. The disease is usually caused by internal damage due to intemperance of seven emotions, dysfunction of liver dispersion, improper diet, generation of endogenous dampness and heat, or intake of unclean food and stagnation of turbid qi. The location of this disease is in the liver and gallbladder, but it usually involves the spleen and stomach.

〔辨证论治〕 Syndrome differentiation and treatment

1. 肝胆气滞

11.1 Syndrome of qi stagnation in the liver and gallbladder

【症状】右胁隐隐作痛，时轻时重，时作时止，胃脘胀满，恶心，饮食减少，厌油，嗳气频频，舌苔薄白，脉象弦滑或弦细。

【分析】本证由肝气不舒，失于条达，胆失通降，木郁犯土所致。肝之脉络布于两胁，肝郁不舒，气结胁下，故右胁隐隐作痛，并反复发作；肝郁不解，克伐脾胃，则见胃脘胀满；胃气不降，则见恶心、嗳气频频；脾胃被困，湿浊不化，故有厌油、饮食减少之症；脉舌表现为肝郁脾湿等所致。

【治法】疏肝利胆，健脾和胃。

【方药】逍遥散加味。方取柴胡、薄荷疏肝理气，以解肝郁；当归、川芎、白芍养血柔肝，有利于肝气的条达；白术、茯苓健脾和胃；甘草、生姜调和营卫之气。另加生麦芽疏肝健脾，加半夏降逆，加神曲、鸡内金开胃进食。若胃痛不能缓解时，可加木香、川楝子理气疏肝止痛。

Clinical manifestations: Dull pain in the right hypochondrium, occasional alleviation and aggravation of the pain as well as occasional onset or disappearance, epigastric distention and fullness, nausea, reduced appetite, aversion to greasy food, frequent belching, thin whitish fur as well as taut and slippery pulse or taut and thin pulse.

Analysis：This syndrome is caused by qi depression in the liver, dysfunction of liver dispersion as well as failure of the gallbladder to disperse and descend stagnated qi, thus, qi depression in the liver invading into the spleen. The liver collaterals are distributed in the hypochondrium, liver qi depression results in accumulation of stagnated qi below the hypochondrium, which brings about frequent onset of dull pain in the right hypochondrium; epigastric distention and fullness are due to unrelieved depression of liver qi attacking the spleen and stomach; nausea and frequent belching are due to failure to descend stomach qi; reduced appetite and aversion to greasy food are caused by obstruction of qi in the spleen and stomach and failure to resolve turbid qi and dampness; thin whitish fur and taut and slippery pulse or taut and thin pulse are manifestations of liver depression and splenic dampness.

Prescription：Soothe the liver to promote circulation of bile, invigorate the spleen and harmonize the stomach.

Formulas：Xiaoyao San Jiawei (Modified Xiaoyao Powder). In the formula, Chaihu (*Radix Bupleuri*) and Bohe (*Herba Menthae*) can soothe the liver and regulate qi to eliminate liver depression; Danggui (*Radix Angelicae Sinensis*), Chuanxiong (*Rhizoma Ligustici Chuanxiong*) and Baishao (*Radix Paeoniae Alba*) have an action of nourishing blood and softening the liver, which is helpful for liver qi to move freely and disperse normally; Baizhu (*Rhizoma Atractylodis Macrocephalae*) and Fuling (*Herba Menthae*) have an action of invigorating the spleen and harmonizing the stomach; Gancao (*Radix Glycyrrhizae*) and Shengjiang (*Rhizoma Zingiberis Recens*) can reconcile nutrient qi and defensive qi. Besides, Maiya (*Fructus Hordei Germinatus*) is combined to soothe the liver and invigorate the spleen. Banxia (*Rhizoma Pinelliae*), with a function of descending adverse flow of qi, Shenqu (*Massa Medicata Fermentata*) and Jineijin (*Endothelium Corneum Gigeriae Galli*) are added to promote appetite. For failure to alleviate stomachache, Muxiang (*Radix Aucklandiae*) and Chuanlianzi (*Fructus Meliae Toosendan*) could be combined to regulate qi and soothe the liver to stop pain.

2. 湿热蕴结
11.2 Syndrome of damp heat accumulation

【症状】右胁痛甚，腹满拒按，发热畏寒，身目黄染，大便秘结，小便黄赤，或伴有恶心呕吐，脘腹胀满，口苦咽干，舌苔黄腻，脉象弦滑数。

【分析】本证由湿热内蕴，肝胆脾胃均失其职所致。湿热蕴结肝胆，肝胆失其疏泄，则见胁痛拒按；湿热之浊气蒸于外，则见发热畏寒、身目黄染；湿热蕴结脾胃，上蒸则口苦咽干、恶心呕吐，下迫则大便秘结、小便黄赤；舌苔黄腻与滑数之脉，是脾胃湿热的表象，也是鉴别湿热的依据。

【治法】清热化湿，利胆通腑。

【方药】茵陈蒿汤合大柴胡汤加味。方取茵陈、栀子、大黄清热通腑；柴胡、枳实疏肝利胆；半夏和胃止呕；黄芩解热化湿；白芍能泻肝火，使木不克土，前人说是"安脾敛阴"；姜枣调和营卫而行津液。发热重者，加金银花、连翘、败酱草、龙胆草加强清热解毒作用；有胆石者，加金钱草、鸡内金利胆排石；疼痛拒按难忍者，加延胡索、川楝子行气活血止痛；便秘重者，加芒硝冲服。

Clinical manifestations: Severe pain in the right hypochondrium, unpressable abdominal fullness, fever and aversion to cold, yellow coloration of the skin and eyes, constipation, yellowish or brownish urine, or accompanied with nausea and vomiting, epigastric and abdominal distention and fullness, bitter taste and dry throat, greasy yellowish fur as well as taut, slippery and fast pulse.

Analysis: This syndrome is caused by internal accumulation of damp heat and dysfunction of the liver, gallbladder, spleen and stomach. Unpressable hypochondriac pain is due to failure of the liver and gallbladder to disperse because of accumulation of dampness and heat in the liver and gallbladder; fever, aversion to cold and yellow coloration of the skin and eyes are due to outward fumigation of turbid qi of dampness and heat; bitter taste and dry throat as well as nausea and vomiting are caused by upward fumigation of accumulated dampness and heat in the spleen and stomach, and constipation and yellowish or brownish urine are due to downward migration of accumulated dampness and heat; yellowish greasy fur and slippery fast pulse are manifestations of dampness and heat in the spleen and stomach, which could be regarded as an evidence to discern the syndrome of dampness and heat.

Prescription: Clear away heat and dissolve dampness, promote circulation of bile and dredge the intestines.

Formulas: Yinchenhao Tang (Decoction) combined with Large Chaihu Tang (Decoction) Jiawei. In the formula, Yinchen (*Herba Artemisiae Scopariae*), Zhizi (*Fructus Gardeniae*) and Dahuang (*Radix et Rhizoma Rhei*) have an action of clearing away heat and promoting qi circulation in fu-organs; Chaihu (*Radix Bupleuri*) and Zhishi (*Fructus Aurantii Immaturus*) can soothe the liver and promote the normal circulation of bile; Banxia (*Rhizoma Pinelliae*) has the function of harmonizing the stomach and stopping vomiting; Huangqin (*Radix Scutellariae*) could relieve heat and resolve dampness; Baishao (*Radix Paeoniae Alba*) can purge liver fire so that wood (the liver) will not restrain earth (the spleen), which is known as "calming the spleen to astringe yin"; Shengjiang (*Rhizoma Zingiberis Recens*) and Dazao (*Fructus Jujubae*) can reconcile nutrient qi and defensive qi to activate body fluid. For high fever, Jinyinhua (*Flos Lonicerae*), Lianqiao (*Fructus Forsythiae*), Baijiangcao (*Herba Patriniae*) and Longdancao (*Radix Gentianae*) could be combined to reinforce the effect of clearing away heat as well as eliminating toxic pathogens; for gallstones, Jinqiancao (*Herba Lysimachiae*) and Jineijin (*Endothelium Corneum Gigeriae Galli*) may be used to promote circulation of bile to eliminate gallstones; for unpressable and unbearable pain, Yanhusuo (*Rhizoma Corydalis*) and Chuanlianzi (*Fructus Meliae Toosendan*) should be combined to activate qi and blood and stop pain; for severe constipation, Mangxiao (*Natrii Sulfas*) could be used as infusion for oral taking.

十二、黄疸

12 Jaundice

〔概说〕 Summary

黄疸，是指以目黄、身黄、小便黄为主要症状的传染病的总称。凡传染性肝炎、肝硬化、钩端螺旋体病，以及胆石症等出现黄疸，均可依此进行辨证论治。

中医学认为，黄疸与脾胃虚弱、湿热外袭、饮食不洁、七情郁结等因素有密切关系。特别是湿热外袭、饮食不洁，皆可使湿从热化，湿热郁蒸，发为黄疸。其辨证论治主要从黄疸分类入手，即从阳黄、阴黄辨证，治疗从"湿"字着眼，并以小便通利与否为出发点，进行诊治。

Jaundice is defined as an infectious disease with the pathological condition marked by symptoms such as yellow coloration of the eyes, skin as well as urine. According to the above symptoms, all diseases with the appearance of jaundice such as infectious hepatitis, hepatocirrhosis, leptospirosis as well as cholelithiasis, could be differentiated and treated.

In TCM, it is held that jaundice is closely related to outward invasion of pathogenic dampness and heat due to asthenia of the spleen and stomach, intake of unclean food as well as emotional depression. And it is particularly related to outward invasion of pathogenic dampness and heat as well as intake of unclean food, which could result in heat transformation from dampness, thus, fumigation of dampness and heat brings about jaundice. Syndrome differentiation of jaundice generally starts from classification of jaundice which includes yang jaundice and yin jaundice, and treatment should be based on "dampness" and whether urination is smooth or not so as to figure out an overall diagnostic and treating plan.

〔辨证论治〕 Syndrome differentiation and treatment

（一）阳黄

12.1 Yang jaundice

1. 湿热郁蒸

12.1.1 Syndrome of stagnation and fumigation of dampness and heat

湿热郁蒸黄疸又分热重于湿和湿重于热两种类型。

【症状】①热重于湿者，症见身目俱黄，如橘子色，发热口渴，恶心呕吐，心中懊恼，大便秘结，小便短赤，或腹部胀满，两胁不适，舌苔黄腻，脉象弦数；②湿重于热者，症见发热不高或不明显，身黄不鲜明，兼有头重身困，胸脘痞满，口淡不渴，小便淡黄，大便稀软，舌苔白腻或微黄，脉象濡缓。

【分析】①热重于湿者，湿热交蒸，胆汁外泄于肌肤，热为阳邪，故黄色鲜明；湿热熏蒸，胃浊上逆，则见恶心呕吐、心中懊恼；热势弛张，故发热口渴；膀胱热盛，则小便短赤；大肠热盛，则大便秘结；病发于肝脾，肝脾两经气机不利，故见腹部胀满，两胁不适；舌苔与脉象均为热盛之象。②湿重于热者，湿遏热伏，故热势不高，且黄色不鲜明；湿困清阳，阳气不展，则头重身困；脾被湿困，则胸脘痞满，口淡不渴；其他如二便、舌脉，均为湿胜热伏之象。

【治法】清利湿热。

【方药】热重于湿者，用茵陈蒿汤加味。湿重于热者，用茵陈五苓散加味。

茵陈蒿汤由茵陈、大黄、栀子三味组成。茵陈为清热利湿退黄之要品，大黄、栀子清热解毒，导热下行，可使湿热之毒从二便排出。可酌加车前子、猪苓淡渗利湿，增强方药的排尿作用；呕吐不能食者，可加半夏、陈皮、竹茹降逆开胃止呕；腹部胀满者，可加厚朴、代代花、大麦芽行气解郁消胀。

茵陈五苓散由五苓散加茵陈组成。方取五苓散（茯苓、猪苓、泽泻、桂枝、白术）健脾利湿、利尿祛湿，茵陈清热利湿退黄。全方的利湿作用大于清热作用，以便使湿邪快速地排出体外，解除湿困脾阳之苦。

Stagnation and fumigation of dampness and heat can be divided into syndrome of severe heat with mild dampness and syndrome of severe dampness with mild heat.

Clinical manifestations:

a. Syndrome of severe heat with mild dampness: Yellow coloration of the skin and eyes like the color of orange, fever and thirst, nausea and vomiting, vexation, dry feces, scanty and brownish urine, or abdominal distention and fullness, discomfort in the hypochondrium, greasy yellowish fur as well as taut and fast pulse.

b. Syndrome of severe dampness with mild heat: Dull fever or unobvious fever, unobvious yellow coloration of the skin, accompanied with heavy sensation of the head and tiredness of the head and body, distention and fullness in the chest and hypochondrium, bland taste without thirst, light yellowish urine, thin loose stool, greasy whitish or slight yellowish fur as well as soft and moderate pulse.

Analysis:

a. Syndrome of severe heat with mild dampness: Obvious yellow coloration of the skin and eyes is due to extravasation of the bile in the skin and muscles because of stagnation and fumigation of dampness and heat, and heat is a pathogenic yang factor; nausea, vomiting and vexation are due to adverse flow of turbid stomach qi resulting from stagnation and fumigation of dampness and heat; fever with thirst is due to spreading tendency of heat; scanty and brownish urine is due to exuberant heat in the bladder; dry feces is due to superabundance of heat in the large intestine; the disease breaks out from the liver and spleen, qi disorder in the meridians of the liver and spleen causes abdominal distention and fullness and discomfort in the hypochondrium; greasy yellowish fur and taut and fast pulse are signs of hyperactive heat.

b. Syndrome of severe dampness with mild heat: Mild fever and unobvious yellow coloration of the skin and eyes are due to retention of heat because of blockage of dampness; heavy sensation and tiredness over the head and body is due to stagnation of yang qi because of dampness encumbering lucid yang; distention and fullness in the chest and hypochondrium and bland taste without thirst are caused by stagnation of dampness in the spleen; other manifestations such as light brownish urine, thin and loose stool and greasy and whitish fur are signs of exuberance of dampness and retention of heat.

Prescription: Eliminate dampness and heat.

Formulas: Yinchenhao Tang Jiawei (Modified Yinchenhao Decoction) for the syndrome of severe heat with mild dampness; Yinchen Wuling San Jiawei (Modified Yinchen Wuling Powder) for severe dampness with mild heat.

Yinchenhao Tang consists of Yinchen (*Herba Artemisiae Scopariae*), Dahuang (*Radix et Rhizoma Rhei*) and Zhizi (*Fructus Gardeniae*), of which, Yinchen is an essential drug to eliminate heat and dampness so as to relieve jaundice, Dahuang and Zhizi can clear away heat relieve toxic factors and guide heat to migrate downward so as to discharge dampness and heat through urination and defecation. Cheqianzi (*Semen Plantaginis*) and Zhuling (*Polyporus Umbellatus*), bland in flavor, can be added to induce diuresis with their action of resolving dampness; for vomiting and nausea, Banxia (*Rhizoma Pinelliae*), Chenpi (*Pericarpium Citri Reticulatae*) and Zhuru (*Caulis Bambusae in Taenia*) could be added to descend adverse flow of qi, promote appetite and stop vomiting; for abdominal distention and fullness, Houpohua (*Flos Magnoliae Officinalis*), Daidaihua (*Cirus aurantium anara Engl*) and Damaiya (*Fructus Hordei Germinatus*) may be added to activate qi and resolve stagnation to eliminate distention and fullness.

Yinchen Wuling San (Powder) is the combination of Yinchen with Wuling San, made up of Fuling (*Poriae Cocos*), Zhuling (*Polyporus Umbellatus*), Zexie (*Rhizoma Alismatis*), Guizhi (*Ramulus Cinnamomi*) and Baizhu (*Rhizoma Atractylodis Macrocephalae*), with an action of invigorating the spleen, inducing diuresis, resolving as well as eliminating dampness. And Yinchen can clear away heat, remove dampness through urination and eliminate jaundice. Because the action of removing dampness of this recipe is stronger than its function of heat-clearing, so it could drive dampness pathogen out of the body quickly and relieve the syndrome of dampness obstructing splenic yang.

2. 热毒炽盛
12.1.2 Syndrome of exuberant pathogenic heat toxin

【症状】黄疸突起, 既然加重, 身黄如金, 高热烦渴, 呕吐频频, 脘腹胀满, 腹痛拒按, 大便秘结, 小便短赤, 烦躁不安, 舌苔黄腻粗糙, 舌边尖红, 脉象弦数, 或滑大。

【分析】热毒内侵, 毒势猛烈, 熏灼肝胆, 胆汁外溢, 发黄如金; 热毒内炽, 耗灼津液，则高热烦渴、小便短赤；热毒结于阳明，则大便秘结；热毒上扰，心神不宁，则烦躁不安；热毒伤津，则舌边尖红、苔黄粗糙；脉象弦数或滑大，有热极生风之象，故对此证不可怠慢。

【治法】清热解毒，泻火退黄。

【方药】茵陈蒿汤、黄连解毒汤、五味消毒饮三方加减。方用茵陈清热利湿退黄，黄芩清上焦之火，黄连清中焦之火，黄柏清下焦之火，栀子清三焦之火，大黄清解肠胃之瘀热；配合五味消毒饮，是增强清热解毒的功效。这三个方子清解气分热毒的力大，若热毒侵入血分，可加入生地黄、牡丹皮、紫草等，以凉血清营，败毒救阴。

Clinical manifestations：Sudden outbreak of jaundice, aggravation of it with golden coloration of the skin, high fever and polydypsia, frequent vomiting, gastric and abdominal distention and fullness, unpressable pain in the abdomen, dry feces, scanty and brownish urine, restlessness, rough and yellowish and greasy fur, reddish tongue tip and margin as well as taut and fast pulse or large and slippery pulse.

Analysis：Yellow coloration of the skin like gold is due to internal invasion of severe toxin of heat scorching and steaming the liver and gallbladder, which results in extravasation of the bile in the skin; high fever and polydypsia and scanty and brownish urine are caused by scorching consumption of body fluid due to internal retention of heat toxin; dry feces is due to accumulation of heat toxin in yangming meridian; restlessness is caused by up-disturbance of heat toxin into the heart; reddish tongue tip and margin as well as rough and greasy and yellowish fur is due to heat toxin impairing fluid; taut and fast pulse or large and slippery pulse is the sign of generation of endogenous wind due to hyperactive heat, which should not be neglected.

Prescription：Clear away heat, relieve toxin and purge fire to eliminate jaundice.

Formulas：Yinchenhao Tang （ Decoction ） combined with Huanglian Jiedu Tang （ Decoction ） and Wuwei Xiaodu Yin （ Decoction ） Jiajian. In these recipes, Yinchen （ *Herba Artemisiae Scopariae* ） can clear away heat, resolve dampness and eliminate jaundice, Huangqin （ *Radix Scutellariae* ） has an action of clearing away fire from upper energizer, Huanglian （ *Rhizoma Coptidis* ） can clear away fire from middle energizer, and Huangbo （ *Cortex Phellodendri* ） can purge fire from lower energizer, Zhizi （ *Fructus Gardeniae* ） could eliminate fire in triple energizer, Dahuang （ *Radix et Rhizoma Rhei* ） has a function of clearing away stagnated heat in the intestines and stomach; Wuwei Xiaodu Yin is combined to reinforce the effect of clearing away heat and eliminating toxin. The three formulas have strong action in removing heat and toxin in qi phase. For invasion of heat toxin in blood phase, Shengdihuang （ *Radix Rehmanniae Recens* ）, Mudanpi （ *Cortex Moutan Radicis* ） and Zicao （ *Radix Arnebiae* ） can be added to cool blood and clear away heat in nutrient phase and to relieve toxin so as to rescue yin.

（二）阴黄

12.2 Yin jaundice

1. 寒湿郁滞

12.2.1 Syndrome of stagnation of cold and dampness

【症状】黄疸色泽暗晦，食欲不振，胃脘闷胀，神疲畏寒，大便不实，舌体胖而质淡，苔白腻，脉象沉细而缓。

【分析】本证由湿胜阳微或中阳不振所致。黄疸色泽暗晦，是因寒湿郁滞中焦，阳气不振，胆汁不循常道而外泄；食欲不振、胃脘闷胀、大便不实，皆是脾阳不振，运化失常的表现；神疲畏寒，是阳气虚弱，气血不足所致。舌体胖是阳气不足，舌质淡是气血亏虚，脉象沉细而缓为阳气不能运行血脉所致。总之，本证是阳气不足，寒湿郁滞于内，不能正常运化所形成的。

【治法】健脾和胃，温化寒湿。

【方药】茵陈术附汤加味。方中茵陈、附子并用，温阳化气，以祛寒湿；白术、干姜、甘草健脾和胃，可使湿邪消散。临证可加茯苓、泽泻渗湿之品，以加快祛湿作用。

Clinical manifestations：Sallow and tarnished complexion, poor appetite, epigastric distention and fullness, dispiritedness and aversion to cold, loose stool, pale bulgy tongue with whitish greasy fur as well as sunken, thin and moderate pulse.

Analysis：The syndrome is caused by superabundant dampness impairing yang, or due to weakening of yang in middle energizer. Sallow and tarnished complexion is due to abnormal extravasation of the bile because of stagnation of cold and dampness and weakness of yang in middle energizer; poor appetite, epigastric distention and fullness and loose stool are manifestations of weakness of yang in middle energizer and dysfunction of the spleen in transportation and transformation; dispiritedness and aversion to cold are caused by weakening of yang and insufficiency of qi and blood. Bulgy tongue is due to deficiency of yang qi, pale tongue is due to deficiency of qi and blood, sunken, thin and moderate pulse is caused by failure of yang qi to circulate in blood vessels. In general, the syndrome is caused by dysfunction of the spleen in transportation and transformation due to insufficiency of yang qi and internal stagnation of cold and dampness.

Prescription：Invigorate the spleen, harmonize the stomach and resolve cold and dampness by warming.

Formulas：Yinchen Zhu Fu Tang Jiawei (Modified Yinchen Zhu Fu Decoction). In the formula, Yinchen (*Herba Artemisiae Scopariae*) and Fuzi (*Radix Aconiti Lateralis Preparata*) are used to promote transformation of qi by warming yang so as to expel cold and dampness; Baizhu (*Rhizoma Atractylodis Macrocephalae*), Ganjiang (*Rhizoma Zingiberis*) and Gancao (*Radix Glycyrrhizae*) have the action of invigorating the spleen and harmonizing the stomach to disperse pathogenic damp factors. Fuling (*Poriae Cocos*) and Zexie (*Rhizoma Alismatis*) could be combined to promote resolving dampness in some specific cases.

2. 脾虚血亏

12.2.2 Syndrome of asthenic spleen and deficient blood

【症状】面目与肌肤发黄，黄色较淡，肢软乏力，心悸气短，食欲不振，大便溏薄，舌质淡红，苔薄白，脉象濡细。

【分析】脾胃虚弱，气血不足，不能荣华于面与肌肤，故面目发黄，肌肤不泽，肢软乏力；血不足则心悸，气不足则气短；脾胃虚弱，纳运无力，则食欲不振，大便溏薄；舌与脉象均为脾虚血亏之象。

【治法】健脾温中，补养气血。

【方药】黄芪建中汤加味。方中黄芪为补气温中之上品，不唯补气，且可补气生血；桂枝配合生姜、大枣辛甘化合生阳；白芍配甘草酸甘化阴；饴糖缓中补脾。全方虽仅七味，但阴阳并济，气血俱生。气血旺盛，黄色自退。若气虚甚者，加党参、白术；血虚甚者，加当归、熟地黄；阳虚甚者，可改桂枝为肉桂，或少加附子，以促阳生。

Clinical manifestations: Light sallow complexion and pale yellowish coloration of the eyes and skin, weakness of limbs and lack of energy, palpitation and shortness of breath, poor appetite, loose stool, pale reddish tongue with thin whitish fur as well as soft and thin pulse.

Analysis: Lusterless and sallow complexion, yellowish coloration of the eyes and skin and weakness of limbs are due to asthenic spleen and stomach and insufficiency of qi and blood, which fails to nourish the face and skin; palpitation is due to insufficiency of blood, and shortness of breath is due to qi deficiency; poor appetite and loose stool are caused by failure of asthenic spleen and stomach to transport and transform qi and blood; pale reddish tongue with thin whitish fur and soft and thin pulse are signs of splenic asthenia and blood deficiency.

Prescription: Invigorate the spleen, warm middle energizer and nourish qi and blood.

Formulas: Huangqi Jianzhong Tang Jiawei (Modified Huangqi Jianzhong Decoction). In the recipe, Huangqi (*Radix Astragali seu Hedysari*) is the best drug to supplement qi and warm middle energizer. Besides its action of supplementing qi, Huangqi can promote production of blood; Guizhi (*Ramulus Cinnamomi*), together with Shengjiang (*Rhizoma Zingiberis Recens*) and Dazao (*Fructus Jujubae*), can transform yang with their pungent and sweet nature; Baishao (*Radix Paeoniae Alba*) and Gancao (*Radix Glycyrrhizae*), sweet and sour in nature, can promote transformation of yin; Yitang (*Saccharum Granorum*) has an action of relieving spasm and pain in middle energizer and tonify the spleen. Although made up of only seven medicinal herbs, the formula could strengthen both yin and yang and promote production of qi and blood. With exuberant qi and blood, yellow coloration of the skin could be relieved. For severe qi asthenia, Dangshen (*Radix Codonopsis*) and Baizhu (*Rhizoma Atractylodis Macrocephalae*) should be added; for severe blood asthenia, Danggui (*Radix*

Angelicae Sinensis) and Shudihuang (*Radix Rehmanniae Preparata*) may be added; for yang asthenia, Guizhi (*Ramulus Cinnamomi*) could be replaced by Rougui (*Cortex Cinnamomi*), or a small amount of Fuzi (*Radix Aconiti Lateralis Preparata*) can be added to promote transformation of yang.

十三、慢性肝炎

13　Chronic hepatitis

〔概说〕 Summary

慢性肝炎是由病毒引起的病程持续超过 6 个月的炎症性肝脏疾病，多数是由乙型肝炎病毒感染所致。另外，机体自身免疫功能紊乱，长期服用某些肝脏毒性药物、酗酒、生活质量下降等，均可导致本病的发生。

慢性肝炎属于中医学"胁痛""癥瘕"及"黄疸"等范畴。其形成的病机主要是肝气郁结、湿热积聚、脾胃不和、血脉瘀滞所致。治疗应重视疏肝健脾、理气化瘀、清热化湿、滋养肝肾等。饮食调养、适当休息、谨慎房事对疾病的控制也是十分重要的。

Chronic hepatitis is a disease characterized by inflammation of the liver, and its duration is generally more than six months. In many cases, chronic hepatitis is caused by infection of hepatitis B virus. In addition, other factors such as dysfunction of immune system, intake of some medicines with toxic substance for a long time, alcoholism as well as declined living quality could lead to the outbreak of it.

In TCM, chronic hepatitis pertains to "hypochondriac pain" "abdominal mass" "jaundice", etc. Generally speaking, pathogenesis of it is liver qi stagnation, accumulation of dampness and heat, disharmony of the spleen and stomach as well as blood stasis in vessels. Therefore, much stress should be attached to its therapeutic methods such as soothing the liver, invigorating the spleen, regulating qi and dissolving stasis, clearing away heat and resolving dampness, moistening the liver and nourishing the kidney. Furthermore, in order to keep the disease under control, recuperation with proper diet, appropriate rest and temperate sexual life are very essential.

〔辨证论治〕 Syndrome differentiation and treatment

1. 湿热内蕴

13.1　Internal retention of damp heat

【症状】右胁胀痛，食欲不振，恶心，腹胀，精神倦怠，面色如油垢所涂，舌苔黄腻，脉象弦紧。

【分析】外感湿热之邪，同气相求，归于脾胃，使湿热内蕴；或因饮食不节，饥饱无常，或因酗酒过度，或因劳倦伤脾，致使脾胃运化水谷和升清降浊的功能发生障碍，清者不升，浊者不降，郁于中焦，酿成湿热内结之候。湿热阻遏肝气的舒条，则右胁胀痛、精神倦怠；浊气不降，故食欲不振、恶心、腹胀；湿热之气上蒸，则见面色如油垢所涂；舌苔黄腻是湿热的明证，脉象弦者肝气不舒也，带有紧象为久郁不解之兆。

【治法】清热利湿。

【方药】龙胆泻肝汤加味。方用龙胆草苦寒清泻肝热，柴胡疏达肝胆气机；黄芩、栀子清泻三焦之热；泽泻、木通、车前子清热利湿，可使从小便而解；苦寒之药有伤肝之弊，故取当归、生地黄养血以补肝；甘草清热缓急，调和诸药。若湿热较重，可加茵陈、滑石加强清热利湿作用；若湿热伤及营血，见齿衄、鼻衄、肌衄，可加金银花、藕节、牡丹皮清营凉血；若口气秽浊，舌苔白腻，可加藿香、佩兰、苏叶芳香化浊，以开胃气。

Clinical manifestations: Distention and pain in the right hypochondrium, poor appetite, nausea, abdominal distention, lassitude, tarnished complexion like being coated with oil dirt, yellowish greasy tongue fur as well as taut and tense pulse.

Analysis: Internal accumulation of dampness and heat is caused by exogenous dampness and heat pathogens in the lung, acting in unison with stagnated dampness and heat in the spleen and stomach, which results in internal retention of dampness and heat; or dysfunction of the spleen and stomach to transport and transform digested food as well as failure to lift lucid yang and descend turbid qi, give rise to stagnation of dampness and heat in middle energizer because of improper diet, or alcoholism, or impairment of the spleen with overstrain. Distention and pain in the right hypochondrium and lassitude are due to failure of the liver to disperse because of damp heat obstruction; poor appetite, nausea and abdominal distention is due to failure to descend turbid qi; tarnished complexion like being coated with oil dirt is due to up-steaming of damp heat; yellowish greasy tongue fur is an obvious manifestation of damp heat, taut pulse indicates stagnation of qi in the liver, taut and tense pulse is a sign of unrelieved qi stagnation for a long time.

Prescription: Clear away heat and relieve dampness.

Formuals: Longdan Xiegan Tang Jiawei (Modified Longdan Xiegan Decoction). In the formula, Longdancao (*Radix Geutianae*), cold and bitter in nature, can purge heat from the liver, Chaihu (*Radix Bupleuri*) can soothe the liver and promote qi circulation; Huangqin (*Radix Scutellariae*) and Zhizi (*Fructus Gardeniae*) could clear away heat in triple energizer; Zexie (*Rhizoma Alismatis*), Mutong (*Caulis Akebiae*) and Cheqianzi (*Semen Plantaginis*) have an action of clearing away heat and inducing diuresis to remove dampness. Because medicinal herbs with cold and bitter nature are harmful to the liver, so Danggui (*Radix Angelicae Sinensis*) and Shengdihuang (*Radix Rehmanniae Recens*) can be combined to nourish blood and tonify the liver; Gancao (*Radix Glycyrrhizae*) can be added to reconcile the above herbs by clearing away heat and relieving spasm and pain. For severe dampness and heat, Yinchen (*Herba Artemisiae Scopariae*) and Huashi (*Talcum*) may be combined to strengthen the action of purging fire and relieving dampness; for symptoms such as gringival and nasal hemorrhage and muscular bleeding because dampness heat impair nutrient qi and blood, Jinyinhua (*Flos Lonicerae*), Oujie (*Nodus Nelumbinis Rhizomatis*) and Mudanpi (*Cortex Moutan Radicis*) could be combined to clear away nutrient qi and cool blood; for foul and turbid odor of the mouth, Huoxiang (*Herba Agastachis,*), Peilan (*Herba Eupatoril*) and Suye (*Folium Perillae*), aromatic in flavor, should be added to eliminate turbidity so as to regulate stomach qi.

2. 肝郁脾虚
13.2　Syndrome of liver depression and splenic asthenia

　　【症状】右胁隐隐作痛，腹胀，饮食减少，倦怠无力，大便溏薄，舌苔薄白，脉象弦缓无力。

　　【分析】肝郁脾虚多由情绪不遂，气机不畅，肝郁日久，克伐脾胃所引起。病发于肝，故右胁隐隐作痛；脾失健运之力，则腹胀、食欲不振；脾不化湿，故大便溏薄；舌苔白腻为脾湿之象；脉象弦缓为肝气舒条无力之征。

　　【治法】疏肝健脾。

　　【方药】逍遥散合香砂六君子丸。逍遥散以柴胡、薄荷疏肝解郁，以助肝用；当归、白芍养血柔肝，以养肝体；白术、茯苓、甘草益气健脾；甘草益气和胃。以此煎汤，送服香砂六君子丸，香砂六君子丸是健脾理气之名方，具有益气健脾、化湿和胃、理气消胀的作用。

Clinical manifestations: Dull pain in the right hypochondrium, abdominal distention, reduced appetite, weakness and lassitude, loose stool, thin whitish tongue fur as well as taut, moderate and weak pulse.

Analysis: The syndrome is mainly caused by impairment of the spleen and stomach due to emotional upset, qi stagnation and prolonged liver depression. Dull pain in the right hypochondrium is because the disease originates from the liver; abdominal distention and reduced appetite are due to dysfunction of the spleen in transportation and transformation; loose stool is due to stagnation of unresolved dampness in the spleen; whitish greasy tongue fur is a sign of splenic dampness, taut and moderate pulse indicates failure of liver qi to act freely and disperse normally.

Prescription: Soothe the liver and invigorate the spleen.

Formulas: Xiaoyao San (Powder) combined with Xiang Sha Liujunzi Wan (Pill). In Xiaoyao San, Chaihu (*Radix Bupleuri*) and Bohe (*Herba Menthae*) have the action of soothing the liver to relieve qi stagnation; Danggui (*Radix Angelicae Sinensis*) and Baishao (*Radix Paeoniae Alba*) could nourish blood and soften and tonify the liver; Baizhu (*Rhizoma Atractylodis Macrocephalae*), Fuling (*Poriae Cocos*) and Gancao (*Radix Glycyrrhizae*) have an action of benefiting qi and invigorating the spleen; Gancao could benefit qi and harmonize the stomach. As a well-known recipe for invigorating the spleen and regulating qi, Xiang Sha

Liujunzi Wan, with an action of benefiting qi, invigorating the spleen and resolving dampness to harmonize the stomach as well as regulating qi to eliminate abdominal distention, should be combined with the above one.

3. 气滞血瘀
13.3 Syndrome of qi stagnation and blood stasis

【症状】两胁刺痛，固定不移，肝脾肿大，面色晦滞，舌质晦暗，苔白腻或黄腻，脉象弦紧。

【分析】气郁日久，病邪必然由气及血，由经及络，由气郁证转化为气滞血瘀证。血瘀者，血络不通也，"不通则痛"，痛必刺痛，痛处固定不移；血瘀日久，则肝脾肿大；血不荣面，则面色晦滞；舌质晦暗，血瘀之象；苔腻，气滞之征；脉象弦紧，乃肝经气血郁滞所为。

【治法】行气活血。

【方药】膈下逐瘀汤加味。方中当归、川芎、赤芍、桃仁、红花、五灵脂、牡丹皮、延胡索为活血化瘀之佳品；香附、乌药、枳壳为行气解郁常用之药；甘草缓急和中。全方配伍，具有行气活血、通络止痛的功效。可加三棱、莪术、川楝子等以增强化瘀软坚之力。在服用期间，还可间服香砂六君子丸，以健脾和中，增进食欲，实为攻补兼施之法。

Clinical manifestations: Stabbing pain in the hypochondrium with fixed region, swollen liver and spleen, dull and tarnished complexion, darkish and tarnished tongue with whitish greasy fur or yellowish greasy fur as well as taut and tense pulse.

Analysis: Prolonged qi stagnation must cause pathogenic factors to transmit from qi phase into blood phase, and from meridians to collaterals, and the syndrome of qi stagnation could transform into qi stagnation coupled with blood stasis. Blood stasis indicates obstruction of blood vessels, which, would surely result in stabbing pain in fixed area; prolonged blood stasis would give rise to swollen liver and spleen; dull and tarnished complexion is due to failure of blood to nourish the face; darkish and tarnished tongue suggests blood stasis; greasy fur is a sign of qi stagnation; taut and tense pulse is caused by qi stagnation and blood stasis in liver meridian.

Prescription: Activate qi and promote blood circulation.

Formulas: Gexia Zhuyu Tang Jiawei (Modified Gexia Zhuyu Decoction). In the formula, Danggui (*Radix Angelicae Sinensis*), Chuanxiong (*Rhizoma Ligustici Chuanxiong*), Chishao (*Radix Paeoniae Rubra*), Taoren (*Semen Persicae*), Honghua (*Flos Carthami*), Wulingzhi (*Faeces Togopteri*), Mudanpi (*Cortex Moutan Radicis*) and Yanhusuo (*Rhizoma Corydalis*) are the best drug for activating qi and resolving blood stasis, Xiangfu (*Rhizoma Cyperi*), Wuyao (*Radix Linderae*) and Zhiqiao (*Fructus Aurantii*) are the common herbs for activating qi and relieving stagnation; Gancao (*Radix Glycyrrhizae*) can relieve spasm and pain and regulate middle energizer. The whole formula has the action of activating qi and promoting blood circulation and dredge blood vessels to stop pain. To reinforce the effect of resolving stasis and softening dry feces, Sanling (*Rhizoma Sparganii*), Ezhu (*Rhizoma Curcumae*) and Chuanlianzi (*Fructus Meliae Toosendan*) could be added. Xiang Sha Liujunzi Wan (Pill) may be used to combine with the above recipe to invigorate the spleen, harmonize middle energizer and promote appetite, therefore, it is actually a therapeutical method of purgation and tonifying.

4. 肝肾阴亏
13.4 Syndrome of yin asthenia of the liver and kidney

【症状】胁痛隐隐，腰膝酸软，口干咽燥，五心烦热，舌质嫩暗或青暗，脉象虚数。

【分析】肝阴不足，则肝失所养，故肝之所属部位（以右胁为重）胁痛隐隐；肾阴不足，则腰膝酸软；阴不足则口干咽燥；阴虚日久，则心阴亦显亏虚，故有五心烦热；肝阴不足以养肝，则舌质嫩暗，甚则青暗；"阴虚生内热"，故脉象虚数。

【治法】滋养肝肾。

【方药】一贯煎加味。方中生地黄、当归、沙参、枸杞子、麦冬滋阴养血以补益肝肾；川楝子性虽苦寒，但能理气解郁，配入大量甘寒养阴之品，则不会伤津，反而疏泄肝气；另加女贞子、旱莲草滋阴清热；还可少佐砂仁芳香开胃醒脾，并防滋阴之药过于甘寒生湿伤脾。

Clinical manifestations: Dull pain in the hypochondrium, aching and weakness of the loins and knees, dry mouth and throat, feverish sensation over the palms, soles and chest, tender darkish or even dark cyanotic tongue as well as weak and fast pulse.

Analysis: Insufficient liver yin causes malnutritioum of the liver, which gives rise to dull pain over the region where the liver is located (especially the right hypochondrium); aching and weakness of the loins and knees is due to insufficiency of kidney yin; dry mouth and throat are due to deficiency of yin; feverish sensation over the palms, soles and chest is due to prolonged yin deficiency involving asthenia of heart yin; tender darkish or even dark cyanotic tongue is caused by failure of insufficient liver yin to nourish the liver; weak and fast pulse indicates "yin asthenia generating endogenous heat".

Prescription: Moisten the liver and nourish the kidney.

Formulas: Yiguan Jian Jiawei (Modified Yiguan Dectoction). In the formula, Shengdihuang (*Radix Rehmanniae Recens*), Danggui (*Radix Angelicae Sinensis*), Shashen (*Adenophora stricta*), Gouqizi (*Fructus Lycii*) and Maidong (*Radix Ophiopogonis*) can moisten yin and nourish blood to benefit the liver and kidney; Chuanlianzi (*Fructus Meliae Toosendan*), though bitter in flavor and cold in nature, can regulate qi and relieve stagnation, combined with large amount of sweet-cold natured herbs, it could not impair body fluid but soothe the liver and remove qi stagnation; Nuzhenzi (*Fructus Ligustri Lucidi*) and Hanliancao (*Eclipta Alba*) can be added to nourish yin and clear away heat, and a little amount of aromatic natured Sharen (*Fructus Amomi Villosi*) could be combined to promote appetite, refresh the spleen, and prevent yin-nourishing herbs from impairing the spleen because of their excessive sweet-cold nature.

十四、肝硬化

14 Liver cirrhosis

〔**概说**〕 Summary

肝硬化是一种慢性全身性疾病。其病理特点为广泛的肝细胞变性和坏死，纤维组织弥漫性增生并有再生小结节的形成。临床上的主要表现为肝功能减退，门静脉高压，从而引起脾肿大、腹水、腹壁静脉曲张、食管和胃底静脉曲张破裂、肝性昏迷等。

肝硬化属于中医学"臌胀""单腹胀""积聚"等病范畴，认为该病由情志不遂、酒食不节、劳欲过度、湿热郁滞所致。治疗上针对病因病机以及病人的体质而拟定治法。肝硬化是一种比较难以治疗的疾病，中医中药对该病具有缓解症状、改善体质、提高生命质量的效果。

Liver cirrhosis is a chronic systemic disease with a pathological condition characterized by denaturation or necrosis of liver cells in a wide range, diffusive regeneration of fibre tissue as well as new formation of regenerative nodules. Its main clinical manifestations are as follows: swollen spleen, abdominal dropsy, varicosity over abdominal wall, broken varicosity of oesophagus and of stomach fundus as well as hepatic coma due to dysfunction of the liver and hypertension on portal vein.

In TCM, liver cirrhosis is classified into "tympanites" "abdominal distention" "abdominal mass", and so on. It is generally believed that liver cirrhosis is mainly caused by emotional upset, alcoholism, overstrain, intemperance of sexual life as well as stagnation of dampness and heat. Treatment for the disease should be based on its etiology, pathogenesis as well as a patient's constitution. Liver cirrhosis is difficult to cure, and TCM plays an undeniable role in alleviating some symptoms of it and in improving the constitution as well as the living quality of patients.

〔**辨证论治**〕 Syndrome differentiation and treatment

1. 肝郁脾虚

14.1 Syndrome of liver depression and splenic asthenia

【症状】两胁胀痛，面色萎黄，食欲不振，胃脘痞满，时时肠鸣，大便溏薄，身困乏力，精神疲倦，舌质淡暗，苔薄白，脉象弦缓。

【分析】肝郁脾虚多为肝硬化的初起证候，由于肝气郁结，故见两胁胀痛；脾虚则面色萎黄；肝郁使胃气受阻，故食欲不振、胃脘痞满；脾虚则运化水湿的能力下降，故有时时肠鸣、大便稀薄；肝郁则筋脉不舒，脾虚则气血难生，故精神疲倦、身困乏力；舌质淡暗者，乃肝郁所致；苔薄白为脾虚之象；脉象弦缓，弦为肝郁，缓为脾虚，合见则为肝脾不和之征。

【治法】疏肝理气，健脾利湿。

【方药】柴胡疏肝散加味。柴胡疏肝散由四逆散加香附、陈皮、川芎组成。四逆散为疏肝理脾的常用方，方以柴胡透邪舒郁，枳实下气散结，白芍益阴养血，炙甘草益气健脾，四味配伍，可使气血调畅，肝舒脾健。药味简练，但经历代医家临床证实，该方收效甚捷。加入香附、陈皮、川芎，增强行气疏肝、和血止痛之效，服后可使肝气条达，血脉通畅，营卫自和，痛止而胀满消除。

Clinical manifestations: Distending pain in the hypochondrium, sallow complexion, poor appetite, epigastric distention and fullness, frequent borborygmus, loose stool, heavy body and lack of energy, lassitude, dull darkish tongue with thin whitish fur as well as taut and moderate pulse.

Analysis: The initial syndrome of liver cirrhosis is marked by liver depression and splenic asthenia. Distending pain in the hypochondrium is due to stagnation of liver qi; sallow complexion is due to spleen asthenia; poor appetite, epigastric distention and fullness are due to inhibited stomach qi because of liver stagnation; frequent borborygmus and loose stool are caused by failure of asthenic spleen to transport and transform dampness; stagnation of liver qi results in inflexibility of the tendons and obstruction of vessels; lassitude, heavy body and lack of energy are due to failure of asthenic spleen to promote generation of qi and blood; dull darkish tongue is caused by qi depression of the liver; thin whitish fur indicates asthenic spleen; taut pulse suggests liver depression, moderate pulse is a sign of asthenic spleen, taut and moderate pulse indicates disharmony of the liver and spleen.

Prescription: Soothe the liver to regulate qi and invigorate the spleen to resolve dampness.

Formulas: Chaihu Shugan San Jiawei (Modified Chaihu Shugan Powder). Chaihu Shugan San is made up of Sini San (Powder) in combination with Xiangfu (*Rhizoma Cyperi*), Chenpi (*Pericarpium Citri Reticulatae*) and Chuanxiong (*Rhizoma Ligustici Chuanxiong*). Sini San is a common recipe for soothing the liver and regulating the spleen, in which, Chaihu (*Radix Bupleuri*) can remove pathogenic factors to relieve qi stagnation of the liver, Zhishi (*Fructus Aurantii Immaturus*) could descend qi and dissolve masses, Baishao (*Radix Paeoniae Alba*) may benefit yin and nourish blood, and stir-baked Gancao (*Radix Glycyrrhizae*) can benefit qi and invigorate the spleen. Combined together, the four herbs could promote qi and blood circulation, soothe the liver and invigorate the spleen. Having been confirmed by ancient TCM practitioners, the simple recipe could achieve a rapid effect. Xiangfu (*Rhizoma Cyperi*), Chenpi (*Pericarpium Citri Reticulatae*) and Chuanxiong (*Rhizoma Ligustici Chuanxiong*) could be combined to strengthen the function of activating qi, soothing the liver, harmonizing blood circulation as well as arresting pain. After intake of the drug, liver qi could act freely and disperse normally, blood vessels could keep smooth circulation, and nutrient qi and defensive qi could be reconciled naturally. As a result, pain could get relieved and distention and fullness be eliminated.

2. 气滞血阻
14.2　Syndrome of qi stagnation and blood obstruction

【症状】肝脾积块，软而不坚，固定不移，胀痛并见，不欲饮食，舌苔薄腻，脉象弦紧。

【分析】这里用"血阻"二字，反映其证候比"血瘀"严重，是由于气滞血瘀日久所致。气滞血阻，脉络不通，故积而成块；肝气不舒，脾气不运，浊气不降，故胀痛并见；脾胃被克，纳运失常，故不欲饮食；舌苔薄腻，脾不运化；脉象弦紧，乃肝气拘紧不舒之象。

【治法】理气活血，通络消积。

【方药】金铃子散合失笑散加味。金铃子散中的金铃子即川楝子，以疏肝理气见长，延胡索以活血止痛作用突出。失笑散由蒲黄、五灵脂组成，蒲黄（炒）与五灵脂都是活血化瘀药，但一个侧重于气分，一个侧重于血分。蒲黄侧重于气分，五灵脂侧重于血分，两药配伍，互相促进，作用加强，适用于心腹剧痛，有气滞血瘀之"积聚"者。腹胀甚者，加青皮、陈皮、藿香、香附以行气散血；不欲饮食者，加鸡内金、生麦芽、谷芽、神曲以开胃进食；大便不通者，加大黄（后下）、牵牛子以通腑祛积。

Clinical manifestations: Soft lumps in the liver and spleen with fixed region without migration, accompanied with distending pain, anorexia, thin greasy fur as well as taut and tense pulse.

Analysis: The syndrome is caused by prolonged qi stagnation and blood stasis. "Blood obstruction" here shows that the syndrome is more serious than "blood stasis". Lumps in the liver and spleen are due to obstructed blood vessels and collaterals because of accumulation of stagnated qi and blood; distending pain is due to failure to soothe liver qi, dysfunction of splenic qi to transport as well as failure to descend turbid qi; anorexia is due to dysfunction of the spleen and stomach because they are restrained; thin greasy fur indicates dysfunction of the spleen in transformation; taut and tense pulse is a sign of failure to disperse qi stagnation in the liver.

Prescription: Regulate qi to promote blood circulation, dredge collaterals and resolve lumps of blood stasis.

Formulas: Jinlingzi San (Powder) combined with Shixiao San (Powder) Jiawei. In Jinlingzi San, Jinlingzi, also known as Chuanlianzi (*Fructus Meliae Toosendan*), has an action of soothing the liver and regulating qi, Yanhusuo (*Rhizoma Corydalis*) is featured by its function of activating blood and arresting pain; Shixiao San consists of stir-baked Puhuang (*Pollen Typhae*) and Wulingzhi (*Faeces Togopteri*), both of them could activate blood and resolve stasis, but the former is prone to exerting its function in qi phase, while the latter tends to activate blood in blood phase. Combined together, both herbs could improve and strengthen their actions mutually, and they are usually used for acute pain of the heart and abdomen, in particular, for "abdominal mass" of the syndrome of qi stagnation and blood stasis. For abdominal distention, Qingpi (*Pericarpium Citri Reticulatae Viride*), Chenpi (*Pericarpium Citri Reticulatae*), Huoxiang (*Herba Agastachis*) and Xiangfu (*Rhizoma Cyperi*) could be added to activate qi and dissolve blood stasis; for anorexia, Jineijin (*Endothelium Corneum Gigeriae Galli*), Maiya (*Fructus Hordei Germinatus*), Guya (*Fructus Setariae Germinatus*) and Shenqu (*Massa Medicata Fermentata*) can be combined to promote appetite; for constipation, Qianniuzi (*Semen Pharbitidis*) and Dahuang (*Radix et Rhizoma Rhei*) (decocted later) may be added to dredge fu-organs and remove masses.

3. 水湿内阻
14.3　Syndrome of internal retention of dampness

【症状】腹部胀大，按之坚满，胃痞纳呆，恶心呕吐，小便短少，舌苔薄白而滑，脉象弦细或弦紧。

【分析】本证候以脾虚水湿内阻为病机。"诸腹胀满，皆属于脾。"脾失运化，气机不顺，故腹部胀大，按之坚满；水湿内阻，胃气不得通降，故恶心呕吐；气不化湿，则小便短少；舌苔白滑为脾湿不化，脉象弦细或弦紧，为肝气不舒之征。

【治法】健脾利湿，理气行水。

【方药】胃苓汤。胃苓汤由平胃散与五苓散组成。平胃散由陈皮、苍术、厚朴、甘草组成，作用为健脾和胃、行气散湿；五苓散由茯苓、猪苓、泽泻、白术、桂枝组成，功效为温阳健脾、散湿利水。两方合用，重在健脾和胃、理气行水。若小便不利者，可加车前子、陈葫芦瓢利尿消肿；若见阳虚恶寒者，可加干姜、附子以助阳化阴；若腹水多不易消退者，可加牵牛子、大黄以通便消水。

Clinical manifestations: Abdominal distention and fullness, hard and full sensation under pressure, indigestion in the spleen and stomach, nausea and vomiting, scanty urine, thin slippery whitish fur as well as taut and thin pulse or taut and tense pulse.

Analysis: Pathogenesis for this syndrome is internal retention of dampness due to splenic asthenia. "All symptoms of abdominal distention and fullness originate from the spleen." Abdominal distention with hard and full sensation under pressure is caused by dysfunction of the spleen and qi disorder; nausea and vomiting are due to failure to descend stomach qi because of internal retention of dampness; scanty urine is due to failure of splenic qi to resolve dampness; greasy whitish fur indicates failure of the spleen to resolve dampness; taut and thin pulse or taut and tense pulse is a sign of stagnation of liver qi.

Prescription: Invigorate the spleen to resolve dampness and regulate qi to induce diuresis.

Formulas: Weiling Tang (Decoction). Weiling Tang is made up of Pingwei San (Powder) and Wuling San (Powder). Pingwei San consists of Chenpi (*Pericarpium Citri* reticulatae）, Cangzhu （*Rhizoma Atractylodis*）, Houpo （*Cortex Magnoliae Officinals*）and Gancao （*Radix Glycyrrhizae*）, having an action of invigorating the spleen, harmonizing the stomach and activating qi to dispel dampness. Wuling San （Powder）, made up of Fuling （*Poriae Cocos*）, Zhuling （*Polyporus Umbellatus*）, Zexie （*Rhizoma Alismatis*）, Baizhu （*Rhizoma Atractylodis Macrocephalae*）and Guizhi （*Ramulus Cinnamomi*）, has an action of warming yang, invigorating the spleen, dispelling dampness and inducing diuresis. Combined together, both recipes could exert the function of invigorating the spleen, harmonizing the stomach and activating qi to dispel dampness. For unsmooth urination, Cheqianzi （*Semen Plantaginis*）and bottle gourd planted in the previous year can be used to induce diuresis and relieve dropsy; for yang asthenia and aversion to cold, Ganjiang （*Rhizoma Zingiberis*）and Fuzi （*Radix Aconiti Lateralis Preparata*）should be used to assist yang to transform yin; for abdominal dropsy with difficulty to eliminate, Qianniuzi （*Semen Pharbitidis*）and Dahuang （*Radix et Rhizoma Rhei*）may be used to relax the bowels and resolve dropsy.

4. 肝肾阴虚
14.4 Syndrome of yin asthenia of the liver and kidney

【症状】面色枯槁，消瘦无力，两颧泛红，心中烦躁，手足心热，持续低热，时有鼻衄、齿衄，腹大胀满，小便短赤，舌质红绛少津，苔少，脉象弦细数。

【分析】肝肾阴虚多为肝硬化的晚期证候。肝郁日久，气郁化火，火灼肝肾之阴，形成一派阴液枯槁之象。"阴虚生内热"，故见两颧泛红，心中烦躁，手足心热，持续低热；时有火动伤络，故有鼻衄、齿衄；阴液消耗，故消瘦无力；肝阴亏耗，肝气必然失于约束，过于克伐脾胃，则见腹大胀满；阴虚内热，则小便短赤；其舌质、舌苔、脉象，均显示阴虚内热之征。

【治法】滋养肝肾，育阴利水。

【方药】一贯煎合猪苓汤加味。一贯煎为养肝阴之主剂，猪苓汤为育阴利水之主剂。一贯煎的药物效应已在"慢性肝炎"一节中叙述。猪苓汤由猪苓、茯苓、泽泻、滑石、阿胶五味组成，为育阴利水之主方。猪苓、茯苓、泽泻、滑石为利水之剂，而甘寒的滑石兼有生津的作用，唯阿胶为滋阴补血之剂，使其利水而不伤阴，滋阴而不腻窍。此方与五苓散相比，仅两味之差，但其作用却不相同。本方为育阴利水，而五苓散为化气利水，切不可因方中利水之药相同而混用。

Clinical manifestations: Withered complexion, emaciation and lack of energy, flushed cheek, restlessness, feverish sensation over the palms and soles, persistent mild fever, occasional nasal and gringival hemorrhage, abdominal distention and fullness, scanty brownish urine, deep reddish tongue with scanty fluid, scanty fur as well as taut, thin and fast pulse.

Analysis: The syndrome usually occurs at the advanced stage of cirrhosis. Prolonged qi depression in the liver can transform into fire, which scorches liver yin and kidney yin, thus giving rise to exhaustion of yin fluid. Flushed cheek, restlessness, feverish sensation over the palms and soles and persistent mild fever are caused by endogenous heat due to yin asthenia; nasal and gringival hemorrhage are caused by hyperactive fire scorching the collaterals; emaciation and lack of energy are due to consumption of yin fluid; abdominal distention and fullness are due to uncontrolled hyperactive liver qi restraining the spleen and stomach because of deficiency and consumption of liver-yin; scanty brownish urine is caused by yin asthenia generating endogenous heat; deep reddish tongue with scanty fluid, scanty fur and taut, thin and fast pulse are signs of endogenous heat due to yin asthenia.

Prescription: Moisten the liver, nourish the kidney and benefit yin to induce diuresis.

Formulas: Yiguan Jian (Decoction) combined with Zhuling Tang (Decoction) Jiawei. Yiguan Jian is a principal recipe for nourishing liver yin, its medicinal action has been discussed in *Chronic Hepatitis*. Zhuling Tang is a main recipe for benefiting yin and inducing diuresis, which consists of Zhuling (*Polyporus Umbellatus*), Fuling (*Poriae Cocos*), Zexie (*Rhizoma Alismatis*), Huashi (*Talcum*) and Ejiao (*Colla Corii Asini*). In the recipe, the first four herbs can induce diuresis, Huashi, cold and sweet in nature, has an action of promoting production of body fluid, and Ejiao is the only one with the effect of nourishing yin and tonifying blood, so it could help the whole recipe induce diuresis without impairing yin, nourish yin without obstructing the orifices. Compared with Wuling San which focuses on warming yang and resolving dampness, this formula has a different action of nourishing yin and inducing diuresis. Both formulas should not be confused with each other just because of containing the the same medicinal herbs for inducing diuresis.

5. 脾肾阳虚
14.5 Syndrome of yang asthenia of the spleen and kidney

【症状】面色晦暗，畏寒喜温，神疲无力，口淡食少，脘腹胀满，两胁坠痛，下肢浮肿，大便溏薄，舌质胖淡，苔白腻，脉象沉细无力。

【分析】脾肾阳虚亦为肝硬化之重证。阳虚不能温运气血，故面色晦暗，神疲无力；"阳虚则外寒"，故其形寒肢冷喜温；脾阳虚则口淡食少，脘腹胀满；脾肾阳虚，肝气不得生发，故有两胁坠痛之感；阳虚则水湿不化，水性就下，故下肢浮肿，大便溏薄；舌质胖淡，为阳气不能温养之象，脾阳虚则苔腻不运，脉象沉细无力为阳虚不能鼓动脉搏之征。

【治法】健脾补肾，温阳利水。

【方药】实脾饮合济生肾气丸。实脾饮由附子、干姜、白术、厚朴、木香、草果、槟榔、木瓜、茯苓、生姜、大枣、甘草组成。是方具有温阳健脾、行气利水的功效，为治疗阴水的主要方剂。而济生肾气丸由金匮肾气丸加牛膝、车前子组成，是治疗肾阳虚弱、邪水潴留的代表方剂。一个方抓脾阳虚，一个方抓肾阳虚，两方用于温阳的药物主要是附子、干姜、桂枝等，而健脾利水的药物为白术、茯苓、木瓜等，其他药物多为行气之品，更有生姜、大枣、甘草三味，可调和营卫、缓和诸药的副作用。两方合用，脾湿兼顾，温阳为本，利水为标。但对于附子、干姜等辛温药物的用量，要从小剂量开始，不可猛然从大剂量开始，特别是附子，以炮制过的为宜。"少火生气"，用过量了，就会造成"壮火食气"的弊端。

Clinical manifestations：Tarnished complexion, aversion to cold and preference for warmth, dispiritedness and lack of energy, bland taste and poor appetite, distention and fullness in the epigastrium and abdomen, prolapsing pain of the hypochondrium, dropsy of the lower limbs, thin loose stool, pale bulgy tongue with greasy whitish fur as well as sunken, thin and weak pulse.

Analysis：Syndrome of yang asthenia of the spleen and kidney is a serious syndrome of cirrhosis. Tarnished complexion, dispiritedness and lack of energy are due to failure of asthenic yang to warm and transport qi and blood; cold limbs and body with preference for warmth indicates "yang asthenia generating stagnation of cold on the exterior"; bland taste and poor appetite as well as distention and fullness in the epigastrium and abdomen are due to yang asthenia of the spleen; prolapsing pain of the hypochondrium is caused by failure to disperse liver qi due to yang asthenia of the spleen and kidney; dropsy of lower limbs and thin loose stool indicate failure to resolve dampness and susceptibility of dampness to flowing downward; pale bulgy tongue suggests failure of asthenic yang qi to warm and nourish, greasy fur indicates kidney yang asthenia and failure to transport, sunken, thin and weak pulse is a sign of failure of asthenic yang to rise in blood vessels.

Prescription：Invigorate the spleen, tonify the kidney and induce diuresis by warming yang.

Formulas：Shipi Yin (Decoction) combined with Jisheng Shenqi Wan (Pill). Shipi Yin, consisting of Fuzi (*Radix Aconiti Lateralis Preparata*), Ganjiang (*Rhizoma Zingiberis*), Baizhu (*Rhizoma Atractylodis Macrocephalae*), Houpo (*Cortex Magnoliae Officinals*), Muxiang (*Radix Aucklandiae*), Caoguo (*Fructus Tsaoko*), Binlang (*Semen Arecae*), Mugua (*Fructus Chaenomelis*), Fuling (*Poriae Cocos*) Shengjiang (*Rhizoma Zingiberis Recens*), Dazao (*Fructus Jujubae*) and Gancao (*Radix Glycyrrhizae*), has an action of invigorating the spleen by warming yang, activating qi and resolving dampness, so it is the principal recipe for yin edema. While Jisheng Shenqi Wan (or Decoction), made up of Jingui Shenqi Wan (Pill), Niuxi (*Radix Achyranthis Bidentatae*) and Cheqianzi (*Semen Plantaginis*), is a typical formula for yang asthenia of the kidney and retention of pathogenic dampness. The former formula aims at treating splenic yang asthenia, while the latter aims at curing kidney yang asthenia. In both formulas, the herbs for warming yang are mainly Fuzi, Ganjiang and Guizhi, the herbs for invigorating the spleen and inducing diuresis include Baizhu, Fuling, Mugua, and other herbs are used for activating qi. Besides, Shengjiang, Dazao and Gancao are combined to reconcile nutrient qi and defensive qi so as to alleviate the side effect of all herbs. Combined together, both formulas can treat the syndrome of dampness in the spleen, with taking warming yang being the fundamental therapeutic principle, and inducing diuresis being the secondary one. The amount of pungent-warm herbs, such as Fuzi and Ganjiang, should not be large, in particular, Fuzi (a poisonous herb), because soaked

Fuzi has decreased toxicity, so it should be the most suitable in the formula. "Mild fire (appropriate dose) warms qi", dosage beyond appropriate degree can give rise to "sthenic fire", which will surely "consume qi".

十五、便秘

15　Constipation

〔**概说**〕 Summary

便秘是指粪便在肠内停留过久，以致大便干结，排出困难或不尽，为临床常见的症状。可伴有一些自觉症状，如下腹部胀满，直肠排空迟缓，有矢气，甚则食欲不振，口中有秽浊之气，头痛头晕等；但亦有大便秘结而无自觉症状者。多数病人是由于局部机械作用而引起神经反射的结果。本病多见于妊娠妇女、老年人以及不大运动的人。根据病理可分为功能性便秘和器质性便秘，本文主要讨论功能性便秘。

便秘在中医古籍中早有记载，如汉代张仲景《金匮要略》中麻子仁丸所治的"脾约"证，《伤寒论》中的"阳结"与"阴结"等，都是指的便秘。中医治疗便秘，从辨证论治入手，方证对应，丝丝入扣，常能取得良好效果。

Constipation refers to a disease with the common pathological symptoms such as dry feces, difficulty in defecation or incomplete defecation due to prolonged retention of feces in the large intestine. Constipation is accompanied by some symptoms that a patient can feel by himself, for instance, distention and fullness of the lower abdomen, slowness of evacuation in the rectum, flatus, or even poor appetite, foul and turbid odor in the mouth as well as headache and vertigo. In some cases, constipation is not accompanied with the above symptoms that could be felt by patients themselves. For most patients, constipation is caused by neural reflex to regional mechanism, and the disease is usually seen in pregnant women, aging people as well as those who lack of exercise. According to its different pathological changes, constipation can be divided into structural constipation and functional constipation, with the latter being the focus of this chapter.

Constipation has been recorded in ancient TCM classics, for instance, Zhang Zhongjing from the Han Dynasty has mentioned treatment for "the syndrome of spleen constipation" with Maziren Wan (Pill) in *Jingui Yaolue* (*Synopsis of Golden Chamber*), yang constipation and yin constipation in *Shanghan Lun* (*Treatise on Cold Pathogenic and Miscellaneous Diseases*). All of the syndromes mentioned above are constipation. Treatment for it by means of TCM medication should start with syndrome differentiation, every syndrome must get its corresponding formula, and every step must be taken carefully without any confusion or mistake. Only in this way can perfect curative effect be achieved.

〔辨证论治〕 Syndrome differentiation and treatment

1. 燥热内结

15.1 Syndrome of internal accumulation of dryness and heat

【症状】大便干结，小便短赤，口干口苦，口臭，腹胀或痛，舌红苔黄，脉象滑数。

【分析】胃肠积热，暗耗津液，致使大便干结；热伏于内熏蒸于上，故有口干口苦、口臭；热积于内，腑气不通，故腹胀或痛；舌红苔黄、脉象滑数，为燥热内盛之象。

【治法】清热润肠通便。

【方药】麻子仁丸加减。麻子仁丸为治疗燥热内盛、津亏便秘之主方。方由小承气汤加火麻仁、杏仁、白芍、蜂蜜组成。方以火麻仁润肠通便为君药；大黄通便泻热，杏仁降气润肠，白芍养阴和里，共为臣药；枳实、厚朴下气破结，加强降气通便力量，蜂蜜润燥滑肠，共为佐使药。诸药合而为丸，具有润肠泻热、行气通便的作用。见肝火上炎，面红目赤者，可加芦荟、龙胆草、牡丹皮凉血泻火。

Clinical manifestations: Dry feces, scanty brownish urine, dry mouth and bitter taste, foul odor of the mouth, abdominal distention or pain, reddish tongue with yellowish fur as well as slippery and fast pulse.

Analysis: Dry feces is caused by accumulation of heat in the stomach and intestines, which consumes body fluid; dry mouth, bitter taste and foul odor in the mouth are due to up-fumigation of internal heat retention; abdominal distention or pain is due to stagnation of large intestinal qi because of internal heat accumulation; reddish tongue with yellowish fur and slippery and fast pulse are signs of internal exuberance of dry heat.

Prescription: Clear away heat and relax bowels by relieving constipation.

Formulas: Maziren Wan Jiajian (Modified Maziren Pill). Maziren Wan is a major formula for treating fluid-deficient constipation because of internal exuberance of dry heat. The formula is the combination of Small Chengqi Tang with Huomaren (*Fructus Cannabis*), Xingren (*Semen Armeniacae Amarum*), Baishao (*Radix Paeoniae Alba*) and Fengmi (*Mel*). In the formula, Huomaren, with its action of moistening the intestines and relieving constipation, is used as sovereign drug. Dahuang (*Radix et Rhizoma Rhei*) has an function of relieving constipation and purging heat, Xingren can descend adverse flow of qi and moisten the bowels, Baishao can nourish yin and harmonize the interior. Combined together, the three herbs are used as ministerial drug. Zhishi (*Fructus Aurantii Immaturus*) and Houpo (*Cortex Magnoliae Officinalis*) could send down qi and break lumps to reinforce the action of descending qi and relaxing the bowels, and Fengmi has an effect of moistening dryness of the intestines, the three herbs are used together as assistant and courier drug. After being processed and made into pill, all the above medicinal herbs could bring the action of moistening the intestines, purging heat, activating qi and relieving constipation into full play. For flushed cheek and ears caused by liver fire hyperactivity, Luhui (*Aloe*), Longdancao (*Radix Gentianae*) and Mudanpi (*Cortex Moutan Radicis*) may be added to cool blood and purge fire.

2. 气机郁滞
15.2 Syndrome of qi stagnation

【症状】大便秘结，嗳气食少，胁腹胀满或疼痛，舌质红，苔薄黄，脉象沉弦。

【分析】情志不遂，肝气郁结，郁而生热，热耗阴津，故大便秘结；肠道失去传导之功，气逆而上，故嗳气频作；肝脏位于腹内而经脉布于两胁，肝气不舒，则胁腹胀满或疼痛；脾气失运，食难消化，故饮食减少；舌红苔黄、脉象沉弦，为气郁化热之象。

【治法】顺气导滞。

【方药】六磨汤加减。六磨汤出自《证治准绳》，由木香、沉香、乌药、大黄、槟榔、枳实组成。方中木香、沉香、乌药顺气宽肠；大黄、槟榔、枳实导滞通腑。口苦咽干，可加芦荟、黄芩清肺胃之热；腹胀可加莱菔子、青皮、陈皮，以加强理气消胀的作用。

Clinical manifestations: Dry feces, belching and reduced appetite, distention and fullness or pain of the abdomen and hypochondrium, reddish tongue with thin yellowish fur as well as sunken and taut pulse.

Analysis: Dry feces or constipation is caused by heat generated from liver qi depression because of emotional upset consuming yin fluid of the body; frequent belching is due to dysfunction of the intestines in transportation, which causes adverse flow of qi; the liver is located in the abdomen but the liver meridians are distributed in the area of the hypochondrium, therefore, qi stagnation of the liver brings about distention and fullness or pain of the abdomen and hypochondrium; reduced appetite is due to dysfunction of splenic qi in transportation and failure to digest food; reddish tongue with thin yellowish fur and sunken and taut pulse are signs of transformation of heat from stagnated qi.

Prescription: Facilitate qi flow and relieve dyspepsia.

Formulas: Liumo Tang Jiajian (Modified Liumo Decoction). It is quoted from *Zhengzhi Zhunsheng* (*Standards for Diagnosis and Treatment*), consisting of Muxiang (*Radix Aucklandiae*), Chenxiang (*Lignum Aquilariae Resinatum*), Wuyao (*Radix Linderae*), Dahuang (*Radix et Rhizoma Rhei*), Binlang (*Semen Arecae*) and Zhishi (*Fructus Aurantii Immaturus*). Among them, the first three can facilitate qi flow and relax the bowels; Dahuang, Binlang and Zhishi have an action of relieving dyspepsia and dredging the Fu-organs. For bitter taste and dry throat, Luhui (*Aloe*) and Huangqin (*Radix Scutellariae*) can be combined to clear away heat from the lung and stomach; for abdominal distention, Laifuzi (*Semen Raphani*), Qingpi (*Pericarpium Citri Reticulatae Viride*) and Chenpi (*Pericarpium*

Citri Reticulatae) can be combined to regulate qi and remove distention.

3. 气虚不运
15.3 Syndrome of qi asthenia and dysfunction of transportation

【症状】欲排便而难出，临厕努挣而无力，汗出短气，排便后身感疲惫，舌质淡红，苔薄白，脉象细弱。

【分析】由于肺气虚而导致大肠传导无力，故欲排便而难出；临厕用力排便，易感乏力、汗出、短气；排便后，气不接续，故身感疲惫；舌淡与脉象，均为气虚之象。

【治法】益气润肠。

【方药】黄芪润肠汤（经验方）。方由黄芪、白术、黄精、肉苁蓉、火麻仁、柏子仁、郁李仁组成。方中黄芪、白术、黄精补气健脾，脾气健大肠传导有力；肉苁蓉有补肾润肠之功；火麻仁、柏子仁、郁李仁，均为种子类药物，内含油脂，有润肠通便作用。若口干，可加北沙参、玄参等滋阴润肠。

Clinical manifestations: Difficulty and weakness in defecation, obstructive defecation, sweating and short breath, tiredness after defecation, pale reddish tongue with thin whitish fur and thin and feeble pulse.

Analysis: Difficulty and weakness in defecation and obstructive defecation are due to asthenic lung qi and dysfunction of the large intestine in transportation; lack of energy, sweating and short breath are due to exhaustion of energy in defecation; tiredness after defecation is due to failure to keep continuous circulation of qi; pale reddish tongue with thin whitish fur and thin and weak pulse are signs of qi asthenia.

Prescription: Benefit qi and moisten the large intestine.

Formulas: Huangqi Runchang Tang (Decoction) (an empirical formula for the syndrome). It is made up of Huangqi (*Radix Astragali seu Hedysari*), Baizhu (*Rhizoma Atractylodis Macrocephalae*), Huangjing (*Rhizoma Polygonati*), Roucongrong (*Herba Cistanches*), Huomaren (*Fructus Cannabis*), Baiziren (*Semen Platycladi*) and Yuliren (*Semen Pruni*). Among them, Huangqi, Baizhu and Huangjing have an action of tonifying qi and invigorating the spleen to strengthen splenic qi and improve the function of the large intestine in transportation; Roucongrong can strengthen the kidney and moisten the large intestine; Huomaren, Baiziren and Yuliren are all seeds containing oil, so they can moisten the bowels and promote defecation. For dry mouth, Beishashen (*Radix Glehniae*) and Xuanshen (*Radix Scrophulariae*) can be added to nourish yin and moisten the large intestine.

4. 血虚肠燥
15.4 Syndrome of blood asthenia and dryness of the large intestine

【症状】大便秘结，面色无华，头晕目眩，心悸，失眠多梦，舌质淡红，脉细弱。

【分析】本证因血虚津少，不能泽润大肠，故大便秘结；血虚不能上荣，故面色无华，头晕目眩；血虚心失所养，故心悸、失眠、多梦；舌质淡、脉细弱，为血虚之明证。

【治法】养血润燥。

【方药】润肠丸加减。方由大黄、当归、羌活、桃仁、火麻仁组成。方中当归养血，桃仁化瘀，火麻仁润肠，羌活祛风，大黄泻下。五味药物，共奏养血、润肠、化瘀、通腑的作用。阴虚火旺，可加知母、玄参、天花粉；兼有气虚者，可加党参、黄芪、白术，以补气增力。

Clinical manifestations：Dry feces, sallow and lusterless complexion, dizziness and vertigo, palpitation, insomnia and dreaminess, pale reddish tongue as well as thin and feeble pulse.

Analysis：Dry feces is due to blood asthenia and failure of scanty fluid to moisten the large intestine; sallow and lusterless complexion, dizziness and vertigo are due to failure of asthenic blood to nourish the face; palpitation, insomnia and dreaminess are due to failure of asthenic blood to nourish the heart; pale reddish tongue and thin and weak pulse are obvious manifestations of blood asthenia.

Prescription：Nourish blood and moisten dryness.

Formulas：Runchang Wan Jiajian (Modified Runchang Pill). The formula is made up of Dahuang (*Radix et Rhizoma Rhei*), Danggui (*Radix Angelicae Sinensis*), Qianghuo (*Rhizoma et Radix Notopterygii*), Taoren (*Semen Persicae*) and Huomaren (*Fructus Cannabis*). Of them, Danggui and Taoren can invigorate blood and resolve stasis, Huomaren has an action of moistening intestine, Qianghuo can dispel wind, Duhuang has a function of purging fire. Combined together, the five herbs can bring nourishing blood, moistening intestine, invigorating blood, resolving stasis as well as relaxing bowels into full play. For hyperactive fire due to yin asthenia, Zhimu (*Rhizoma Anemarrhenae*), Xuanshen (*Radix Scrophulariae*) and Tianhuafen (*Radix Trichosanthis*) could be combined; for the complicated syndrome of qi asthenia, Dangshen (*Radix Codonopsis*), Huangqi (*Radix Astragali seu Hedysari*) and Baizhu (*Rhizoma Atractylodis Macrocephalae*) should be added to supplement qi and strength.

5. 阳虚寒凝

15.5　Syndrome of yang asthenia and cold stagnation

【症状】大便艰涩，排出困难，腹中冷痛，肢冷怯寒，或腰膝酸冷，舌淡苔白，脉象沉迟。

【分析】体质阳虚，寒从内生，肠道传导无力，故大便艰涩，排出困难；阴寒内盛，气机阻滞，故腹中冷痛；阳虚不能温煦肢体，故肢冷怯寒，或腰膝酸冷；舌淡苔白、脉象沉迟，为阳虚寒凝之征。

【治法】温阳润肠。

【方药】济川煎加减。济川煎出自《景岳全书》，由当归、牛膝、肉苁蓉、泽泻、升麻、枳壳组成。方中肉苁蓉温肾助阳，暖腰润肠，为君药；当归养血和血，润肠通便，牛膝补肾壮腰，性善下行，共为臣药；枳壳宽肠下气而助通便，泽泻渗利小便而泄肾浊，共为佐药；尤妙在用升麻升清阳，清阳升则浊阴自降，与诸药配合，以利于气机通畅，以加强通便作用，是为使药。

Clinical manifestations：Obstructive defecation with difficulty, cold and pain sensation of the abdomen, cold limbs with aversion to cold, or aching and cold loins and knees, pale tongue with whitish fur as well as sunken and slow pulse.

Analysis：Obstructive defecation with difficulty is due to yang asthenic constitution which generates endogenous cold and dysfunction of the intestines in transportation；cold and pain sensation of the abdomen is due to superabundance of endogenous cold obstructing qi circulation；cold limbs with aversion to cold, or aching and cold loins and knees is due to failure of yang asthenia to warm the limbs and body；pale tongue with whitish fur and sunken and slow pulse indicate yang asthenia and cold stagnation.

Prescription：Warm yang and moisten the intestines.

Formulas：Jichuan Jian Jiajian (Modified Jichuan Decoction). Jichuan Jian is quoted from *Jingyue Quanshu* (*Jingyue's Complete Works*), consisting of Danggui (*Radix Angelicae Sinensis*), Niuxi (*Radix Achyranthis Bidentatae*), Roucongrong (*Herba Cistanches*), Zexie (*Rhizoma Alismatis*), Shengma (*Rhizoma Cimicifugae*) and Zhiqiao (*Fructus Aurantii*). In the formula, Roucongrong, with an action of warming the kidney to strengthen yang and warming the loins to moisten the large intestine, is used as sovereign drug；Danggui can nourish blood, activate blood circulation, moisten the intestines and relieve constipation, Niuxi, with a descending direction of action, may tonify the kidney and strengthen the loins, both of them are used as ministerial drug；Zhiqiao and Zexie are used as assistant drug, for Zhiqiao can relax the bowels, descend qi and relieve constipation and Zexie has an action of resolving dampness and promoting diuresis to purge turbidity in the kidney；Shengma is used as courier drug here, for it has an effect of lifting lucid yang, resulting in turbid yin descending automatically, which is also the advantage of this recipe. The above herbs, combined with Shengma can improve qi circulation to reinforce the action of relieving constipation.

十六、脂肪肝

16　Fatty liver

〔概说〕 Summary

脂肪肝是指各种原因引起的肝细胞内脂肪堆积的临床现象。绝大多数脂肪肝是由甘油三酯的堆积所致，其中肝脏内的脂肪含量可高达肝脏重的 40%~50%。本病多见于肥胖、大量饮酒及其他因素者。轻度脂肪肝可无临床症状，但大多数病人有不同程度的肝区疼痛或不适，少数病人可伴有黄疸。严重者可有蜘蛛痣、乳房发育、月经过多、闭经、睾丸萎缩、阳痿等。

脂肪肝属于中医"肝着""胁痛""肝壅"等病证。本病以痰湿内停、瘀阻气机为其发病机理。多因饮食失调、肝气郁结、湿热壅积等因素而发病。病位在肝，但与胆、胃、脾等脏功能失调有关。临床治疗多以标本兼治为法，健脾、疏肝、化湿、逐瘀为其主要治疗法则。

Fatty liver refers to accumulation of excess fat in liver cells for various reasons. In vast majority of cases, it is the result of accumulation of large vacuoles of triglyceride fat in the liver, and sometimes fat may account for 40% ~ 50% of the weight of the liver. Obesity and alcoholism can cause fatty liver, and other factors may influence the chances of developing into it. For patients with unsevere fatty liver, there may be no clinical manifestations, but most patients have varying degrees of pain or discomfort in the liver area, and a few patients may have jaundice. In serious cases, the following manifestations will appear, such as spider angioma, mamary development, profuse menstrual flow, amenorrhoea, orchiatrophy as well as sexual impotence.

In terms of TCM, fatty liver pertains to "pain in the liver" "hypochondriac pain" and "obstruction of liver qi". Pathogenesis for it is internal retention of damp phlegm obstructing qi circulation. The disease is generally caused by improper diet, liver qi stagnation, accumulation of dampness and heat, etc. The region of the disease is in the liver, but dysfunction of the gallbladder, stomach and spleen could also affect the outbreak of fatty liver. Clinically, therapeutic methods for fatty liver is marked by treating both its symptoms and root cause, and invigorating the spleen, soothing the liver, resolving dampness and eliminating blood stasis are taken as the principal methods.

〔**辨证论治**〕 Syndrome differentiation and treatment

1. 湿热蕴结
16.1 Accumulation of dampness and heat

【症状】右胁胀痛或胀满不适，口苦咽干，形体肥胖，肢体重着，腹部胀满，食欲减退，舌质红，苔腻，脉象滑数。

【分析】本证由湿热蕴结，肝失条达，疏泄无权所致。肝脉布于两胁，肝郁则胁痛或胀满；湿热内蕴，阻滞胆汁的排泄，故口苦咽干；湿盛瘀阻，故肢体重着；肝失疏泄，克伐脾土，脾失运化，故腹部胀满、食欲减退；舌质红、苔腻、脉象滑数，均为湿热蕴结之象。

【治法】清利湿热，疏肝通络。

【方药】龙胆泻肝汤加减。龙胆泻肝汤为清利肝胆湿热之主剂，其方义见"慢性肝炎"篇。在具体应用时，可加丝瓜络、荷叶清化湿气；加丹参、赤芍化瘀通络；纳呆不食者，可加生山楂、生麦芽开胃进食；口苦甚者，可加茵陈、虎杖清热化瘀。

Clinical manifestations：Distending pain or distention, fullness and discomfort in the right hypochondrium, bitter taste and dry throat, obesity, heavy sensation of the body, abdominal distention, reduced appetite, reddish tongue with greasy whitish fur as well as slippery and fast pulse.

Analysis：The syndrome is caused by dysfunction of the liver in dispersion due to accumulation of dampness and heat. The liver meridians are distributed in the area of hypochondrium, so depression of liver qi gives rise to pain or distention and fullness of the hypochondrium; bitter taste and dry throat are due to accumulation of dampness and heat which inhibits bile from normal excretion; heavy sensation of the body is due to stagnation of exuberant dampness; abdominal distention, fullness, and reduced appetite are due to failure of the liver in dispersing qi which restrains the spleen, thus, leading to dysfunction of the spleen in transportation and transformation; reddish tongue with greasy fur and slippery and fast pulse are signs of accumulation of dampness and heat.

Prescription：Clear away heat, induce diuresis, soothe the liver and dredge the collaterals.

Formulas：Longdan Xiegan Tang Jiajian （Modified Longdan Xiegan Decoction）. Longdan Xiegan Tang is a principal recipe for purging dampness and heat in the liver and gallbladder, its action and ingredients have been introduced in the chapter of *Chronic hepatitis*. In clinical practice, Sigualuo （*Retinervus Luffae Fructus*） and Heye （*Folium Nelumbinis*） can be added to resolve dampness; Danshen （*Radix Salviae Miltiorrhizae*） and Chishao （*Radix Paeoniae Rubra*） can be combined to dissolve stasis and dredge blood vessels; for reduced appetite, Shengshanzha （*Fructus Crataegi*） and Shengmaiya （*Fructus Hordei Germinatus*） may be added to promote appetite; for severe bitter taste, Yinchen （*Herba Artemisiae Scopariae*） and Huzhang （*Rhizoma Polygoni Cuspidati*） could be added to clear away heat and dissolve blood stasis.

2. 肝郁脾虚
16.2　Syndrome of liver depression and spleen asthenia

【症状】肝区隐隐作痛，倦怠无力，头晕，大便溏泄，口黏，腹部胀痛，舌质淡红、舌体胖大，脉象沉细或弦细。

【分析】肝气郁结，加之脾虚，是本证的主要病机。由于肝气郁结，故而肝区隐隐作痛；脾虚运化无权，故大便溏泄，腹部胀痛；肝郁则清阳不升，故头晕；舌脉之象皆为肝郁脾虚之征。

【治法】疏肝理气，益气健脾。

【方药】补中益气汤合四逆散加减。补中益气汤为补益中气、健脾养胃的主方，其方义见"胃下垂"篇。四逆散为疏肝理气的常用方，其方义见"肝硬化"篇。两方合用，可以使肝脾同时得到和解，郁结自然解除。

Clinical manifestations: Dull pain in the liver, lassitude, dizziness, loose stool or diarrhea, sticky taste of the mouth, abdominal distending pain, bulgy and pale reddish tongue as well as sunken and thin pulse or taut and thin pulse.

Analysis: Pathogenesis for this syndrome is qi stagnation in the liver as well as spleen asthenia. Dull pain in the liver is due to qi stagnation in the liver; loose stool or diarrhea and abdominal distending pain are due to dysfunction of the spleen to transport; dizziness is due to failure to lift lucid yang because of liver depression; bulgy and pale reddish tongue and sunken and thin pulse or taut and thin pulse are signs of liver depression and spleen asthenia.

Prescription: Soothe the liver, regulate qi and benefit qi to invigorate the spleen.

Fornulas: Buzhong Yiqi Tang (Decoction) combined with Sini San (Powder) Jiajian. Buzhong Yiqi Tang is a principal formula for tonifying qi in middle energizer, invigorating the spleen and nourishing the stomach (it has been discussed in the chapter of *Gastroptosi*). Sini San is a common recipe for soothing the liver and regulating qi, which has been introduced in *Liver Cirrhosis*. Combined together, the liver and spleen could be reconciled simultaneously, and liver depression could be relieved naturally.

3. 痰瘀阻滞
16.3 Syndrome of phlegmatic obstruction and blood stasis

【症状】肝气刺痛或胀痛，面色晦暗，精神疲倦，嗜睡，腹胀，舌质紫暗，或有瘀点，舌苔白腻，脉象沉涩。

【分析】本证由痰湿阻滞日久，致使气滞血瘀所致。痰湿与瘀血皆是有形的病理产物，为阴邪，容易阻滞肝经络脉不通，故见右胁刺痛或胀痛；瘀血阻滞，气血不能上荣于面，故面色晦暗；痰湿郁滞，气血不畅，无以上荣元神之府，故精神疲倦、嗜睡；肝失疏泄，影响脾胃之消化，则舌苔白腻，脉象沉涩，为瘀阻之象。

【治法】祛湿化痰，活血通络。

【方药】温胆汤合桃红四物汤加减。温胆汤为理气化痰、清利肝胆的方剂，由二陈汤加枳实、竹茹而成。二陈汤之陈皮、半夏、茯苓、甘草健脾祛湿，化痰理气；枳实、竹茹清泻痰热。桃红四物汤（由当归、白芍、熟地黄、川芎、桃仁、红花组成）为养血活血的方剂，具有养血活血、攻补兼施的作用。两方合用，可以攻逐痰瘀互结的顽症，如脂肪肝、各种囊肿、包块、息肉、结节等。肝胆肿大者，可加生牡蛎、穿山甲破坚散结；肝区疼痛明显者，可加丹参、泽兰、延胡索等。

Clinical manifestations: Stabbing pain or distending pain due to liver qi, tarnished complexion, dispiritedness, somnolence, abdominal distention, dark purplish tongue with greasy whitish fur as well as sunken and astringent pulse.

Analysis: This syndrome is caused by qi stagnation and blood stasis due to prolonged obstruction of phlegmatic dampness. Phlegmatic dampness and blood stasis are tangible substance produced by pathological changes, belonging to pathogenic yin factors with susceptibility to obstructing liver meridians and collaterals, which brings about stabbing pain or distending pain in the right hypochondrium; tarnished complexion is due to obstruction of blood stasis which fails to nourish the face; dispiritedness and somnolence are due to failure of inhibited qi and blood circulation to nourish the brain, the "house of mental activity"; greasy whitish fur is due to dysfunction of the spleen and stomach because of failure of liver dispersion; sunken and astringent pulse is a sign of blood obstruction.

Prescription: Expel dampness, resolve phlegm, invigorate blood circulation and dredge collaterals.

Formulas: Wendan Tang (Decoction) combined with Tao Hong Siwu Tang (Decoction) Jiajian. Wendan Tang is a recipe for regulating qi, resolving phlegm, clearing the liver and promoting production of bile in the gallbladder, and it consists of Erchen Tang (*Decoction*), Zhishi (*Fructus Aurantii Immaturus*) and Zhuru (*Caulis Bambusae in Taenia*). In Erchen Tang, Chenpi (*Pericarpium Citri Reticulatae*), Banxia (*Rhizoma Pinelliae*), Fuling (*Poriae Cocos*) and Gancao (*Radix Glycyrrhizae*) can invigorate the spleen, dispel dampness, resolve phlegm and regulate qi; Zhishi and Zhuru have an action of purging phlegmatic heat. Tao Hong Siwu Tang, made up of Danggui (*Radix Angelicae Sinensis*), Baishao (*Radix Paeoniae Alba*), Shudihuang (*Radix Rehmanniae Preparata*), Chuanxiong (*Rhizoma Ligustici Chuanxiong*), Taoren (*Semen Persicae*) and Honghua (*Flos Carthami*), is a recipe for nourishing blood and promoting blood circulation, therefore, it can bring purgation and supplementing into full play. Combined together, both recipes can be used for persistent ailments caused by coagulation of phlegm and blood stasis, for instance, fatty liver, cystides, enclosed mass, polypus, nodules, etc. For swollen liver and gallbladder, Shengmuli (*Concha Ostreae*) and Chuanshanjia (*Squama Manis*) can be combined to remove stasis and disperse mass; for obvious pain in the liver, Danshen (*Radix Salviae Miltiorrhizae*), Zelan (*Herba Lycopi*) and Yanhusuo (*Rhizoma Corydalis*) may be added.

4. 肝肾阴虚
16.4　Syndrome of yin asthenia of the liver and kidney

【症状】胁肋疼痛，腰膝酸软，头晕目眩，视物不清，善太息，舌质淡，苔薄白，脉象沉细。

【分析】本证由肝肾阴血不足，致使肝失条达所致。肝肾阴精不足，则所主之经脉失养，故胁肋疼痛；肝肾亏虚，脑与腰失其所养，故头晕目眩、腰膝酸软；肝失疏泄，故善太息；舌质淡、脉象沉细，为肝肾亏损之象。

【治法】养肝益肾，补益精血。

【方药】左归丸加减。左归丸为滋阴补肾，"阳中求阴"的代表方剂。方中重用熟地黄滋补肾阴，枸杞子益精养肝，山茱萸补肝涩精；龟鹿二胶为血肉有情之品，鹿角胶偏于补阳，龟板胶偏于滋阴，两胶合力，沟通任督二脉，有利于全身气血阴阳的调和；菟丝子配牛膝强腰膝、壮筋骨，山药滋补脾肾。全方以滋补为主，待肝肾之阴精充足，其多余的脂浊就会被软化。腰膝酸软可加桑寄生、续断；头晕不适可加决明子、茺蔚子；胁肋疼痛可加延胡索、川楝子。

Clinical manifestations：Pain in the chest and hypochondrium, aching and weakness of the loins and knees, dizziness and vertigo, blurred vision, frequent sigh, pale tongue, thin whitish fur as well as sunken and thin pulse.

Analysis：This syndrome is caused by failure of the liver to disperse because of insufficiency of yin and blood in the liver and kidney. Pain in the chest and hypochondrium is due to failure of insufficient yin and essence in the liver and kidney to nourish the meridians associated with the liver and kidney; dizziness and vertigo and aching and weakness of the loins and knees are due to malnutrition of the cerebral marrow and the loins because of asthenia of the liver and kidney; frequent sigh is due to failure of the liver to disperse; pale tongue, thin whitish fur and sunken and thin pulse are signs of deficiency and consumption of the liver and kidney.

Prescription：Nourish the liver, benefit the kidney and supplement kidney essence and blood.

Formulas：Zuogui Wan Jiajian（Modified Zuogui Pill）. Zuogui Wan can nourish yin and tonify the kidney by combining a small amount of herbs that could replenish yang with the yin-nourishing drug. Of the formula, large amount of Shudihuang（*Radix Rehmanniae Preparata*）is used to nourish and tonify kidney yin, Gouqizi（*Fructus Lycii*）can supplement kidney essence and nourish the liver, Shanzhuyu（*Fructus Corni*）has an action of tonifying the liver and astringing essence; Guibanjiao（*Plastrum Testudinis Praeparatae*）could nourish yin, while Lujiaojiao（deer horn glue, *Colla Corni Cervi*）tends to supplement yang, combined together, both of them can communicate governor vessel and conception vessel, and promote reconciling qi, blood, yin and yang of the whole body; Tusizi（*Semen Cuscutae*）and Niuxi（*Radix Achyranthis Bidentatae*）can strengthen the loins, knees, tendons and bones, Shanyao（*Rhizoma Dioscoreae*）has an action of tonifying the spleen and kidney. The main function of the formula is to nourish and supplement, once yin and essence in the liver and kidney are sufficient, the surplus turbid fat could be softened. For aching and weakness of the loins and knees, Sangjisheng（*Herba Taxilli*）and Xuduan（*Radix Dipsaci*）can be added; for dizziness and discomfort, Juemingzi（*Semen Cassiae Torae*）and Chongweizi（*Fructus Leonuri*）should be combined; for pain in the chest and hypochondrium, Yanhusuo（*Rhizoma Corydalis*）and Chuanlianzi（*Fructus Meliae Toosendan*）should be added.

十七、急性肾小球肾炎
17　Acute glomerulonephritis

〔**概说**〕 Summary

急性肾小球肾炎又称急性肾炎，多数是由急性链球菌感染后引起的免疫反应所致。

其临床特点是起病急、浮肿、高血压、蛋白尿、血尿、管型尿等。

中医学将急性肾小球肾炎归属于 "水肿" 范畴。人体的水液代谢依靠肺气的通调，脾气的转输，肾气的开阖；而三焦的决渎作用，膀胱的气化通畅，对水液代谢也起着十分重要的作用。若有风邪外袭、水湿内停等因素的影响，就会使肺、脾、肾三脏的功能失调，引发水液潴留，发为水肿疾患。依据以上所述，对水肿的治疗，必须调节肺、脾、肾以及三焦、膀胱的气化作用，使之发挥通调、转输、开阖、决渎等功效，这样才能使水肿很快消失，不致形成慢性疾患，难以治疗。

Acute glomerulonephritis, also known as acute nephritis, is caused by acute immunoreaction to the infection of streptococcus in vast majority of cases. Clinically, glomerulonephritis is marked by sudden onset, edema, hypertension, albuminuria, urination with blood, cylindruria and so on.

In terms of TCM, acute glomerulonephritis belongs to "edema". Water or fluid metabolism of human body depends on the regulating function of lung qi, transporting function of splenic qi as well as discharging and retention function of kidney qi. Besides, the function of triple-energizer in regulating the waterways and transporting fluid and that of the bladder in qi transformation are very essential for fluid metabolism. Some factors, for instance, invasion of pathogenic wind factor into the superficies and internal retention of dampness, can cause dysfunction of the liver, spleen and kidney, which could give rise to diseases like edema due to fluid retention. Accordingly, treatment for edema, to a great extent, is to reconcile the liver, spleen and kidney, triple-energizer, as well as the bladder in qi transformation in order that they could bring their normal functions into full play. Only in this way, could edema be relieved quickly and it would not develop into chronic or incurable disease.

〔辨证论治〕 Syndrome differentiation and treatment

1. 风寒风水
17.1　Edema due to wind and cold

【症状】恶寒发热，头痛无汗，身重腰痛，骨节酸痛，浮肿从颜面开始，继而遍及全身，或见咳嗽喉痒，小便不利，舌苔薄白，脉象沉紧。

【分析】风寒外袭，卫阳被遏，故恶寒发热、头痛无汗；风寒属阴，其性不扬，故有身重、骨节酸痛；腰为肾之府，风寒由表入里，由经入络，伤及肾府，故腰部疼痛明显；"伤于风者，上先受之"，肺气不能通调水道，故先从颜面出现水肿，渐之伤及脾肾，则水肿也会遍及全身；若风邪干扰咽喉不退，则有咳嗽喉痒；膀胱气化不利，则小便量少；其舌苔、脉象为气虚水湿不化之象。

【治法】辛温解表，宣肺利水。

【方药】麻黄加术汤合五皮饮加味。麻黄加术汤由麻黄汤加白术而成。麻黄汤的作用是发汗解表，宣肺利水，加白术意在益气护卫，健脾化湿。"脾土为肺金之母"，培土生金，脾土强壮了，肺金之气有了来源，自然有能力散寒解表，祛除外邪。但本方利水作用较弱，故加五皮饮，即五加皮、地骨皮、茯苓皮、大腹皮、生姜皮，功效为行气利水消肿，在本证治疗中起到辅助作用。

Clinical manifestations：Aversion to cold and fever, headache and no sweating, heavy sensation of the body and aching loins, aching sensation of the bones and knuckles, edema starting from the cheek involving the whole body, or cough and itching throat, unsmooth urine, thin whitish fur as well as sunken and tense pulse.

Analysis：Aversion to cold, fever, headache and no sweating are due to pathogenic wind and cold factors invading the superficies and inhibiting defensive yang; wind and cold are pathogenic yin factors and they posses a feature of descending, which results in heavy sensation of the body and aching bones and knuckles; the loins are the house of the kidney, invasion of pathogenic wind and cold from the exterior to the interior, from meridians to collaterals impairs the house of the kidney, bringing about obvious pain in the loins. "Impairment resulting from wind invasion could transmit the upper limbs first", failure of lung qi to regulate water passage gives rise to edema of the face, then, gradually, edema spreads to the spleen, kidney, even the whole body. If pathogenic wind factor impairs the throat persistently, it could cause itchy sensation in the throat; scanty urine is due to dysfunction of the bladder in qi transformation; thin whitish fur and sunken and tense pulse are signs of failure of asthenic qi to resolve dampness.

Prescription：Relieve the superficies with pungent-warm natured herbs and disperse the lung to promote diuresis.

Formulas：Mahuang Jia Zhu Tang (Decoction) combined with Wupi Yin (Decoction) Jiawei. Mahuang Jia Zhu Tang consists of Mahuang Tang and Baizhu (*Rhizoma Atractylodis Macrocephalae*). Mahuang Tang has an action of inducing sweating, relieving the superficies and dispersing the lung to promote diuresis. The combination of Baizhu is for the sake of benefiting qi, protecting defensive qi, invigorating the spleen and resolving dampness. The spleen (earth) is the mother of the lung (metal), consolidating earth aims at generating metal, if the spleen is strong, lung qi will acquire its source and it is surely able to dispel cold, relieve the superficies and expel exogenous pathogenic factors. Because the action of the formula in inducing diuresis is slightly weak, so Wupi Yin, including Wujiapi (*Cortex Acanthopanax Radicis*), Digupi (*Cortex Lycii*), Fulingpi (peel of *Poriae Cocos*), Dafupi (*Pericarpium Arecae*) and Shengjiangpi (peel of *Rhizoma Zingiberis Recens*), is combined to activate qi, induce diuresis and eliminate edema.

2. 风热风水
17.2 Edema due to wind and heat

【症状】发热，微恶风寒，口渴，心烦，咳嗽，咽痛，颜面浮肿，渐至全身，小便不利、色黄，舌苔薄黄，脉象浮数。

【分析】风热外袭，影响肺卫的开阖，故有发热；邪热为阳，故恶风寒较轻；热伤津液，则见口渴、心烦；肺气失于肃降，则咳嗽；肺气失肃，不能很好地通调水道，则见颜面浮肿，渐至全身；膀胱气化失司，则小便不利，色黄为热；舌苔与脉象均表示为风热所致。

【治法】辛凉解表，清热利水。

【方药】麻黄连翘赤小豆汤加味。麻黄连翘赤小豆汤由麻黄、连翘、赤小豆、桑白皮、杏仁、生姜、甘草、大枣组成。方中麻黄、杏仁、桑白皮宣肺解表，连翘、赤小豆清热利水，生姜、甘草、大枣三味调和营卫。全方意在辛凉开腠理，清热以透邪，利尿消水肿。临证可加车前子、石韦、白茅根清肺利尿；若有血尿，可加藕节、茜草清热凉血止血。

Clinical manifestations: Fever and slight aversion to wind and cold, thirst, vexation, cough and painful throat, edema involving the cheek as well as the whole body, unsmooth urination with yellowish color, thin yellowish fur as well as floating and fast pulse.

Analysis: Fever is due to wind and heat pathogens invading the superficies, which affects the function of the lung in governing dispersing of qi; yang-natured pathogenic heat results in slight aversion to wind and cold; thirst and vexation are due to heat impairing the body fluid; cough is due to failure to depurate and descend lung qi; edema involving the cheek and the whole body is due to failure of the lung to regulate water passage; unsmooth urination is due to dysfunction of the bladder in qi transformation, yellowish urine is caused by heat scorching; thin yellowish fur and floating and fast pulse are caused by wind and heat.

Prescription: Relieve the superficies with pungent-cold natured herbs, clear away heat and induce diuresis.

Formulas: Mahuang Lianqiao Chixiaodou Tang Jiawei (Modified Mahuang Lianqiao Chixiaodou Decoction). It is made up of Mahuang (*Herba Ephedrae*), Lianqiao (*Fructus Forsythiae*), Chixiaodou (*Semen Phaseoli*), Sangbaipi (*Cortex Mori*), Xingren (*Semen Armeniacae Amarum*), Shengjiang (*Rhizoma Zingiberis Recens*), Gancao (*Radix Glycyrrhizae*) and Dazao (*Fructus Jujubae*). Of them, Mahuang, Xingren and Sangbaipi can disperse the lung and relieve the superficies; Lianqiao and Chixiaodou can clear away heat and induce diuresis; Shengjiang, Gancao and Dazao have the action of reconciling nutrient qi and defensive qi. The whole formula aims at clearing away heat to erupt pathogens, opening sweat pores by cooling as well as inducing diuresis to eliminate edema. Clinically, Cheqianzi (*Semen Plantaginis*), Shiwei (*Folium Pyrrosiae*) and Baimaogen (*Rhizoma Imperatae*) can be added to purge heat from the lung and induce diuresis; for urine with blood, Oujie (*Nodus Nelumbinis Rhizomatis*) and Qiancao (*Radix Rubiae*) can be combined to cool blood and stop bleeding.

3. 阴虚风水

17.3　Edema due to yin asthenia

【症状】身热，微恶风寒，头痛，咽干，五心烦热，腰膝酸软，浮肿，小便短赤，或见血尿，舌红少苔，脉象细滑数。

【分析】阴虚风水与体质有密切关系，多见于阴虚之体，或热病伤阴之后。"阴虚生内热"，咽干、五心烦热，乃为阴虚内热之象；身热、微恶风寒、头痛，为阴虚感受外邪的表证；外邪入里，内及于肾，使其气化不利，则见浮肿、小便短赤；伤及血络，可见尿血；舌与脉象，均显示阴虚内热之征。

【治法】育阴清热，宣肺利水。

【方药】青蒿鳖甲汤加味。方中鳖甲滋阴清热；青蒿清热透络，引邪外出；生地黄、牡丹皮养阴凉血，与青蒿配伍，透解阴分邪热；知母养阴清热。可加桑白皮、浮萍以宣肺利水，茯苓皮、白茅根利尿消肿。

Clinical manifestations: Fever and slight aversion to wind cold, headache, dry throat, feverish sensation over the palms, soles and the chest, aching and weakness of the loins and knees, dropsy, scanty brownish urine, or urine with blood, reddish tongue with scanty fur as well as thin, slippery and fast pulse.

Analysis: Edema due to yin asthenia is closely related to a patient's constitution, usually seen in those of yin asthenic constitution, or after impairment of yin due to fever. Dry throat and feverish sensation over the palms, soles and chest indicate endogenous heat due to asthenic yin; fever, slight aversion to wind cold and headache are manifestations of yin asthenia complicated by exogenous pathogens; dropsy and scanty brownish urine are due to exogenous pathogens invading from the superficies internally and even the kidney, resulting in inhibited transformation of qi; urine mingled with blood is due to invasion of exogenous pathogens impairing blood vessels; reddish tongue with scanty fur and thin, slippery and fast pulse are indication of yin asthenia and endogenous heat.

Prescription: Nourish yin, clear away heat and disperse the lung to induce diuresis.

Formulas: Qinghao Biejia Tang Jiawei (Modified Qinghao Biejia Decoction). In the formula, Biejia (*Carapax Trionycis*) has an action of nourishing yin and clearing away heat; Qinghao (*Herba Artemisiae Annuae*) can purge heat and relax the collaterals by letting out pathogenic heat; Shengdihuang (*Radix Rehmanniae Recens*) and Mudanpi (*Cortex Moutan Radicis*) may nourish yin and cool blood, combined with Qinghao, they can resolve latent pathogenic heat in yin phase; Zhimu (*Rhizoma Anemarrhenae*) has an action of nourishing yin and clearing away heat. Sangbaipi (*Cortex Mori*) and Fuping (*Herba Spirodelae*) can be added to disperse heat of the lung and induce diuresis, Fulingpi (peel of *Poriae Cocos*) and Baimaogen (*Rhizoma Imperatae*) may be added to induce diuresis and eliminate edema.

4. 阳虚风水

17.4 Edema due to yang asthenia

【症状】发热恶寒，头身重痛，面色㿠白，四肢不温，腰膝凉痛，颜面及下肢浮肿，小便不利，舌质淡红，苔淡白，脉象沉缓。

【分析】阳虚风水是由体质所决定的，素体阳虚的人感受外邪，很容易邪从寒化。恶寒发热、头身重痛，是风寒袭表的症状；面色㿠白、四肢不温、腰膝凉痛，乃是阳气不能温运，肢体表面失于温养的表现；风寒之邪内及于肾，肾阳对水液不能温化，小便不利，使水湿下注或上逆于面部，即出现浮肿；阳虚则舌质淡红、舌苔淡白；脉象沉缓为阳虚无力运行血脉之象。

【治法】宣肺解表，温阳利水。

【方药】麻黄附子细辛汤合五苓散。方用麻黄辛温解表，附子温养补肾，两味合用，起到温经助阳、散寒解表之效；细辛辛温通络，以散寒邪；桂枝温通卫阳；泽泻、茯苓、猪苓淡渗利湿；白术健脾运化湿邪。两方合用，表里双解，可使水湿之邪从诸窍中导流下注，从小便排出。

Clinical manifestations: Fever and aversion to cold, heavy and painful sensation over the head and body, pale complexion, cold limbs, cold and pain over the loins and knees, edema of the face and lower limbs, unsmooth urination, pale reddish tongue with pale whitish fur as well as sunken and moderate pulse.

Analysis: Edema due to yang asthenia depends on a patient's constitution. For those with yang asthenic constitution, exogenous pathogens are susceptible to transforming into cold. Fever and aversion to cold and heavy painful sensation over the head and body are symptoms of pathogenic wind and cold attacking the superficies; pale complexion, cold limbs, cold and painful sensation over the loins and knees are indications of malnutrition of the superficial skin due to failure of yang qi to warm and transport; invasion of pathogenic wind and cold into the kidney and failure of kidney yang to warm and transform the fluid result in unsmooth urination, which causes downward migration of dampness, or adverse flow of fluid onto the face, thus bringing about edema; pale reddish tongue and pale whitish fur indicate yang asthenia, sunken and moderate pulse suggests failure of asthenic yang to rise up in blood vessel.

Prescription: Disperse the lung, relieve the superficies and induce diuresis by warming yang.

Formulas: Mahuang Fuzi Xixin Tang (Decoction) combined with Wuling San (Powder). Mahuang (*Herba Ephedrae*) has an action of relieving the superficial syndrome with its pungent and warm nature, Fuzi (*Radix Aconiti Lateralis Preparata*) can tonify the kidney by warming and nourishing, combined together, both herbs can warm the meridians and supplement yang, dispel cold and relieve superficial syndrome; Xixin (*Herba Asari*) can dredge the collaterals to dispel pathogenic cold factor with its warm and pungent nature; Guizhi (*Ramulus Cinnamomi*) can warm defensive yang; Zexie (*Rhizoma Alismatis*), Fuling (*Poriae Cocos*) and Zhuling (*Polyporus Umbellatus*) can resolve dampness and induce diuresis；Baizhu（*Rhizoma Atractylodis Macrocephalae*）can invigorate the spleen and promote its function in transportation and transformation. The combination of both formulas can expel pathogens from the exterior as well as the interior and discharge pathogenic dampness from the orifices with urine.

十八、慢性肾小球肾炎

18　Chronic glomerulonephritis

〔**概说**〕　Summary

慢性肾小球肾炎又称慢性肾炎，可由急性肾小球肾炎转化而来，但多数慢性肾炎并无急性期，即一开始就呈现出慢性症状。本病可发生于不同年龄，但以中青年为多，男性发病率比女性高。临床表现为蛋白尿或血尿，伴有管型尿，病至后期多数有浮肿、贫血、高血压和肾功能不全。其发病原因，认为是变态反应，自身免疫因素是导致疾病迁延不愈的主要原因。

慢性肾炎属于中医学"水肿""虚劳"等病范畴。其发病机理与肺、脾、肾三脏的气化功能失调有关。先天肾气不足，后天调护失度，使得肺气失于护卫，脾气失于健运，肾气失于温化，三焦和膀胱疏通水道的功能亦受到影响，这样就会使精气不能内守，流于体外；浊气不能外泄，乱于体内，形成清浊不分。水湿之毒内蕴，阳损及阴，还会伤及血络，久而久之，就会使肾脏虚损，开阖完全不能自主，最后阴阳离决，危及生命。依据以上病程发展，中医多从气化入手，从益肺、健脾、温肾，以及滋阴、化瘀、疏导方面考虑，对缓解病情、改善体质、逆转病程的发展，有着较好的效果。

Chronic glomerulonephritis, also known as chronic nephritis, can be transformed from acute glomerulonephritis. However, in most cases, chronic nephritis has no acute stage, namely, chronic glomerulonephritis presents some chronic manifestations from its outbreak. People of different ages, mostly, young and middle-aged people can contract this disease, and the ratio among male patients is higher than female. The clinical manifestation of chronic glomerulonephritis is albuminuria or blood urine, accompanied with cylindruria. At the advanced stage of the disease, symptoms such as edema, anemia, hypertension as well as hypofunction of the kidney can appear. The cause for the disease is regarded as abnormal reaction, and prolonged pathological condition concerning immune system is one of the primary causes of the disease.

In terms of TCM, chronic nephritis pertains to "edema" "consumptive disease" (diabetes) and so on. Pathogenesis of it is related to dysfunction of the lung, spleen and kidney in qi transformation. Congenital insufficiency of kidney qi and acquired imbalanced regulation and nursing during a patient's convalescence give rise to loss of defensive protection of lung qi, failure of the spleen qi to transport, failure of kidney qi to warm and transform, as well as affected function of triple energizer and bladder in dredging and regulating water passage, which could result in failure of essence and qi to be stored internally, thus, bringing about outward discharge. Internal disturbance of turbid qi causes inability to separate lucidity from turbidity, internal retention of toxic dampness, impairment of yang involving yin and blood vessel, which, gradually, causes consumption and deficiency of the kidney, failure of the kidney's function in discharge and retention, separation of yin from yang, at last, endangering the patient's life. Based on the development of the course of the disease, its concerning TCM therapeutic methods should start from qi transformation, taking benefiting the lung, invigorating the spleen, warming the kidney, nourishing yin, dissolving stasis as well as dredging collaterals into consideration, which could be of great curative effect in alleviating the disease, improving constitution as well as restraining the disease from further development.

〔**辨证论治**〕 Syndrome differentiation and treatment

1. 肺脾两虚
18.1　Asthenia of the lung and spleen

【症状】面色萎黄，身疲乏力，少气懒言，食欲不振，大便溏薄，有轻度水肿，偶见蛋白尿，舌淡苔白，脉象细弱。

【分析】本症见于病变之初期，仅有肺脾气血虚弱症状，如脾经气血不足，血不荣面，则见面色萎黄、身疲乏力；肺气虚则少气懒言；脾虚及胃，则不欲饮食；脾经气陷则大便溏薄；肺主调节水道，脾主运化水湿，两经虚弱，水湿不循常道，则会发生水肿；精微外泄，则有蛋白尿出现；舌苔与脉象均为虚弱之象。

【治法】益肺健脾，渗湿利水。

【方药】参苓白术散加味。参苓白术散是在四君子汤的基础上，加山药、白扁豆、薏苡仁、砂仁、桔梗而成，是一个以调补脾胃功能为主的方子。它的作用是补气健脾、运化水湿。脾的运化功能恢复了，停留在体内的水湿之邪，才能通过三焦的疏导和膀胱的气化，经过分别清浊，将多余的水湿排出体外；另外，脾胃的气血充足了，主管宗气的肺才能得到补益，这就是"培土生金"一举两得的效果。

Clinical manifestations: Sallow complexion, dispiritedness and lack of energy, shortness of breath and no desire to speak, poor appetite, loose stool, slight edema, occasional albuminuria, pale tongue with whitish fur as well as thin and feeble pulse.

Analysis: The syndrome occurs at the initial stage of chronic nephritis with the single symptom of asthenia of qi and blood in the lung and spleen. Sallow complexion, dispiritedness and lack of energy are due to insufficiency of qi and blood in the spleen meridian and failure of blood to nourish the face; lack of energy and no desire to speak are due to qi asthenia of the lung; poor appetite is due to asthenic spleen involving the function of the stomach; loose stool is caused by qi sinking of spleen meridian; the lung regulates water passage, the spleen governs transportation and transformation of dampness, asthenia of both meridians causes edema because of abnormal dampness transportation; albuminuria is caused by outward discharge of food essence; pale tongue with whitish fur and thin and feeble pulse are signs of asthenia.

Prescription: Benefit the lung, invigorate the spleen, resolve dampness and induce diuresis.

Formulas: Shen Ling Baizhu San Jiawei (Modified Shen Ling Baizhu Powder). Shen Ling Baizhu San is the combination of Sijunzi Tang with Shanyao (*Rhizoma Dioscoreae*), Baibiandou (*Semen Dolichoris Album*), Yiyiren (*Semen Coicis*), Sharen (*Fructus Amomi Villosi*) and Jiegeng (*Radix Platycodonis*), used for reconciling and supplementing the function of the spleen and stomach. It has the action of supplementing qi and invigorating the spleen, transporting and transforming dampness. Only by restoring the function of the spleen in transportation and transformation, could internal retention of surplus dampness be eliminated by means of dredging function of triple energizer and qi transformation of the bladder as well as separation of lucidity from turbidity; furthermore, the lung which dominates pectoral qi could get reinforced in this way, which is the effect achieved by "consolidating earth (the spleen) to generate metal (the lung)".

2. 脾肾阳虚
18.2 Yang asthenia of the spleen and kidney

【症状】水肿明显，遍及头面与四肢，面色㿠白，形寒肢冷，腰膝酸软，小便量少，大便溏薄，精神疲倦，尿中大量蛋白，舌体胖大，边有齿痕，苔白滑，脉象沉细。

【分析】本证是病变的严重阶段，由肺脾气虚发展到脾肾阳虚，显然由轻到重，由较表的一层发展到较深的一层，因此症状比较严重。脾的运化功能与肾的气化功能均呈现弱势，所以水湿之浊就会弥漫，水肿较为严重，头面、四肢都会出现浮肿；阳气不能卫外，则形寒肢冷，面色也呈㿠白色；肾阳虚弱，不能温养其府，则出现腰膝酸软，不能主司二便，则二便呈乖逆状态；肾阳虚不能统摄精微，精微外露，会有大量蛋白尿；舌体胖大，为阳气虚弱之态；边有齿痕，为脾气虚弱之象；阳气不能鼓动脉搏，则脉象沉细。

【治法】温补脾肾，化气行水。

【方药】济生肾气丸合六君子汤加味。济生肾气丸是在金匮肾气丸的基础上加牛膝、车前子而成，以治疗肾阳虚弱，气化不行，水湿潴留证。金匮肾气丸是补益肾阳的方子，加牛膝与车前子以利小便。这里还要说明一下，牛膝行血分之水，车前子行气分之水，有气分药，有血分药，就能使停留在体内的水浊从小便排出。六君子汤是健脾行气的方子，药性是温和的。人参、白术、茯苓、甘草为四君子汤，是补益脾胃之气的主方，加入半夏、陈皮二味，可增强脾的运化能力，有利于消散脾经的湿浊。这样两张方子合用，有补肾的，有健脾的，相得益彰。如水肿比较严重，还可加入猪苓、泽泻、泽兰、益母草等利水之药，大剂量黄芪也可考虑使用，它的补气利水作用比较强，这是许多医家的经验。

Clinical manifestations: Obvious edema involving the head, face as well as limbs, pale complexion, cold limbs and body, aching and weakness of the loins and knees, scanty urine, loose stool, dispiritedness and fatigue, profuse albumen mingled with urine, bulgy tooth-marked tongue with slippery whitish fur as well as sunken and thin pulse.

Analysis: The syndrome is the advanced stage of chronic nephritis. Development of the disease from qi asthenia of the lung and spleen into yang asthenia of the spleen and kidney and from the superficial level to the deep level indicates obvious worsening of it. Weakening function of the spleen in transportation and transformation and that of the kidney in qi transformation result in diffusive turbid dampness and severe edema involving the head, face as well as the limbs; cold body and limbs and pale complexion are due to failure of yang qi to defend the superficies; aching and weakness of the loins and knees result from failure of asthenic kidney yang to warm and nourish its residence, the loins, and abnormal condition of urination and defecation is caused by failure of asthenic kidney yang to dominate urination and defecation; profuse albumen mingled with urine is due to failure of asthenic kidney yang to govern the receiving of food essence, causing outward discharge of food essence; enlarged tongue indicates yang qi asthenia; tooth-marked tongue is a sign of splenic qi asthenia; sunken and thin pulse is due to failure of yang qi to rise up in the blood vessel.

Prescription: Warm and tonify the spleen and kidney and transform qi and promote diuresis.

Formulas: Jisheng Shenqi Wan (Pill) combined with Liujunzi Tang (Decoction) Jiawei. The former is the combination of Jingui Shenqi Wan with Niuxi (*Radix Achyranthis Bidentatae*) and Cheqianzi (*Semen Plantaginis*), it is used for syndromes of kidney yang asthenia, failure to transform qi and retention of dampness. Jingui Shenqi Wan is used for supplementing kidney yang, the combination with Niuxi and Cheqianzi can promote smooth urination. Besides, Niuxi can drain dampness in blood phase, and Cheqianzi can eliminate dampness in qi phase, both herbs could eliminate retention of turbid dampness through urination. The latter, Liujunzi Tang, made up of Renshen (*Radix Ginseng*), Baizhu (*Rhizoma Atractylodis Macrocephalae*), Fuling (*Poriae Cocos*), Gancao (*Radix Glycyrrhizae*), Banxia (*Rhizoma Pinelliae*) and Chenpi (*Pericarpium Citri Reticulatae*), is adopted to invigorate the spleen and activate qi with its warm nature. The first four herbs, also known as Sijunzi Tang, is a principal formula for supplementing and benefiting the spleen and stomach, while the last two can strengthen the function of the spleen in transportation and transformation, helping dispel dampness and turbidity in spleen meridian. The combination of both formulas can not only supplement the kidney, they can also invigorate the spleen. For severe edema, Zhuling (*Polyporus Umbellatus*), Zexie (*Rhizoma Alismatis*), Zelan (*Herba Lycopi*) and Yimucao (*Herba Leonuri*) may be added to relieve dampness retention, or large amount of Huangqi (*Radix Astragali seu Hedysari*), with its stronger action of tonifying qi and resolving dampness retention, can be added, which is also the experience of many TCM experts.

3. 阴虚湿热
18.3 Syndrome of dampness and heat due to yin asthenia

【症状】全身浮肿，小便不利，或有尿血，低热，手足心热，夜间盗汗，口苦口黏，纳呆，舌质红赤，苔黄燥，脉象细数。

【分析】此为慢性肾炎的复合证候，比较复杂。湿热之邪以湿浊为本，热邪为标。湿浊不散，弥漫三焦，则全身浮肿；湿热下注，则小便不利，伤及血络，会有尿血现象；湿热内蕴，伤阴耗液，则出现低热、手足心热；湿热熏蒸，会有盗汗出；脾胃被湿热所困，则不欲饮食、口苦口黏；舌质红赤，为阴虚内热之象，苔黄燥是湿热伤阴所致；脉象细数，阴虚内热也。

【治法】滋阴清热，利湿消肿。

【方药】知柏地黄丸（汤）合五皮饮。知柏地黄丸是在六味地黄丸的基础上加知母、黄柏而成。六味地黄丸为滋阴补肾的要药，它对慢性阴虚证候是常用的首选药物，对慢性肾炎也是不可或缺的。但它有点滋腻，不利于清热，加上知母、黄柏两味，对于阴虚引起的内热证，非常合拍。还有一个问题，就是水湿内停的水肿，知柏地黄丸是难以消除的。所以就加上五皮饮，加强行气利尿作用，以利于消除水肿。这样的组合，知柏地黄丸是主要的，而五皮饮是辅助的，或者说知柏地黄丸是治本的，五皮饮是治标的，标本合治，补而不滞，利而不耗，是比较恰当的方剂配伍。

Clinical manifestations: Edema all over the body, unsmooth urination, or urine mingled with blood, mild fever, feverish sensation over the palms and soles, night sweating, bitter or sticky taste, anorexia, reddish tongue with dry yellowish fur as well as thin and fast pulse.

Analysis: This is a complicated syndrome of chronic nephritis. As far as the syndrome of dampness and heat is concerned, turbid dampness is the fundamental aspect, and pathogenic heat is the secondary aspect. Edema all over the body is due to damp turbidity permeating in triple energizer because of failure to disperse it; unsmooth urination is due to downward migration of dampness and heat; urine mingled with blood is caused by downward migration of damp heat impairing blood vessels; mild fever and feverish sensation over the palms and soles are due to internal stagnation of dampness and heat which impairs yin and consumes body fluid; night sweating is due to fumigation of dampness and heat; poor appetite and bitter or sticky taste are caused by dampness and heat encumbering the spleen and stomach; reddish tongue is a sign of yin asthenia and endogenous heat, dry yellowish fur is caused by damp-heat impairing yin; thin and fast pulse indicates yin asthenia and endogenous heat.

Prescription: Nourish yin, clear away heat, remove dampness through diuresis and eliminate edema.

Formulas: Zhi Bo Dihuang Wan (pill) (or Decoction) combined with Wupi Yin (Decoction). Zhi Bo Dihuang Wan is the combination of Liuwei Dihuang Wan with Zhimu

(*Rhizoma Anemarrhenae*) and Huangbo (*Cortex Phellodendri*). Liuwei Dihuang Wan, as an essential formula for nourishing yin and supplementing the kidney, is the best choice for the syndrome of chronic yin asthenia, and it is also indispensible for chronic nephritis. However, because of its side effect of generating dampness and its stagnant nature which are unhelpful for clearing away heat, so the combination of Zhimu and Huangbo is very suitable to deal with the syndrome of yin asthenia and endogenous heat. Besides, it is very hard for Liuwei Dihuang Wan to eliminate edema due to internal retention of dampness, therefore, Wupi Yin is combined to activate qi and induce diuresis so as to eliminate edema. Of the combination of both formulas, Zhi Bo Dihuang Wan is primary, Wupi Yin plays an assistant role; or in other words, Zhi Bo Dihuang Wan is used to treat the fundamental aspect of the disease, Wupi Yin is used for the secondary aspect of the disease. Treating the fundamental together with the secondary aspect of the disease, supplementing without causing stagnation, and inducing diuresis without consuming yin and body fluid, are very suitable combination of formulas.

4. 血脉瘀阻

18.4　Syndrome of obstruction of blood vessels

【症状】浮肿明显，小便不利，面色黧黑，肌肤甲错，蛋白尿，舌暗有瘀点，脉象沉涩。

【分析】本证亦是慢性肾炎比较难以治疗的证候。由于它已由气分转入血分，由经入络，所以一旦证候形成，就难以在短时间内消除。血分已瘀，水分自然不可能流通，小便不利，头面及下肢浮肿就比较明显。血瘀于面部，必然黧黑；肌肤得不到营养，就显得粗糙如鱼鳞一样。肾脏的血液循环不利，统摄精微物质无力，蛋白尿就会出现。舌质有瘀点，脉象沉涩，是瘀血的特点，在诸多瘀血证中都会显露。

【治法】活血化瘀，利水消肿。

【方药】桃红四物汤加味。桃红四物汤是由四物汤加桃仁、红花而成。四物汤即当归、芍药、川芎、地黄，是养血、活血的主方，有的书上说它是单纯补血剂，这是不全面的。因为仅当归一味就有养血活血的作用，其他如川芎更是活血药，地黄既能补血，又能润燥；如果用于活血，芍药就要选赤芍，加强整个方剂的活血作用。所加药物以益母草、牛膝、泽兰为好。因为这几味药既活血又利水，是活血利水的常用药物，不像五皮饮那样，只行气利水，不入血分。

Clinical manifestations: Obvious edema, unsmooth urination, darkish complexion, squamous skin, albuminuria, darkish tongue with petechiae as well as sunken and astringent pulse.

Analysis: This is one syndrome of chronic nephritis with difficulty to cure. Because it has transmitted from qi phase into blood phase, from meridians to collaterals, so once the syndrome has been developed, it will be difficult to get rid of it. Blood stasis in blood phase will surely inhibit dampness or fluid from circulating freely, which gives rise to unsmooth urination and obvious edema over the head and face as well as lower limbs. Blood stasis on the face causes darkish complexion; rough and squamous skin is due to malnutrition of the skin. Albuminuria is caused by failure of the kidney to control intake of food essence due to unsmooth blood circulation of the kidney. Darkish tongue with petechiae and sunken and astringent pulse are signs of blood stasis, which could appear in many syndromes of blood stasis.

Prescription: Activate blood circulation, resolve stasis, induce diuresis and eliminate edema.

Formulas: Tao Hong Siwu Tang Jiawei (Modified Tao Hong Siwu Decoction). It is made up of Siwu Tang combined with Taoren (*Semen Persicae*) and Honghua (*Flos Carthami*). Siwu Tang, consisting of Danggui (*Radix Angelicae Sinensis*), Shaoyao (*Radix Paeoniae*), Chuanxiong (*Rhizoma Ligustici Chuanxiong*) and Dihuang (*Radix Rehmanniae Recens*), is a principal recipe for nourishing blood and activating blood circulation. The statement quoted form some books that the recipe is only used for blood supplementation is not correct, for Danggui itself can not only nourish blood, but it can also promote blood circulation, other herbs like Chuanxiong is for activating blood, Dihuang can not only replenish blood, but it can also moisten dryness; Chishao (*Radix Paeoniae Rubra*) is preferable to Baishao (*Radix Paeoniae Alba*) in promoting blood circulation, for it can reinforce the action of the whole formula in activating blood. Yimucao (*Herba Leonuri*), Niuxi (*Radix Achyranthis Bidentatae*) and Zelan (*Radix Achyranthis Bidentatae*), as the common medicinal herbs for promoting blood circulation and inducing diuresis, can be added to the formula. In this aspect, the formula is not like Wupi Yin, which with the single function of activating qi and resolving dampness, can not transmit into blood phase.

十九、急性膀胱炎
19　Acute cystitis

〔**概说**〕 Summary

急性膀胱炎以尿频、尿急、尿痛和尿意不尽等膀胱激惹症状为突出临床表现,有的还伴有腰痛、腰酸、小腹拘急等不适症状。

急性膀胱炎隶属于中医"淋证""癃闭"等病范畴。究其原因,多与肾气亏虚、膀胱湿热、肝脉郁滞有关,有的则是由不洁的生活习惯所引起的。治疗上依据致病因素和体质状况,拟定针对性的方药,多能获得良效。

中医内科学对淋证的辨别是以临床主要症状为标准,常见的淋证有热淋、血淋、气淋、膏淋、石淋五种,但其中的膏淋、石淋应与西医学乳糜尿、膀胱结石等相对照,而本文所叙述的则以热淋、血淋、气淋为主要内容。

The clinical manifestations of acute cystitis are marked by inflammatory symptoms of the bladder such as frequent and urgent urination, pain in urination as well as obstructive urination. In some cases, it is accompanied with sensation of discomfort such as lumbago, aching of the loins, and pain and spasm of the lower abdomen.

Acute cystitis pertains to the scope of "stranguria" and "dysuria" in terms of TCM. The cause of the disease is related to kidney qi asthenia, dampness and heat in the bladder as well as qi stagnation in liver meridian or collaterals. In some cases, it is caused by improper living habit. Treatment for acute cystitis should be based on its etiology or the patient's constitution. To achieve a better curative effect, suitable formulas can be worked out accordingly.

The differentiation of "stranguria" in internal medicine of TCM is based on its main clinical manifestations. And common syndromes of it include pyretic stranguria, bloody stranguria, qi stranguria, chyloid stranguria as well as stony stranguria, among which, the latter two should be contrasted with albiduria and cystic calculus in Western medicine. This chapter focuses on the first three types.

〔辨证论治〕 Syndrome differentiation and treatment

1. 热淋
19.1 Pyretic stranguria

【症状】小便频数，点滴而下，急迫不爽，灼热刺痛，痛引脐中，尿色黄赤，或伴有腰痛，或伴有寒热口苦，恶心呕吐，或大便秘结，舌苔黄腻，脉象濡数。

【分析】湿热之毒客于膀胱，气化失司，水道不利，致使小便频数，点滴而下，急迫不爽；湿热之毒，蕴而不发，故尿道灼热刺痛，痛引脐中；湿热蕴蒸，则尿色黄赤；腰为肾之府，湿热内侵于肾，则腰痛明显；上犯少阳，则现寒热口苦、恶心呕吐；若热及大肠，则大便秘结；舌苔黄腻与脉象濡数，均为湿热为病之象。

【治法】清热除湿，通淋解毒。

【方药】八正散加味。八正散为治疗热淋之主方，方中木通、灯芯草清肺热而降心火；车前子通膀胱而络阴器；瞿麦、萹蓄降三焦之火而通淋；滑石利窍散结，栀子、大黄苦寒下行，皆泻热而兼利湿之品；甘草合滑石为六一散，通利三焦，引水下行。若腹胀、便秘者，加大大黄用量，并加枳实以通腑气；小腹坠胀者，加川楝子、乌药以行气止痛。

Clinical manifestations: Frequent urination, dripping discharge with urgent and unsmooth sensation, scorching sensation and stabbing pain involving the navel, yellowish or brownish urine, or accompanied with lumbago, or aversion to cold, fever and bitter taste, nausea and vomiting, or dry feces, greasy yellowish fur as well as soft and fast pulse.

Analysis: Pathogenic dampness and heat factors attacking the bladder and dysfunction of the bladder in transformation of qi give rise to frequent urination and dripping discharge with urgent and unsmooth sensation; scorching sensation and stabbing pain in the urethra involving the navel are due to stagnated toxic dampness and heat pathogens, which can not be discharged; yellowish or brownish urine is due to fumigation of stagnation of dampness and heat; the kidney is the house of the loins, invasion of dampness and heat into the kidney results in obvious lumbago, and up-attack of dampness and heat in shaoyang meridian gives rise to aversion to cold, fever, bitter taste, nausea and vomiting; dry feces is due to dampness and heat attacking the large intestine; greasy yellowish fur and soft and fast pulse are manifestations of dampness and heat.

Prescription: Clear away heat and eliminate dampness, treat stranguria and relieve toxin.

Formulas: Bazheng San Jiawei (Modified Bazheng Powder). It is a principal recipe for pyretic stranguria, of which, Mutong (*Caulis Akebiae*) and Dengxincao (*Medulla Junci*) can clear away heat in the lung and purge heart fire; Cheqianzi (*Semen Plantaginis*) has an action of dredging the bladder and external genitals, Qumai (*Herba Dianthi*) and Bianxu (*Herba Polygoni Avicularis*) could treat stranguria by purging fire in triple energizer; Huashi (*Talcum*) has an action of promoting defecation and urination and scattering mass, Zhizi (*Fructus Gardeniae*) and Dahunag (*Radix et Rhizoma Rhei*), bitter and cold in nature, have the function of descending fire, purging heat and removing dampness through diuresis; Gancao (*Radix Glycyrrhizae*), in combination with Huashi, makes up Liuyi San (Powder), and has an effect of clearing away damp-heat in triple energizer, and guiding dampness to descend down. For abdominal distention and constipation, the amount of Dahunag should be increased, and Zhishi (*Fructus Aurantii Immaturus*) could be added to relieve qi stagnation in the large intestine; for prolapse and distending sensation of the lower abdomen, Chuanlianzi (*Fructus Meliae Toosendan*) and Wuyao (*Radix Linderae*) should be combined to activate qi and arrest pain.

2. 血淋
19.2 Bloody stranguria

【症状】
①实证：尿色红赤，尿频拘急，灼热痛剧，滞涩不利，甚则尿道满急疼痛，牵引脐腹，舌尖红，苔薄黄，脉象数而有力。
②虚证：尿色淡黄红，尿痛略有涩滞，腰膝酸软，手足心热，舌红少苔，脉象细数。

【分析】血淋是热伤血络，渗入膀胱所致。前人有血淋为热淋之甚的说法，不无道理。多与心和小肠的病变有关。心为火脏，主血脉而合小肠，心火炽盛，移热于小肠，下注膀胱，热迫血络，则形成血淋。但此证为血淋之实证。

若体质阴虚火旺，或患热病之后，可以形成阴虚血淋，由于阴液不足，热势不甚，所以尿色不那么红赤，虽有尿痛，但不若实证那样痛剧；肾阴不足，不足以养护肾府，所以腰膝酸软；舌苔与脉象均为阴虚内热之象。

【治法】实证当清热通淋，凉血止血；虚证当滋阴补肾，清热止血。

【方药】实证用小蓟饮子。小蓟、藕节退热散瘀，生地黄凉血，蒲黄止血，木通降心火于小肠，栀子散三焦之火由小便而出，竹叶凉心而清肺，滑石祛热通窍，当归养阴，甘草调和中气。便秘加大黄以清热通腑；有瘀血加三七、琥珀粉化瘀止血；若茎中疼痛欲死者，可加一味川牛膝以化瘀止痛。

虚证则用知柏地黄丸（汤），加女贞子、旱莲草、龟板、鳖甲等，以养阴清热。若虚证尿血者，可加阿胶育阴止血。若病势不重，则可用小蓟、白茅根煎汤，送服知柏地黄丸。

Clinical manifestations：

a. Sthenic bloody stranguria：Brownish urine，frequent urination with spasm and pain，scorching sensation with severe pain，obstructive urination，even distention and scorching pain in the urethra involving peri-navel region，reddish tongue tip with thin yellowish fur as well as fast and powerful pulse.

b. Asthenic bloody stranguria：Light yellowish or light brownish urine，painful urination with slight obstructive sensation，aching and weakness of the loins and knees，feverish sensation over the palms and soles，reddish tongue with scanty fur as well as thin and fast pulse.

Analysis：Bloody stranguria is caused by heat impairing blood vessels and permeating into the bladder. The view in ancient time that blood stranguria is more serious than pyretic stranguria is reasonable. It is related to pathological changes of the heart and small intestine. The heart is the viscus of fire，governing blood vessels and associated with the small intestine. Exuberant fire in the heart transmits into the small intestine，migrates into the bladder and scorches blood vessels，giving rise to bloody stranguria. This syndrome is sthenia syndrome of blood stranguria.

Bloody stranguria could be caused by hyperactivity of fire due to yin asthenic constitution too，or by suffering from pyrexia. In such cases，fever is not high and urine is not brownish because of insufficient yin fluid. Although odynuria is accompanied，it is not so acute as that in sthenic blood stranguria；aching and weakness of the loins and knees are due to failure of insufficient kidney yin to nourish the kidney；reddish tongue with scanty fur and fast pulse are signs of endogenous heat resulting from yin asthenia.

Prescription：（for sthenic bloody stranguria）Clear away heat to eliminate stranguria，cool blood and stop bleeding；（for asthenic bloody stranguria）nourish yin，supplement the kidney，clear away heat and stop bleeding.

Formulas：（for sthenic bloody stranguria）Xiaoji Yinzi（Decoction）. In the formula，Xiaoji（*Herba Cirsii*）and Oujie（*Nodus Nelumbinis Rhizomatis*）have an action of dispelling heat and dispersing stasis of blood，Shengdihuang（*Radix Rehmanniae Recens*）can cool blood，Puhuang（*Pollen Typhae*）can stop bleeding，Mutong（*Caulis Akebiae*）could descend heart fire to the small intestine，Zhizi（*Fructus Gardeniae*）has an effect of dispersing fire from triple energizer and discharging it through urination，Zhuye（*Herba Lophatheri*）can cool heat in the heart and clear away lung heat，Huashi（*Talcum*）could purge pathogenic heat and dredge the orifices, Danggui (*Radix Angelicae Sinensis*) could nourish yin and Gancao (*Radix Glycyrrhizae*) may regulate qi in middle energizer. For constipation, Dahuang (*Radix et Rhizoma Rhei*) can be added to purge heat and relieve qi stagnation in the intestines; for blood stasis, Sanqi (*Radix Notoginseng*) and powder of Hupo (*Succinum*) may be combined to stop bleeding; for severe pain in the penis, Chuanniuxi (*Radix Cyathulae*) can be added to dissolve stasis and stop pain.

For asthenia syndrome of bloody stranguria, Zhi Bo Dihuang Wan (Pill) (or decoction) combined with Nuzhenzi (*Fructus Ligustri Lucidi*), Hanliancao (*Eclipta Alba*), Guiban (*Plastrum Testudinis*) and Biejia (*Carapax Trionycis*) can be used to nourish yin and clear away heat. For hematuria of asthenia, Ejiao (*Colla Corii Asini*) could be added to nourish yin and stop blood. For unserious disease, Xiaoji (*Herba Cirsii*) and Baimaogen (*Rhizoma Imperatae*) may be added to make into decoction, and Zhi Bo Dihuang Wan (Pill) should be taken with it.

3. 气淋
19.3　Qi stranguria

【症状】
①实证：小便滞涩，淋沥不畅，余沥难尽，脐腹憋闷，甚则胀痛难忍，舌苔薄白，脉象沉弦。

②虚证：尿频，但不红赤，滞涩不甚，余沥难尽，小腹空痛，喜按，不耐劳累，面色㿠白，少气懒言，舌苔薄白，脉象沉细无力。

【分析】肝主疏泄，其经脉循少腹，络阴器，肝脉郁滞，郁而化火，火邪郁于下焦，不得宣通，浸淫膀胱，则小便滞涩，腹痛难忍，余沥难尽。若病久不愈，或过用苦寒之药，伤及中气，脾虚气陷，不得统摄，则小便频数；气虚不能温养，则空痛喜按；其他均为气虚之象。

【治法】实证宜理气和血，通淋利尿；虚证宜补中健脾，益气升陷。

【方药】实证用沉香散。本方以石韦、冬葵子、滑石、甘草清利湿热；沉香、陈皮、王不留行理气活血；当归、白芍养血和血，标本兼顾。小腹胀满难忍，可加青皮、乌药、木香开郁消胀；有刺痛感者，可加川牛膝、赤芍、红花活血化瘀。

虚证以补中益气汤为主方。若气血双虚者，可用八珍汤双补气血。只是在用补益气血的时候，要加一些行气活血的药物，如青皮、乌药、木香、赤芍、柴胡、王不留行等，以免单纯补益而造成药物壅塞之弊。

Clinical manifestations:

a. Sthenia syndrome of qi stranguria: Obstructive and unsmooth urination with endless dripping discharge, oppression over the peri-navel region, even unbearable distending pain, thin whitish fur as well as sunken and taut pulse.

b. Asthenia syndrome of qi stranguria: Frequent urination, pale brownish urine, unserious obstructive urination with endless dripping discharge, vacuous pain over the lower abdomen, preference for pressing, tiredness with overstrain, pale complexion, lack of energy and no desire to speak, thin whitish fur as well as sunken, thin and weak pulse.

Analysis: The liver dominates dispersion liver meridian travels around the lower abdomen as well as the external genitals. Transformation of fire from qi depression in liver meridian and failure to disperse stagnation of pathogenic fire in lower energizer result in fire permeating into the bladder, which gives rise to obstructed and unsmooth urination, unbearable abdominal pain and endless dripping urination. Prolonged incurable diseases or excess intake of bitter-and-cold natured drugs impairs qi in middle energizer, giving rise to asthenic spleen and sunken qi with failure to be controlled, which brings about frequent urination; vacuous pain with preference for pressing is due to failure of asthenic qi to warm and nourish; other manifestations indicate qi asthenia.

Prescription: (for sthenia syndrome) Regulate qi and blood circulation, eliminate stranguria and induce diuresis; (for asthenia syndrome) supplement qi in middle energizer, invigorate the spleen, benefit qi and lift sunken qi.

Formulas: (for sthenia syndrome) Chenxiang San (Powder). In the formula, Shiwei (*Folium Pyrrosiae*), Dongkuizi (*Fructus Malvae*), Huashi (*Talcum*) and Gancao (*Radix Glycyrrhizae*) can clear away dampness and heat; Chenxiang (*Lignum Aquilariae Resinatum*), Chenpi (*Pericarpium Citri Reticulatae*) and Wangbuliuxing (*Semen Vaccariae*) can regulate qi and activate blood circulation, Danggui (*Radix Angelicae Sinensis*) and Baishao (*Radix Paeoniae Alba*) may nourish blood, regulate blood circulation. treating the fundamental and secondary aspects of the disease simultaneously. For unbearable distending fullness over the lower abdomen, Qingpi (*Pericarpium Citri Reticulatae Viride*), Wuyao (*Radix Linderae*) and Muxiang (*Radix Aucklandiae*) can be added to disperse qi depression and eliminate distention; for piercing pain, Chuanniuxi (*Radix Cyathulae*), Chishao (*Radix Paeoniae Rubra*) and Honghua (*Flos Carthami*) can be combined to activate blood and dissolve stasis.

(For asthenia syndrome) Buzhong Yiqi Tang (Decoction) should be used as the principal formula. For qi and blood asthenia, Bazhen Tang (Decoction) can be combined to tonify qi and blood. And some herbs that could activate qi and blood such as Qingpi (*Pericarpium Citri Reticulatae Viride*), Wuyao (*Radix Linderae*), Muxiang (*Radix Aucklandiae*), Chishao (*Radix Paeoniae Rubra*), Chaihu (*Radix Bupleuri*) and Wangbuliuxing (*Semen Vaccariae*) should be added to avoid congestion of the drug with pure tonifying function.

二十、糖尿病

20 Diabetes

〔**概说**〕 Summary

　　糖尿病是由于机体胰岛素相对或绝对分泌不足，引起糖、脂肪及蛋白质的代谢紊乱而致血糖增高和排泄糖尿的一种慢性疾病。早期无症状，典型症状为多尿、多饮、多食、消瘦。并发症为酮症酸中毒、感染、动脉硬化，肾和视网膜微血管病变，以及神经病变等。

　　糖尿病属于中医学"消渴""虚劳"等病范畴。认为与先天肾气不足、饮食不节、情志失调、房劳过多等因素有关。阴虚为本，燥热为标。病变虽与五脏有关，但主要在肺、脾（胃）、肾三脏，三脏之中尤以肾为主。治疗上以滋阴为本，清热为标，并发症出现后，活血化瘀是必不可少的。病变后期，阴虚日久，还会出现阳虚证候，因此扶阳救逆也是治疗晚期糖尿病的主要措施。

Diabetes is a chronic disease with pathological condition of metabolic disturbance of sugar, fat and protein which causes increase of blood glucose as well as discharge of glycosuria due to comparative or complete insufficient excretion of insulin in human body. Its typical symptoms are diuresis, polydipsia, polyphagia and emaciation. However, no manifestations can appear at the initial stage of the disease. The complicated syndromes of diabetes are diabetic ketoacidosis, infection, arteriosclerosis and pathological changes of the kidney, micrangium of the retina as well as the nerves.

In terms of TCM, diabetes pertains to "wasting-thirst" and "consumptive disease", and it is believed that it is related to lots of factors such as congenital insufficiency of kidney qi, improper diet, emotional upset as well as intemperate sexual life. Yin asthenia is its fundamental cause, and dryness and heat are its secondary cause. Although diabetes is connected with five-zang organs, its pathological changes are mainly located in the lung, spleen (stomach) and kidney, of which, the kidney is the primary one. As far as its treating method is concerned, nourishing yin should be placed at the primary place so as to treat the root cause of the disease, and clearing away heat at the secondary place to deal with superficial symptoms. After the onset of its complicated syndrome, activating blood circulation to resolve stasis is indispensible. At the advanced stage of diabetes, prolonged yin asthenia will bring about yang asthenia, therefore, supplementing yang to save patients from collapse is a principal therapeutic method.

〔**辨证论治**〕 Syndrome differentiation and treatment

1. 肺胃燥热

20.1 Syndrome of dryness and heat in the lung and stomach

【症状】烦渴多饮，消谷善饥，形体消瘦，口干舌燥，小便频数、量多，舌红少苔，脉象洪数。

【分析】饮食不节，积热于胃，胃热灼于肺，肺热阴亏，津液耗伤，故烦渴引饮；饮水虽多，但不能敷布全身，水性润下，肾不能固摄，则水谷精微从小便泄出，故小便频数，且量多；津液的耗伤，必然使口干舌燥；水谷精微大量外泄，机体得不到营养，故人体日渐消瘦；舌苔与脉象均为津液耗伤，燥热炽盛的表现。

【治法】清热生津止渴。

【方药】白虎人参汤加味。白虎人参汤是白虎汤加人参而成。方中生石膏辛甘大寒，清泻肺胃之热而除烦渴，为主药；知母苦寒，清泻肺胃之热且润燥，为辅药。石膏与知母相配，其清热除烦之力更强。人参、甘草、粳米益胃护津，使大寒之剂无伤脾胃之弊。全方配伍，共奏清热生津之效。此外，本证还可以选用玉泉丸（葛根、天花粉、生地黄、麦冬、五味子、甘草）。

Clinical manifestations: Polydipsia with profuse drink, polyorexia and frequent eating, emaciation, dry mouth and tongue, frequent urination, profuse urine, reddish tongue with scanty fur as well as full and fast pulse.

Analysis: Accumulation of heat in the stomach due to intemperate diet scorching the lung results in lung heat and yin and deficiency, consumption and impairment of body fluid, giving rise to polydipsia with desire to drink; frequent urination with profuse amount of urine is due to failure of profuse drink to distribute and spread to the whole body, and body fluid is characterized by moistness and down-flowing, thus causing failure of the kidney to store food essence which causes discharge of food essence from urination; dry mouth and tongue are due to impairment and consumption of body fluid; emaciation is due to malnutrition of the body because of discharge of food essence in large amount; reddish tongue with scanty fur and full and fast pulse are signs of impairment and consumption of body fluid as well as superabundance of dryness and heat.

Prescription: Clear away heat, promote production of body fluid and stop thirst.

Formulas: Baihu Renshen Tang Jiawei (Modified Baihu Renshen Decoction). Baihu Renshen Tang is made up of Baihu Tang combined with Renshen (*Radix Ginseng*). In the formula, Shengshigao (*Gypsum Fibrosum*), pungent and sweet in flavor and cold in nature, is used as the principal drug to clear away heat in the lung and stomach so as to eliminate polydipsia; Zhimu (*Rhizoma Anemarrhenae*), bitter and cold in nature, is used as adjuvant drug to purge heat in the lung and stomach and moisten dryness. Shigao combined with Zhimu has a stronger action of clearing away heat and eliminating restlessness. Renshen, Gancao

(*Radix Glycyrrhizae*) and Jingmi (*Semen Oryzae Sativae*) can benefit the stomach and protect body fluid to prevent excessive cold-natured recipe from impairing the spleen and stomach. The whole formula brings the action of clearing away heat and promoting production of body fluid into full play. Additionally, Yuquan Wan (Pill), which consists of Gegen (*Radix Puerariae*), Tianhuafen (*Radix Trichosanthis*), Shengdihuang (*Radix Rehmanniae Recens*), Maidong (*Radix Ophiopogonis*), Wuweizi (*Fructus Schisandrae Chinensis*) and Gancao, can be adopted to treat this syndrome.

2. 肝肾阴虚
20.2　Syndrome of yin asthenia of the liver and kidney

【症状】尿频量多，混浊如脂膏，或尿甜，腰膝酸软，疲乏无力，头晕耳鸣，多梦遗精，皮肤干燥，全身瘙痒，舌红少苔，脉象细数。

【分析】肝肾阴虚是糖尿病常见证候，虽然不像所叙述的那样症状典型，但或多或少都可以找到肝肾阴虚的特点。由于肝之疏泄太过，肾之封藏失司，津液直泄膀胱，故尿频量多；大量水谷精微下注，使尿如脂膏，或有甜味；腰为肾之府，为肾所主，膝为筋之府，筋为肝所主，肝肾失养，故腰膝酸软；肝肾阴精不能上布于头及清窍，故头晕耳鸣；水谷之精不能营养皮肤与四肢，故皮肤干燥、全身瘙痒；多梦、遗精为阴虚火旺所致；舌红少苔，脉象细数，为阴虚火旺之征。

【治法】滋养肝肾，润燥止渴。

【方药】六味地黄丸（汤）为主方。方中熟地黄滋肾填精，为主药，辅以山茱萸养肝肾而益精，山药补脾阴而摄精微。三药合用，以达到三脏并补之效。另一方面，又以泽泻清泻肾火，以防熟地黄之滋腻；牡丹皮清泻肝火，以制约山茱萸之温；茯苓淡渗脾湿，以防山药过于收敛。这样"三补""三泄"，使滋补而不留邪，降泻而不伤正，适合糖尿病病人长期服用。若阴虚火旺，骨蒸潮热、遗精盗汗，可加知母、黄柏，即知柏地黄丸，以滋阴降火。

Clinical manifestations: Frequent urination with profuse urine, turbid urine like cream, or sweet-smell urine, aching and weakness of the loins and knees, dispiritedness and lassitude, dizziness and tinnitus, dreaminess and seminal emission, dry skin with itching sensation, reddish tongue with scanty fur as well as thin and fast pulse.

Analysis: Syndrome of yin asthenia of the liver and kidney is a common one of diabetes. Although it is not typical, the syndrome is marked by yin asthenia of the liver and kidney to some degree. Frequent urination with profuse urine is due to excessive dispersion and conveyance of the liver and dysfunction of the kidney in storing essence, causing body fluid to discharge directly into the bladder. Turbid urine like cream or sweet flavored urine is due to downward migration of food essence in large amount. The loins, the house of the kidney, are dominated by the kidney; the knees, the residence of tendons, are associated with the liver, malnutrition of the liver and kidney gives rise to aching and weakness of the loins and knees. Dizziness and tinnitus are caused by failure of yin essence of the liver and kidney to distribute in the head as well as in lucid orifices. Dry skin with itching sensation over the whole body is due to failure of food essence to nourish the skin and limbs. Dreaminess and seminal emission are caused by yin asthenia and fire hyperactivity. Reddish tongue with scanty fur and thin and fast pulse are manifestations of yin asthenia and fire hyperactivity.

Prescription: Nourish the liver and kidney, moisten dryness and stop thirst.

Formulas: Liuwei Dihuang Wan (or Decoction) is used as a major recipe. In the recipe, Shudihuang (*Radix Rehmanniae Preparata*), with the action of nourishing the kidney and replenishing essence, is the principal drug, Shanzhuyu (*Fructus Corni*) is used as the adjuvant drug to nourish the liver and kidney and benefit essence, Shanyao (*Rhizoma Dioscoreae*) can replenish spleen yin and astringe food essence, combined together, the three could tonify the three viscera; besides, Zexie (*Rhizoma Alismatis*) can purge kidney fire to prevent Shudihuang from generating dampness, Mudanpi (*Cortex Moutan Radicis*) has an action of clearing away liver fire to restrict the warming function of Shanzhuyu, Fuling (*Poriae Cocos*), bland in flavor, can resolve dampness to stop Shanyao from astringing too much. The formula, with its "triple tonifying" and "triple purging" functions, could nourish without leaving pathogenic factors and descend and purge fire without impairing healthy qi, so it is very suitable for patients of diabetes. For yin asthenia and fire hyperactivity, bone steaming, tidal fever and seminal emission, Zhimu (*Rhizoma Anemarrhenae*) and Huangbo (*Cortex Phellodendri*) (the main ingredients of Zhi Bo Dihuang Wan) may be combined with this formula to nourish yin and descend fire.

3. 脾胃气阴两虚
20.3 Syndrome of qi and yin asthenia in the spleen and stomach

【症状】口渴引饮，能食与便溏并见，或饮食减少，精神不振，四肢酸软，舌质淡红，苔薄白而干，脉象细弱无力。

【分析】脾胃气阴两虚证，在糖尿病的进程中并不少见。它的病理基础是病人体质显示脾胃气阴两虚，或者过用清热苦寒之药味，伤及脾胃之气阴，胃阴不足则口渴引饮，能食与脾虚便溏并见；若脾胃气阴耗伤过重，则食欲减少，精神不振；脾胃之精微失于濡养，则所主之四肢酸软；舌质淡红，为脾虚之征；薄白而干之苔，为阴亏之象；脉象细弱无力，是气阴两虚之兆。总之，显示一派虚象。

【治法】健脾养胃，生津止渴。

【方药】七味白术散合益胃汤。七味白术散由四君子汤加木香、藿香、葛根组成。四君子汤为补益脾胃之气的主方，方中人参、白术、茯苓、甘草健脾益气，木香、藿香醒脾散津，葛根生津止渴。益胃汤由沙参、麦冬、生地黄、玉竹组成，是滋阴养胃之主方。前方偏于补脾经之气，后方偏于养胃经之阴，两方合用，相得益彰，对脾胃气阴两虚之证，颇为适宜。

Clinical manifestations: Thirst with desire for drink, normal appetite and loose stool, or reduced appetite, dispiritedness, aching and weakness of limbs, pale reddish tongue with dry thin whitish fur as well as thin and weak pulse.

Analysis：Syndrome of qi and yin asthenia of the spleen and stomach is very common during the developing process of diabetes. Pathogenesis of the disease is constitutional asthenia of qi and yin in the spleen and stomach, or impairment of qi and yin in the spleen and stomach due to excessive intake of bitter-and-cold natured drug which has the action of clearing away heat, thus, insufficient stomach yin gives rise to thirst with desire to drink as well as good appetite and loose stool; reduced appetite and dispiritedness are due to severe consumption and impairment of qi and yin in the spleen and stomach; aching and weakness of limbs are due to hypofunction of asthenic spleen and stomach to transform food, which fails to nourish the limbs; pale reddish tongue is a sign of spleen asthenia, dry thin whitish fur indicates yin deficiency; thin and weak pulse signifies qi and yin asthenia. In a word, all manifestations indicate asthenia.

Prescription：Invigorate the spleen, nourish the stomach, promote production of body fluid and stop thirst.

Formulas：Qiwei Baizhu San (Powder) combined with Yiwei Tang (Decoction). Qiwei Baizhu San is made up of Sijunzi Tang, Muxiang (*Radix Aucklandiae*), Huoxiang (*Herba Agastachis*) and Gegen (*Radix Puerariae*). Sijunzi Tang is a major recipe for tonifying qi in the spleen and stomach, of which, Renshen (Radix Ginseng), Baizhu (*Rhizoma Atractylodis Macrocephalae*), Fuling (*Poriae Cocos*) and Gancao (*Radix Glycyrrhizae*) can invigorate the spleen and benefit qi, Muxiang and Huoxiang have an action of refreshing the spleen and scattering body fluid, Gegen can promote production of fluid to stop thirst. Yiwei Tang, consisting of Shashen (*Radix Glehniae*), Maidong (*Radix Ophiopogonis*), Shengdihuang (*Radix Rehmanniae Recens*) and Yuzhu (*Rhizoma Polygonati Odorati*), is a principal formula for nourishing yin and the stomach. The former is prone to supplementing qi in spleen meridian, and the latter is susceptible to nourishing stomach yin. Combined together, both formulas are very suitable for the syndrome of asthenic qi and yin in the spleen and stomach.

4. 阴阳两虚

20.4 Syndrome of yin and yang asthenia

【症状】小便频数，混浊如膏，甚则饮一溲一，手足心热，咽干烦躁，耳轮干枯，面色黧黑，腰膝酸软，四肢欠温，畏寒怕冷，性冷淡，舌淡苔白干，脉象沉细无力。

【分析】阴阳两虚证是糖尿病的严重阶段，在经过了肺、肝、肾阴虚燥热病程以后，阴损及阳，或过用苦寒之药，伤及机体的阳气，形成了阴阳两虚的局面。本证之手足心热、咽干烦躁、耳轮干枯等为阴虚证候；而四肢欠温、恶寒怕冷、性冷淡等为阳虚证候；面色黧黑、腰膝酸软，阴阳两虚均可以见到此症状，舌苔与脉象为正气虚弱之象。

【治法】滋阴温阳补肾。

【方药】金匮肾气丸（汤）为主方。本方的组成可以分为两部分，即六味地黄丸，另加附子、桂枝。六味地黄丸是滋补肝肾之阴的主方，另加附子、桂枝温养补肾，意在微微生火，以鼓舞肾气，取"少火生气"之意。用金匮肾气丸治疗消渴（糖尿病），始于汉代张仲景，后代又有发挥。至于治疗消渴病为什么要用温热之药，是否有耗伤阴液的副作用，这个问题应当从气化学说上来理解。前人认为，肾为水脏，肾暖则气上腾而润肺，肾冷则气不升而枯萎；若肾不能气化阴液，那么阴液就会成为"一潭死水"，对身体只会有害处，绝无好处。

Clinical manifestations: Frequent urination, even right after drinking, urine like turbid cream, feverish sensation over the palms and soles, dry throat and restlessness, dry and withered helix of the ear, darkish complexion, aching and weakness of the loins and knees, cold limbs, aversion to cold, sexual hypofunction, pale tongue with whitish dry fur as well as sunken, thin and weak pulse.

Analysis: Syndrome of yin and yang asthenia occurs at the advanced stage of diabetes. After the course of dryness and heat due to yin asthenia in the lung, liver and kidney, impairment of yin involves yang, or intake of excessive cold-and-bitter natured drug impairs yang qi of the body, thus, giving rise to the condition of yin and yang asthenia. Such symptoms as feverish sensation over the palms and soles, dry throat and restlessness as well as dry and withered helix of the ear belong to the syndrome of yin asthenia; while cold limbs, aversion to cold and sexual dysfunction are symptoms of yang asthenia; darkish complexion as well as aching and weakness of the loins and knees can be seen in both syndromes of yin and yang asthenia; pale tongue with whitish dry fur and sunken, thin and weak pulse are signs of deficiency of healthy qi.

Prescription: Nourish yin, warm yang and tonify the kidney.

Formulas: Jingui Shenqi Wan (or Decoction) (used as the major formula). It is the combination of Liuwei Dihuang Wan with Fuzi (*Radix Aconiti Lateralis Preparata*) and Guizhi (*Ramulus Cinnamomi*). Liuwei Dihuang Wan is a major recipe for nourishing and supplementing yin in the liver and kidney, Fuzi and Guizhi can warm yang and tonify the kidney, aiming at "invigorating qi in the kidney with mild fire".Treating consumptive disease (namely, diabetes) by means of Jingui Shenqi Wan is handed down from Zhang Zhongjing from the Han Dynasty. Later, the recipe has been improved. Why are warm natured medicinal herbs adopted to treat consumptive disease? Is there any side effect of consuming and impairing yin fluid? This topic should be approached from the theory of qi transformation. Ancient TCM experts hold that the kidney is the viscus of water, if it is warm, qi will rise up and moisten the lung; if it is cold, qi will not lift and it withers; if it fails to transform yin fluid into qi, yin fluid will become uncirculated, which will do harm to human body.

附：并发症
Complications

（1）肺痨

【症状】先病消渴（糖尿病），后病咳嗽，呈现干咳少痰，痰中带血，五心烦热，潮热盗汗，舌红少苔，脉象细数。

【分析】糖尿病多由肺、脾、肾阴虚所致，若体质素弱，肺阴不足，患糖尿病后很容易引发肺痨，肺阴不足，阴虚内热，肺气开阖不利，则干咳少痰，或血络有伤，会痰中带血；"阴虚生内热"，内热熏蒸，则五心烦热，潮热盗汗；舌苔与脉象为阴虚内热之明证。

【治法】养阴清热，润肺止咳。

【方药】百合固金汤。方中百合、生地黄和熟地黄滋肺肾之阴，为本方之主药；麦冬助百合以润肺止咳，玄参助生地黄和熟地黄以滋阴清热，当归、白芍养血滋阴，贝母、桔梗清肺化痰止咳，共为辅药；甘草调和诸药，为佐使之剂。

（1）Tuberculosis complicated with diabetes

Clinical manifestations: Outbreak of tuberculosis at the initial stage of diabetes, dry cough with scanty sputum mingled with blood, feverish sensation over the palms, soles and the chest, tidal fever and night sweating, reddish tongue with scanty fur as well as thin and fast pulse.

Analysis: Diabetes is caused by yin asthenia in the lung, spleen and kidney. Constitutional asthenia and insufficient lung yin lead to development of tuberculosis from diabetes. Insufficiency of lung yin and yin asthenia due to endogenous heat cause dry cough with scanty sputum because of disorder of lung qi, sputum mingled with blood is due to impairment of blood vessels; feverish sensation over the palms, soles and the chest, tidal fever and night sweating are caused by fumigation of superabundant endogenous heat generated from yin asthenia; reddish tongue with scanty fur and thin and fast pulse are clear signs of yin asthenia and endogenous heat.

Prescription: Nourish yin, clear away heat and moisten the lung to stop cough.

Formulas: Baihe Gujin Tang (Decoction). In the formula, Baihe (*Bulbus Lilii*), Shengdihuang (*Radix Rehmanniae Recens*) and Shudihuang (*Radix Rehmanniae Preparata*), with an action of nourishing yin in the lung and kidney, are used as the major drug; Maidong (*Radix Ophiopogonis*) can assist Baihe to moisten the lung and stop cough, Xuanshen (*Radix Scrophulariae*) can help Shengdihuang and Shudihuang nourish yin and clear away heat, Danggui (*Radix Angelicae Sinensis*) and Baishao (*Radix Paeoniae Alba*) may nourish blood and promote production of yin, Beimu (*Bulbus Fritillaria*) and Jiegeng (*Radix Platycodonis*), with an action of clearing away lung heat, resolving phlegm and stopping cough, are used as adjuvant drug; Gancao (*Radix Glycyrrhizae*) is used as courier drug to harmonize the above herbs.

（2）瘀血证

【症状】消渴病（糖尿病）兼见舌质瘀暗，舌上有瘀点或瘀斑，舌下静脉粗张，或静脉旁有许多紫色珠粒（络脉瘀阻），或胸中刺痛，或半身不遂，脉象涩滞。

【分析】消渴病（糖尿病）的并发症，瘀血证是最常见的。瘀血证最明显的指征是舌质瘀暗和有瘀点或瘀斑。若瘀于心肺经脉，则会出现胸中刺痛；瘀于足三阳经，则会有半身不遂等症状。其脉象表现为不流利的涩滞象。

【治法】活血化瘀。

【方药】降糖活血方。方由木香、当归、益母草、赤芍、川芎、葛根、丹参组成。方中丹参、赤芍、川芎、益母草活血化瘀；当归养血活血；木香行气导滞，可增强活血化瘀药物的药力；葛根生津止渴。若兼见气阴两虚者，可加生脉饮益气养阴；若下肢瘀血比较重者，可加川牛膝、鸡血藤、穿山龙等通经活络。

（2）Blood stasis complicated with diabetes

Clinical manifestations：Consumptive disease（diabetes）complicated with dark spots or petechia on the tongue，varicose vein under the tongue，or obstruction of blood like purplish beads in the collaterals，or piercing pain in the chest，or hemiplegia and astringent pulse.

Analysis：Blood stasis is a common complicated syndrome of diabetes，and the most obvious manifestation of blood stasis is dark spots on the tongue，or petechiae on the tongue. Piercing pain in the chest indicates blood stasis stagnating in heart and lung meridians；hemiplegia suggests blood stasis stagnating in three yang meridians of the feet. Astringent and unsmooth pulse is a sign of blood stasis.

Prescription：Activate blood circulation and resolve blood stasis.

Formulas：Jiangtang Huoxue Formula. The formula is made up of Muxiang（*Radix Aucklandiae*），Danggui（*Radix Angelicae Sinensis*），Yimucao（*Herba Leonuri*），Chishao（*Radix Paeoniae Rubra*），Chuanxiong（*Rhizoma Ligustici Chuanxiong*），Gegen（*Radix Puerariae*）and Danshen（*Radix Salviae Miltiorrhizae*），among which，Danshen，Chishao，Chuanxiong and Yimucao can activate blood circulation and resolve blood stasis；Danggui has an action of nourishing blood and activating blood circulation；Muxiang can activate qi，disperse stagnation and reinforce the effect of activating blood circulation and resolving blood stasis；Gegen can promote production of body fluid and stop thirst. For the complicated syndrome of asthenia of qi and yin，Shengmai Yin（Decoction）can be added to benefit qi and nourish yin；for severe blood stasis in lower limbs，Chuanniuxi（*Radix Cyathulae*），Jixueteng（*Caulis Spatholobi*）and Chuanshanlong（*Ningpo Yam Rhizome*）can be combined to promote blood circulation by removing blood stasis in meridans and collaterals.

（3）痈疽

【症状】消渴病（糖尿病）并发痈疽，症见皮肤痈疽或牙龈脓肿，久久不愈，或伴发高热，神昏谵语，舌红苔黄，脉象滑数。

【分析】消渴病并发痈疽，是内热炽盛所致。加之小便过多，津液亏耗，营卫不行，热邪滞留，更易形成痈疽。邪热攻心，则神昏谵语；舌苔与脉象均呈现热势弛张的本象。

【治法】清热解毒。

【方药】五味消毒饮。方中金银花清热解毒、消散痈疽为主药；紫花地丁、天葵子、蒲公英、野菊花均可清热解毒，是治疗外科疮疖的要药。大便秘结者，可加大黄（后下）、芒硝（冲服）通腑泻热。

(3) Ulcer complicated with diabetes

Clinical manifestations：Ulcer on the skin or gingival abscess with a long duration, or accompanied by high fever, unconsciousness and delirious speech, reddish tongue with yellowish fur as well as slippery and fast pulse.

Analysis：Ulcer complicated with consumptive disease (diabetes) is caused by superabundance of endogenous heat. Profuse urination, deficiency and consumption of body fluid, failure to activate nutrient qi and defensive qi as well as retention of pathogenic heat factors give rise to susceptibility to ulcer. Pathogenic heat factors attacking the heart results in unconsciousness and delirious speech; reddish tongue with yellowish fur and slippery and fast pulse are signs of internal retention of heat.

Prescription：Clear away heat and relieve toxic pathogen.

Formulas：Wuwei Xiaodu Yin (Decoction). In the formula, Jinyinhua (*Flos Lonicerae*) is used as the principal drug to clear away heat, relieve toxic heat and eliminate ulcer; Zihuadiding (*Herba Violae*), Tiankuizi (*Semiaquilegia adoxoides*), Pugongying (*Herba Taraxaci*) and Yejuhua (*Flos Chrysanthemi Indici*) are the essential drug to clear away heat and relieve toxic heat, and they are used for the treatment of surgical sore and furuncle. For dry feces, Dahuang (*Radix et Rhizoma Rhei*) can be added (decocted) later, and Mangxiao (*Natrii Sulfas*) can be taken for oral use after being infused in boiled water to eliminate stagnation of intestinal qi and purge heat.

(4) 泄泻

【症状】食欲减退，精神不振，大便溏泻，或完谷不化，日渐消瘦，舌淡苔白，脉象沉细。

【分析】消渴病日久，常常使脾肾阳气衰弱，形成脾不能运化，肾不能温化，导致水谷不分，大便溏泻，体质下降，舌苔、脉象也呈虚弱状态，为消渴病发展过程中的阶段性疾病，若不及时治疗，会使阳气日渐衰败，难以挽回。

【治法】温补脾肾。

【方药】理中汤。由人参、白术、干姜、甘草组成。人参甘温健脾，补中益气，是强壮脾胃的要药；白术苦温燥湿健脾，是温中止泻的要药；干姜辛热，温中扶阳；甘草甘缓扶正。四药合用，共奏温阳驱寒、健脾止泻之效。根据历代医家的经验，本方不但是治疗脾虚泄泻的主方，而且还是治疗消渴病的良方之一。若泄泻严重，可加肉豆蔻、补骨脂温肾止泻。

(4) Diarrhea complicated with diabetes

Clinical manifestations：Reduced appetite, dispiritedness, loose stool or diarrhea with indigested food, emaciation, pale tongue with whitish fur as well as sunken and thin pulse.

Analysis: Prolonged diabetes causes deficiency of yang qi in the spleen and kidney, which results in indigested food mixed with water, loose stool and diarrhea, even deteriorated health condition due to dysfunction of the spleen in transportation and transformation as well as failure of the kidney to warm and transform qi; pale tongue with whitish fur and sunken and thin pulse indicate weak constitution. The syndrome occurs in the developing process of diabetes, and delayed treatment can lead to irretrievable condition because of gradual decline of yang qi.

Prescription: Warm and supplement the spleen and kidney.

Formulas: Lizhong Tang (Decoction). It consists of Renshen (*Radix Ginseng*), Baizhu (*Rhizoma Atractylodis Macrocephalae*), Ganjiang (*Rhizoma Zingiberis*) and Gancao (*Radix Glycyrrhizae*), among which, Renshen, sweet and warm in nature, is the essential drug to strengthen the spleen and stomach with the action of invigorating the spleen, tonifying middle energizer and benefiting qi; Baizhu, bitter and warm in nature, with an action of drying dampness and invigorating the spleen, is an important herb to warm middle energizer and stop diarrhea; Ganjiang, pungent and hot in nature, can warm middle energizer and strengthen yang; Gancao, sweet in flavor, has the action of harmonizing and strengthening healthy qi. Combined together, the four medicinal herbs can bring the effect of warming yang, dispelling cold, invigorating the spleen and stopping diarrhea into full play. Ancient TCM experts hold that the formula is not only a major recipe for treating diarrhea due to spleen asthenia, but it is also an effective one for treating diabetes. For severe diarrhea, Roudoukou (*Semen Myristicae*) and Buguzhi (*Fructus Psoraleae*) can be added to warm the kidney and stop diarrhea.

(5) 白内障、雀目、耳鸣

【症状】白内障可见视物模糊，眼前黑花缭乱，或蚊虫飞舞；有的表现为雀目，入夜即视物不清，至天明则视觉恢复；有的表现为耳鸣、耳聋。

【分析】消渴日久，消耗阴精，致使肝肾阴血亏虚，肝开窍于目，肾开窍于耳，精血不能上承，濡养目与耳，故形成白内障和雀目、耳鸣等。

【治法】滋补肝肾。

【方药】明目地黄丸。由六味地黄丸加当归、柴胡、五味子组成。六味地黄丸滋补肝肾之阴精，加当归养血，柴胡疏肝，五味子收敛精气，不使其耗散。也可选择杞菊地黄丸养肝明目；或可用石斛夜光丸平肝熄风，滋阴明目；或可用耳聋左慈丸滋补肝肾，镇肝潜阳，以疗耳聋、耳鸣。

(5) Cataract, night blindness and tinnitus complicated with diabetes

Clinical manifestations: As for cataract, the manifestations are blurred vision, or dazzling vision like some small insects such as mosquitoes or flies dancing before the eyes; the manifestations of night blindness are unclear sight at dusk, sight recovering to normal at dawn; in other cases, tinnitus or deafness can appear with diabetes.

Analysis：Consumption of yin essence due to prolonged diabetes causes yin asthenia and blood deficiency of the liver and kidney. The liver opens at the eyes, the kidney opens at the ears, failure of essence and blood to flow upward to nourish the eyes and ears results in cataract, night blindness and tinnitus.

Prescription：Nourish and supplement the liver and kidney.

Formulas：Mingmu Dihuang Wan (Pill). The recipe is made up of Liuwei Dihuang Wan in combination with Danggui (*Radix Angelicae Sinensis*), Chaihu (*Radix Bupleuri*) and Wuweizi (*Fructus Schisandrae Chinensis*). Liuwei Dihuang Wan can nourish and tonify yin and essence in the liver and kidney, Danggui has an action of nourishing blood, Chaihu can soothe the liver, Wuweizi may astringe essence and qi to avoid being consumed. Qiju Dihuang Wan can also be adopted to nourish the liver and improve visual acuity, or Shihu Yeguang Wan can be used to suppress hyperactive liver for calming endogenous wind and nourish yin to improve eyesight, or Erlong Zuoci Wan could be used to nourish liver and kidney and suppress hyperactive liver yang so as to treat deafness and tinnitus.

（6）水肿

【症状】腹部胀满，四肢水肿，甚则全身浮肿，小便不利，舌淡苔白，脉象沉迟。

【分析】消渴日久，肾气虚衰，不能蒸化水液，水液潴留，则演变成水肿。这种水肿多由阳气虚亏，或阴阳俱虚所致。

【治法】温肾化气行水。

【方药】济生肾气丸合真武汤。济生肾气丸在"慢性肾小球肾炎"篇中已经论述，请参考。真武汤是张仲景用来治疗阳虚水肿的一张名方。方由附子、茯苓、白术、芍药、生姜组成。附子是温阳的，温阳才能化气行水；茯苓是健脾渗湿的，有利于使水邪从小便排出；白术是健脾主导运化的，生姜走而不守，以利于消散水邪；芍药在这里的作用是滋阴的，以防利尿伤阴，也可以说是固摄正气的，我常常是白芍与赤芍并用，一方面护阴扶正，一方面疏通经脉，以利水邪的排泄。

（6）Edema

Clinical manifestations：Abdominal distention and fullness, edema over the limbs, even over the whole body, unsmooth urination, pale tongue with whitish fur as well as sunken and slow pulse.

Analysis：Consumption of kidney qi due to prolonged diabetes results in failure to fumigate and transform body fluid and retention of body fluid, giving rise to edema. This type of edema is caused by yang qi asthenia or asthenia of yin and yang.

Prescription：Warm the kidney, transform qi and induce diuresis.

Formulas：Jisheng Shenqi Wan (Pill) and Zhenwu Tang (Decoction). The former Wan has been introduced in *Chronic Glomerulonephritis*. The latter, Zhenwu Tang is a famous recipe of Zhang Zhongjing for treating edema due to yang asthenia, consisting of Fuzi (*Radix Aconiti Lateralis Preparata*), Fuling (*Poriae Cocos*), Baizhu (*Rhizoma Atractylodis Macrocephalae*), Shaoyao (*Radix Paeoniae*), and Shengjiang (*Rhizoma Zingiberis Recens*).

Fuzi is used to warm yang so as to transform qi and induce diuresis; Fuling can invigorate the spleen and resolve dampness to help pathogenic dampness discharge through urine; Baizhu has the action of invigorating the spleen and dominating transportation and transformation, Shengjiang is very helpful to expel pathogenic dampness factor; Shaoyao, including Chishao (*Radix Paeoniae Rubra*) and Baishao (*Radix Paeoniae Alba*), has an action of nourishing yin to prevent excessive diuresis from impairing yin, namely, to help consolidate healthy qi. The combination of Chishao with Baishao, on one hand, can strengthen yin and healthy qi, on the other hand, it can dredge meridians and collaterals to promote discharge of pathogenic dampness.

（7）肢体麻木
【症状】肌肉消瘦，肢体麻木不仁，行走时如踏于棉花之上。
【分析】消渴日久，耗伤气血，气血精气不能濡养肢体，故麻木不仁。
【治法】补益气血。
【方药】黄芪六一汤合四物汤。黄芪六一汤，即黄芪与甘草两味。黄芪大补元气，补气才能生血；甘草甘温和中，以利于健脾生血。四物汤即当归、熟地黄、川芎、白芍，是补益阴血的主方，两个方子配合起来，补气生血，阳中生阴，药味虽少，但功力较宏。

（7）Syndrome of numb limbs complicated with diabetes

Clinical manifestations: Emaciation, numb limbs, and flaccid sensation like walking on cotton mat.

Analysis: Prolonged diabetes consuming and impairing qi and blood causes failure of qi, blood and essence to nourish the body, leading to numb limbs.

Prescription: Benefit qi and supplement blood.

Formulas: Huangqi Liuyi Tang (Decoction) combined with Siwu Tang (Decoction). The former consists of Huangqi (*Radix Astragali seu Hedysari*) and Gancao (*Radix Glycyrrhizae*). Huangqi has an action of tonifying promordial qi to generate blood; Gancao, sweet in flavor and warm in nature, has an action of harmonizing middle energizer to help invigorate the spleen and promote production of blood. The latter, Siwu Tang, made up of Danggui (*Radix Angelicae Sinensis*), Shudihuang (*Radix Rehmanniae Praeparata*), Chuanxiong (*Rhizoma Ligustici Chuanxiong*), and Baishao (*Radix Paeoniae Alba*), is a major recipe for tonifying yin and blood. The combination of both formulas, though with few herbs, can bring supplementing qi, promoting production of blood and generation of yin from yang into full play.

二十一、甲状腺功能亢进

21 Hyperthyroidism

〔**概说**〕 Summary

甲状腺功能亢进，简称"甲亢"，是以甲状腺肿大、基础代谢增加，自主神经功能失常为基本生理、病理特点，以弥漫型、结节型、混合型为病理解剖特征，以怕热多汗、静时心动过速、食欲亢进、体重下降、甲状腺肿大、突眼、甲状腺局部震颤及血管杂音为典型临床表现的一种常见内分泌疾病。

"甲亢"属于中医"瘿""瘿气"病范畴。认为本病与地理环境、个人情绪、饮食结构等有关。初期多实证，病机有气滞、肝火、痰凝、血瘀之分；久病则以阴虚居多。临床应从理气、化痰、泻火、养阴着手，辅以活血化瘀、平肝熄风、扶正补虚等法。

Hyperthyroidism is a disease featured by thyroid enlargement, increase of basal metabolism and dysfunction of autonomic nerve. From the anatomic angle, the disease can be physiologically classified into diffusive, nodular as well as mixed type of goiter. As a common disease concerning internal secretion, hyperthyroidism has the following typical clinic manifestations: aversion to heat, profuse sweating, tachycardia (fast heart beat) in tranquility, bulimia (good appetite), decline of weight, enlargement of thyroid, ocular proptosis, tremor in part of the thyroid gland as well as vascular murmur.

In terms of TCM, hyperthyroidism is categorized as "Ying" (goiter) or "Ying qi" (scrofula). It is believed that the disease is related to geographical environment, personal mood, improper dietary habit, etc. At the primary stage, the disease pertains to a syndrome of sufficiency, and its pathogenesis falls into qi stagnation, liver fire, phlegm coagulation and blood stasis. Most cases of prolonged hyperthyroidism belong to yin deficiency, and clinically, the main therapeutic methods should be regulating qi, dissolving phlegm, purging pathogenic fire and nourishing yin. Activating blood and dissolving stasis, calming liver wind and strengthening body resistance to replenish deficiency can be used as its supplementary treatment.

〔**辨证论治**〕 Syndrome differentiation and treatment

1. 肝郁气滞

21.1 Stagnation of qi due to liver depression

【症状】性情急躁，心烦易怒，失眠多梦，夜寐不安，胸闷胁胀，善太息，口干口苦，多伴咽哽如炙，舌苔白腻或薄黄，脉象弦数。

【分析】"甲亢"初期，多情志不遂，出现胸闷、急躁、心烦、失眠，忧郁不畅，这些症状与小柴胡汤主症相似，是以肝胆气机不利所致，故以清解少阳郁热为主。有的病人会有痰热夹杂，所以有口干口苦、咽哽如炙、舌苔薄黄之症。在此阶段，应积极疏肝理气，和解少阳。

【治法】疏肝理气，和解少阳，并佐以化痰之品。

【方药】小柴胡汤加减。方取柴胡舒达肝气，和解少阳；黄芩清热，半夏除痰，党参益气生津，甘草中和诸药，大枣与生姜调和营卫。另加紫苏梗、郁金开三焦郁结；酸枣仁、夜交藤宁心安神。若有大便干结者，加决明子、火麻仁。

Clinical manifestations: Irritability, susceptibility to rage, insomnia and dreaminess, restlessness at night, distending pain in the chest and hypochondrium, chest oppression with frequent sigh, bitter taste and dryness of the mouth, scorching sensation of obstruction in the throat, whitish and greasy tongue fur, or thin and yellowish fur as well as taut and rapid pulse.

Analysis: Emotional upset at the primary stage of hyperthyroidism results in distending pain in the chest and hypochondrium, irritability and restlessness, insomnia and depression. These symptoms, similar to the leading symptoms which could be cured with Small Chaihu Tang (Decoction), are caused by qi depression in the liver and gallbladder. Thus, the main treating methods should be clearing and dissolving heat stagnation in Shaoyang meridian. In some cases, heat of phlegm can be combined with the above symptoms, it might bring about bitter taste and dryness of the mouth, scorching sensation of obstruction in the throat, as well as thin and yellowish tongue. In this period, alleviating liver depression, regulating qi and harmonizing Shaoyang should be adopted as its therapeutic methods.

Prescription: Alleviating liver depression to regulate qi, relieving Shaoyang disorder, and resolving phlegm can be taken as the supplementary method.

Formulas: Small Chaihu Tang Jiajian (Modified Small Chaihu decoction). In the formula, Chaihu (*Radix Bupleuri*) has a function of relieving qi depression in the liver as well as disorder in Shaoyang; Huangqin (*Radix Scutellariae*) is able to clear heat, Banxia (*Rhizoma Pinelliae*) can resolve phlegm, Dangshen (*Radix Codonopsis*) has the ability of tonifying qi and promoting the secretion of saliva or body fluid, Gancao (*Radix Glycyrrhizae*) can regulate all the other herbs, Dazao (*Fructus Jujubae*) and Shengjiang (*Rhizoma Zingiberis Recens*) have the effect of keeping nutrient qi and defensive qi in balance. Zisugeng (*Caulis Perllae*) and Yujin (*Radix Curcumae*) can relieve qi stagnation in Sanjiao; Suanzaoren (*Semen Ziziphi Spinosae*) and Yejiaoteng (*Tuber Fleeceflower Stem*) can be added to tranquilize uneasiness of the mind. For constipation, Juemingzi (*Semen Cassiae*) and Huomaren (*Fructus Cannabis*) can be added.

2. 肝郁化火
21.2　Stagnated liver-qi transforming into liver fire

【症状】瘿肿突眼，畏热多汗，面红耳赤，心烦易怒，消谷善饥，手抖舌颤，舌红苔黄，脉象弦数。

【分析】由于肝失疏泄，木失条达，肝气内郁日久，化火冲逆。冲于心，则心烦易怒；冲于肺，则肺失清肃，腠理不密，而畏热汗多；冲于胃府，则消谷善饥；热极生风，故会出现手抖舌颤；病本在肝，累及他脏，也会出现其他意想不到的症状。

【治法】清肝泻火，佐以育阴潜阳。

【方药】龙胆泻肝汤加减。方中龙胆草直折肝胆实热；栀子、黄芩清泻心肺胃肠之郁火；加入钩藤、石决明以镇惊、缓急、达郁；肝体阴而用阳，故加生地黄、女贞子清热养阴；柴胡清解肝郁，顺其条达之性；甘草调和诸药。全方泻中有补，滋中含疏。便秘者，加大黄；心火甚，加黄连；干渴甚，加天花粉、芦根；突眼者，加贝母、胆南星。

Clinical manifestations：Enlargement of goiter, ocular proptosis, aversion to heat and profuse sweating, flushed complexion and ears, irritability and susceptibility to rage, rapid digestion of food and polyorexia, tremor of the hands and tongue, reddish tongue and yellowish tongue fur, and taut and rapid pulse.

Analysis：Prolonged stagnation of liver-qi transforms into liver fire due to failure of the liver to disperse. Irritability and susceptibility to rage are caused by liver fire attacking the heart. Aversion to heat and profuse sweating are due to loose interspaces of the skin and muscles because of dysfunction of the lung to depurate caused by liver fire attacking the heart. Rapid digestion of food and polyorexia result from liver fire attacking the stomach. Tremor of the hands and tongue is caused by excessive heat generating wind. And other unexpected symptoms might originate from diseases in the liver, which can impair other organs of the body.

Prescription：Purge liver fire, nourish yin and suppress exuberance of yang.

Formulas：Longdan Xiegan Tang Jiajian (Modified Longdan Xiegan decoction). In the formula, Longdancao (*Radix Geutianae*) can purge the excessive heat in the liver and gallbladder; Zhizi (*Fructus Gardeniae*) and Huangqin (*Radix Scutellariae*) have an effect of clearing stagnated fire in the heart, lung, stomach and intestines; Gouteng (*Ramulus Uncariae cum Uncis*) and Shijueming (*Concha Haliotidis*) can be able to relieve convulsion, alleviate critical symptoms and disperse suppressed fire; the liver pertains to yin while it has the function of yang, therefore, Shengdihuang (*Radix Rehmanniae Recens*) and Nuzhenzi (*Fructus Ligustri Lucidi*) can be used to clear heat and nourish yin; Chaihu (*Radix Bupleuri*) can clear and purge suppressed fire in the liver and enhance the liver's function of dispersing stagnation; and Gancao (*Radix Glycyrrhizae*) can regulate the above herbs. This formula contains herbs with the function of tonifying, purging, nourishing as well as dispersing. For constipation, Dahuang (*Radix et Rhizoma Rhei*) can be added; for exuberant heart fire, Huanglian (*Rhizoma Coptidis*) should be used; as for dry and thirsty sensation, Tianhuafen (*Radix Trichosanthis*) and Lugen (*Rhizoma Phragmitis*) can be combined; for ocular proptosis, Beimu (*Bulbus Fritillaria*) and Dannanxing (*Rhizoma Arisaematis Cum Bile*) should be added to the formula.

3. 阴虚火旺
21.3　Hyperactivity of fire due to yin deficiency

【症状】心烦易怒，易激动，怕热出汗，易饥多食，四肢抖动，突眼，颈部肿大，舌质红赤，苔薄黄，脉象细数。

【分析】阴虚火旺，有多种因素，以肝经阴虚火旺为多，但也可以伤及心肺之阴，出现心肺阴虚火旺证。此条证候，既有肝火之突眼、四肢抖动，颈部肿大；又有心阴不足之心烦易怒，以及肺阴虚之怕热出汗；还有胃阴虚之易饥多食等。其舌质、脉象，均为阴虚火旺之征。

【治法】滋阴、凉血、清热。

【方药】百合地黄汤合百合知母汤加减。方以百合为主药，清解气分之热，且清金制木，使金气清肃，木火受抑，则肝火之势自然有所消退；生地黄滋阴以配阳，养心阴而清血热；更以知母清肺胃之热，其清肃之气下行，邪热从小便而出。三味协力，共奏清肺金、抑肝火、养阴津之效。口渴失眠，加天花粉、生龙骨、生牡蛎；烦躁，加鸡子黄、栀子；小便黄赤，加滑石、竹叶。

Clinical manifestations: Irritability and susceptibility to rage and excitement, aversion to heat and profuse sweating, rapid digestion of food and polyorexia, tremor of the limbs, ocular proptosis, swollen and enlarged neck, reddish tongue with thin yellowish fur, thready and rapid pulse.

Analysis: Hyperactivity of fire due to yin deficiency can be caused by many factors, and the most important one is yin deficiency and fire hyperactivity in liver meridian which can impair heart yin and lung yin, bringing about the syndrome of fire hyperactivity due to yin deficiency in the heart and lung. This syndrome contains not only symptoms such as ocular proptosis, trembling limbs and swollen neck caused by liver fire, but it also involves irritability and susceptibility to rage due to deficiency of heart yin as well as the symptoms of aversion to heat and sweating due to yin asthenia of the lung, and digestion of food and polyorexia which result from yin deficiency of the stomach. Reddish tongue with thin yellowish fur and thready and rapid pulse are signs of hyperactivity of fire due to yin deficiency.

Prescription: Nourish yin, cool blood and clear heat.

Formulas: Baihe Dihuang Tang (Decoction) combined with Baihe Zhimu Tang (Decoction) Jiajian. Baihe (*Bulbus Lilii*) is the basic herb in the formula, it can clear and dissolve heat in qi phrase and purge heat in the lung (the lung pertains to metal according to the five-element theory) so as to check the liver (which pertains to wood). This herb can get lung qi depurated and liver fire restrained, thus, liver fire could be eliminated. Shengdihuang

(*Radix Rehmanniae Recens*) has an effect of nourishing heart yin and clearing heat in the blood. Zhimu (*Rhizoma Anemarrhenae*) can purge heat in the lung and stomach, therefore, depurated qi and heat can be brought downward and discharged from urine. Combined together, the three herbs have the function of clearing lung heat, inhibiting liver fire and nourishing yin fluid. For sensation of thirst and insomnia, Tianhuafen (*Radix Trichosanthis*), Shenglonggu (*Os Draconis*) and Shengmuli (*Concha Ostreae*) should be used; as to irritability, Jizihuang (hen egg yolk) and Zhizi (*Fructus Gardeniae*) could be added; for yellowish and brownish urine, Huashi (*Talcum*) and Zhuye (*Folia Bambosae*) can be combined.

4. 阴虚重证
21.4　Critical syndrome of yin deficiency

【症状】咽干口燥，心烦易怒，烘热上火，舌质红绛。或兼有夜寐不安，心悸；或兼有头痛、口苦、便秘等。

【分析】甲亢病多以肝肾阴虚为本，他脏虚热为标，所以见证以阴虚与虚热并见。此类证候可以累及多个脏器，总以肝肾阴虚为本，舌质红绛为主要指征。肺胃阴虚者，见咽干口燥；心阴虚者，见心烦易怒；胃阴虚热者，见烘热上火；肝阴虚者，见头痛、脑涨；大肠燥结者，见便秘难解。

【治法】滋阴降火，益气养阴。

【方药】甲亢重方（上海中医药大学附属曙光医院）。黄芪45克，鳖甲20克，生地黄20克，白芍20克，夏枯草30克，制香附12克。心阴虚火旺者，加黄连6克；肝阴虚火旺者，加龙胆草6克、黄芩10克，并加重夏枯草分量。

Clinical manifestations: Dryness of the throat and mouth, irritability, susceptibility to rage, inflaming sensation in the throat, and deep-reddish tongue, or combination with symptoms such as unease sleep and palpitation, or with headache, bitter sensation of the mouth and constipation.

Analysis: Generally, the fundamental cause of hyperthyroidism is yin deficiency in the liver and kidney, with asthenic heat in other viscera as its manifest feature, therefore, yin deficiency and asthenic heat can appear simultaneously in one disease. This syndrome can involve several other Zang-fu organs, and deep-reddish tongue is its main symptom. Dryness of throat and mouth indicates yin deficiency of the lung and stomach. Irritability and susceptibility to rage are the main character of yin deficiency in the heart. Inflaming sensation in the throat signifies yin deficiency and heat in the stomach. Headache and distending sensation suggest asthenia of liver yin. And constipation indicates accumulation of dry feces in the large intestine.

Prescription: Nourish yin to suppress fire and tonify qi to replenish yin.

Formulas: Compound recipe for hyperthyroidism (produced by Affiliated Shuguang Hospital of Shanghai University of TCM). The formula includes Huangqi (*Radix Astragali seu*

Hedysari）45 g, Biejia （*Carapax Trionycis*）20 g, Shengdihuang （*Radix Rehmanniae Recens*）20 g, Baishao （*Radix Paeoniae Alba*）20 g, Xiakucao （*Spica Prunellae*）30 g and Zhixiangfu （processed *Rhizoma Cyperi*）12 g. For hyperactivity of fire caused by yin deficiency in the heart, add Huanglian （*Rhizoma Coptidis*）6 g；for hyperactivity of fire caused by yin deficiency in the liver, add Longdancao （*Radix geutianae*）6 g and Huangqin （*Radix Scutellariae*）10 g, and increase the dosage of Xiakucao.

5. 痰瘀互结
21.5 Coagulation of phlegm and blood stasis

【症状】精神抑郁, 心烦失眠, 咽部有堵塞感, 两眼突出, 颈前瘿肿, 按之有结节, 舌苔薄黄, 脉象弦滑。

【分析】甲亢有一种证候, 为痰瘀互结证, 也是比较严重的证候之一。由于气滞、血瘀、痰聚, 形成几种致病因素搅和在一起, 所以呈现出咽部堵塞、颈前结节明显, 以及精神抑郁状态。

【治法】理气化痰, 软坚散结。

【方药】四海舒郁汤加减。四海舒郁汤出自顾世澄《疡医大全》。方由海带、海藻、海螵蛸、昆布、青木香、陈皮、海蛤粉组成。此方集理气化痰、软坚散结、却瘀活血于一方, 对甲亢突眼、瘿肿明显, 属痰瘀互结者, 效果最优。另加柴胡、青皮疏肝解郁；浙贝母清热化痰；枳壳、香附、莪术理气却瘀。综合诸药, 此方对甲亢突眼症有回缩软坚之功效。

Clinical manifestations：Mental depression, irritability, insomnia, sensation of obstruction in the throat, ocular proptosis, goiter in the front neck, nodules detected when pressed, thin and yellowish tongue fur and taut and slippery pulse.

Analysis：Coagulation of phlegm and blood stasis is a serious syndrome of hyperthyroidism. Combined together, several factors, such as qi stagnation, blood stasis and phlegm coagulation, can cause the sensation of obstruction in the throat, obvious nodules in the front neck as well as emotional depression.

Prescription：Regulate qi for eliminating phlegm, soften and resolve goiter.

Formulas：Sihai Shuyu Tang Jiajian （Modified Sihai Shuyu Decoction）. The formula originates from *Complete Work of Royal Surgeons* by Gu Shicheng, composed of Haidai （*Laminaria japonica*）, Haizao （*Sargassum*）, Haipiaoxiao （*Os Sepiellae seu Sepiae*）, Kunbu （*Thallus Laminariae*）, Qingmuxiang （*Radix Aristolochiae*）, Chenpi （*Pericarpium Citri Reticulatae*）and Haigefen （powder of sea clam）. The formula has a function of regulating qi to eliminate phlegm, softening and resolving goiter and dissolving stasis to invigorate blood circulation. It has an obvious curative effect for treating ocular proptosis, thyroid enlargement and goiter and it is particularly effective for coagulation of phlegm and blood stasis. For soothing liver qi depression, add Chaihu （*Radix Bupleuri*）and Qingpi （*Pericarpium Citri Reticulatae Viride*）；for clearing heat and eliminating phlegm, combine

Zhebeimu (*Bulbus Fritillariae Thunbergii*); and Zhiqiao (*Fructus Aurantii*), Xiangfu (*Rhizoma Cyperi*) and Ezhu (*Rhizoma Curcumae*) can be used to regulate qi and dissolve stasis. Combined together, all the above herbs can astringe swelling, soften and resolve goiter.

6. 突眼症

21.6 Syndrome of ocular proptosis

【症状】以突眼为主要症状。突眼是甲亢病的一个重要合并症状，中医西医治疗都比较棘手。而控制突眼是治疗甲亢的重要指标，因此将突眼列为一个证候，以便在临床上有针对性地选用。

【分析】甲亢突眼症，主要是淋巴细胞、巨噬细胞等炎症浸润、水肿所致。中医学认为，突眼是肝气郁久，生风生火，致使属于肝经的眼睛脉络郁结不开，形成气血郁滞，久而突出眼眶，是甲亢病情加重的一种表现，不可忽视。

【治法】滋阴养血，祛风泄浊。

【方药】突眼秘方（徐福松方）。熟地黄 30 克，当归 15 克，枸杞子 15 克，羌活 1.5 克，泽泻 5 克。水煎服。方以熟地黄、当归养血活血；枸杞子养阴补血，益精明目；羌活止痛，且有抗免疫反应作用；泽泻起阴气，聪耳明目。诸药合力，共达益精明目、舒络止痛，以愈突眼之效。若能外用熏洗法，疗效更好。熏洗剂：蒲公英 60 克，水煎熏洗。

Clinical manifestations: As a leading feature, ocular proptosis is a developed complication, difficult to be treated whether by means of TCM or Western medicine. A significant target for treating hyperthyroidism is to bring ocular proptosis under control, which is, therefore, regarded as a syndrome of hyperthyroidism so that specific therapeutic methods could be adopted to cure it clinically.

Analysis: Ocular proptosis is caused by inflammatory infiltration of the lymphocyte and macrophage in organs of the body, which results in dropsy or edema. In terms of TCM, prolonged depression of liver qi causes liver wind and fire, which brings about stagnation of eye veins in liver meridian, thus, resulting in qi stagnation and blood stasis, and eyes will pop out of the eye socket if this syndrome lasts for a long time. The syndrome indicates aggravation of hyperthyroidism, hence, it can not be ignored.

Prescription: Nourish yin to tonify blood and dispel pathogenic wind and turbidity.

Formulas: Secret recipe for ocular proptosis (Recipe from Xu Fusong). The formula is composed of Shudihuang (*Radix Rehmanniae Preparata*) 30 g, Danggui (*Radix Angelicae Sinensis*) 15 g, Gouqizi (*Fructus Lycii*) 15 g, Qianghuo (*Rhizoma et Radix Notopterygii*) 1.5 g, and Zexie (*Rhizoma Alismatis*) 5 g. All the herbs should be decocted. Of the formula, Shudihuang and Danggui can nourish and invigorate blood; Gouqizi has a function of nourishing yin and replenishing blood, tonifying essence and enhancing eyesight; Qianghuo can relieve pain and resist immune reaction; Zexie is able to clear yin qi and promote the function of ears and eyes. Combined together, all medicinal herbs can have a function of tonifying essence, enhancing eyesight, activating collaterals and stopping pain, hence, ocular proptosis could get cured. If external fumigating therapy is adopted, it will have a better curative effect. Fumigating therapy: Decoct 60 g of Pugongying (*Herba Taraxaci*) in water and use the hot decoction to fumigate the eyes.

二十二、高血压病
22　Hypertension

〔**概说**〕 Summary

高血压是一种常见的慢性疾病，又称"原发性高血压病"，以持续性动脉血压增高为主要特征，可伴有心脏、血管、脑、肾脏等器质性改变的全身性慢性疾病。影响动脉压的主要因素是左心室搏出量、外周血管阻力以及血流动力学等。近年来发病率有所增高，这除了与年龄、职业、家庭史等因素有关外，还与环境污染、心理压力增大等因素有关。

中医学将高血压病归属于"眩晕""头痛""中风""肝阳"等病证范畴。认为该病的致病原因与风、火、痰、瘀等有密切关系，发病部位与心、肝、肾及脾等有关。历代医家有"无风不作眩""无虚不作眩""无痰不作眩"等说。说明本病的形成病机有两大类，即虚与实，或虚中夹实，或实中夹虚等。治疗上或从本，以滋补肝肾为主，或从标，以熄风、化痰、活瘀为主；但多半是补虚与祛邪并用，对减轻临床症状有着明显效果。

Hypertension is a common chronic disease, also known as "primary hypertension". It is characterized by continuous elevation of blood pressure in the arteries, accompanied by chronic diseases of the whole body with organic changes in the heart, blood vessels, brain as well as kidney. The factors that affect artery pressure include output volume of the left ventricle, periphery blood vessel resistance as well as hemodynamic change and so on. In recent years, incidence of the disease has increased, which may be related to environment pollution, mental pressure, age, profession, family history of a patient, etc.

Hypertension has the following symptoms such as "vertigo" "headache" "wind stroke" and "hyperactive liver yang" in TCM. Pathogenesis of the disease is closely related to pathogenic wind, fire, phlegm, blood stasis and so on. And location of the disease is mainly in the heart, liver, kidney, spleen, etc. Ancient practitioners hold that the symptom of vertigo is caused mainly by pathogenic wind factor, asthenia and phlegm, which indicates that pathogenesis for the disease is classified into asthenia, sthenia, or asthenia mingled with sthenia, or sthenia mixed with asthenia. Treatment for it should either start from the root cause of the disease, focusing on nourishing and tonifying the liver and kidney, or give priority to its superficial manifestations, namely, concentrating on suppressing endogenous wind, resolving phlegm, activating blood circulation and dissolving stasis. In most cases, its treatment should be the combination of tonifying asthenia with expelling pathogenic factors, which can achieve an obvious curative effect in alleviating clinical manifestations.

〔辨证论治〕 Syndrome differentiation and treatment

1. 肝肾阴亏
22.1 Syndrome of yin asthenia of the liver and kidney

【症状】眩晕，精神萎靡，腰膝酸软，或有耳鸣，脱发，齿摇，或遗精，早泄，咽干、口燥、五心烦热，舌质红赤，苔少，脉象细数。

【分析】肝肾阴精不足，无以生精充髓，脑髓失养，故眩晕，精神萎靡；"腰为肾之府"，"齿为骨之余"，肾主骨，精虚骨失所养，则腰膝酸软、牙齿松动；"肾开窍于耳"，肾虚则耳鸣；肾之华在发，肾虚则发易脱落；肾精不固，则遗精、早泄；阴虚则内热，则见咽干、口燥、五心烦热；阴精不足，内热上炎，则舌脉均呈虚热之象。

【治法】补益肝肾，充养脑髓。

【方药】左归丸。此方为滋补肝肾阴精的首选方剂。方中熟地黄、山茱萸、枸杞子、山药、菟丝子为滋补肝肾阴精的要药，另有龟板胶填精生髓，鹿角胶扶阳固精，怀牛膝补肾强筋壮骨。本方是张景岳"善补阴者，必于阳中求阴，则阴得阳升，而泉源不竭"的代表方剂。阴虚内热者，可加知母、黄柏、菊花、女贞子、旱莲草等，以滋阴清热，不使肝肾阴精内耗。

Clinical manifestations: Vertigo, dispiritedness, aching and weakness of the loins and knees, or accompanied with tinnitus, trichomadesis, loose tooth, or seminal emission, premature ejaculation, dry throat and mouth, feverish sensation over the palms, soles and chest, reddish tongue with scanty fur as well as thin and fast pulse.

Analysis: Vertigo and dispiritedness are due to insufficient yin essence in the liver and kidney which fails to generate essence and supplement brain marrow, thus causing malnutrition of the brain; the loins are the house of the kidney, the teeth are surplus part of the bone, which is controlled by the kidney, deficiency of essence results in malnutrition of the bone which gives rise to aching and weakness of the loins and knees as well as loose tooth; the kidney opens at the ears, asthenia of the kidney brings about tinnitus; the kidney manifests its condition on the hair, and kidney asthenia results in susceptibility to trichomadesis; insufficiency of kidney essence results in seminal emission and premature ejaculation; dry throat and mouth, feverish sensation over the palms, soles and chest are due to yin asthenia and endogenous heat; reddish tongue with scanty fur and thin and fast pulse indicate asthenic heat due to deficiency of yin essence.

Prescription: Benefit the liver and kidney, supplement and nourish brain marrow.

Formulas: Zuogui Wan (Pill). The formula is the first choice for tonifying yin essence in the liver and kidney, in which, Shudihuang (*Radix Rehmanniae Preparata*), Shanzhuyu (*Fructus Corni*), Gouqizi (*Fructus Lycii*), Shanyao (*Rhizoma Dioscoreae*) and Tusizi (*Semen Cuscutae*) are the essential drug for nourishing and supplementing the liver, the kidney and yin essence, Guibanjiao (*Colla Plastri Testudinis*) can supplement essence and generate brain marrow, Lujiaojiao (*Colla Corni Cervi*) has an action of strengthening yang and reinforcing essence, Huainiuxi (*Radix Achyranthis Bidentatae*) can strengthen the tendons and bones. This formula typically represents Zhang Jingyue's theory that "Those who are skilled at supplementing yin must resort to yang in order that yin be acquired and yang be lifted, consequently, the fountain of essence could not get exhausted and be supplied." For yin asthenia and endogenous heat, Zhimu (*Rhizoma Anemarrhenae*), Huangbo (*Cortex Phellodendri*), Juhua (*Flos Chrysanthemi*), Nuzhenzi (*Fructus Ligustri Lucidi*) and Hanliancao (*Eclipta Alba*) can be added to nourish yin and clear away heat to avoid consuming yin essence in the liver and kidney.

2. 肝阳上亢
22.2 Syndrome of liver yang hyperactivity

【症状】眩晕，头涨痛，耳鸣，易怒，失眠多梦，常伴有口苦，目赤，面色红赤，大便秘结，小便短赤，舌红苔黄，脉象弦数有力。或眩晕，泛泛欲呕，肢麻震颤，语言不利，步履不稳。或眩晕，腰膝酸软，健忘，精神萎靡，舌红少苔，脉象细数。

【分析】肝阳上亢证是高血压病最为常见的证候，也是比较危重的证候之一。肝阳上亢，上冒颠顶，干扰清窍，故有眩晕、头涨痛、耳鸣等症状；肝阳上亢无制，则易怒；心神被扰，则失眠多梦；阳亢则阴液不足，故见大便秘结、小便短赤；肝阳上亢为阳证、实证，故舌苔、脉象均呈现阳热之象。若肝阳亢极，呈肝阳化风之兆，则见眩晕、泛泛欲呕、肢麻震颤等症，这是非常危险的征兆。若肝阳上亢，水不涵木，会有腰膝酸软、健忘、精神萎靡等症状，这是在肝阳上亢的基础上，又见肝肾阴精不足的症状。

【治法】平肝潜阳，泻火熄风。

【方药】天麻钩藤饮。本方以天麻、钩藤平肝熄风为主药，配以石决明镇肝潜阳；牛膝、益母草化瘀，引上亢之肝阳下行；黄芩、栀子以清肝火，以使肝火、肝风得到平息；杜仲、桑寄生补益肝肾；夜交藤、茯神安神宁心。若出现肝阳化风，中风先兆时，可用羚角钩藤汤，此方被医家评为"平肝熄风第一方"。方中羚羊角与钩藤作用为熄风止痉；桑叶、菊花可使热邪外透；鲜生地黄与白芍合用，清肝养阴；川贝母、茯神、竹茹清热化痰，以防止神昏不语；甘草与白芍酸甘化阴，能够舒筋缓急。如果没有羚羊角，可用大剂量水牛角或石决明代替，以砸碎先煎 1 小时，后下其他药为宜。若肝肾阴精不足，呈现腰膝酸软等症状，可考虑加用左归丸辅之。

Clinical manifestations: Vertigo, distending headache, tinnitus, susceptibility to rage, insomnia and dreaminess, accompanied with bitter taste, red eyes, dry feces, scanty brownish urine, reddish tongue with yellowish fur and taut, fast and powerful pulse; or vertigo, occasional nausea and vomiting, numbness and tremor of limbs, slurred speech, and staggering gait; or vertigo, aching and weakness of the loins and knees, forgetfulness, dispiritedness, reddish tongue with scanty fur as well as thin and fast pulse.

Analysis: Liver yang hyperactivity is the most common syndrome of hypertension, and one of its critical syndromes too. Up-attack of hyperactive liver yang on the head disturbs upper orifices and results in such symptoms as vertigo, distending headache and tinnitus; susceptibility to rage is due to failure to control hyperactive liver yang; insomnia and dreaminess are due to mind and spirit being disturbed; dry feces and scanty brownish urine are due to insufficiency of yin fluid because of liver yang hyperactivity; liver yang hyperactivity is yang syndrome and sthenia syndrome, therefore, tongue fur and pulse condition present manifestations of syndromes of yang and heat. Vertigo, occasional nausea and vomiting, numbness and tremor of limbs indicate liver yang transforming into wind due to hyperactivity of liver yang, a very critical sign. Aching and weakness of the loins and knees, forgetfulness and dispiritedness are due to failure of water (the kidney) to nourish wood (the liver) because of hyperactivity of liver yang. It is a syndrome of insufficient the liver and kidney yin and essence based on hyperactivity of liver yang.

Prescription: Suppress hyperactive liver yang and purge fire for calming endogenous wind.

Formulas: Tianma Gouteng Yin (Decoction). In the formula, Tianma (*Rhizoma Gastrodiae*) and Gouteng (*Ramulus Uncariae Cum Uncis*) are used as the principal drug to suppress hyperactive liver yang and calm endogenous wind, Shijueming (*Concha Haliotidis*) is combined to arrest hyperactive liver yang; Niuxi (*Radix Achyranthis Bidentatae*) and Yimucao (*Herba Leonuri*) can resolve blood stasis to guide hyperactive liver yang to descend; Huangqin (*Radix Scutellariae*) and Zhizi (*Fructus Gardeniae*) can calm liver fire and liver wind by clearing away liver fire; Duzhong (*Cortex Eucommiae*) and Sangjisheng (*Herba Taxilli*) can replenish the liver and kidney; Yejiaoteng (*Tuber Fleeceflower Stem*) and Fushen (*Sclerotium Poriae Circum Radicem*) have an action of tranquilizing the mind. For the precursor of wind stroke, hyperactive liver yang transforming into wind, Lingjiao Gouteng Tang, which is regarded as "the first formula for suppressing liver yang to calm wind" can be adopted. In the formula, Lingyangjiao (*Cornu Saigae Tataricae*) and Gouteng (*Ramulus Uncariae Cum Uncis*) have an action of calming wind and stopping convulsion; Sangye (*Folium Mori*) and Juhua (*Florist's chrysanthemum*) can let out pathogenic heat; Shengdihuang (*Radix Rehmanniae Recens*) combined with Baishao (*Radix Paeoniae Alba*) can clear away liver fire and nourish yin; Chuanbeimu (*Bulbus Fritillaria*), Fushen and Zhuru (*Bulbus Fritillaria*) could clear away heat and resolve phlegm to prevent coma and delirium; Gancao (*Radix Glycyrrhizae*) and Baishao, sour and sweet in flavor, can nourish yin to relieve stiffness of tendons and alleviate spasm and pain. Shuiniujiao (*Cornu Bubali*) or

Shijueming in large amount can replace Lingyangjiao by breaking them into pieces and decocting first for an hour, then other medicinal herbs can be decocted later. For aching and weakness of the loins and knees due to insufficiency of yin essence in the liver and kidney, Zuogui Wan (Pill) can be combined.

3. 痰浊壅盛
22.3　Syndrome of exuberant turbid phlegm

【症状】眩晕，头重如裹，胸闷，或时时欲呕，口淡纳呆，舌体胖大，苔白腻，或白厚而腻，脉象弦滑，或兼结代。有的呈现头目涨痛，心烦易怒，口苦而干黏，舌苔黄腻，脉象滑数。

【分析】此证一般见于形体肥胖者。痰浊中阻，上蒙清窍，故眩晕；痰为湿邪，湿邪重浊，阻遏清阳，故头重如裹；清阳不展，故胸闷不舒；胃气不降，故泛泛欲呕；湿困中焦，则口淡纳呆；舌体胖大、舌体白腻、脉象弦滑等，均为痰浊内蕴之象。若痰浊热化，痰热上攻，则头目涨痛，心烦易怒；热化伤津，则口苦而干黏；舌体黄腻和脉象滑数，为痰浊热化之明证。

【治法】燥湿化痰，健脾和胃。

【方药】半夏天麻白术汤（《医学心悟》）为主方。方中半夏燥湿化痰，白术健脾祛湿，天麻熄风止痛，共为主药；辅以陈皮理气化痰，茯苓健脾渗湿；生姜、甘草、大枣为健脾和胃、调和营卫之药。脾胃健运，痰湿不留，眩晕自去。若眩晕较甚，呕吐频频，可加旋覆花、代赭石、胆南星等除痰降逆。若眩晕较轻、泛泛欲呕、口苦、苔薄黄，可改用黄连温胆汤清热除痰和胃。若寒饮内停，眩晕，舌苔白滑，浮有一层水分，可用苓桂术甘汤加干姜、附子、白芥子等，温阳化其寒饮。

Clinical manifestations: Vertigo, heavy sensation of head like being wrapped, chest oppression, or frequent nausea and vomiting, bland taste and poor appetite, enlarged tongue, greasy whitish fur, or thick greasy whitish fur as well as taut and slippery pulse, or complicated by slow-intermittent-regular pulse. In some cases, symptoms such as distending headache, painful eyes, vexation and susceptibility to rage, bitter, dry and sticky taste, yellowish, greasy fur as well as slippery and fast pulse can appear.

Analysis: The syndrome is usually seen in those obese patients. Vertigo is due to obstructive turbid phlegm invading upper orifices; phlegm is a pathogenic dampness factor, heavy and turbid phlegm obstructing lucid yang from rising results in heavy sensation of head like being wrapped; chest oppression is due to failure of lucid yang to rise up; occasional nausea and vomiting are due to failure to descend stomach qi; bland taste and poor appetite are due to accumulation of dampness in middle energizer; enlarged tongue, greasy whitish fur or thick greasy whitish fur and taut and slippery pulse are signs of internal retention of turbid phlegm. Distending headache, painful eyes, vexation and susceptibility to rage are caused by upward invasion of heat transformed from turbid phlegm; bitter, dry and sticky taste indicates heat transformed from phlegm impairing body fluid; yellowish greasy fur and slippery and fast pulse are obvious manifestations of transformation of heat from turbid phlegm.

Prescription: Dry dampness, resolve phlegm, invigorate the spleen and harmonize the stomach.

Formulas: Banxia Tianma Baizhu Tang (Decoction) (cited from *Medicine Comprehended*). In the formula, Banxia (*Rhizoma Pinelliae*) can dry dampness and resolve phlegm, Baizhu (*Rhizoma Atractylodis Macrocephalae*) can invigorate the spleen and expel dampness, Tianma (*Rhizoma Gastrodiae*) can suppress endogenous wind and stop pain, so they are used as the principal drug; Chenpi (*Pericarpium Citri Reticulatae*), with an action of regulating qi and resolving phlegm, and Fuling (*Poriae Cocos*), having an effect of invigorating the spleen and resolving dampness, are used as adjuvant drug; other herbs such as Shengjiang (*Rhizoma Zingiberis Recens*), Gancao (*Radix Glycyrrhizae*) and Dazao (*Fructus Jujubae*) can strengthen the spleen, harmonize the stomach and reconcile nutrient qi and defensive qi. The restored normal function of the spleen and stomach in transportation can eliminate retention of dampness, therefore, vertigo can disappear itself. For severe vertigo and frequent vomiting, Xuanfuhua (*Flos Inulae*), Daizheshi (*Haematitum*) and Dannanxing (*Rhizoma Arisaematis Cum Bile*) can be added to eliminate phlegm and descend adverse qi. For mild vertigo, occasional nausea and vomiting, bitter taste and thin yellowish fur, Huanglian Wendan Tang (Decoction) can be used to replace the above formula to clear away heat, disperse phlegm and harmonize the stomach. For internal retention of cold fluid, vertigo and whitish slippery fur like being coated with a layer of water, Ling Gui Zhu Gan Tang (Decoction), combined with Ganjiang (*Rhizoma Zingiberis*), Fuzi (*Radix Aconiti Lateralis Preparata*) and Baijiezi (*Semen Sinapis Albae*) can be adopted to warm yang and resolve retention of cold fluid.

4. 瘀血阻络
22.4 Syndrome of blood stasis obstructing collaterals

【症状】眩晕时作，头痛，健忘，失眠，心悸，精神不振，面部或唇色紫暗，舌有紫斑或瘀点，脉象弦细兼涩。

【分析】瘀血阻络与病人的体质有关，也与病程的长短有一定关联。疾病初期多在气分与经脉，病久则入血分与络脉，导致瘀血阻络，经络不通。瘀血阻络，气血不得正常运行，脑失所养，故眩晕时作；头部络脉瘀阻，则头痛、健忘；瘀血不去，新血不生，则心悸、精神不振；血不养心，故失眠；舌质与脉象均具瘀血特点。

【治法】祛瘀生新，活血清脑。

【方药】补阳还五汤加减。方中以大量黄芪补益宗气，"气为血之帅"，宗气不虚，则可贯心脉而鼓动血行；当归、川芎、赤芍、桃仁、红花养血活血；地龙活血通络。全方共奏益气活血、祛瘀生新之效。若肢体不利，可加豨莶草、透骨草、怀牛膝通经活络利关节；眩晕甚者，可加天麻、钩藤以平肝潜阳。

Clinical manifestations: Frequent vertigo, headache, forgetfulness, insomnia, palpitation, dispiritedness, dark purplish complexion and lips, purple spots or petechiae on the tongue as well as taut, thin and astringent pulse.

Analysis: The syndrome is connected with a patient's constitution as well as with the course of the disease. At its initial stage, pathogenic factors are in qi phase and in the meridians, prolonged course of the disease results in transmission of pathogenic factors into blood phase and collaterals, causing stasis of blood obstructing collaterals, which results in failure of qi and blood to circulate normally and malnutrition of the brain, thus, giving rise to frequent vertigo; headache and forgetfulness are due to blood stasis obstructing collaterals in the head; palpitation and dispiritedness are due to failure to generate new blood because blood stasis has not been eliminated; insomnia is due to inability of blood to nourish the heart; purple spots or petechiae on the tongue as well as taut, thin and astringent pulse are indications of blood stasis.

Prescription: Remove blood stasis for promoting blood regeneration, invigorate blood circulation and refresh the brain.

Formulas: Buyang Huanwu Tang Jiajian (Modified Buyang Huanwu Decoction). In the formula, large amount of Huangqi (*Radix Astragali seu Hedysari*) can tonify pectoral qi, "qi is the commander of blood", sufficient pectoral qi passes through the heart meridians and rises up blood vessels to promote blood circulation; Danggui (*Radix Angelicae Sinensis*), Chuanxiong (*Rhizoma Ligustici Chuanxiong*), Chishao (*Radix Paeoniae Rubra*), Taoren (*Semen Persicae*) and Honghua (*Flos Carthami*) can nourish blood and activate blood; Dilong (*Lumbricus*) has an action of invigorating blood circulation and dredging collaterals. The whole formula can bring benefiting qi, activating blood and removing blood stasis for promoting blood regeneration into full play. For inflexible limbs, Xixiancao (*Herba Siegesbeckiae*), Tougucao (*Caulis Impatientis*) and Huainiuxi (*Radix Achyranthis Bidentatae*) can be added to activate meridians and collaterals and ease movement of joints; for severe vertigo, Tianma (*Rhizoma Gastrodiae*) and Gouteng (*Ramulus Uncariae Cum Uncis*) can be combined to calm the liver and suppress yang.

二十三、冠心病

23　Coronary heart disease

〔概说〕 Summary

　　冠心病是"冠状动脉粥样硬化心脏病"的简称，是由于多种原因引起冠状动脉粥样硬化，导致血管腔的狭窄或梗阻，使心肌缺氧、缺血所造成的常见的心脏病。它包括心绞痛、心律不齐、心肌梗死、心力衰竭、心脏猝死等。

　　冠心病属于中医学"胸痹""心痛"等病证范畴。认为本病的发生与七情内伤、饮食不节、元气不足等因素有关。其发病部位虽然在心，但与肝、肾、脾、肺等脏器有密切关联。治疗上以辨证论治为原则，不单纯有活血化瘀法，还有益气养阴、疏肝理气、健脾化痰、温阳散寒等法。近年来对冠心病的治疗有长足的进步，许多新的中成药被病人所接受，同时也走出国门，使许多病人的病情得到缓解和好转。

本文主要探讨冠心病心绞痛的辨证论治。

Coronary heart disease is the abbreviation of "coronary atherosclerotic cardiopathy". There are many factors contributing to coronary atherosclerosis, causing narrowing or blockage of the coronary arteries, which results in common heart disease due to heart muscle starved of oxygen and blood. The disease includes angina pectoris, arrhythmia, myocardial infarction, heart failure as well as cardiac sudden death.

Coronary heart disease pertains to "thoracic obstruction" and "heartache" in terms of TCM. It is believed that the disease is related to internal injury of seven emotions, intemperance of diet and insufficient primordial qi. Although the location of the disease is in the heart, it is closely connected with the liver, kidney, spleen and lung. On basis of syndrome differentiation, treating principles for the disease not only involves activating blood to dissolve stasis, it also includes the following methods such as benefiting qi to nourish yin, soothing liver to regulate qi, invigorating the spleen to resolve phlegm and dispelling cold by warming. Recently, great achievements have been accomplished in treating the disease, lots of new Chinese-patent drugs have been gradually accepted by Chinese patients, meanwhile, they have been introduced into western world, and consequently alleviated many patients' suffering and some of them even get recovered from the ailment. This chapter mainly deals with syndrome differentiation of angina pectoris of coronary disease.

〔辨证论治〕 Syndrome differentiation and treatment

（一）实证
23.1 Sthenia syndrome

1. 寒凝心脉
23.1.1 Syndrome of cold coagulation in heart vessels

【症状】猝然心痛如绞，心痛彻背，背痛彻心，形寒肢冷，寒冷天气心痛易发作或加重，甚则出冷汗，心悸气短，舌苔薄白，脉象沉紧。

【分析】胸背为阳气集散之地，心阳不振，复受寒邪，以致寒邪集于胸中，心脉不和，营血运行不畅，故发作心绞痛；"背为胸中之府"，心脉不通，则心痛彻背；阳气不能温养肢体，故形寒肢冷，每遇寒冷天气病情发作或加重；甚则卫阳失护，可见冷汗出；心中阳气不能接续，则心悸气短；舌苔与脉象为寒邪凝于心脉之象。

【治法】祛寒活瘀，通阳宣痹。

【方药】当归四逆汤为主方。方以当归、芍药养血活血；桂枝、细辛温散寒邪，通阳止痛；通草入经通脉；大枣健脾和营。诸药共奏祛寒活瘀、通阳止痛之功。若疼痛发作剧烈彻背者，可用乌头赤石脂丸。方以乌头辛温雄烈之性，散寒通络止痛；附子、干姜温经逐寒；恐辛温之品大辛大热，大开大散，故用赤石脂入心经固涩而收阳气。若痛剧、冷汗出、四肢不温，可加用苏合香丸，芳香化浊，温开通窍，常能收到较快痛止寒散之效。

Clinical manifestations：Abrupt colic pain of the heart involving the back, cold body and limbs, high incidence or aggravation of heart pain in cold weather, even cold sweating, palpitation and short breath, thin whitish tongue fur as well as sunken and tense pulse.

Analysis：The chest and back are the area where yang qi converges, hypoactivity of heart yang complicated with invasion of pathogenic cold factor results in accumulation of cold pathogen in the chest and disharmony of heart vessels, and unsmooth circulation of nutrient qi and blood, causing the onset of angina pectoris; "the back is the house of the heart and lung", obstruction of heart vessels brings about colic pain of the heart involving the back; cold body and limbs and high incidence or aggravation of heart pain in cold weather are due to failure of yang qi to warm and nourish the body; aggravation of colic heart pain results in failure to protect defensive yang, which manifests cold sweating; palpitation and short breath are due to failure to supplement yang qi; thin whitish tongue fur and sunken and tense pulse indicate coagulation of cold in heart vessels.

Prescription：Dispel cold, dissolve stasis and activate yang by eliminating obstruction in heart vessels.

Formulas：Danggui Sini Tang (Decoction) used as the principal formula. In the formula, Danggui (*Radix Angelicae Sinensis*) and Shaoyao (*Radix Paeoniae*) can nourish blood and activate blood circulation; Guizhi (*Ramulus Cinnamomi*) and Xixin (*Herba Asari*) have an action of dispersing cold pathogen by warming and activating yang to stop pain; Tongcao (*Medulla Tetrapanacis*) can permeate into the meridians to dredge blood vessels; Dazao (*Fructus Jujubae*) has an action of invigorating the spleen and reconciling nutrient qi and blood. Combined together, both of them can expel cold, dissolve blood stasis and activate yang to stop pain. For severe pain involving the back, Wutou Chishizhi Wan (Pill) can be adopted, of which, Wutou (*Radix Aconiti*), strong pungent and warm in nature, can expel cold and dredge blood vessels to alleviate pain; Fuzi (*Radix Aconiti Lateralis Preparata*) and Ganjiang (*Rhizoma Zingiberis*) can warm the meridians to dispel cold; in order to prevent pungent-warm medicine from excessive dispersing, Chishizhi (*Halloysitum Rubrum*) can be used as astringent drug to permeate into heart meridians so as to astringe yang qi. For severe pain, cold sweating and cold limbs, Suhexiang Wan (Pill) can be used to dissolve turbidity with its aromatic flavor and dredge the orifices by warming in order to achieve the effect of alleviating pain and dispelling cold in a short time.

2. 气滞心胸

23.1.2　Syndrome of qi stagnation in the heart and chest

【症状】 心胸满闷，阵阵隐痛，痛无定处，每遇情绪不舒则诱发，或加剧，或可兼有胃脘痞满，得嗳气、矢气则隐痛缓解，舌苔白腻，脉象弦细。

【分析】 本证多见于情绪不稳定者，情绪抑郁，气滞胸中，宗气郁滞，血脉不和，故胸闷隐痛；气走无着，故痛无定处；肝气郁结，每易横逆中焦，出现胃脘痞满之症，得嗳气或矢气则暂得缓解；脉舌为肝郁克脾之象。

【治法】 疏肝理气，调理气血。

【方药】 柴胡疏肝散。本方由四逆散加香附、川芎、陈皮组成。四逆散能疏肝理气，解除胸胁气机之郁滞。其中柴胡与枳壳相配，可升降气机；白芍与甘草相配，可缓急止痛。香附为理气之要药，川芎为气中之血药，以活血而助调气；陈皮辛温，为理气健脾之品，且有解除胸闷之效。若胸闷、心痛明显者，可加失笑散，以增强活血止痛之功；若舌苔厚腻，可加丹参饮，以活血调气，化湿畅中。

Clinical manifestations: Distention and fullness of the chest, frequent dull pain without fixed position, pain induced from qi depression and emotional discomfort or aggravation of pain, or complicated with epigastric distention and fullness, alleviation with belching and flatus, greasy and whitish fur as well as taut and thin pulse.

Analysis: The syndrome is usually seen with emotional upset. Depression and qi stagnation of the chest, especially stagnation of pectoral qi causes disharmony of blood and vessels, which gives rise to chest oppression and dull pain; unfixed position of qi results in pain with unfixed position; epigastric distention and fullness are due to depressed qi in the liver invading middle energizer, alleviation of qi depression is due to belching and flatus; greasy whitish fur and taut and thin pulse are signs of liver depression restraining the spleen.

Prescription: Soothe the liver, regulate qi and reconcile qi and blood.

Formulas: Chaihu Shugan San (Powder). The formula is the combination of Sini San (Powder) with Xiangfu (*Rhizoma Cyperi*), Chuanxiong (*Rhizoma Ligustici Chuanxiong*) and Chenpi (*Pericarpium Citri Reticulatae*). Sini San can remove qi depression in the chest and hypochondrium by soothing the liver and regulating qi, of which, Chaihu (*Radix Bupleuri*), together with Zhiqiao (*Fructus Aurantii*) can lift and descend qi; Gancao (*Radix Glycyrrhizae Alba*) and Baishao (*Radix Paeoniae Alba*) can relax spasm and relieve pain. Xiangfu is an essential herb to regulate qi, Chuanxiong has an action of activating blood circulation to help regulate qi; Chenpi, pungent and warm in nature, has an effect of regulating qi, invigorating the spleen as well as relieving chest oppression. For obvious chest oppression and heart pain, Shixiao San (Powder) can be combined to reinforce the function of activating blood circulation and relieving pain; for thick greasy fur, Danshen Yin (Decoction) may be added to promote blood circulation and regulate qi so as to resolve dampness and relieve qi stagnation in middle energizer.

3. 痰浊痹阻

23.1.3 Syndrome of turbid phlegm obstruction

【症状】胸闷而兼心痛时作，痰黏而不易咳出，口黏而乏味，苔白腻偏干，或淡黄腻，脉象滑而缓，或兼数。

【分析】痰为脾湿所生，湿聚为浊，故痰浊较痰饮为重。若痰浊布于胸中，阻遏胸中阳气的温煦，就会出现胸闷而痛；痰性黏腻，不易咳出，且影响口中的气味；痰浊舌苔偏腻，有热化者，兼黄腻，或见数脉。

【治法】健脾祛湿，宣痹通阳。

【方药】温胆汤合瓜蒌薤白半夏汤主之。温胆汤乃二陈汤加枳实、竹茹而成。二陈汤之陈皮、半夏、茯苓、甘草健脾祛湿，化痰理气；枳实、竹茹清泻痰热。加瓜蒌薤白半夏汤，意在宣痹通阳，开结散浊。若痰热明显者，可加郁金、黄连清热，解痰热之郁；若痰热伤阴者，可加麦冬、生地黄、沙参等，以滋阴泻热。

Clinical manifestations：Chest oppression coupled with frequent heart pain, sticky sputum with difficulty to expectorate, sticky and bland taste of the mouth, greasy, dry and whitish fur, or greasy and yellowish fur as well as slippery and moderate pulse or fast pulse.

Analysis：Turbid phlegm generates from accumulation of dampness in the spleen, therefore, turbid phlegm is more serious than fluid retention. Accumulation of turbid phlegm in the chest obstructing warm yang qi gives rise to chest oppression and heart pain; sticky and greasy phlegm results in difficulty to expectorate, which, in turn, affects the taste of the mouth; turbid phlegm brings about greasy fur, transformation of heat from phlegm is accompanied with yellowish fur or fast pulse.

Prescription：Invigorate the spleen, dispel dampness and activate yang by eliminating obstruction.

Formulas：Wendan Tang (Decoction) combined with Gualou Xiebai Banxia Tang (Decoction). Wendan Tang consists of Erchen Tang (Decoction), Zhishi (*Fructus Aurantii Immaturus*) and Zhuru (*Caulis Bambusae in Taenia*). In Erchen Tang, Chenpi (*Pericarpium Citri Reticulatae*), Banxia (*Rhizoma Pinelliae*), Fuling (*Poriae Cocos*) and Gancao (*Radix Glycyrrhizae*) can invigorate the spleen, dispel dampness, resolve phlegm and regulate qi; Zhishi and Zhuru have an action of purging phlegmatic heat. The formula combined with Gualou Xiebai Banxia Tang aims at activating yang by eliminating obstruction and dispersing accumulation of phlegm. For obvious phlegmatic heat, Yujin (*Radix Curcumae*) and Huanglian (*Rhizoma Coptidis*) may be added to remove stagnation of phlegmatic heat; for yin impairment due to phlegmatic heat, Maidong (*Radix Ophiopogonis*), Shengdihuang (*Radix Rehmanniae Recens*) and Shashen (*Radix Adenophorae*) can be combined to nourish yin and purge heat.

4. 瘀血痹阻

23.1.4 Syndrome of blood obstruction

【症状】心胸疼痛较剧，如绞如刺，痛有定处，平时胸闷不已，表情烦躁，唇舌暗红或紫暗，舌下静脉迂曲严重，脉象沉涩或结代。

【分析】瘀血痹阻证多见于性格暴躁之人，或长期郁闷不解者，一般是由气郁衍变而来。由于瘀血久结，所以疼痛比较严重，痛有定处，如绞如刺；平时气郁不解，则会胸闷不已；由于瘀血较重，心神亦不得安宁，表现出烦躁；瘀血久居，故唇舌会呈紫暗色；脉象亦不流畅，或呈结代脉象。

【治法】活血化瘀，通脉止痛。

【方药】血府逐瘀汤为主方。本方基本上是以桃红四物汤合四逆散加牛膝、桔梗组成。当归、川芎、赤芍、桃仁、红花活血祛瘀以通血脉；柴胡、桔梗与枳壳、牛膝配伍，一升一降，调畅气机，行气活血，开胸通阳；生地黄是一味凉血消瘀药，《神农本草经》说它能"逐血痹"。全方共奏活血化瘀、通脉止痛之功效。心痛较剧者，加乳香、没药或失笑散，活血止痛的延胡索、郁金也可考虑加大剂量使用。身体疲惫，可加黄芪、山茱萸、太子参等补益之味。

Clinical manifestations: Acute colic pain or piercing pain in the chest and heart, pain with fixed position, persistent chest oppression, restlessness, dark reddish or dark purplish lips and tongue, severe varicosity under the tongue, sunken and astringent pulse, or slow and intermittent pulse, or slow-intermittent-regular pulse.

Analysis: The syndrome is usually seen in those people with restless temper, or in those with prolonged chest oppression. Generally, it evolves from qi stagnation. Prolonged blood stasis brings about severe colic pain or piercing pain with fixed position; unrelieved qi stagnation gives rise to frequent chest oppression; restlessness is caused by severe blood stasis which results in restless heart and mind; dark purplish lips and tongue, unsmooth pulse condition such as slow and intermittent pulse or slow-intermittent-regular pulse are due to prolonged blood stasis.

Prescription: Activate blood circulation by dissolving blood stasis and dredge blood vessels to relieve pain.

Formulas: Xuefu Zhuyu Tang (Decoction). The formula is made up of Tao Hong Siwu Tang (Decoction) combined with Sini San (Powder), Niuxi (*Radix Achyranthis Bidentatae*) and Jiegeng (*Radix Platycodonis*). In the formula, Danggui (*Radix Angelicae Sinensis*), Chuanxiong (*Rhizoma Ligustici Chuanxiong*), Chishao (*Radix Paeoniae Rubra*), Taoren (*Semen Persicae*) and Honghua (*Flos Carthami*) can activate blood and dissolve blood stasis to dredge blood vessels; Chaihu (*Radix Bupleuri*), Jiegeng, Zhiqiao (*Fructus Aurantii*) and Niuxi can lift and descend qi to regulate qi movement, activate qi and blood to soothe the chest and activate yang qi circulation; according to *Shennong Bencao Jing* (*Shennong's Classic of Materia Medica*), Shengdihuang (*Radix Rehmanniae Recens*) has an action of cooling blood and dispelling blood obstruction. The whole formula can bring the action of activating blood, dissolving blood stasis to dredge blood vessels and stopping pain into full play. For acute pain in the heart, Ruxiang (*Olibanum*), Moyao (*Myrrha*) or Shixiao San (Powder) can be added, Yanhusuo (*Rhizoma Corydalis*) and Yujin (*Radix Curcumae*) can be added in large amount to promote blood circulation and stop pain. For exhaustion and lassitude, Huangqi (*Radix Astragali seu Hedysari*), Shanzhuyu (*Fructus Corni*) and Taizishen (*Radix Pseudostellariae*), with the action of tonifying and benefiting, can be added.

（二）虚证
23.2　Asthenia syndrome

1. 气阴两虚
23.2.1　Asthenia syndrome of qi and yin

【症状】胸闷隐痛，时作时止，心悸气短，遇劳则甚，自汗，口干少津，舌质嫩红，苔少，脉象弦细无力，或结代。

【分析】由于素体气阴两虚，或心痛日久，伤及气阴，气虚则无以行血，阴虚则脉络不利，均可使血脉不畅，气血郁滞，故见胸闷隐痛，时作时止；心脉失养，故见心悸气短，劳则气阴耗散更甚；气不固摄，则见自汗；阴亏则口干少津；舌质嫩红为气阴两虚之象；脉象弦细为气阴两虚所形成，虚甚则脉结代。

【治法】益气养阴，活血通络。

【方药】生脉饮合丹参饮加味。生脉饮由人参、麦冬、炙甘草组成，为益气养阴的代表方剂。人参益气，麦冬养阴，炙甘草益气和中。阴虚甚者，可用西洋参；气虚甚者，可用移山参；一般气虚者，可用党参。丹参饮由丹参、檀香、砂仁三味组成，丹参养血活血，檀香理气散结，砂仁芳香化浊。两方合用，具有益气养阴、活血通络的效用。心悸不宁，可加酸枣仁、五味子、远志；痛甚，可加三七、五灵脂、郁金。

Clinical manifestations: Occasional outbreak of chest oppression with dull pain, palpitation and short breath, aggravation with overstrain, spontaneous sweating, dry mouth with scanty fluid, tender reddish tongue with scanty fur and taut, thin and weak pulse or slow-intermittent-regular pulse.

Analysis: Constitutional qi and yin asthenia or prolonged pain in the heart causes impairment of qi and yin, qi asthenia results in failure to activate blood circulation, yin asthenia gives rise to obstructive collaterals and blood vessels, which causes qi and blood stagnation, bringing about occasional chest oppression and dull pain in the heart; palpitation and short breath and aggravation with overstrain are due to malnutrition of heart vessels; spontaneous sweating is due to qi failing to astringe; dry mouth with scanty fluid is due to yin asthenia; tender reddish tongue indicates asthenic qi and yin; taut, thin and weak pulse is a sign of asthenic qi and yin; slow-intermittent-regular pulse suggests severe asthenia syndrome.

Prescription：Benefit qi to nourish yin and activate blood to dredge blood vessels.

Formulas：Shengmai Yin（Decoction）combined with Danshen Yin（Decoction）. Shengmai Yin, consisting of Renshen（*Radix Ginseng*）, Maidong（*Radix Ophiopogonis*）and Zhigancao（*Radix Glycyrrhizae Preparata*）, is a representative formula for benefiting qi and nourishing yin. Renshen can benefit qi, Maidong may nourish yin, Zhigancao has an action of supplementing qi and harmonizing middle energizer. For yin asthenia, Xiyangshen（*Radix Panacis Quinquefolii*）can be adopted；for qi asthenia, Yishanshen（wild *Radix Ginseng*）can be used to take the place of Xiyangshen；for the common qi asthenia, Dangshen（*Radix Codonopsis*）may be used. Danshen Yin is made up of Danshen（*Radix Salviae Miltiorrhizae*）, Tanxiang（*Lignum Santali Albi*）and Sharen（*Fructus Amomi Villosi*）, of which, Danshen can nourish blood and activate blood circulation, Tanxiang has an action of regulating qi and scattering lumps, Sharen can resolve turbid dampness with its aromatic flavor. Combined together, both formulas have an action of benefiting qi, nourishing yin and activating blood to dredge blood vessels. For palpitation, Suanzaoren（*Semen Ziziphi Spinosae*）, Wuweizi（*Fructus Schisandrae Chinensis*）and Yuanzhi（*Radix Polygalae*）can be added；for severe pain, Sanqi（*Radix Notoginseng*）, Wulingzhi（*Faeces Togopteri*）and Yujin（*Radix Curcumae*）can be added.

2. 阳气欲脱
23.2.2 Syndrome of yang qi collapse

【症状】胸闷气短, 甚则胸痛彻背, 心悸, 汗出不止, 畏寒肢冷, 面色苍白, 极度乏力, 唇甲淡白或青紫, 舌质淡白或紫暗, 脉象沉细欲绝。

【分析】阳气欲脱证为冠心病的危重证候, 是阳气极度虚弱所出现的。阳气主温煦, 主运行, 是人体的动能。阳气虚衰, 血脉运行无力, 即血行淤滞, 故见胸闷气短, 甚则胸痛彻背；心阳不振, 故见心悸、汗出；肾阳虚衰, 则见畏寒肢冷、面色苍白、极度乏力；由于阳气虚衰, 血脉运行不畅, 故见唇甲、舌质淡白或紫暗, 脉象也不流畅了。

【治法】益气温阳, 活血通络。

【方药】参附汤合右归饮加减。方中人参大补元气, 附子、肉桂温阳补肾, 熟地黄、山茱萸、枸杞子、山药、杜仲补益肾精, 炙甘草益气和中；加入当归、赤芍、红花活血化瘀, 通络止痛。若四肢厥冷, 脉微欲绝, 可重用红参, 并用龙骨、牡蛎, 以回阳救逆固脱；若阳气虚弱, 不能温阳制水, 水气凌心, 症见心悸、气喘、肢体浮肿, 可改用真武汤加猪苓、车前子、防己, 以温阳利水。

Clinical manifestations：Chest oppression with short breath, even chest pain involving the back, palpitation, non-stop sweating, aversion to cold and cold limbs, pale complexion, exhaustion and lack of energy, pale whitish or cyanotic lips and nails, pale whitish tongue or dark purplish tongue, sunken and thin pulse and even insensible pulse.

Analysis：Syndrome of yang qi collapse is a critical syndrome of coronary disease, indicating extreme asthenia of yang qi. Yang qi is the dynamic energy of human body, dominating warming and transportation. Asthenic yang qi results in weak blood circulation, namely, blood stagnation, which, in turn, gives rise to chest oppression and short breath even chest pain involving the back; palpitation and sweating are due to hypoactivity of heart yang; aversion to cold and cold limbs, pale complexion and lack of energy are due to kidney yang asthenia; pale whitish lips and nails, pale whitish tongue or dark purplish tongue and sunken and thin pulse are due to obstructive blood circulation in the vessels.

Prescription: Benefit qi by warming yang and activate blood by dredging blood vessels.

Formulas: Shen Fu Tang (Decoction) combined with Yougui Yin (Decoction) Jiajian. In the formula, Renshen (*Radix Ginseng*) can tonify primordial qi, Fuzi (*Radix Aconiti Lateralis Preparata*) and Rougui (*Cortex Cinnamomi*) can warm yang and tonify the kidney; Shudihuang (*Radix Rehmanniae Preparata*), Shanzhuyu (*Fructus Corni*), Gouqizi (*Fructus Lycii*), Shanyao (*Rhizoma Dioscoreae*) and Duzhong (*Cortex Eucommiae*) can replenish kidney essence; Zhigancao (*Radix Glycyrrhizae Preparata*) has an action of benefiting qi and harmonizing middle energizer. The combination of Danggui (*Radix Angelicae Sinensis*), Chishao (*Radix Paeoniae Rubra*) and Honghua (*Flos Carthami*) can activate blood and dissolve blood stasis to dredge blood vessels. For cold limbs and indistinct pulse, Hongshen (*Radix Ginseng Rubra*) can be used in large amount together with Longgu (*Os Draconis*) and Muli (*Concha Ostreae*) to save from collapse by restoring yang. For failure of asthenic yang qi to warm yang and restrain dampness as well as fluid attacking the heart with such manifestations as palpitation, polypnea and swollen body and limbs, Zhenwu Tang (Decoction) can be used to replace the above formula in combination with Zhuling (*Polyporus Umbellatus*), Cheqianzi (*Semen Plantaginis*) and Fangji (*Radix Stephaniae Tetrandrae*) to warm yang and induce diuresis.

二十四、心律失常

24　Arhythmia

〔**概说**〕　Summary

临床上常见的心律失常，包括窦性心动过缓、窦性心动过速、窦性心律不齐、早搏、阵发性心动过速、心房扑动、心房颤动、心脏传导失常等。心律失常形成的原因比较复杂，在这里不做叙述。

心律失常属于中医学"心悸""怔忡""昏厥"等范畴。其主要临床表现在脉象上，诸如数脉、迟脉、促脉、结脉、代脉等。其形成原因有外因侵袭、七情刺激，以及饮食失节，或嗜好烟、酒、浓茶等。故其治疗有祛除外邪法、疏肝理气法、宁心安神法、健脾和胃法、活血化瘀法等，经过对症治疗，多数能得到缓解或痊愈。

Clinically, arhythmia includes sinus bradycardia, nodal tachycardia, sinus arhythmia, premature beat, paroxysmal tachycardia, atrial flutter, auricular fibrillation and abnormal cardiac conducting system. The complex causes for arrhythmia are omitted here.

Arhythmia belongs to "palpitation" "severe palpitation" and "syncope" in terms of TCM. Changes of pulse conditions are its main clinical manifestations, such as fast pulse, slow pulse, rapid-intermittent pulse, slow-intermittent pulse as well as slow-intermittent-regular pulse, etc. The pathogenesis includes external invasion, stimulation of seven emotions, intemperate diet, or addiction to smoking and strong tea as well as alcoholism. Therefore, treatment for the disease involves dispelling exogenous pathogenic factors, soothing the liver to regulate qi, tranquilizing the heart and mind, invigorating the spleen, reconciling the stomach, and activating blood to dissolve blood stasis. In vast majority of cases, arrhythmia can be relieved or cured by means of the treatment according to the concerning differentiation of syndromes.

〔辨证论治〕 Syndrome differentiation and treatment

1. 热毒内蕴
24.1 Syndrome of internal accumulation of heat toxin

【症状】发热或已无发热，心悸，胸闷，时时烦躁，汗出，咽干痛，舌质红赤，苔薄黄而干，脉象数而促。

【分析】此证多见于热病之余，或仍有余热，或已无热象，但热毒未散，并内侵心脉，心脉不得宁静，故心悸、胸闷；热扰心神，故时时烦躁；阴液不得内藏，故汗出；热邪久羁，则咽干痛；其舌脉之象，均为热毒内蕴之征。

【治法】清热凉营，养阴安神。

【方药】清营汤合加减生脉散。清营汤与加减生脉散均出自《温病条辨》上焦篇。清营汤以治邪热内侵营阴之证而设。方中用犀角咸寒、生地黄甘寒，清营凉血，为君药；玄参、麦冬配生地黄以养阴清热，为臣药；佐以金银花、连翘、黄连、竹叶清热解毒以透解邪热，使其邪热透出气分而解；丹参以活血消除瘀热。加减生脉散由沙参、麦冬、五味子、牡丹皮、生地黄组成，意在酸甘化阴，宁心安神。除去重复药物外，所用方药仅在清营汤中加入了沙参、五味子、牡丹皮三味。如果心悸明显，还可加入酸枣仁、夜交藤以增强养阴安神作用。犀角已被列为禁用之药，可以用水牛角代替。

Clinical manifestations: Fever or no fever, palpitation, chest oppression, frequent restlessness, sweating, dry and sore throat, reddish tongue with thin dry yellowish fur as well as fast and rapid and intermittent pulse.

Analysis: The syndrome usually occurs after outbreak of fever or accompanied with residual fever, or with no manifestation of fever but with unrelieved toxic heat, which invades, and disturbs heart vessels, resulting in palpitation and chest oppression; frequent restlessness is due to heat disturbing the heart and mind; sweating is caused by failure to astringe yin fluid; dry and painful throat is due to prolonged retention of heat pathogen; reddish tongue with thin dry yellowish fur and fast and rapid-intermittent pulse are signs of internal accumulation of toxic heat.

Prescription: Clear away heat to cool nutrient qi and nourish yin to tranquilize the mind.

Formulas: Qingying Tang (Decoction) combined with Jiajian Shengmai San (Modified Shengmai Powder), quoted from the chapter on upper energizer in *Wenbing Tiaobian* (*Detailed Analysis of Epidemic Warm Diseases*). Qingying Tang is designed to treat invasion of pathogenic heat into nutrient qi and yin, in which, Xijiao (*Cornu Rhinoceri*), salty and cold in nature, and Shengdihuang (*Radix Rehmanniae Recens*), with its sweet and cold nature, can clear away heat from nutrient phase and cool blood, they are used as sovereign drug; Xuanshen (*Radix Scrophulariae*) and Maidong (*Radix Ophiopogonis*), combined with Shengdihuang, with an action of nourishing yin and clearing away heat, are used as ministerial drug; Jinyinhua (*Flos Lonicerae*), Lianqiao (*Fructus Forsythiae*), Huanglian (*Rhizoma Coptidis*) and Zhuye (*Folia Bambosae*), are used as adjuvant drug to clear away toxic heat so as to erupt pathogenic heat from qi phase and to resolve it; Danshen (*Radix Salviae Miltiorrhizae*) is combined to activate blood and relieve stagnation of heat. Jiajian Shengmai San is made up of Shashen (*Radix Adenophorae*), Maidong, Wuweizi (*Fructus Schisandrae Chinensis*), Mudanpi (*Cortex Moutan Radicis*) and Shengdihuang, aiming at resolving yin to tranquilize the mind with its sweet and sour nature. Besides the same medicinal herbs in both formulas, Qingying Tang is combined with Shashen, Wuweizi and Mudanpi. For obvious palpitation, Suanzaoren (*Semen Ziziphi Spinosae*) and Yejiaoteng (*Caulis Polygoni Multiflori*) can be added to reinforce the action of nourishing yin and tranquilizing the mind. Xijiao (*Rhinoceros Horn*) can be replaced by Shuiniujiao (*Cornu Bubali*), for it has been listed as banned drug.

2. 气阴两虚

24.2　Syndrome of qi and yin asthenia

【症状】心悸怔忡，自汗，神疲乏力，或心神恍惚，坐卧不安，食欲不振，舌红，苔薄，脉象细数，或结代。

【分析】气阴两虚证与病人体质有密切关系。体质素虚，气阴两亏，心脉不得充盈，久而久之，就会出现心悸怔忡；气虚不能护卫，故有自汗；心神不得营养，则有心神恍惚；周身血脉不和，则坐卧不安；"火者土之母"，心脉虚，则脾胃磨谷不力，食欲不振；舌质红者，阴虚也；舌苔薄者，气虚也；阴虚者，脉细数；气虚者，脉结代。综观全症，呈现一派虚象，而又以阴虚比较明显。

【治法】益气养阴，佐以活络。

【方药】炙甘草汤合甘麦大枣汤。炙甘草汤又名"复脉汤"，为治疗心律失常的常用方药。方中以炙甘草为主药，甘温补气，同时还用人参、大枣补气生阴，以助炙甘草补气之力；麦冬、生地黄、阿胶、麻仁滋阴生血；桂枝、生姜助阳，以鼓动血脉的通畅。全方温阳而不燥，补气而不壅，滋阴补血而不腻，补气与养血配合，温阳与滋阴配合，所以后人称它是"气血阴阳俱补"的方剂。所取甘麦大枣汤实际仅用一味小麦，但它与甘草、大枣配合，具有养心安神、和中缓急的作用。这样两个方剂组合，就起到了滋阴扶阳、宁心安神、缓急和中的功效。一般加入丹参、赤芍活血化瘀药，以促进血脉的流通，更有助于于滋阴扶阳药物发挥作用。

Clinical manifestations：Palpitation, spontaneous sweating, dispiritedness and lack of energy, or unconsciousness, restlessness, poor appetite, reddish tongue with thin fur, thin and fast pulse, or slow-intermittent pulse, or slow-intermittent-regular pulse.

Analysis：Syndrome of qi and yin asthenia is closely connected with a patient's constitution. Congenital asthenic constitution causes qi and yin asthenia, which fails to fill up heart vessels, thus, giving rise to palpitation; spontaneous sweating is due to failure of asthenic qi to protect defensive qi; unconsciousness is due to malnutrition of the heart and mind; restlessness is caused by disharmony of blood vessels of the whole body; "fire (the heart) is the mother of earth (the spleen)", asthenic heart vessels cause dysfunction of the spleen and stomach in digesting food and poor appetite; reddish tongue and thin and fast pulse indicate yin asthenia, thin fur and slow-intermittent-regular pulse are signs of qi asthenia. The manifestations of the whole syndrome suggest asthenia, in particular, obvious yin asthenia.

Prescription：Benefit qi, nourish yin, and activate blood vessels.

Formulas：Zhigancao Tang (Decoction) combined with Gan Mai Dazao Tang (Decoction). Zhigancao Tang is known as "Fumai Tang"(Decoction for Restoring blood vessels), of which, Zhigancao (*Radix Glycyrrhizae Preparata*), sweet and warm in nature, can be used as the principal drug to supplement qi, Renshen (*Radix Ginseng*) and Dazao (*Fructus Jujubae*) can tonify qi and promote production of yin so as to help Zhigancao to tonify qi; Maidong (*Radix Ophiopogonis*), Shengdihuang (*Radix Rehmanniae Recens*), Ejiao (*Colla Corii Asini*) and Maziren (*Fructus Cannabis*) have an action of nourishing yin and producing blood; Guizhi (*Ramulus Cinnamomi*) and Shengjiang (*Rhizoma Zingiberis Recens*) can strengthen yang to rise up blood vessels and promote smooth blood circulation. The whole formula can warm yang without causing dryness, supplement qi without obstruction, nourish yin and supplement blood without generating stagnation of dampness. It combines tonifying qi with nourishing blood, warming yang with replenishing yin, therefore, the formula is regarded as "a formula of supplementing qi, blood, yin and yang". In Gan Mai Dazao Tang, Xiaomai (*Fructus Tritici Aestivi*), combined with Gancao and Dazao, has an action of nourishing the heart to tranquilize the mind, harmonizing middle energizer and relieving spasm. The combination of both formulas can bring the action of nourishing yin to strengthen yang, calming the heart to tranquilize the mind, and relieving spasm to reconcile middle energizer into full play. Danshen (*Radix Salviae Miltiorrhizae*) and Chishao (*Radix Paeoniae Rubra*) are added to activate blood and dissolve blood stasis to promote smooth blood circulation, which is very helpful to improve the effect of nourishing yin to strengthen yang.

3. 阴虚火旺
24.3 Syndrome of asthenia of yin and superabundance of fire

【症状】心悸怔忡，心烦少眠，头晕目眩，腰酸耳鸣，舌质红赤，苔少津，脉象细数。

【分析】阴虚火旺证与体质亦有一定关系，或发生于热病之后。阴虚失养，故心悸怔忡；"阴虚则内热"，故心烦少眠；若肝阴虚则头晕目眩，肾阴虚则腰酸耳鸣；舌质红赤、苔少津，为阴虚之兆；脉象细数，为阴虚火旺之象。阴虚火旺证，必见细数之脉，若非细数之脉，而为缓或迟，则非阴虚火旺之证。

【治法】滋阴降火，宁心安神。

【方药】天王补心丹。天王补心丹为滋补心阴的代表方剂。方以生地黄滋补肾水并制火，为其主药；玄参、麦冬、天冬有甘寒滋润以清虚火之效；丹参、当归补血、养血；人参、茯苓益气宁心；酸枣仁、五味子以收敛心气而安心神；柏子仁、远志、朱砂养心安神。以上皆为滋阴降火，宁心安神而设。方中桔梗为载药上行而用。是方若改为汤剂，朱砂可以不用。若头晕目眩甚者，可加杭菊花、枸杞子清肝明目；腰酸耳鸣甚者，可加知母、黄柏滋肾泻火。

Clinical manifestations: Palpitation, irritancy and insomnia, dizziness and vertigo, aching sensation of the loins and tinnitus, reddish tongue with scanty saliva as well as thin and fast pulse.

Analysis: The syndrome of yin asthenia and fire superabundance is related to a patient's constitution to some extent, or it outbreaks after fever. Palpitation is due to malnutrition of the heart vessels because of yin asthenia; irritancy and insomnia are due to yin asthenia and endogenous heat; dizziness and vertigo are caused by yin asthenia of the liver; aching sensation of the loins and tinnitus are caused by yin asthenia of the kidney; reddish tongue and scanty saliva indicate yin asthenia and fire superabundance, which surely gives rise to thin and fast pulse; appearance of moderate or slow pulse rather than thin nor fast pulse suggests the syndrome is not superabundance of fire due to yin asthenia.

Prescription: Nourish yin, descend fire and calm the heart to tranquilize the mind.

Formulas: Tianwang Buxin Dan (Pill). It is a representative formula for nourishing heart yin, in which, Shengdihuang (*Radix Rehmanniae Recens*) is used as the essential drug to nourish kidney essence so as to curb fire, Xuanshen (*Radix Scrophulariae*), Maidong (*Radix Ophiopogonis*) and Tiandong (*Radix Asparagi*), which are sweet, cold and moist in nature, can clear away asthenic fire, Danshen (*Radix Salviae Miltiorrhizae*) and Danggui (*Radix Angelicae Sinensis*) may tonify and nourish blood; Renshen (*Radix Ginseng*) and Fuling (*Poriae Cocos*) have an action of benefiting qi and tranquilizing the heart; Suanzaoren (*Semen Ziziphi Spinosae*) and Wuweizi (*Fructus Schisandrae Chinensis*) could astringe qi to calm the heart and mind; Baiziren (*Semen Platycladi*), Yuanzhi (*Radix Polygalae*) and Zhusha (*Cinnabaris*) have an action of nourishing the heart and tranquilizing the mind. The above herbs are all used to nourish yin, descend fire and tranquilize the heart and mind. Jiegeng (*Radix Platycodonis*) has an effect of lifting. If this formula is changed into decoction, Zhusha can be removed. For severe dizziness and vertigo, Hangjuhua (*Flos Chrysanthemi* from Hangzhou) and Gouqizi (*Fructus Lycii*) can be added to clear away heat in the liver and improve sight; for severe tinnitus and poor appetite, Zhimu (*Rhizoma Anemarrhenae*) and Huangbo (*Cortex Phellodendri*) can be combined to nourish kindey yin and purge fire.

4. 心脾两虚
24.4 Asthenia syndrome of the heart and spleen

【症状】心悸，气短，面色无华，健忘，失眠，头晕目眩，食欲不振，舌质淡红，脉象结代，或迟缓无力。

【分析】心主血脉，脾主统血并主水谷精华之营运，心脾两虚，即心脾气血不足。气血失养，则心悸、气短；血不荣面，则面色无华；记忆虽在大脑，但心血不足，无力养脑，则见健忘、头晕、目眩；脾失健运，则食欲不振；舌质淡红，为气血不足之象；心脾之气血不能充盈血脉，则会出现结代或缓迟脉。总之，呈现出一派气血虚亏之证。

【治法】益气养血，补益心脾。

【方药】归脾汤加味。归脾汤为补益心脾气血的代表方剂，特别是思虑过度所引起的心脾两伤，首选此方。是方以人参、黄芪、白术、甘草、大枣、生姜甘温补脾益气；当归养肝而生心血，茯神、酸枣仁、龙眼肉养心安神；远志交通心肾而定志宁心，木香理气醒脾，以防益气补血之药腻胃滞气。故本方为养益心脾，补气补血相融之剂。

Clinical manifestations: Palpitation, short breath, sallow or lusterless complexion, forgetfulness, insomnia, dizziness and vertigo, poor appetite and pale reddish tongue with slow-intermittent pulse or slow-intermittent-regular pulse , or slow or moderate and weak pulse.

Analysis: The heart dominates blood vessels. The spleen governs blood, and it also controls transportation of food essence. Asthenia of the heart and spleen causes insufficient qi and blood of the heart and spleen. Palpitation and short breath are due to malnutrition of qi and blood; sallow or lusterless complexion is caused by failure of blood to nourish the face; forgetfulness, insomnia, dizziness and vertigo are due to failure of insufficient heart blood to nourish the brain; poor appetite is due to dysfunction of the spleen in transportation; pale reddish tongue indicates insufficiency of qi and blood; slow-intermittent pulse or slow-intermittent-regular pulse , or slow or moderate weak pulse suggests failure of qi and blood of the heart and spleen to enrich the vessels. Generally speaking, all manifestations indicate qi and blood asthenia.

Prescription: Benefit qi, nourish blood and tonify the heart and spleen.

Formulas: Guipi Tang Jiawei (Modified Guipi Decoction). It is a typical formula for tonifying qi and blood of the heart and spleen, and the best choice for impairment of the heart and spleen due to excessive thinking. In the formula, Renshen (*Radix Ginseng*), Huangqi (*Radix Astragali seu Hedysari*), Baizhu (*Rhizoma Atractylodis Macrocephalae*), Gancao (*Radix Glycyrrhizae*), Dazao (*Fructus Jujubae*) and Shengjiang (*Rhizoma Zingiberis Recens*), sweet and warm in nature, have an action of tonifying the spleen and benefiting qi; Danggui (*Radix Angelicae Sinensis*) may nourish the liver and promote production of heart blood, Fushen (*Sclerotium Poriae Circum Radicem*), Suanzaoren (*Semen Ziziphi Spinosae*) and Longyanrou (*Arillus Longan*) can nourish the heart and tranquilize the mind; Yuanzhi (*Radix Polygalae*) may restore normal coordination between the heart and kidney to calm the spirit and tranquilize the heart, Muxiang (*Radix Aucklandiae*) has an action of regulating qi and refreshing the spleen so as to prevent herbs with function of tonifying qi and blood from stagnating in the stomach. Therefore, the formula has an action of nourishing the heart and spleen as well as tonifying qi and blood.

5. 气滞血瘀
24.5 Syndrome of qi stagnation and blood stasis

【症状】心悸，胸闷，时有胸痛，善太息，睡眠不安宁，头晕或头痛，舌质紫暗，舌下静脉迂曲，脉象弦涩。

【分析】本证多见于性情乖逆之人，或郁闷不解，或时时急躁，致使气滞血瘀，血脉运行不顺。心脏血脉瘀而不畅，心血不得及时补充，则心悸、胸闷，郁滞甚者，会胸痛；气滞不行，则善太息；睡眠不安宁者，血瘀不和也；头晕或头痛，为血瘀不能布散所致；舌质紫暗，舌下静脉迂曲，以及脉象弦涩，均为血瘀之明证。

【治法】活血化瘀，宁心安神。

【方药】血府逐瘀汤加味。血府逐瘀汤为治疗心肺瘀血之主剂。其方药分析见于本书"冠心病"篇。在具体应用时，可加酸枣仁、柏子仁、合欢皮、降香等，增强其宁心安神、解郁理气的作用。

Clinical manifestations: Palpitation, chest oppression with occasional pain, frequent sigh, disturbed sleep, dizziness, or headache, dark purplish tongue, varicosity under the tongue as well as taut and astringent pulse.

Analysis: The syndrome is usually seen in those with eccentric and disobedient character, or with gloomy mood, or frequent restlessness, which causes qi stagnation, blood stasis and obstructive blood circulation. Blood of the heart cannot be supplemented in time, bringing about palpitation and chest oppression, severe qi stagnation can give rise to occasional chest pain; frequent sigh is due to failure of stagnated qi to activate; disturbed sleep is caused by disharmony of blood due to blood stasis; dizziness or headache is due to failure of blood stasis to distribute blood; dark purplish tongue, varicosity under the tongue and taut and astringent pulse are obvious signs of blood stasis.

Prescription: Activate blood circulation to dissolve blood stasis and calm the heart to tranquilize the mind.

Formulas：Xuefu Zhuyu Tang Jiawei (Modified Xuefu Zhuyu Decoction). It is a major formula for treating blood stasis in the heart and lung and it has been introduced in the chapter of *Coronary Disease*. Clinically, Suanzaoren (*Semen Ziziphi Spinosae*), Baiziren (*Semen Platycladi*), Hehuanpi (*Cortex Albiziae*) and Jiangxiang (*Lignum Dalbergiae Odoriferae*) can be added to strengthen the action of calming the heart to tranquilize the mind and relieving stagnation to regulate qi.

二十五、头痛

25 Headache

〔概说〕 Summary

头痛是临床上常见的症状，常以主诉出现，也可见于多种急慢性疾病之中。本文所讨论的头痛，是以内科杂病为主。若在其他疾病过程中出现，只能以兼症对待。本文不做讨论。

中医学对头痛分两大类，即外感头痛和内伤头痛。外感头痛多因起居不慎，感受风、湿、寒、热等外邪，尤以感受风邪为主。内伤头痛以情志内伤为主，与肝、脾、肾三脏有关。头痛的辨证除病因辨证、脏腑辨证外，还与经络辨证有关。如太阳经头痛多在头后部，阳明经头痛多在前额及眉棱处，少阳经头痛多在头之两侧，并连及耳部，厥阴经头痛则在颠顶部位。只有明了头痛的病因及所患部位与经络的关系，才能进行正确的治疗。

Headache is a common clinical syndrome, usually mentioned in the chief complaint of a patient. It always occurs in various acute or chronic diseases. Headache that will be discussed in this chapter is mainly about miscellaneous diseases of internal medicine department. Outbreak of it in other diseases can be regarded as a complicated disease, which is not approached here.

In terms of TCM, pathogenesis of headache is divided into exogenous pathogenic factors and internal impairment. The former is caused by invasion of exogenous pathogenic wind, dampness, cold as well as heat factors, in particular, exogenous pathogenic wind. The latter is mainly caused by emotional upset, connected with the liver, spleen and kidney. Syndrome differentiation of headache is related to its etiology, its concerning viscera and meridians and collaterals. For instance, headache of taiyang meridian usually occurs in the rear of the head, headache of yangming meridian usually appears at the forehead and at the eyebrows, headache of shaoyang meridian appears at the lateral sides of the head involving the ears, headache of jueyin meridian is on the top of head. Only by clearly understanding the causes of various types of headache and the relationship between its location and the concerning meridians and collaterals can doctors take the most effective therapeutic methods.

〔辨证论治〕Syndrome differentiation and treatment

（一）外感头痛
25.1　Headache due to exogenous pathogenic factors

1. 风寒头痛

25.1.1　Headache due to pathogenic wind and cold factors

【症状】头痛时作，痛连项背，腰酸，恶风畏寒，遇风寒尤剧，口淡不渴，舌苔薄白，脉象浮而紧。

【分析】头为诸阳之会，风寒外袭，循足太阳经上犯颠顶，清阳之气被遏，疼痛乃作；足太阳经出于目内眦，"上额交颠……入络脑……还出别下项……夹脊抵腰中"，风寒束于太阳经肌表，故痛连项背，并有腰酸；卫阳被遏，不得宣达，则恶风畏寒；风寒为阴邪，不伤阴液，故口不渴而淡；舌苔薄白、脉象浮紧，为风寒袭表的明证。

【治法】疏散风寒。

【方药】川芎茶调散加减。方中川芎、荆芥、防风、羌活、白芷、细辛等均为辛温药，具有疏风散寒、通络止痛的作用。其中川芎为血中之气药，祛血中之风，上行头目，为临床治疗外感头痛的要药。如兼有瘀热，薄荷必须同用。

Clinical manifestations: Frequent outbreak of headache involving the neck and back, aching sensation of the loins, aversion to wind cold, aggravation with invasion of wind cold, bland taste and no thirst, thin whitish fur as well as floating and tense pulse.

Analysis: The head is the region where all yang meridians converge, pathogenic wind cold factors transmit from the superficies along foot taiyang meridian up to the top of the head, causing obstruction of lucid yang qi, which brings about headache; foot taiyang meridian starts form the inner canthus, converges at the forehead and passes through the cranial cavity, the curved line of occipital bone, the neck, the spine and to the waist. Encumbrance of wind cold on muscular superficies of taiyang meridian gives rise to headache involving the neck and back, accompanied by aching sensation of the loins; aversion to wind and cold is due to failure of obstructed defensive yang to disperse; wind and cold are yin pathogens, which cannot cause impairment of yin fluid, therefore, resulting in bland taste with no thirst; thin whitish fur and floating and tense pulse are obvious manifestations of wind cold attacking the superficies.

Prescription: Expel wind and cold.

Formulas: Chuanxiong Chatiao San Jiajian (Modified Chuanxiong Chatiao Powder). In the formula, Chuanxiong (*Rhizoma Ligustici Chuanxiong*), Jingjie (*Herba Schizonepetae*), Fangfeng (*Radix Saposhnikoviae*), Qianghuo (*Rhizoma et Radix Notopterygii*), Baizhi (*Radix Angelicae Dahuricae*) and Xixin (*Herba Asari*), pungent and warm in nature, have an action of expelling wind cold and dredging the collaterals to stop pain. Chuanxiong, with the action of promoting qi and blood circulation and expelling wind from the blood which flows upward onto the head, is an essential herb for headache due to exogenous wind cold. For heat stagnation, Bohe (*Herba Menthae*) must be used together with Chuanxiong.

2. 风热头痛
25.1.2　Headache due to wind heat

【症状】头痛而涨，甚则头痛如裂，发热或恶风，面目红赤，口渴引饮，大便秘结，小便黄赤，舌质红赤，苔黄，脉象浮数。

【分析】热为阳邪，其性炎上，风热中于阳经，上扰清窍，故疼痛而涨，甚则头痛如裂；热邪炎上，则面目红赤；风热为患，卫阳失护，故发热恶风；热盛伤津，则口渴引饮；阴液耗伤，不能润泽二便，故便秘溲黄；舌与脉象均为风热炽盛之征。

【治法】疏风清热。

【方药】芎芷石膏汤加减。方中用石膏清热泻火，菊花散风清热，川芎、白芷祛风止痛，寓“火郁发之”之意，不用原方羌活、藁本之辛温，而加金银花、连翘、黄芩辛凉清热。若兼口渴、舌红少津，可加天花粉、石斛生津止渴；大便干结，可加大黄泻热通腑。

Clinical manifestations: Distending headache, aggravation of it like being split, fever or aversion to wind, flushed complexion and eyes, thirst with desire to drink, dry feces, yellowish urine, reddish tongue with yellowish fur and floating and fast pulse.

Analysis: Heat, with a nature of flaring-up, is a yang pathogen, wind cold attacking yang meridians and disturbing the upper orifices, gives rise to distending headache and aggravation of it like being split; flushed complexion and eyes are due to heat pathogen flaming up; fever or aversion to wind is due to failure to protect defensive yang because of invasion of wind heat; thirst with desire to drink is due to exuberance of heat impairing body fluid; dry feces and yellowish urine are caused by consumption and impairment of yin fluid failing to moisten urine and stool; reddish tongue with yellowish fur and floating and fast pulse are signs of superabundance of wind heat.

Prescription: Expel wind and clear away heat.

Formulas: Xiong Zhi Shigao Tang Jiajian (Modified Xiong Zhi Shigao Decoction). In this formula, Shigao (*Gypsum Fibrosum*) can clear away heat and purge fire, Juhua (*Flos Chrysanthemi*) has an action of dispersing wind and clearing away heat, Chuanxiong (*Rhizoma Ligustici Chuanxiong*) and Baizhi (*Radix Angelicae Dahuricae*) can expel wind to stop pain, that is, "fire stagnation can be dispelled", Qianghuo (*Rhizoma et Radix Notopterygii*) and Gaoben (*Rhizoma Ligustici*) can be removed due to their pungent and warm nature, and Jinyinhua (*Flos Lonicerae*), Lianqiao (*Fructus Forsythiae*) and Huangqin (*Radix Scutellariae*), pungent and cool in nature, may be added to clear away heat. For complicated symptoms as thirst and reddish tongue with scanty saliva, Tianhuafen (*Radix Trichosanthis*) and Shihu (*Herba Dendrobii*) can be combined to promote production of fluid to stop thirst; for dry feces, Dahuang (*Radix et Rhizoma Rhei*) can be added to purge heat and remove stagnation of intestinal qi.

3. 风湿头痛
25.1.3 Headache due to wind and dampness

【症状】头痛如裹，身体困重，纳呆胸闷，大便不成形，小便或不利，舌苔白腻，脉濡。

【分析】为感受风湿而致。风湿上犯颠顶，清窍为湿邪所困，故疼痛如裹；脾司运化并主四肢，脾阳被湿浊所困，故见四肢困重、纳呆胸闷；湿浊下注二便，则大便不成形，小便或不利；舌苔白腻与脉濡为湿浊中阻之象。

【治法】祛风胜湿。

【方药】羌活胜湿汤加减。方用羌活、独活、川芎、防风、蔓荆子、藁本等辛温药物，意在祛风胜湿，为治疗风湿外感之主药。若湿浊中阻，胸闷不饥、便溏，可加苍术、厚朴、陈皮、枳壳等燥湿宽中；若恶心呕吐，可加半夏、生姜以降逆止呕。

Clinical manifestations: Headache like being wrapped, heavy sensation of the body, anorexia and chest oppression, loose stool, or dysuria, greasy whitish fur as well as soft pulse.

Analysis: This syndrome is caused by exogenous wind and dampness. Headache like being wrapped is caused by invasion of exogenous wind and dampness onto the top of the head and obstruction of upper orifices by pathogenic dampness factors; the spleen dominates transportation and transformation, obstruction of spleen yang by turbid dampness gives rise to heavy sensation of the limbs, anorexia and chest pain; loose stool and dysuria are due to downward migration of turbid dampness; greasy and whitish fur and soft pulse are signs of obstruction of turbid dampness in middle energizer.

Prescription: Expel wind and eliminate dampness.

Formulas: Qianghuo Shengshi Tang Jiajian (Modified Qianghuo Shengshi Decoction). In the formula, Qianghuo (*Rhizoma et Radix Notopterygii*), Duhuo (*Radix Angelicae Pubescentis*), Chuanxiong (*Rhizoma Ligustici Chuanxiong*), Fangfeng (*Radix Saposhnikoviae*), Manjingzi (*Fructus Viticis*) and Gaoben (*Rhizoma Ligustici*), pungent and warm in nature, with an action of expelling wind and eliminating dampness, are used as the principal drug to treat the syndrome of exogenous wind dampness. For obstruction of turbid dampness in middle energizer, anorexia and chest oppression and loose stool, Cangzhu (*Rhizoma Atractylodis*), Houpo (*Cortex Magnoliae Officinalis*), Chengpi (*Pericarpium Citri Reticulatae*) and Zhiqiao (*Fructus Aurantii*) can be combined to dry dampness and ease middle energizer; for nausea and vomiting, Banxia (*Rhizoma Pinelliae*) and Shengjiang (*Rhizoma Zingiberis Recens*) may be added to descend adverse qi and arrest vomiting.

（二）内伤头痛
25.2 Headache due to internal impairment

1. 肝阳头痛
25.2.1 Headache due to liver yang hyperactivity

【症状】头痛且眩晕，心烦易怒，夜眠不安，或常做噩梦，口苦，咽干，耳鸣，面部红赤，舌苔薄黄，脉弦有力。

【分析】"诸风掉眩，皆属于肝。"肝阳偏亢，上扰清窍，故疼痛而眩晕；肝阳内藏相火，火性炎上，扰乱心神，则心烦易怒、夜眠不安；肝火伤阴，故口苦、咽干；肝阳化风，时有耳鸣；面部红赤，为阳亢之象；舌苔薄黄、脉弦有力，为肝阳亢胜之征。

【治法】平肝潜阳。

【方药】天麻钩藤饮加减。方中天麻、钩藤、石决明均为平肝熄风之药，为本方之主药；黄芩、栀子清热泻火，使肝经之热不易偏亢，为辅药；益母草活血利水，牛膝引血下行，杜仲、桑寄生补益肝肾，夜交藤、茯神安神定志，共为佐使药。病重者，可加羚羊角（研粉冲服）。

Clinical manifestations: Headache with vertigo, vexation with susceptibility to rage, disturbed sleep or frequent nightmare, bitter taste, dry throat, tinnitus, flushed complexion, thin yellowish fur as well as taut and powerful pulse.

Analysis: "The symptoms of convulsion and dizziness belong to the syndrome of liver yang transforming into wind." Hyperactive liver yang disturbs the upper orifices, which gives rise to headache and vertigo; vexation with susceptibility to rage and disturbed sleep are due to internal storage of ministerial fire because of up-flaring of liver yang which disturbs the heart and mind; bitter taste and dry throat are due to liver fire impairing yin fluid; occasional tinnitus is caused by liver yang transforming into wind; flushed complexion is a sign of hyperactivity of liver yang; thin yellowish fur and taut and powerful pulse are manifestations of hyperactivity of liver yang.

Prescription: Calm the liver and suppress yang.

Formulas: Tianma Gouteng Yin Jiajian (Modified Tianma Gouteng Decoction). In the formula, Tianma (*Rhizoma Gastrodiae*), Gouteng (*Ramulus Uncariae Cum Uncis*) and Shijueming (*Concha Haliotidis*) are principal drug for suppressing hyperactive liver to calm endogenous wind; Huangqin (*Radix Scutellariae*) and Zhizi (*Fructus Gardeniae*) are used as adjuvant drug to clear away heat and purge fire; Yimucao (*Herba Leonuri*) can activate blood circulation to induce diuresis, Niuxi (*Radix Achyranthis Bidentatae*) can guide blood to flow down, Duzhong (*Cortex Eucommiae*) and Sangjisheng (*Herba Taxilli*) can replenish the liver and kidney, Yejiaoteng (*Tuber Fleeceflower Stem*) and Fushen (*Sclerotium Poriae Circum Radicem*) can tranquilize the spirit and mind. The above six herbs are used as assistant and courier drug. For aggravation of the disease, Lingyangjiao (*Cornu Saigae Tataricae*) may be grinded into powder and taken orally as infusion.

2. 肾虚头痛
25.2.2　Headache due to kidney asthenia

【症状】头痛有空虚感，每兼眩晕，腰膝酸软，神疲乏力，男子遗精，女子带下，耳鸣少眠，舌红少苔，脉细无力。

【分析】此证与病人体质有密切关系。或者精神压力过大，暗耗肾阴，或者过用辛辣之品，灼伤肾阴。肾主骨，骨生髓，髓充脑，肾阴不足，则髓不能充脑，故头痛有空虚感，并每兼眩晕；"腰为肾之府"，肾精不足，故腰膝酸软；男子精关不固则遗精，女子带脉不束则带下；精髓不足，自然神疲乏力；耳为肾之窍，肾精不充，故耳鸣少眠；舌红少苔，脉细无力，为肾阴不足所出现的阴虚内热证。

【治法】滋阴补肾。

【方药】大补元煎加减。大补元煎为明代张景岳所拟定的名方。方由人参、山药、熟地黄、山茱萸、枸杞子、杜仲、当归、甘草组成。方中熟地黄、山药、山茱萸、枸杞子滋补肝肾之阴，人参、当归补益气血，杜仲益肾强腰，甘草调和气血。男子遗精可加金樱子、桑螵蛸补肾固精；女子带下可加茯苓、牡蛎渗湿止带。

Clinical manifestations: Headache with vacuous sensation complicated by dizziness, aching and weakness of the loins and knees, dispiritedness and lack of energy, seminal emission in male, morbid leucorrhea in female, tinnitus and less sleep, reddish tongue with scanty fur as well as thin and weak pulse.

Analysis: The syndrome is closely connected with a patient's constitution. Mental stress consumes kidney yin, or excessive intake of pungent food scorches kidney yin. The kidney dominates the bone, and the bone generates marrow, which enriches the brain, insufficiency of kidney yin results in failure of marrow to be filled in the brain, thus, giving rise to headache with vacuous sensation complicated by occasional dizziness and vertigo; "the loins are the house of the kidney", insufficiency of kidney essence causes aching and weakness of the loins and knees; seminal emission in male is due to failure to reinforce sperm house, morbid leucorrhea in female is due to dysfunction of belt vessel; dispiritedness and lack of energy are due to insufficiency of kidney essence and cerebral marrow; the ears are the orifices of the kidney, insufficiency of kidney essence gives rise to tinnitus and less sleep; reddish tongue with scanty fur and thin and weak pulse are signs of yin asthenia generating endogenous heat due to asthenic kidney yin.

Prescription: Nourish yin and supplement the kidney.

Formulas: Large Buyuan Jian Jiajian (Modified Large Buyuan Decoction). This is a famous formula designed by Zhang Jingyue from the Ming Dynasty, consisting of Renshen (*Radix Ginseng*), Shanyao (*Rhizoma Dioscoreae*), Shudihuang (*Radix Rehmanniae Preparata*), Shanzhuyu (*Fructus Corni*), Gouqizi (*Fructus Lycii*), Duzhong (*Cortex Eucommiae*), Danggui (*Radix Angelicae Sinensis*) and Gancao (*Radix Glycyrrhizae*), of them, Shudihuang, Shanyao, Shanzhuyu and Gouqizi can nourish and tonify liver yin and kidney yin, Renshen and Danggui can supplement qi and blood, Duzhong has an action of strengthening the function of the kidney and loins, Gancao may regulate qi and blood. For seminal emission, Jinyingzi (*Fructus Rosae Laevigatae*) and Sangpiaoxiao (*Ootheca Mantidis*) can be combined to tonify the kidney and control nocturnal emission; for morbid leucorrhea, Fuling (*Poriae Cocos*) and Muli (*Concha Ostreae*) may be added to resolve dampness and arrest morbid leucorrhea.

3. 血虚头痛
25.2.3　Headache due to blood asthenia

【症状】头痛而晕，心悸不宁，面色㿠白，神疲乏力，舌质淡红，苔薄白，脉象沉细。

【分析】血虚也与体质有关。血虚不能养脑，故头痛而晕；血不足以养心，则心悸不宁；血虚不足上荣，故面色㿠白；阴血为体，精神为用，体不足则用不能，今阴血亏耗，故精神疲倦而乏力；舌质淡红、苔薄白、脉象沉细，为血虚之象。

【治法】养心滋阴。

【方药】四物汤加味。四物汤为补血之主剂，方中当归、熟地黄、白芍养血，川芎活血行气；加入菊花、蔓荆子平肝熄风，清头明目。若肝血不足，出现头晕、虚烦、少眠，加入何首乌、枸杞子、黄精滋肾养肝；若血虚导致气虚，出现气短乏力、恶风怕冷，加入党参、黄芪、桂枝、甘草补益中气。

Clinical manifestations: Headache and dizziness, palpitation and restlessness, pale complexion, dispiritedness and lack of energy, pale reddish tongue, pale whitish fur as well as sunken and thin pulse.

Analysis: Blood asthenia is related to a patient's constitution. Headache and dizziness are due to failure of asthenic blood to nourish the brain; palpitation and restlessness are due to failure of insufficient blood to nourish the heart; pale complexion is due to inability of asthenic blood to nourish the face; yin and blood are inherent basis, spirit is external presentation of human body, deficiency of yin and blood brings about inability of spirit, therefore, deficiency and consumption of yin and blood results in dispiritedness and lack of energy; pale reddish tongue, pale whitish fur and sunken and thin pulse are signs of blood asthenia.

Prescription: Nourish the heart and moisten yin.

Formulas: Siwu Tang Jiawei (Modified Siwu Decoction). Siwu Tang is a principal recipe for supplementing blood, of which, Danggui (*Radix Angelicae Sinensis*), Shudihuang (*Radix Rehmanniae Preparata*) and Baishao (*Radix Paeoniae Alba*) can nourish blood, Chuanxiong (*Rhizoma Ligustici Chuanxiong*) has an action of activating blood and qi; Juhua (*Flos Chrysanthemi*) and Manjingzi (*Fructus Viticis*) can calm the liver to suppress endogenous wind and clear away heat in the head to improve sight. For dizziness, dysphoria and insomnia due to insufficiency of liver blood, Heshouwu (*Radix Polygoni Multiflori*), Gouqizi (*Fructus Lycii*) and Huangjing (*Rhizoma Polygonati*) can be added to nourish the kidney and liver; for short breath, lack of energy, aversion to wind and cold due to blood asthenia which results in qi asthenia, Dangshen (Radix Codonopsis), Huangqi (*Radix Astragali seu Hedysari*), Guizhi (*Ramulus Cinnamomi*) and Gancao (*Radix Glycyrrhizae*) may be combined to tonify qi in middle energizer.

4. 痰浊头痛
25.2.4 Headache due to phlegmatic turbidity

【症状】头痛昏蒙，胸脘痞闷，呕恶痰涎，舌苔白腻，脉象弦滑。

【分析】痰浊的产生与脾不化湿有关。脾失健运，湿浊中阻，清阳不振，上蒙清窍，故头痛昏蒙；痰浊阻膈，故胸脘痞闷；痰浊上逆，则呕恶痰涎；舌苔白腻与脉象弦滑，均为痰浊中阻之征。

【治法】化痰降逆。

【方药】半夏白术天麻汤加减。本方取自清代程钟龄《医学心悟》，方由二陈汤加白术、天麻而成。二陈汤为治痰基本方；天麻甘微温，入肝经，功能熄风镇痉，古有"定风草"之称，是治疗内风引起头痛、眩晕的佳品；白术健脾益气，助运化而祛湿浊，并可增强化痰的作用。还可加入蔓荆子，此药体轻上浮而散，主治头面风虚之证，与天麻配合，散风化痰清头目，但用量不宜过大，以免虚风上扰。

Clinical manifestation: Headache and dizziness, oppression and distension in the chest and hypochondrium, nausea and vomiting sputum and saliva, greasy whitish fur as well as taut and slippery pulse.

Analysis: Production of phlegmatic turbidity is connected with failure of the spleen to resolve dampness. Headache and dizziness are due to dysfunction of the spleen in transportation, which results in obstruction of turbidity and dampness in middle energizer, hypofunction of lucid yang and invasion of phlegm in upper orifices; oppression and distension in the chest and hypochondrium are caused by obstruction of turbid phlegm in the diaphragm; nausea and vomiting sputum and saliva are due to upward invasion of turbid phlegm; greasy whitish fur and taut and slippery pulse are signs of obstruction of turbidity and dampness in middle energizer.

Prescription: Resolve phlegm and descend adverse qi.

Formulas: Banxia Baizhu Tianma Tang Jiajian (Modified Banxia Baizhu Tianma Decoction). This formula is quoted from *Yixue Xinwu* (*Medicine Comprehended*) by Cheng Zhongling from the Qing Dynasty, consisting of Erchen Tang combined with Baizhu (*Rhizoma Atractylodis Macrocephalae*) and Tianma (*Rhizoma Gastrodiae*). Erchen Tang is a basic recipe for phlegm syndrome; Tianma, known as "the grass of calming wind" in ancient time, is slight warm in nature and attributive to liver meridian, having an action of calming endogenous wind to suppress spasm, and it is the best drug for treating headache and dizziness caused by endogenous wind; Baizhu has an action of invigorating the spleen to benefit qi, removing turbid dampness by improving transportation and transformation as well as strengthening the action of resolving phlegm. Manjingzi (*Fructus Viticis*), with its action of floating and dispersing due to its light weight, can be combined for treating asthenia coupled with invasion of pathogenic wind factors, and it can be combined with Tianma to disperse wind, resolve phlegm and eliminate dizziness. But the amount of both herbs should not be large so as to avoid up-disturbance of asthenic wind.

5. 瘀血头痛
25.2.5　Headache due to blood stasis

【症状】头痛经久不愈，痛处固定不移，痛如锥刺，舌质紫暗，苔薄白，脉象细涩。

【分析】中医学有"初病在经，久病入络"之说，此证多为病久所见，有的是头部外伤所致。病久邪从经入络，由气入血，络脉不通，所以头痛难以速愈；瘀血固定于一处，则疼痛固定不移，且痛如锥刺；舌质紫暗与脉象细涩，为瘀血内阻之明证。

【治法】活血化瘀。

【方药】通窍活血汤加减。方取桃红四物汤去当归、地黄，另取麝香、生姜、葱白辛温通络。还可加入石菖蒲、郁金、细辛、白芷理气通窍，活络止痛。头痛甚者，可加虫类药，如全蝎、蜈蚣、地鳖虫等入络搜风。头痛缓解后可加补益肝肾之品，如何首乌、枸杞子、熟地黄等。头痛还要注意选择引经药，如太阳经头痛，加羌活、蔓荆子；阳明经头痛，加葛根、白芷、知母；少阳经头痛，加柴胡、黄芩、川芎；厥阴经头痛，加吴茱萸、藁本等。

Clinical manifestation: Prolonged headache, fixed position of headache, pain like being pierced with a wimble, dark purplish tongue with thin whitish fur as well as thin and astringent pulse.

Analysis: In TCM, it is held that the location of a disease at its initial stage is in meridians, gradually, the prolonged disease penetrates into the collaterals. And this syndrome is usually seen in prolonged or chronic diseases. In some cases, headache is caused by trauma in the head. As far as a chronic disease is concerned, pathogenic factors transmit from the meridians into the collaterals, and through qi phase into blood phase; headache that cannot be cured quickly is caused by obstruction of collaterals and blood vessels; fixed position of headache and pain like being pierced with a wimble are due to fixed position of blood stasis; dark purplish tongue with thin whitish fur and thin and astringent pulse are obvious manifestations of internal obstruction of blood stasis.

Prescription: Activate blood circulation and resolve blood stasis.

Formulas: Tongqiao Huoxue Tang Jiajian (Modified Tongqiao Huoxue Decoction). The formula is composed by removing Danggui (*Radix Angelicae Sinensis*) and Dihuang (*Radix Rehmanniae*) from Tao Hong Siwu Tang (Decoction), and adding pungent-and-warm natured Shexiang (*Moschus*), Shengjiang (*Rhizoma Zingiberis Recens*) and Congbai (*Allium Fislulosum*) to dredge blood vessels. And Shichangpu (*Rhizoma Acori Tatarinowii*), Yujin

(*Radix Curcumae*), Xixin (*Herba Asari*) and Baizhi (*Radix Angelicae Dahuricae*) can be added to regulate qi to open the upper orifices and activate blood circulation to stop pain. For severe headache, Quanxie (*Scorpio*), Wugong (*Scolopendra*) and Tubiechong (*Eupolyphaga Seu Steleophaga*) may be added to remove endogenous wind by penetrating into blood vessels. After alleviation of headache, Heshouwu (*Radix Polygoni Multiflori*), Gouqizi (*Fructus Lycii*) and Shudihuang (*Radix Rehmanniae Preparata*) can be combined to supplement the liver and kidney. As far as headache is concerned, the selection of some meridian-ushering drug should not be neglected, for instance, for taiyang meridian headache, Qianghuo (*Rhizoma et Radix Notopterygii*) and Manjingzi (*Fructus Viticis*) should be combined; as for yangming meridian headache, Gegen (*Radix Puerariae*), Baizhi (*Radix Angelicae Dahuricae*) and Zhimu (*Rhizoma Anemarrhenae*) can be added; as for shaoyang meridian headache, Chaihu (*Radix Bupleuri*), Huangqin (*Radix Scutellariae*) and Chuanxiong (*Rhizoma Ligustici Chuanxiong*) could be added; for jueying meridian headache, Wuzhuyu (*Fructus Evodiae*) and Gaoben (*Rhizoma Ligustici*) can be combined.

二十六、眩晕

26　Dizziness and vertigo

〔概说〕　Summary

　　眩晕是目眩与头晕的总称。目眩即眼花，或眼前发黑，视物不清；头晕即感觉自身或外界景物旋转，站立不稳。二者常同时并见，故称眩晕。

　　眩晕一词，在中医学的典籍中很早就有记载。《黄帝内经》对此论述颇多，后世医家多有发挥。如金代朱丹溪认为眩晕与痰浊有关，李东垣则认为与后天脾胃失和有关，而刘河间则认为"六气皆从火化"，与火毒有关；到了清代，唐容川与王清任认为眩晕与瘀血相关。医家各述其词，并行不悖，不可固定于一种模式。总的治疗原则是，有什么证候，选用什么方药。

Dizziness refers to blurred vision, or darkness before the eyes; vertigo means that the patient subjectively feels that his body or the things in sight are swirling and he cannot stand steadily. Dizziness and vertigo usually appear simultaneously.

Statements on dizziness and vertigo have been recorded in early TCM classic works, for example, there are many remarks about them in *Huangdi Neijing* (*Huangdi's Internal Classic*). Later on, lots of TCM experts have talked about their own understanding on them. For instance, in the Jin Dynasty, Zhu Danxi claims that dizziness and vertigo are connected with phlegmatic turbidity, Li Dongyuan holds that they are related to acquired disharmony of the stomach and spleen, but Liu Hejian insists that the six factors, wind, cold, summer heat, dampness, dryness and fire in nature can transform into exuberant fire of human body, that is, dizziness and vertigo are associated with toxic fire pathogen; Tang Rongchuan and Wang Qingren in the Qing Dynasty think that they are caused by blood stasis. These views about dizziness and vertigo are not against one another, however, treatments for the diseases should not be confined to one of them. The general therapeutic principle is that application of formulas should be based on various syndromes of the diseases.

〔辨证论治〕 Syndrome differentiation and treatment

1. 肝阳上亢
26.1 Hyperactivity of liver yang

【症状】眩晕耳鸣，头痛且涨，每因烦劳或恼怒而加剧，面色潮红或暗红，急躁易怒，少眠多梦，口苦而干，舌质红赤，苔黄，脉象弦而有力。肝阳上亢之甚，则可见眩晕欲仆，泛泛欲呕，头痛如掣，肢体麻木或震颤，语言不利，步履不正等。

【分析】劳则伤肾，怒则伤肝，均可使肝阳上亢，引发头痛、眩晕与耳鸣，且常因烦劳或恼怒而加剧；肝阳亢则火随之上炎，故见面色潮红或暗红；肝火扰动心神，则少眠多梦；阳亢则伤阴，故口苦而干；舌质红、苔黄、脉弦，均为肝阳上亢之征；如见脉弦细数，则为肝肾阴虚内热之象。若肝阳上亢之极，则形成肝阳化风之证，如见眩晕欲仆，泛泛欲呕，头痛如掣，肢体麻木或震颤，语言不利，步履不正，此为中风之先兆，必须严加防范。

【治法】平肝潜阳，滋阴熄风。

【方药】天麻钩藤饮加味。天麻钩藤饮为平肝熄风之首选方剂，其基本方义已在"高血压病"篇中叙述。阴虚可加女贞子、生地黄、何首乌、龟板滋阴熄风；肝阳亢极化风，可加羚羊角、生牡蛎、珍珠母等镇肝熄风；如预防中风，可加服安宫牛黄丸，以平肝熄风、清脑开窍、泻火解毒。

Clinical Manifestations: Dizziness and tinnitus, headache and distention, aggravation of the symptoms with vexation, overstrain or rage, tidal flushed cheek or dark reddish complexion, restlessness with susceptibility to rage, insomnia and dreaminess, bitter taste and dry mouth, reddish tongue with yellowish fur and taut and powerful pulse. Hyperactivity of liver yang gives rise to the following symptoms such as vertigo with tendency to collapse, occasional vomiting, dragging sensation of headache, numb limbs or tremor, slurred speech and staggering gait.

Analysis: Headache, dizziness and tinnitus, aggravation of the symptoms with vexation, overstrain or rage are due to hyperactivity of liver yang, because overstrain impairs the kidney and rage impairs the liver; tidal flushed cheeks or dark reddish complexion is caused by up-flaming of fire due to hyperactivity of liver yang; insomnia and dreaminess are due to disturbance of liver fire in the heart and mind; bitter taste and dry mouth are due to hyperactive liver yang impairing yin; reddish tongue with yellowish fur and taut pulse are manifestations of yin asthenia of the liver and kidney. Vertigo with tendency to collapse, occasional vomiting, dragging sensation of headache and numb limbs or tremor are due to extremely hyperactive liver yang, slurred speech and staggering gait are indications of wind stroke. Therefore, precautions should be taken.

Prescription: Calm the liver to suppress liver yang and nourish yin for calming endogenous wind.

Formulas: Tianma Gouteng Yin Jiawei (Modified Tianma Gouteng Decoction). Tianma Gouteng Yin is the best formula for suppressing hyperactive liver to calm endogenous wind, and it has been approached in the chapter of *Hypertension*. For yin asthenia, Nuzhenzi (*Fructus Ligustri Lucidi*), Shengdihuang (*Radix Rehmanniae Recens*), Heshouwu (*Radix Polygoni Multiflori*) and Guiban (*Plastrum Testudinis*) can nourish yin to calm endogenous wind; for liver yang transforming into wind, Lingyangjiao (*Cornu Saigae Tataricae*), Shengmuli (*Concha Ostreae*) and Zhenzhumu (*Concha Margaritifera*) can be added to suppress the liver and calm wind; for the sake of guarding against wind stroke, Angong Niuhunag Wan (Pill) can be combined to calm the liver and wind, regain consciousness by inducing resuscitation and purge fire to relieve toxic pathogen.

2. 气血亏虚
26.2　Qi and blood asthenia

【症状】时时眩晕，动则加剧，劳则发作，面色萎黄或㿠白，唇甲不华，发色不泽，时有心悸，精神疲惫，饮食减少，舌质淡红，脉象细弱。

【分析】气虚则清阳不展，血虚则脑失所养，故头晕且遇劳加重；心主血脉，其华在面，血虚则面色㿠白；血不养心，则心悸；心肾气虚则精神疲惫，脾胃气虚则饮食减少；舌质淡红，脉象细弱，均为气血亏虚之象。

【治法】补益气血，健脾养心。

【方药】归脾汤加味。归脾汤为补益气血之主方。方中人参、黄芪、白术、甘草、生姜、大枣甘温补脾益气；当归养肝而生心血；茯神、酸枣仁、龙眼肉养心安神；远志交通心肾而定志宁心；木香理气醒脾，以防补益药物滋腻滞气。若血虚甚者，可加熟地黄、阿胶、紫河车粉（另冲服）；如胃口不开，可加砂仁、白蔻仁、神曲；若清阳不升，时时眩晕，便溏下坠，可加柴胡、升麻以升清祛浊。

Clinical manifestations: Frequent dizziness and vertigo, aggravation with movement, outbreak with overstrain, sallow or pale complexion; pale lips and nails; lusterless hair, occasional palpitation, dispiritedness, reduced appetite, pale reddish tongue and thin and weak pulse.

Analysis: Dizziness and aggravation with overstrain are due to failure to lift lucid yang because of qi asthenia and malnutrition of the brain caused by blood asthenia; the heart dominates blood vessels with its outward manifestation on the face, blood asthenia gives rise to pale complexion; palpitation is due to failure of asthenic blood to nourish the heart; dispiritedness is caused by qi asthenia of the heart and kidney; reduced appetite is due to qi asthenia of the spleen and stomach; pale reddish tongue and thin and weak pulse are signs of qi and blood asthenia.

Prescription：Supplement qi and blood, invigorate the spleen and nourish the heart.

Formulas：Guipi Tang Jiawei (Modified Guipi Decoction). It is a main formula for supplementing qi and blood, of which, Renshen (*Radix Ginseng*), Huangqi (*Radix Astragali seu Hedysari*), Baizhu (*Rhizoma Atractylodis Macrocephalae*), Gancao (*Radix Glycyrrhizae*), Shengjiang (*Rhizoma Zingiberis Recens*) and Dazao (*Fructus Jujubae*), sweet and warm in nature, can supplement the spleen and benefit qi; Danggui (*Radix Angelicae Sinensis*) has an action of nourishing the liver and promoting production of heart blood, Fushen (*Sclerotium Poriae Circum Radicem*), Suanzaoren (*Semen Ziziphi Spinosae*) and Longyanrou (*Arillus Longan*) can nourish the heart and tranquilize the mind; Yuanzhi (*Radix Polygalae*) can restore normal coordination between the heart and kidney; Muxiang (*Radix Aucklandiae*) has an action of regulating qi and refreshing the spleen to prevent tonifying medicinal herbs from generating dampness and qi stagnation. For blood asthenia, Shudihuang (*Radix Rehmanniae Preparata*) and Ejiao (*Colla Corii Asini*) can be added, and powder of Ziheche (*Placenta Hominis*) may be used with oral infusion; for poor appetite, Sharen (*Fructus Amomi Villosi*), Baikouren (*Frectus Amomi Rotundus*) and Shenqu (*Massa Medicata Fermentata*) can be combined; for failure to lift lucid yang, frequent dizziness and vertigo, loose stool and prolapsing sensation of the anus, Chaihu (*Radix Bupleuri*) and Shengma (*Rhizoma Cimicifugae*) can be combined to lift lucid yang and dispel turbidity.

3. 肾精不足
26.3　Insufficiency of kidney essence

【症状】眩晕，精神萎靡不振，健忘，少眠多梦，腰膝酸软。偏于阴虚者，遗精、耳鸣，五心烦热，舌质红赤，脉象细数；偏于阳虚者，四肢不温，形寒怯冷，舌质淡，脉象沉细无力。

【分析】精髓不足，不能上充于脑，故眩晕，精神萎靡不振；肾虚则心肾不交，故健忘，少眠多梦；"腰为肾之府"，肾虚精不充养，则腰膝酸软。偏于阴虚者，"阴虚生内热"，故五心烦热；肾开窍于耳，阴虚生风，故耳鸣；阴虚则精关不固，故遗精；舌质红赤，脉象细数，为阴虚内热之象。偏于阳虚者，"阳虚生外寒"，故四肢不温，形寒怯冷；舌质淡，脉象沉细，为阳气不充之征。

【治法】偏于阴虚者，补肾滋阴；偏于阳虚者，补肾扶阳。

【方药】补肾滋阴，左归丸为主方。方中熟地黄、枸杞子、山茱萸补肾以滋真阴；龟鹿二胶为血肉有情之品，鹿角胶偏于补阳，龟板胶偏于补阴，两胶合力，沟通任督二脉，填精益髓，于补阴中含有"阳中求阴"之义；菟丝子配牛膝强腰膝，健筋骨；山药滋补脾肾。全方共奏滋肾填阴、育阴潜阳之效。本方滋补药较多，在具体运用时，可加入砂仁、陈皮理气醒脾之品，防止进补碍运之弊。阴虚内热明显者，可加知母、黄柏、地骨皮、牡丹皮等以滋阴清热。

补肾扶阳，右归丸为主方。方中附子、肉桂配合血肉有情的鹿角胶，温补肾阳，填精补髓；熟地黄、山茱萸、山药、菟丝子、枸杞子、杜仲，具有滋阴补肾、养肝补脾之效；更加当归补血养肝。诸药配伍，共奏温阳补肾、填精补血之功。若阳虚腹泻者，可加五味子、补骨脂补肾止泻；阳痿、遗精者，可加金樱子、桑螵蛸补肾固精。

Clinical manifestations: Dizziness and vertigo, dispiritedness, forgetfulness, insomnia and dreaminess and aching and weakness of the loins and knees. For yin asthenic constitution, manifestations such as seminal emission, tinnitus, feverish sensation over the palms, soles and chest, reddish tongue and thin and fast pulse will appear; for constitution of yang asthenia, the following manifestations such as cold limbs and body, aversion to cold, pale tongue and sunken, thin and weak pulse will appear.

Analysis: Dizziness, vertigo and dispiritedness are due to failure of insufficient essence and marrow to enrich the brain; forgetfulness, insomnia and dreaminess are due to kidney asthenia which gives rise to imbalance between heart-yang and kidney-yin; "the loins are the house of the kidney", aching and weakness of the loins and knees are due to failure of asthenic kidney to nourish kidney essence; feverish sensation over the palms, soles and chest is due to endogenous heat generated from yin asthenia; the kidney opens at the ears, tinnitus is due to "asthenic yin generating endogenous wind"; seminal emission is due to failure of asthenic yin to store sperms; reddish tongue and thin and fast pulse are signs of yin asthenia and endogenous heat; cold limbs and body and aversion to cold are due to "yang asthenia generating exogenous cold"; pale tongue and sunken and thin pulse are manifestations of failure to enrich yang qi.

Prescription: Tonify the kidney and nourish yin for yin asthenia syndrome; for yang asthenia, supplement the kidney and strengthen yang.

Formulas: Zuo Gui Wan used as a main formula to supplement the kidney and nourish yin. In the formula, Shudihuang (*Radix Rehmanniae Preparata*), Gouqizi (*Fructus Lycii*) and Shanzhuyu (*Fructus Corni*) have an action of tonifying the kidney to nourish kidney yin; Lujiaojiao (*Colla Corni Cervi*) is used to supplement yang, Guibanjiao (*Plastrum Testudinis Praeparatae*) is prone to supplementing yin, combined together, both of them can dredge the governor vessel and conception vessel by enriching essence and benefiting marrow, aiming at "achieving the effect of tonifying yin during supplementing yang"; Tusizi (*Semen Cuscutae*), combined with Niuxi (*Radix Achyranthis Bidentatae*) can strengthen the loins and knees and reinforce tendons and bones; Shanyao (*Rhizoma Dioscoreae*) has an action of tonifying the spleen and kidney. All medicinal herbs of the formula bring nourishing the kidney, enriching yin, supplementing yin and suppressing yang into full play. Because of too many medicinal herbs with the action of nourishing in the formula, so in clinical practice, Sharen (*Fructus Amomi Villosi*) and Chenpi (*Pericarpium Citri Reticulatae*) can be added to regulate qi and refresh the spleen so as to prevent drug of nourishing action from obstructing the function of the spleen in transportation. For obvious yin asthenia and endogenous heat, Zhimu (*Rhizoma Anemarrhenae*), Huangbo (*Cortex Phellodendri*), Digupi (*Cortex Lycii*) and Mudanpi

(*Cortex Moutan Radicis*) can be added to nourish yin and clear away heat.

You Gui Wan (Pill) is a principal recipe for supplementing the kidney and strengthening yang, of which, Fuzi (*Radix Aconiti Lateralis Preparata*), Rougui (*Cortex Cinnamomi*), together with Lujiaojiao (*Colla Corni Cervi*), have an action of tonifying kidney yang by warming and enriching essence and marrow; Shudihuang (*Radix Rehmanniae Preparata*), Shanzhuyu (*Fructus Corni*), Shanyao (*Rhizoma Dioscoreae*), Tusizi (*Semen Cuscutae*), Gouqizi (*Fructus Lycii*) and Duzhong (*Cortex Eucommiae*), can nourish yin and tonify the kidney, liver and spleen; Danggui (*Radix Angelicae Sinensis*) can be added to supplement blood and nourish the liver. For diarrhea due to yang asthenia, Wuweizi (*Fructus Schisandrae Chinensis*) and Buguzhi (*Fructus Psoraleae*) can be combined to supplement the kidney and stop diarrhea; for sexual impotence and seminal emission, Jinyingzi (*Fructus Rosae Laevigatae*) and Sangpiaoxiao (*Ootheca Mantidis*) can be combined to replenish the kidney and arrest spontaneous seminal emission.

4. 痰浊中阻
26.4　Obstruction of turbid phlegm in middle energizer

【症状】眩晕而见头重如裹，胸闷恶心，饮食减少，口黏，舌苔白腻，脉象濡滑。

【分析】痰浊中阻证多见于形体肥胖之人。痰浊蒙蔽清窍，则眩晕，头重如裹；痰浊中阻，胸阳不展，则胸闷恶心；痰浊病在中焦，脾湿不运，饮食减少；痰浊者，湿也，湿邪不化，则口黏；舌苔白腻，脉象濡滑，为痰浊不化之象。

【治法】燥湿祛痰，健脾和胃。

【方药】半夏白术天麻汤加味。半夏白术天麻汤出自清代程钟龄《医学心悟》，方义见“头痛”篇。若眩晕较甚，频作呕吐者，可加旋覆花、代赭石、竹茹、生姜以镇逆止呕；若脘闷不饥，可加砂仁、白蔻仁以醒脾开胃；若痰浊郁而化火，症见头目涨痛、心烦口苦、渴不欲饮，苔黄腻，脉弦滑，可改为黄连温胆汤，以清热祛湿，和胃调中。

Clinical manifestations: Dizziness and vertigo together with heavy sensation of the head like being wrapped, chest oppression and nausea, reduced appetite, sticky taste, greasy whitish fur as well as soft and slippery pulse.

Analysis: The syndrome is usually seen in obese patients. Dizziness and vertigo together with heavy sensation of the head like being wrapped are due to invasion of turbid phlegm into the upper orifices; chest oppression and nausea are due to obstruction of turbid phlegm in middle energizer and hypofunction of yang qi in the chest; reduced appetite is due to dysfunction of the spleen in transportation because of dampness in the spleen; turbid phlegm indicates dampness, sticky taste results from unresolved turbid dampness; greasy whitish fur and soft and slippery pulse are signs of unresolved turbid phlegm.

Prescription: Dry dampness to dispel phlegm, invigorate the spleen and harmonize the stomach.

Formulas：Banxia Baizhu Tianma Tang Jiawei (Modified Banxia Baizhu Tianma Decoction). This formula is quoted from *Yixue Xinwu* (*Medicine Comprehended*) by Cheng Zhongling from the Qing Dynasty, and its introduction has been discussed in the chapter of *Headache*. For severe dizziness, vertigo, and frequent vomiting, Xuanfuhua (*Flos Inulae*), Daizheshi (*Haematitum*), Zhuru (*Caulis Bambusae in Taenia*) and Shengjiang (*Rhizoma Zingiberis Recens*) can be added to suppress adverse qi and stop vomiting; for chest oppression and reduced appetite, Sharen (*Fructus Amomi Villosi*) and Baikouren (*Frectus Amomi Rotundus*) may be combined to refresh the spleen and promote appetite; for fire transformed from stagnation of turbid phlegm complicated with symptoms as distending pain of the head and eyes, vexation and bitter taste, thirst without desire to drink, greasy yellowish fur as well as taut and slippery pulse, Huanglian Wendan Tang (Decoction) can replace it to clear away heat, dispel dampness and harmonize the stomach to reconcile middle energizer.

5. 瘀血阻络
26.5 Blood stasis blocking blood vessels

【症状】眩晕，头痛，或见健忘、失眠、心悸，精神不振，面与唇色紫暗，舌有紫斑或瘀点，脉象弦涩。

【分析】病程日久，邪气入络入血，气血不得正常流布，脑失所养，故眩晕时作；瘀血不去，新血不生，心神失养，则可见健忘、失眠、心悸、精神不振等；而头痛，面、唇、舌紫暗或见瘀点，以及脉象弦涩，乃为瘀血内阻之象。

【治法】祛瘀生新，活血通络。

【方药】血府逐瘀汤加味。本方方义见"冠心病"篇。若兼见气虚自汗、气短乏力，可加黄芪补气行血；若形寒肢冷，可加附子、肉桂温经活血；若兼见骨蒸劳热，肌肤甲错，可加知母、黄柏、牡丹皮以清骨热；若精神不振，可加山茱萸、枸杞子以补肾填精；若健忘、失眠重，可加柏子仁、酸枣仁以安神宁心。

Clinical manifestations：Dizziness and vertigo, headache, or accompanied with forgetfulness, insomnia, palpitation, dispiritedness, dark purplish lips and complexion, dark purplish spots or petechiae on the tongue as well as taut and astringent pulse.

Analysis：Prolonged course of diseases causes invasion of pathogenic qi into blood vessels, which results in abnormal flow and distribution of qi and blood, malnutrition of the brain, thus, giving rise to frequent dizziness and vertigo; forgetfulness, insomnia, palpitation and dispiritedness are due to malnutrition of the heart and mind because of failure to generate new blood with unrelieved blood stasis; headache, dark purplish lips and complexion, dark purplish spots or petechiae on the tongue and taut and astringent pulse are signs of internal obstruction of blood stasis.

Prescription：Eliminate blood stasis, generate new blood and activate blood circulation to dredge blood vessels.

Formulas：Xuefu Zhuyu Tang Jiawei (Modified Xuefu Zhuyu Decoction), which has been approached in the chapter of *Coronary Disease*. For spontaneous sweating due to qi asthenia, short breath and lack of energy, Huangqi (*Radix Astragali seu Hedysari*) can be added to supplement qi and activate blood; for cold body and limbs, Fuzi (*Radix Aconiti Lateralis Preparata*) and Rougui (*Cortex Cinnamomi*) could be added to activate blood by warming meridians; for complicated symptoms such as bone steaming, consumptive fever and squamous skin, Zhimu (*Rhizoma Anemarrhenae*), Huangbo (*Cortex Phellodendri*) and Mudanpi (*Cortex Moutan Radicis*) should be combined to clear away heat from the bones; for dispiritedness and lassitude, Shanzhuyu (*Fructus Corni*) and Gouqizi (*Fructus Lycii*) can be added to supplement the kidney and enrich essence; for forgetfulness and insomnia, Baiziren (*Semen Platycladi*) and Suanzaoren (*Semen Ziziphi Spinosae*) can be added to calm the heart and tranquilize the mind.

二十七、抑郁症

27 Emotional depression

〔**概说**〕 Summary

　　抑郁症多有郁怒、多虑、悲哀、忧愁、恐惧等情志内伤病史。

　　中医学认为，抑郁症是由于情志不舒，气机郁滞所致。属于中医学"郁证""脏躁"等病证范畴。其临床表现为忧郁不畅，情绪不宁，表情淡漠，少语少动，或胸闷胁胀，善太息，或多疑多虑，焦急胆怯，或悲忧善哭，或不思饮食，失眠多梦，或易怒善哭等。所谓"郁"，有六，即气郁、血郁、湿郁、热郁、食郁、痰郁。但以气郁最为多见，是"六郁"之首。其发病部位主要在肝、脾、心、肾四脏，尤以肝气不舒为主。治疗上除药物、针灸外，心理开导也是非常重要的。

　　Emotional depression is usually seen in the patients with internal impairment of emotions such as depressed rage, overthought, sadness, melancholy as well as terror.

　　In TCM, the disease is caused by qi stagnation because of emotional discomfort, and it pertains to "depression syndrome" "hysteria" and so on. Clinical manifestations of it are marked by depression and unhappiness, disturbed emotion, indifferent facial expression, hypologia and no desire to move, or chest oppression and hypochondriac distention, frequent sigh, or oversensitivity and overthought, worry and timidity, or susceptibility to weep due to upset, or no appetite, insomnia and dreaminess, or susceptibility to rage and weep, etc. The so-called emotional "depression" or "stagnation" involves six aspects, namely, qi depression, blood stagnancy, stagnation of dampness, stagnation of heat, depression due to food retention as well as phlegmatic stagnation, with qi depression being the most common one, which is regarded as the first among the six aspects. The location of pathological changes of the disease is mainly in the liver, spleen, heart, and kidney, and qi depression in the liver is the primary one. Besides medication and acupuncture, psychological counseling serves as another essential treating method for the disease.

〔**辨证论治**〕 Syndrome differentiation and treatment

1. 肝气郁结

27.1　Stagnation of liver qi

【症状】精神抑郁，情绪不宁，胸部满闷，胁肋胀痛，痛无定处，不思饮食，时有嗳气，大便不调，舌苔薄腻，脉弦。

【分析】肝主疏泄，性喜条达，经脉布于胁肋，贯膈。肝气郁结，经脉不舒，其条达之性失和，故见精神抑郁，情绪不宁；其经脉所过之处，郁而不展，则胸部满闷，胁肋胀痛，且痛无定处；肝郁伤脾，则不思饮食，时有嗳气；脾气运化失常，故大便不调；舌苔与脉象均为肝郁伤脾之征。

【治法】疏肝解郁，理气和中。

【方药】柴胡疏肝散。方以四逆散加川芎、香附、陈皮而成。方中以四逆散疏肝解郁，川芎活血化瘀，香附理气解郁，陈皮健脾和中。若胁肋胀痛，可加郁金、佛手、青皮疏肝理气；肝气犯胃，嗳气频繁，可加旋覆花、紫苏梗、半夏和中降逆；兼有食滞中满，可加焦三仙健脾消食；腹胀明显者，可加代代花、厚朴花、三七花理气消胀；若舌有瘀点，可加桃仁、红花、丹参活血化瘀。

Clinical manifestations: Depression, emotional upset, fullness and oppression in the chest, distending pain in the chest and hypochondrium with unfixed position, poor appetite, occasional belching, irregular defecation, thin greasy tongue fur and taut pulse.

Analysis: The liver dominates dispersion, and it is characterized by growing and acting freely. Liver meridians are distributed in the region of the chest, hypochondrium, passing through the diaphragm. Qi depression in the liver causes faiure to relieve stagnation of qi in liver meridians and dysfunction of the liver in dispersion, which gives rise to depression and emotional upset; fullness and oppression in the chest, distending pain in the chest and hypochondrium with unfixed position are failure to relax the depressed region where liver meridians pass; poor appetite and occasional belching are caused by impairment of the spleen due to liver depression; irregular defecation is due to dysfunction of splenic qi in transportation and transformation; thin greasy tongue and taut pulse are signs of qi depression in the liver impairing the spleen.

Prescription: Sooth the liver by relieving stagnation, regulate qi and reconcile middle energizer.

Formulas: Chaihu Shugan San (Powder), which consists of Sini San in combination with Chuanxiong (*Rhizoma Ligustici Chuanxiong*), Xiangfu (*Rhizoma Cyperi*) and Chenpi (*Pericarpium Citri Reticulatae*). In the formula, Sini San can soothe the liver and relieve depression，Chuanxiong can promote blood circulation by dissolving blood stasis，Xiangfu has an action of regulating qi and relieving stagnation，and Chenpi may invigorate the spleen and harmonize middle energizer. For distending pain in the chest and hypochondrium，Yujin (*Radix Curcumae*) ，Foshou (*Fructus Citri Sarcodactylis*) and Qingpi (*Pericarpium Citri Reticulatae Viride*) can be added to soothe the liver and regulate qi；for liver qi invading the stomach and frequent belching，Xuanfuhua (*Flos Inulae*) ，Zisugeng (*Caulis Perllae*) and Banxia (*Rhizoma Pinelliae*) can be combined to reconcile middle energizer by descending adverse flow of qi；for complicated syndrome such as food retention and fullness and distention in middle energizer，stir-baked Maiya (*Fructus Hordei Germinatus*) ，Shanzha (*Fructus Crataegi*) and stir-baked Shenqu (*Massa Medicata Fermentata*) could be added to invigorate the spleen and eliminate food retention；for obvious abdominal distention，Daidaihua (*Citrus aurantium*) ，Houpohua (*Flos Magnoliae Officinalis*) and Sanqihua (*Flos Notoginseng*) can be added to regulate qi and eliminate abdominal distention；for petechiae on the tongue，Taoren (*Semen Persicae*) ，Honghua (*Flos Carthami*) and Danshen (*Radix Salviae Miltiorrhizae*) should be added to activate blood and dissolve stasis.

2. 痰气郁结
27.2　Stagnation of phlegm and qi

【症状】精神抑郁，胸部闷塞，胁肋胀痛，咽中如有物梗塞，吞之不下，咯之不出，舌苔白腻，脉象弦滑，或弦缓。

【分析】肝郁伤脾，脾气不运，湿聚生痰，痰气阻塞，正气不展，故精神抑郁，胸部闷塞；肝气不舒，其经脉自然郁滞，则出现胁肋胀痛；痰气交阻于胸膈之上，故咽中如有物梗塞，吞吐均不顺利；痰湿停滞，其舌苔白腻；肝气不舒，则脉象弦滑或弦缓。

【治法】行气开郁，化痰散结。

【方药】半夏厚朴汤。半夏厚朴汤出自《金匮要略》，由半夏、厚朴、茯苓、紫苏、生姜组成。方以厚朴、紫苏理气宽胸，开郁调中；半夏、茯苓、生姜化痰散结，和胃降逆。全方共奏辛香散结、行气开郁、降逆化痰之功。若湿痰较重，舌苔厚腻，可加苍术、佛手、橘红理气除湿；若湿痰化热，可加黄芩、竹茹、郁金清热化痰；若舌质有瘀点，可加丹参、降香、姜黄活血化瘀。

Clinical manifestations：Emotional depression，chest oppression，distending pain in the chest and hypochondium，sensation of foreign body being choked in the throat with difficulty to swallow and expectorate，greasy whitish fur and taut and slippery pulse or taut and moderate pulse.

Analysis：Qi depression in the liver impairing the spleen causes dysfunction of splenic qi in transportation，resulting in generation of phlegm due to accumulation of dampness，blockage of qi and phlegm，and stagnation of healthy qi，thus，giving rise to emotional depression and chest oppression；distending pain in the chest and hypochondrium are due to failure to soothe liver qi in liver meridians; sensation of foreign body being choked in the throat with difficulty to swallow and expectorate is due to obstruction of qi and phlegm in the chest and diaphragm; greasy whitish fur is due to internal accumulation of damp phlegm; taut and slippery pulse or taut and moderate pulse is a sign of stagnation of liver qi.

Prescription: Activate qi by dispersing stagnation and resolve accumulation of phlegm.

Formulas: Banxia Houpo Tang (Decocion). It is quoted from *Jingui Yaolue* (*Synopsis of Golden Chamber*), composed of Banxia (*Rhizoma Pinelliae*), Houpo (*Cortex Magnoliae Officinals*), Fuling (*Poriae Cocos*), Zisu (*Folium Perillae*) and Shengjiang (*Rhizoma Zingiberis Recens*). In the formula, Houpo and Zisu can regulate qi and ease the chest, disperse stagnated qi and harmonize middle energizer; Banxia, Fuling and Shengjiang can resolve phlegm and scatter lumps, reconcile the stomach and descend adverse flow of qi. The whole formula can bring the action of scattering lumps, activating qi by dispersing stagnation, descending adverse qi and resolving phlegm into full play with its pungent and aromatic nature. For severe damp phlegm and thick greasy fur, Cangzhu (*Rhizoma Atractylodis*), Foshou (*Fructus Citri Sarcodactylis*) and Juhong (*Exocarpium Citri Rubrum*) can be combined to regulate qi and eliminate dampness; for heat transformed from damp phlegm, Huangqin (*Radix Scutellariae*), Zhuru (*Caulis Bambusae in Taenia*) and Yujin (*Radix Curcumae*) can be added to clear away heat and resolve phlegm; for petechiae on the tongue, Danshen (*Radix Salviae Miltiorrhizae*), Jiangxiang (*Lignum Dalbergiae Odoriferae*) and Jianghuang (*Rhizoma Curcumae Longae*) may be combined to activate blood and dissolve blood stasis.

3. 心脾两虚
27.3 Asthenia of the heart and spleen

【症状】多思善疑，心悸胆怯，头晕如裹，失眠健忘，不思饮食，面色无华，舌质淡红，苔薄白，脉细。

【分析】忧愁思虑，久而不解，则损伤心脾，心主神，脾主思，心脾两伤，故见心悸胆怯、多思善疑、头晕如裹；心不守神，则失眠健忘；脾伤则不思饮食；脾不生化气血，则面色无华；舌质淡红，为气血不足之象；脉细，亦为虚象。总之，本证为心脾虚证，只是在临床上有心虚与脾虚轻重不同之别。

【治法】养心健脾，补气养血。

【方药】归脾汤。方以人参、茯苓、白术、甘草、黄芪补气健脾，当归、龙眼肉养血宁心，酸枣仁、远志、茯苓养心安神，木香理气醒脾。全方补而不滞，温和不寒，是健脾养心的代表方剂。若忧愁不解，可加石菖蒲、郁金解郁开窍；不思饮食，可加生麦芽、鸡内金开胃进食；若心悸、胆怯不解，改用温胆汤加味治疗。

Clinical manifestations: Excess thought and susceptibility to doubt, palpitation and timidity, dizziness with a sensation of like being wrapped, insomnia and forgetfulness, poor appetite, lusterless complexion, pale reddish tongue, thin whitish fur as well as thin pulse.

Analysis: Prolonged and unrelieved overthought and susceptibility to doubt result in impairment of the heart and spleen. The heart governs the mind, and the spleen dominates thought, impairment of the heart and spleen gives rise to palpitation and timidity, overthought and doubt as well as dizziness with a sensation of being wrapped; insomnia and forgetfulness are due to failure of the heart to house the spirit; poor appetite is due to impairment of the spleen; lusterless complexion is due to dysfunction of the spleen in generating and transforming qi and blood; pale reddish tongue is a sign of insufficiency of qi and blood; thin pulse indicates asthenia syndrome. Generally speaking, this syndrome is asthenia of the spleen and heart, which could be differentiated in clinical practice according to the seriousness of heart asthenia or the degree of spleen asthenia.

Prescription: Nourish the heart, invigorate the spleen and tonify qi and blood.

Formulas: Guipi Tang (Decoction). In the formula, Renshen (*Radix Ginseng*), Fuling (*Poriae Cocos*), Baizhu (*Rhizoma Atractylodis Macrocephalae*), Gancao (*Radix Glycyrrhizae*) and Huangqi (*Radix Astragali seu Hedysari*) can supplement qi and invigorate the spleen; Duanggui (*Radix Angelicae Sinensis*) and Longyanrou (*Arillus Longan*) have an action of nourishing blood and tranquilizing the heart; Suanzaoren (*Semen Ziziphi Spinosae*), Yuanzhi (*Radix Polygalae*) and Fuling (*Poriae Cocos*) can nourish the heart and calm the mind; Muxiang (*Radix Aucklandiae*) has an action of regulating qi and refreshing the spleen. The whole recipe, warm but not cold in nature, is a typical one for invigorating the spleen and nourishing the heart by tonifying qi without stagnation. For unrelieved grief and worry, Shichangpu (*Rhizoma Acori Tatarinowii*) and Yujin (*Radix Curcumae*) should be added to eliminate stagnation and awaken consciousness of the orifices; for poor appetite, Shengmaiya (*Fructus Hordei Germinatus*) and Jineijin (*Endothelium Corneum Gigeriae Galli*) can be combined to promote appetite; for unrelieved palpitation and timidity, Wendan Tang Jiawei (Modified Wendan Decoction) can be used to replace Guipi Tang.

4. 阴虚火旺

27.4 Exuberant fire due to yin asthenia

【症状】精神恍惚，心神不宁，五心烦热，手舞足蹈，或走动无常，骂詈号叫，舌质红赤，脉象细数。

【分析】心肝肾阴虚，则会出现阴虚火旺之证。神不守舍，则精神恍惚，心神不宁；"阴虚生内热"，则五心烦热；肝热失于舒条之性，则手舞足蹈，或走动无常；肾阴虚甚，则虚火上炎，使心火更旺，故见骂詈号叫；舌象与脉象为阴虚火旺之征。

【治法】滋阴降火，宁心安神。

【方药】天王补心丹。方以生地黄、天冬、麦冬、玄参滋养心、肾、肝三脏之阴；人参、茯苓、五味子、当归养血益气；柏子仁、酸枣仁、远志、丹参养心安神。若有盗汗，可加牡丹皮、地骨皮、浮小麦、桑叶清热止汗；若走动无常，骂詈号叫，可加生磁石、珍珠母镇肝潜阳；若夜眠不安，可加重酸枣仁的用量，另加夜交藤、莲子心、焦栀子清心火而安心神。

Clinical manifestations：Absent-mindedness, disturbed spirit and mind, feverish sensation over the palms, soles and chest; abnormal or manic movement; shouting with sonorous voice, reddish tongue as well as thin and fast pulse.

Analysis：This syndrome is usually caused by yin asthenia of the heart and liver. Absent-mindedness, disturbed heart and mind are due to failure of the heart to house the mind; feverish sensation over the palms, soles and chest are due to "yin asthenia generating endogenous heat"; abnormal or manic movement is caused by failure to disperse liver qi because of heat in the liver; shouting with sonorous voice is due to up-flaring of asthenic fire because of aggravated yin asthenia of the kidney, which leads to hyperactive heart fire; reddish tongue and thin and fast pulse are signs of yin asthenia and hyperactive fire.

Prescription：Nourish yin, descend fire and tranquilize the heart and mind.

Formulas：Tianwang Buxin Dan (Pill). In the formula, Shengdihuang (*Radix Rehmanniae Recens*), Tiandong (*Radix Asparagi*), Maidong (*Radix Ophiopogonis*) and Xuanshen (*Radix Scrophulariae*) can nourish yin in the heart, kidney and liver; Renshen (*Radix Ginseng*), Fuling (*Poriae Cocos*), Wuweizi (*Fructus Schisandrae Chinensis*) and Danggui (*Radix Angelicae Sinensis*) may nourish blood and benefit qi; Baiziren (*Semen Platycladi*), Suanzaoren (*Semen Ziziphi Spinosae*), Yuanzhi (*Radix Polygalae*) and Danshen (*Radix Salviae Miltiorrhizae*) have an action of calming the heart and tranquilizing the mind. For night sweating, Mudanpi (*Cortex Moutan Radicis*), Digupi (*Cortex Lycii*), Fuxiaomai (*Fructus Tritici Levis*) and Sangye (*Folium Mori*) can be added to clear away heat and stop night sweating; for abnormal or manic movement, shouting and sonorous voice, Shengcishi (*Magnetitum*) and Zhenzhumu (*Concha Margaritifera*) should be combined to calm the liver and suppress yang; for disturbed sleep, Suanzaoren should be added in a large amount, Yejiaoteng (*Caulis Polygoni Multiflori*), Lianzixin (*Plumula Nelumbinis*) and stir-baked Zhizi (*Fructus Gardeniae*) can be combined to purge heart fire and tranquilize the mind.

5. 心胆气虚
27.5   Qi asthenia in the heart and gallbladder

【症状】抑郁善忧，情绪不宁，胆怯恐惧，自卑绝望，难以决断，或易烦善哭，失眠多梦，易于惊醒，咽中异物感，舌质淡，苔薄白，脉沉细或细而无力。

【分析】"心为五脏六腑之大主""胆主决断"，心胆气虚，则心无主事，胆无决断，故人的情绪不宁，抑郁善忧，胆怯绝望；心虚则神不守舍，故失眠多梦，易于惊醒；胆虚则善哭，且自卑易烦，遇事难以决断；胆虚则升降之气失序，故咽中有异物感；其舌与脉均为虚象。

【治法】清胆宁心，化痰理气。

【方药】十味温胆汤。方由温胆汤去竹茹，加人参、熟地黄、五味子、酸枣仁、远志组成。方取温胆汤清胆且化痰，所加人参、熟地黄为补气养血之主药，五味子、酸枣仁宁心安神，远志化痰理气。全方药味虽较平淡，但其功效却不可轻视。对于心胆气虚，痰气郁结所引起的诸多疾病，均有良好效果。

Clinical manifestations：Emotional depression, melancholy, restlessness, timidity and terror, self-contempt and despair, hesitancy, or vexation and frequent upset, insomnia and dreaminess, susceptibility to waking up, sensation of foreign body in the throat, pale tongue, thin whitish fur as well as sunken and thin pulse or thin and weak pulse.

Analysis："The heart is the governor of five-zang and six-fu organs." "The gallbladder dominates the ability of decision." Qi asthenia in the heart and gallbladder results in failure of the heart in governing and failure of the gallbladder in making decision, giving rise to emotional restlessness, depression and worry, timidity and despair; insomnia and dreaminess and susceptibility to waking up are caused by asthenia of the heart, which results in failure of the heart in housing the mind; frequent upset, self-contempt, susceptibility to vexation and hesitancy are due to asthenia of the gallbladder; sensation of foreign body in the throat is due to disorder of lifting and descending; pale tongue, thin whitish fur and sunken and thin pulse or thin and weak pulse are signs of asthenia.

Prescription：Clear the gallbladder and tranquilize the heart, resolve phlegm and regulate qi.

Formulas：Shiwei Wendan Tang (Decoction). The formula is a modified Wendan Tang by removing Zhuru (*Caulis Bambusae in Taenia*) and combining with Renshen (*Radix Ginseng*), Shudihaung (*Radix Rehmanniae Praeparata*), Wuweizi (*Fructus Schisandrae Chinensis*), Suanzaoren (*Semen Ziziphi Spinosae*) and Yuanzhi (*Radix Polygalae*). In the formula, Wendan Tang has an action of clearing away gallbladder and resolving phlegm, the combination of Renshen and Shudihuang are the major drug to supplement qi and nourish blood, Wuweizi and Suanzaoren can tranquilize the heart and mind, Yuanzhi may resolve phlegm and regulate qi. Though the formula is neutral in nature and bland in flavor, it can exert effective function for treating diseases caused by qi asthenia of the heart and gallbladder and accumulation of qi and phlegm.

二十八、老年性痴呆

28　Senile dementia

〔**概说**〕　Summary

老年性痴呆（阿尔茨海默病）是发生在老年期的慢性进行性精神衰退性疾病。一般多见于60岁以上的老年人。其精神症状比较突出，如性格孤僻，多疑自私，主观固执，或缺乏羞辱感和责任感；记忆力缺损，经常失落东西，计算、理解、判断、工作能力下降；甚则生活不能自理，语言杂乱无章，二便失禁等。脑电图与脑CT检查，都有异常变化。

老年性痴呆归属于中医学"痴呆""呆病"等范畴。心藏神，肝藏魂，肾藏志，脾藏意，肺藏魄，痴呆应与五脏功能失调有关，尤以心、肝、肾三脏关系密切。肝肾阴精不足，心血失养，脾湿生痰，血瘀脑络等是其发病机制。治疗上不主张单纯用"补法"，而主张辨证论治，多于补中寓通，或通中寓补，补通兼施；提倡形体锻炼，心理养生，"防患于未然"，这对患病以后的恢复，也是有益的。

Senile dementia (Alzheimer's disease) is a disease usually seen in ageing people over 60 years old, marked by progressive long-term decline of mental ability, with striking symptoms of mental disease such as loneliness, being suspicious and selfish, stubborn personality, or lack of sense of shamefulness and responsibility; loss or decline of memory, forgetfulness, difficulty in communication and understanding, poor judgment and inefficiency, even inability to perform daily activities, confused or disordered language, and abnormal changes of the brain in electroencephalogram and computed tomography.

In terms of TCM, senile dementia pertains to "dementia" "idiocy", and so on. The heart stores Shen (the mind), the liver stores Hun (the soul), the kidney stores Zhi (the emotion), the spleen stores Yi (the thinking), and the lung houses Po (the spirit), dementia is related to dysfunction of five-zang organs, and it is closely connected with the heart, liver and kidney in particular. Pathogenesis for it is insufficient yin and essence in the liver and kidney, which results in malnutrition of heart blood, generation of phlegm due to dampness in the spleen as well as blood stasis in the blood vessels of the brain. Treatment for the disease should not be confined to supplementing but based on syndrome differentiation, which involves mostly, supplementing combined with dredging blood vessels, cultivation of physique and psychologically life nurturing as well as "guarding against future diseases". These therapeutic methods are very beneficial to help patients get restored from diseases.

〔辨证论治〕 Syndrome differentiation and treatment

1. 肝肾亏损
28.1　Deficiency of the liver and kidney

【症状】表情呆板，行动迟缓，头晕眼花，腰膝酸软，健忘失眠，反应迟钝，口干，大便干结，舌质嫩暗，苔薄白，脉象细弱。

【分析】肝主魂，肾主志，肝肾阴精不足，不能主魂主志，故表情呆板、头晕眼花；肝主筋，肾主骨，肝肾亏损，则行动迟缓、腰膝酸软；脑髓空虚，故健忘失眠、反应迟钝；阴不足，则口干、大便干结；阴精失养，故舌质嫩暗、脉象细弱。

【治法】补益肝肾，填精益髓。

【方药】左归丸加减。左归丸为填精益髓之主剂，张景岳称之为"壮水之主，以培左肾之元阴，而精血自足矣"。其方义见"高血压病"篇。伴有干咳者，加百合；夜热者，加地骨皮；大便燥结者，加肉苁蓉；气虚者，加人参；腰膝酸软，加杜仲；夜尿多，肾气不守也，加补骨脂、核桃仁。

Clinical manifestations：Stiffness of facial expression，tardiness of movement，dizziness and blurred vision，aching and weakness of the loins and kness，forgetfulness and insomnia，dull reacting ability，dry mouth，dry feces，tender darkish tongue with thin whitish fur as well as thin and weak pulse.

Analysis：The liver dominates Hun (the soul)，the kidney governs Zhi (the emotion or aspiration)，insufficiency of yin and essence causes failure in dominating the soul and emotion，which gives rise to dull expression，dizziness and blurred vision；the liver dominates tendons and the kidney governs bones，deficiency of the liver and kidney results in tardiness of movement and aching and weakness of the Loins and knees；insomnia and forgetfulness and tardy reaction are due to vacuous or scanty marrow of the brain；dry mouth and constipation are signs of insufficiency of yin；tender darkish tongue and thin and weak pulse are due to malnutrition of yin and essence.

Prescription：Supplement the liver and kidney，enrich essence and tonify marrow.

Formulas：Zuogui Wan Jiajian (Modified Zuogui Pill). Zuo Gui Wan is a principal formula of enriching essence and tonifying marrow，named by Zhang Jingyue as "nourishing yin to enrich primordial qi and yin in the left kidney to ensure sufficiency of essence and blood". And the formula has been discussed in the chapter of *Hypertension*. For dry cough，Baihe (*Bulbus Lilii*) can be added；for fever at night，Digupi (*Cortex Lycii*) should be added；for dry feces，Roucongrong (*Herba Cistanches*) may be combined；for qi asthenia，Renshen (*Radix Ginseng*) can be added；for aching sensation and weakness of the loins and knees，Duzhong (*Cortex Eucommiae*) should be combined；for frequent night urination and failure to astringe kidney qi，Buguzhi (*Fructus Psoraleae*) and Hetaoren (*Juglans Regia*) can be added.

2. 阴虚火旺

28.2 Yin asthenia and fire exuberance

【症状】情绪急躁，烦躁不安，语言颠倒，或盗汗失眠，口干口苦，面色潮红，头昏耳鸣，舌质红，脉象细数。

【分析】肝肾阴虚火旺，火性炎上，扰乱心神，则极易烦躁不安；"言为心声"，心火不宁，故语言颠倒；阴虚内热，故盗汗失眠；阴津不能上润，故口干口苦；"心其华在面"，火旺于上，则面色潮红；头宜宁静，火邪干扰，则头昏耳鸣；舌质红，脉象细数，为阴虚火旺之明证。

【治法】滋阴清热，宁心安神。

【方药】麦味知柏地黄汤加减。麦味知柏地黄汤，即六味地黄汤加麦冬、五味子、知母、黄柏。六味地黄汤为滋阴清热主剂，具有补益肝肾之阴，清泻肝肾虚火的功效。烦躁不安，可加黄连、焦栀子清热除烦；头昏头痛，可加石决明、夏枯草清肝潜阳；盗汗，可加浮小麦、霜桑叶清泻阴火；语言颠倒，可加石菖蒲、炙远志宁心增智，橘红、贝母化痰解郁。

Clinical manifestations: Emotional restlessness, vexation, paraphasia, or night sweating and insomnia, dry mouth and bitter taste, tidal flushed complexion, dizziness and tinnitus, reddish tongue as well as thin and fast pulse.

Analysis: Up-flaring of exuberant fire and disturbance of the heart and spirit are due to yin asthenia of the liver and kidney, which gives rise to susceptibility to restlessness; "speech can indicate condition of the heart", hyperactive fire in the heart causes paraphasia; night sweating and insomnia are due to yin asthenia and endogenous heat; dry mouth and bitter taste are due to failure of yin fluid to moisten the upper part of the body; "the manifestation of the heart is on the face", tidal flushed complexion is due to up-flaring of hyperactive fire; dizziness and tinnitus are due to disturbance of fire pathogen; reddish tongue and thin and fast pulse are obvious signs of yin asthenia and fire exuberance.

Prescription: Nourish yin, clear away heat, calm the heart and tranquilize the mind.

Formulas: Mai Wei Zhi Bo Dihuang Tang Jiajain (Modified Mai Wei Zhi Bo Dihuang Decoction). It is a combination of Liuwei Dihuang Tang with Maidong (*Radix Ophiopogonis*), Wuweizi (*Fructus Schisandrae Chinensis*), Zhimu (*Rhizoma Anemarrhenae*) and Huangbo (*Cortex Phellodendri*). Liuwei Dihuang Tang, with the action of tonifying yin in the liver and kidney and purging asthenic fire in the liver and kidney, is a principal formula for nourishing yin and clearing away heat. For restlessness and vexation, Huanglian (*Rhizoma Coptidis*) and stir-baked Zhizi (*Fructus Gardeniae*) can be combined to clear away heat and eliminate vexation; for dizziness and headache, Shijueming (*Concha Haliotidis*) and Xiakucao (*Spica Prunellae*) may be added to clear away liver fire and suppress yang; for night sweating, Fuxiaomai (*Fructus Tritici Levis*) and frost-stricken Sangye (*Folium Mori*) can be combined to purge yin fire; for paraphasia, Shichangpu (*Rhizoma Acori Tatarinowii*) and stir-baked Yuanzhi (*Radix Polygalae*) can be added to calm the heart and improve intelligence, Juhong (*Exocarpium Citri Rubrum*) and Beimu (*Bulbus Fritillaria*) should be combined to resolve phlegm and relieve depression.

3. 脾虚痰阻
28.3　Obstruction of phlegm due to asthenic spleen

【症状】终日郁闷不乐，呆板迟缓，面色萎黄，表情淡漠，生活不能自理，时而喃喃自语，不知所言，腹胀纳呆，气短乏力，舌质淡胖，苔白腻，脉象细滑。

【分析】脾虚生湿，湿浊生痰，痰浊不化，郁于胸中，心气不展，则终日闷闷不乐；血不华面，故面色萎黄；湿浊为阴邪，阴邪主静，故表情淡漠，行动迟缓而呆板；中气不足，难以发声，故喃喃自语，虽言而不知所言之内容，且显得气短乏力；脾不运化，则腹胀纳呆；舌质淡胖，气虚也，苔白腻，湿也；脉象细滑，湿浊内蕴之象也。

【治法】益气健脾，化痰开窍。

【方药】香砂六君子汤加味。香砂六君子汤为益气健脾化痰的主剂。方以人参、白术、茯苓、甘草补益中气；木香、砂仁理气消胀；陈皮、半夏燥湿化痰，且有降逆祛浊之作用。可加石菖蒲、炙远志醒脑开窍；舌苔黄腻者，可加黄连、郁金清热化痰；腹胀纳呆者，可加鸡矢藤、生麦芽、鸡内金消胀进食。

Clinical manifestations：Emotional depression, dull expression and tardy movement, sallow complexion or indifferent expression, inability to live by oneself, frequent murmuring of nonsense, abdominal distension and poor appetite, short breath and lack of energy, bulgy pale tongue with greasy whitish fur as well as thin and slippery pulse.

Analysis：Asthenic spleen generates dampness, turbid dampness transforms into phlegm, stagnation of unresolved phlegmatic turbidity in the chest results in qi stagnation in the heart and emotional depression; sallow complexion is due to failure of blood to nourish the face; turbid dampness is a pathogenic yin factor indicating quietness, which gives rise to indifferent and dull expression and tardy movement; insufficient qi in middle energizer brings about loss of voice which gives rise to murmuring with nonsense, short breath as well as lack of energy; abdominal distension and poor appetite are due to dysfunction of the spleen in transportation and transformation; bulgy pale tongue indicates qi asthenia; greasy whitish fur suggests dampness; thin and slippery pulse is a sign of internal retention of turbid dampness.

Prescription：Supplement qi, invigorate the spleen, resolve phlegm and induce resuscitation of consciousness.

Formulas：Xiang Sha Liujunzi Tang Jiawei (Modified Xiang Sha Liujunzi Decoction). Xiang Sha Liujunzi Tang is a principal formula for supplementing qi, invigorating the spleen and resolving phlegm. In the formula, Renshen (*Radix Ginseng*), Baizhu (*Rhizoma Atractylodis Macrocephalae*), Fuling (*Poriae Cocos*) and Gancao (*Radix Glycyrrhizae*) can supplement qi in middle energizer; Muxiang (*Radix Aucklandiae*) and Sharen (*Fructus Amomi Villosi*) can regulate qi and eliminate abdominal distension; Chenpi (*Pericarpium Citri Reticulatae*) and Banxia (*Rhizoma Pinelliae*) have an action of drying dampness, resolving phlegm, descending adverse qi and dispelling turbid dampness. Shichangpu (*Rhizoma Acori Tatarinowii*) and stir-baked Yuanzhi (*Radix Polygalae*) can be added to refresh the brain and induce resuscitation of consciousness; for greasy yellowish tongue fur, Huanglian (*Rhizoma Coptidis*) and Yujin (*Radix Curcumae*) may be added to clear away heat and resolve phlegm; for abdominal distension and poor appetite, Jishiteng (*Paederia Foetida*), Shengmaiya (*Fructus Hordei Germinatus*) and Jineijin (*Endothelium Corneum Gigeriae Galli*) can be added to eliminate distension and promote appetite.

4. 气滞血瘀
28.4 Qi stagnation and blood stasis

【症状】表情淡漠，善恐善忘，寡言少语，反应迟钝，头痛如刺如锥，舌质紫暗，苔白腻，脉象细弦或沉涩。

【分析】心主神，其华在面，心血淤滞，则表情淡漠；脑为髓海，气滞血瘀，络脉不和，脑髓空虚，故善恐善忘，反应迟钝；言为心声，心脉淤滞，血不养心，故寡言少语；气滞血瘀，脑络不通，则头痛如刺，或如锥刺；舌质紫暗，脉象细涩，为血瘀必然所见。

【治法】理气活血，通窍健脑。

【方药】通窍活血汤加味。方中赤芍、川芎、桃仁、红花四味以活血化瘀为主药；葱白、生姜、麝香三味为辅药，以通窍建功；并以酒为引，起到增强药力，通经达络的作用。临床应用时，可加石菖蒲、炙远志开窍增智；若血瘀化热，症见夜热早凉，口渴不欲饮，可加牡丹皮、地骨皮、生地黄凉血活血透热。

Clinical manifestations: Emotional indifference, frequent fright and forgetfulness, hypologia, tardy reaction, headache like being pierced with a wimble, purple and darkish tongue with greasy whitish fur as well as thin and taut pulse or sunken and astringent pulse.

Analysis: The heart dominates the spirit with its manifestations on the face, qi stagnation and blood stasis give rise to emotional indifference; the brain is the sea of marrow, qi stagnation and blood stasis, disharmony between collaterals and blood vessels and insufficient marrow in the brain bring about susceptibility to fright, forgetfulness and tardy reaction; speech indicates the activity of the heart, blood stasis of the heart vessels and failure of blood to nourish the heart result in hypologia; headache like being pierced is due to qi stagnation and blood stasis, which results in obstructive blood vessels of the brain; purple and darkish fur and thin and astringent pulse are signs of blood stasis.

Prescription: Regulate qi, activate blood, induce resuscitation of consciousness and strengthen the brain.

Formulas: Tongqiao Huoxue Tang Jiawei (Modified Tongqiao Huoxue Decoction). In the formula, Chishao (*Radix Paeoniae Rubra*), Chuanxiong (*Rhizoma Ligustici Chuanxiong*), Taoren (*Semen Persicae*) and Honghua (*Flos Carthami*) are used as principal drug to activate blood and dissolve stasis; Congbai (*Allium Fistulosum*), Shengjiang (*Rhizoma Zingiberis Recens*) and Shexiang (*Moschus*) are used as assistant drug to induce resuscitation of consciousness; wine can be used as medicinal usher to strengthen function of medicine and dredge meridians and collaterals. In clinic, Shichangpu (*Rhizoma Acori Tatarinowii*) and stir-baked Yuanzhi (*Radix Polygalae*) can be added to awaken consciousness and improve intelligence; for heat transformed from blood stasis with the symptom of worsening fever at night, Mudanpi (*Cortex Moutan Radicis*), Digupi (*Cortex Lycii*) and Shengdihuang (*Radix Rehmanniae Recens*) can be added to cool blood, activate blood and let out heat.

二十九、中风

29　Cerebral apoplexy

〔**概说**〕　Summary

中风又名"卒中"，它包括出血性脑血管病和缺血性脑血管病，临床表现以猝然昏仆、口眼㖞斜、半身不遂为其主要特征，亦有不见猝然昏仆，仅见㖞斜不遂者。本病的发病率、病死率、病残率均较高，严重危害人民的健康。

中医认为本病多由恣酒纵欲、饮食不节、恼怒忧思等因素，以致阴阳失调，气血错乱，经络失和等引起。其病机有心火暴盛、正气虚弱、湿痰生热、气血郁滞等。临床上有中经络、中脏腑，以及闭证、脱证和后遗症等证候区分。中药配合针灸、按摩等治疗，常能取得比较好的效果。

Cerebral apoplexy, known as "blood stroke", includes apoplexy induced by hemorrhagic cerebrovascular disease and by ischemic cerebrovascular disease, with clinical manifestations such as sudden unconsciousness and collapse, facial distortion and hemiplegia. In some cases, individuals may not suddenly collapse or lose consciousness. Instead, they may just suffer from hemiplegia (paralysis on one side of the body) and facial distortion. The disease has a high incidence, fatality and rate of invalidism, so it is very harmful to the health of people.

In terms of TCM, cerebral apoplexy is caused by the following factors such as alcoholism, intemperate sexual life, improper diet as well as excess rage and thought, resulting in disharmony of yin and yang, disordered qi and blood circulation and failure to reconcile meridians and collaterals. Pathogenesis of the disease includes hyperactivity of heart fire, asthenia of healthy qi, transformation of heat from phlegmatic dampness, and stagnation of qi and blood. Clinically, it is classified into stroke involving the meridians and collaterals, apoplexy involving zang-fu organs, apoplexy due to blockage, apoplexy due to collapse as well as apoplexy due to sequelae. Treatment for it by means of TCM can achieve an effective result in combination with therapeutic methods such as acupuncture, moxibustion and massage.

〔**辨证论治**〕　Syndrome differentiation and treatment

（一）中经络

29.1　Apoplexy involving the meridians and collaterals

1. 络脉空虚，风邪入中

29.1.1　Stroke of pathogenic wind in vacant collaterals

【症状】手足麻木，肌肤不仁，或突然口眼㖞斜，语言不利，口角流涎，甚则半身不遂；或兼见恶寒发热，肢体拘急，关节酸痛，舌苔薄白，脉象浮弦。

【分析】卫外不固，络脉空虚，风邪趁虚而入，肌肤气血不畅，筋脉失于濡养，则见手足麻木、肌肤不仁、口眼㖞斜、语言不利，甚则半身不遂等症；若风邪袭于肌表，肌表失于护卫，则见恶寒发热、肢体拘急、关节酸痛等症；舌苔薄白、脉象浮弦，为风邪入表之征。

【治法】祛风通络。

【方药】大秦艽汤加减。大秦艽汤为风邪初入经络而设，清代医学界汪昂称之为"六经中风轻者之通剂也"。方中以秦艽祛风通经活络，为主药；羌活、独活、防风、白芷、细辛，均为辛温之品，能祛风散邪，为辅药；风药多燥，故配以当归、白芍、熟地黄养血柔筋，使风药不伤阴津；又用川芎活血通络；又气能生血，故配以白术、茯苓益气健脾，以助生化之源；至于黄芩、石膏、生地黄凉血清热，是为风邪化热而设；另以甘草调和诸药。诸药合用，共奏祛风清热、养血活血之效。具体应用时，可酌加丹参、鸡血藤、穿山甲活血通络，即"治风先治血，血行风自灭"之意。

Clinical manifestations: Numbness of the hands, feet and skin, or sudden facial distortion, slurred speech, saliva from the mouth, even hemiplegia; or accompanied with fever and aversion to cold, spasm of the limbs, sore and painful sensation of the joints, thin whitish fur as well as floating and taut pulse.

Analysis: Failure of defensive yang to protect the superficies and vacuous collaterals cause invasion of wind pathogen into blood vessels, obstructed qi and blood circulation in the superficial skin and muscles and malnutrition of tendons and vessels, giving rise to numbness of the hands, feet and skin, distorted mouth and eyes, slurred speech, even hemiplegia; fever, aversion to cold, spasm of the limbs and sore and painful sensation of the joints are due to failure of muscles and skin to avoid invasion of wind pathogen; thin whitish fur as well as floating and taut pulse are due to wind pathogen invading the superficial skin.

Prescription: Dispel wind and dredge blood vessels.

Formulas: Da Qinjiao Tang Jiajian (Modified Large Qinjiao Decoction). Da Qinjiao Tang is designed for treating invasion of wind pathogen into meridians and collaterals and named by Wang Ang from the Qing Dynasty as "the common formula for slight apoplexy involving six meridians". In the formula, Qinjiao (*Radix Gentianae Macrophyllae*) is used as principal drug to dredge meridians and activate blood circulation, Qianghuo (*Rhizoma et Radix Notopterygii*); Duhuo (*Radix Angelicae Pubescentis*), Fangfeng (*Radix Saposnikoviae*), Baizhi (*Radix Angelicae Dahuricae*) and Xixin (*Herba Asari*), pungent and warm in nature, are used as assistant drug to dispel wind pathogens; the drug of treating wind pathogen is usually dry in nature, so Danggui (*Radix Angelicae Sinensis*), Baishao (*Radix Paeoniae Alba*) and Shudihuang (*Radix Rehmanniae Preparata*) are combined to nourish blood and soften tendons to avoid impairment of yin fluid because of the adoption of the above herbs; Chuanxiong (*Rhizoma Ligustici Chuanxiong*) can be added to activate blood, dredge blood vessels, promote qi circulation and generate blood, so Baizhu (*Rhizoma Atractylodis Macrocephalae*) and Fuling (*Poriae Cocos*) are added to supplement qi and invigorate the spleen to improve the function of the source of transformation; Huangqin (*Radix Scutellariae*), Shigao (*Gypsum Fibrosum*) and Shengdihuang (*Radix Rehmanniae Recens*) are used to expel heat transformed from wind pathogen with their action of cooling blood and clearing away heat; Gancao (*Radix Glycyrrhizae*) can be added to reconcile the above medicinal herbs. Combined together, the whole formula can bring dispelling wind, clearing away heat, nourishing blood and activating blood into full play. In clinical practice, Danshen (*Radix Salviae Miltiorrhizae*), Jixueteng (*Caulis Spatholobi*) and Chuanshanjia (*Squama Manis*) can be combined to activate blood and dredge blood vessels, which is in accord with the remark "treat apoplexy by activating blood, which, in turn, could eliminate wind pathogen".

2. 肝肾阴虚，风阳上扰

29.1.2 Up-disturbance of wind transformed from liver yang due to yin asthenia of the liver and kidney

【症状】平素头晕头痛，耳鸣耳聋，少眠多梦，突然发生口眼㖞斜、语言謇涩，舌强不利，或手足滞重，甚则半身不遂，舌质红赤，苔腻，脉象弦细数。

【分析】素体肝肾阴虚，易致肝阳上亢，故平时就会头晕头痛、耳鸣耳聋；肾阴不足，心肾不交，则少眠多梦；风阳上扰，干扰脑络，脑络失灵，故突发口眼㖞斜、语言謇涩、半身不遂；脉弦主肝风，数脉主阴虚。脉证合参，乃阴虚阳亢之象。

【治法】滋阴潜阳，熄风通络。

【方药】镇肝熄风汤加减。本方为近代名医张锡纯的经验方，是治疗肝阳偏亢，风阳上扰的主选方药。方中怀牛膝归肝、肾二经，并引血下行，有补益肝肾的功效，为主药；辅以龙骨、牡蛎镇肝熄风，更以龟板、玄参、白芍、天冬滋阴养液，以制阳光；茵陈、川楝子、麦芽三味，配合主药，调达肝经之郁滞，以利于肝阳之平息；甘草调和诸药，与麦芽相配，和胃调中，可以防止金石类药物对胃的刺激。头痛剧烈者，可加羚羊角、夏枯草、珍珠母以熄风潜阳；失眠多梦者，可加珍珠母、夜交藤、茯神以镇肝醒神。

Clinical manifestations: Frequent headache and dizziness, tinnitus and deafness, insomnia and dreaminess, sudden distortion of the mouth and eyes, slurred speech, stiffness of the tongue, or heavy sensation of the hands and feet, even hemiplegia, reddish tongue, greasy fur as well as taut, thin and fast pulse.

Analysis: Constitutional yin asthenia of the liver and kidney results in hyperactive liver yang, which gives rise to frequent dizziness and headache, tinnitus and deafness; insufficiency of kidney yin and disharmony between the heart and kidney cause insomnia and dreaminess; up-attack of wind transformed from liver yang disturbs blood vessels of the brain, which results in dysfunction of brain blood vessels, thus, giving rise to sudden distortion of the mouth and eyes, slurred speech and hemiplegia; taut pulse suggests endogenous wind in the liver, fast pulse indicates yin asthenia, the above manifestations and pulse conditions indicate yin asthenia and yang hyperactivity.

Prescription: Nourish yin, suppress hyperactive yang, calm wind and dredge blood vessels.

Formulas: Zhengan Xifeng Tang Jiajian (Modified Zhengan Xifeng Decoction). This is an empirical formula designed by Zhang Xichun from modern time, and it is also the best choice for treating hyperactive liver yang and up-disturbance of wind transformed from liver yang. In the formula, Huainiuxi (*Radix Achyranthis Bidentatae*), attributive to liver and kidney meridians, is used as principal drug to supplement the liver and kidney with its action of guiding blood to flow downward; Longgu (*Os Draconis*) and Muli (*Concha Ostreae*) are used as assistant drug to calm the liver and suppress wind, Guiban (*Plastrum Testudinis*), Xuanshen (*Radix Scrophulariae*), Baishao (*Radix Paeoniae Alba*) and Tiandong (*Radix Asparagi*) have an action of nourishing yin fluid to restrain yang; Yinchen (*Herba Artemisiae Scopariae*), Chuanlianzi (*Fructus Meliae Toosendan*) and Maiya (*Fructus Hordei Germinatus*) can be combined to disperse stagnation in liver meridian to help calm liver yang; Gancao (*Radix Glycyrrhizae*) can harmonize the above medicinal herbs, combined with Maiya, it can has the action of harmonizing the stomach and reconcile middle energizer so as to avoid harmful stimulation of mineral drug in the stomach. For severe headache, Lingyangjiao (*Cornu Saigae Tataricae*), Xiakucao (*Spica Prunellae*) and Zhenzhumu (*Concha Margaritifera*) can be added to calm wind and suppress liver yang; for insomnia and dreaminess, Zhenzhumu, Yejiaoteng (*Caulis Polygoni Multiflori*) and Fushen (*Sclerotium Poriae Circum Radicem*) may be combined to suppress the liver and refresh the mind.

3. 痰热腑实，风痰上扰
29.1.3 Up-disturbance of phlegm and wind due to phlegmatic heat and sthenia of fu-organ

【症状】突然半身不遂，或半身麻木，口眼㖞斜，头晕头痛，语言不利，口黏有痰，大便秘结，舌苔厚腻，脉象弦滑，偏瘫侧脉象偏大而弦滑。

【分析】本证多见于形体肥胖之人。平时嗜好膏粱肥厚，聚湿生痰，痰聚生热，痰热内蕴，一遇情绪激动，肝阳暴盛，痰热夹风，上扰脑窍，便会发生脑中风。经络阻塞，故见半身不遂或半身麻木，口眼㖞斜；脑络不通，则头晕头痛；痰阻舌本，故语言不利；痰热影响中焦气机升降，使腑实便秘；舌苔厚腻、脉象弦滑，为痰热之明证；"脉大为病进"，偏瘫侧脉象偏大而弦滑，为痰热壅盛，为病情进展之征。

【治法】清热化痰，通腑导滞。

【方药】星蒌承气汤（验方）加减。星蒌承气汤由胆南星、全瓜蒌、生大黄、芒硝组成。方中胆南星、全瓜蒌清化痰热，生大黄、芒硝通腑导滞。此方取效与否在于大便是否通畅，如果服后大便通畅，其半身不遂或麻木就会得到改善。腑气通畅后，可以加一些活血化瘀药，如丹参、鸡血藤、赤芍、稀莶草等。语言不利，可以加一些清心开窍药，如石菖蒲、远志、郁金等。

Clinical manifestations: Sudden hemiplegia, or facial distortion, dizziness and headache, slurred speech, sticky taste and sputum in the mouth, dry feces, thick greasy fur as well as taut and slippery pulse, or large, taut and slippery pulse because of hemiplegic paralysis.

Analysis: The syndrome is usually seen in obese patients who prefer greasy and delicious food. The dietary habit results in internal retention of heat transformed from accumulation of damp phlegm, which causes hyperactivity of liver yang when being excited. Therefore, phlegmatic heat coupled with wind disturbs the brain and gives rise to cerebral apoplexy. Hemiplegia or hemi-numbness and facial distortion are due to obstruction of meridians and collaterals; dizziness and headache are caused by blockage of blood vessels in the brain; slurred speech is due to the root of tongue being obstructed by phlegm; constipation is due to phlegmatic heat preventing qi in middle energizer from ascending and descending; thick greasy fur and taut and slippery pulse are obvious manifestations of phlegmatic heat; "large pulse indicates advancement of diseases", large, taut and slippery pulse suggests stagnation of exuberant phlegmatic heat, a sign of development of hemiplegic paralysis.

Prescription: Clear away heat, resolve phlegm and remove stagnation of intestinal qi.

Formulas: The empirical formula Xing Lou Chengqi Tang Jiajian (Modified Xing Lou Chengqi Decoction). Xing Lou Chengqi Tang is made up of Dannanxing (*Rhizoma Arisaematis Cum Bile*), Gualou (*Fructus Trichosanthis*), Shengdahuang (*Radix et Rhizoma Rhei*) and Mangxiao (*Natrii Sulfas*), of which, Dannanxing and Gualou can resolve phlegmatic heat, Shengdahuang and Mangxiao have an action of removing stagnation of intestinal qi. The formula is effective in dredging the bowels and keeping smooth defecation. In that case, hemiplegia or hemi-numbness will get relieved. With the removal of stagnated intestinal qi, medicinal herbs such as Danshen (*Radix Salviae Miltiorrhizae*), Jixueteng (*Caulis Spatholobi*), Chishao (*Radix Paeoniae Rubra*) and Xixiancao (*Herba Siegesbeckiae*) can be added to activate blood and resolve stasis. For slurred speech, Shichangpu (*Rhizoma Acori Tatarinowii*), Yuanzhi (*Radix Polygalae*) and Yujin (*Radix Curcumae*) could be combined to clear away heart fire and wake up consciousness.

（二） 中脏腑
29.2 Apoplexy involving zang-fu organs

1. 闭证

29.2.1 Apoplexy due to blockage

闭证的主要症状是突然昏仆，不省人事，牙关紧闭，口噤不开，两手握固，大小便闭，肢体强紧。根据有无热象，又分阳闭、阴闭两种证候。

The main manifestations of apoplexy due to blockage are as follows: Sudden collapse, unconsciousness, closed mouth and lock jaw, firm clasping of the fists, constipation and blockage of urine, and stiff and inflexible body and limbs. Apoplexy due to blockage can be divided into yang blockage and yin blockage according to presence of fever.

（1）阳闭

【症状】除有闭证症状外，另有面赤身热，气粗口臭，烦躁不宁，舌苔黄腻，脉象弦滑而数。

【分析】阳闭为肝阳暴张而致。阳升风动，气血上逆，夹痰火上蒙清窍，故突然昏仆，不省人事，这就是《黄帝内经》所说的"大厥"证。风火痰热之邪，内闭经络，则出现一派心、肝、胃等脏腑的实证、热证、阳证，如上见气粗口臭、烦躁不宁，下见大小便闭、肢体强紧等。

【治法】清肝熄风，辛凉开窍。

【方药】牛黄至宝丹或安宫牛黄丸，以灌服或鼻饲法为宜。方以羚羊角汤为主方。方中羚羊角清肝熄风为主药，配菊花、夏枯草、蝉蜕降火熄风，龟板、白芍、石决明育阴潜阳，牡丹皮、生地黄凉血清热。如有抽搐，可加全蝎、蜈蚣、僵蚕熄风止痉；痰多者，可加竹沥、胆南星、天竺黄清化痰热；痰多、昏睡，可加郁金、石菖蒲以增强豁痰开窍之力。

（1）Apoplexy due to yang blockage

Clinical manifestations: Flushed complexion and fever, rapid respiration and foul odor, restlessness, greasy yellowish fur as well as taut, slippery and fast pulse in addition to the above manifestations about apoplexy due to blockage.

Analysis: Apoplexy due to yang blockage is caused by hyperactivity of liver yang. Endogenous liver wind generated from hyperactive liver yang causes adverse flow of qi and blood, which, together with invasion of phlegmatic fire into the upper orifices, brings about sudden collapse and unconsciousness. This is the so-called "coma (severe syncope)" stated in *Huangdi Neijing* (*Huangdi's Internal Classic*). Pathogenic wind, fire and phlegmatic heat blocking meridians and collaterals give rise to sthenia syndrome, heat syndrome, yang syndrome with symptoms such as rapid respiration, halitosis, restlessness, constipation and blockage of urine as well as stiff and inflexible body and limbs.

Prescription: Calm endogenous wind by clearing away liver heat and wake up consciousness with pungent-and-cool natured herbs.

Formulas: Niuhuang Zhibao Dan (Pill) or Angong Niuhuang Wan (Pill) taken by drenching or nasal feeding (nasogastric gavage). In the formulas, Lingyangjiao (*Cornu Saigae Tataricae*) is used as a principal drug to calm endogenous wind by clearing away liver heat; Juhua (*Flos Chrysanthemi*), Xiakucao (*Spica Prunellae*) and Chantui (*Periostracum Cicada*) are combined to send down fire to calm endogenous wind; Guiban (*Plastrum Testudinis*), Baishao (*Radix Paeoniae Alba*) and Shijueming (*Concha Haliotidis*) have an action of nourishing yin and surpressing yang; Mudanpi (*Cortex Moutan Radicis*) and Shengdihuang (*Radix Rehmanniae Recens*) can clear away heat by cooling blood. For convulsion, Quanxie (*Scorpio*), Wugong (*Scolopendra*) and Jiangcan (*Bombyx Batryticatus*) can be combined to calm wind and stop convulsion; for profuse sputum, Zhuli (*Succus Bambusae*), Dannanxing (*Rhizoma Arisaematis Cum Bile*) and Tianzhuhuang (*Tabasheer*) can be added to resolve phlegmatic heat; for lethargy with profuse sputum, Yujin (*Radix Curcumae*) and Shichangpu (*Rhizoma Acori Tatarinowii*) should be combined to improve the action of eliminating phlegm and waking up consciousness.

（2）阴闭

【症状】除有闭证症状外，另有面色苍白，口唇淡暗，静卧不烦，四肢不温，痰涎壅盛，舌苔白腻，脉象沉滑而缓。

【分析】阴闭多为痰湿壅盛所致。痰湿壅盛，风夹痰湿，上蒙清窍，内闭经络，故突然昏仆、不省人事、口噤不开、两手握固、肢体强痉；痰湿属阴，"阴主静"，故静卧不烦；痰湿阻滞经络，阳气不得宣通，故四肢不温、面色苍白、口唇淡暗；苔白腻、脉沉滑缓为痰湿壅盛，内闭不散之象。

【治法】豁痰熄风，辛温开窍。

【方药】急用苏合香丸，温开水化开灌服（或用鼻饲法），以温开透窍；继用涤痰汤煎服。涤痰汤方以半夏、橘红、茯苓、竹茹燥湿化痰；石菖蒲、胆南星开窍豁痰；枳实降气以利风痰下行。加用天麻、钩藤平肝熄风。

（2）Apoplexy due to yin blockage

Clinical manifestations: In addition to the above manifestations of about apoplexy due to blockage, the other symptoms are as follows: pale complexion, slight darkish mouth and lips, preference for lying down quietly and no restlessness, cold limbs, stagnation of profuse sputum and saliva, greasy whitish fur as well as sunken, slippery and moderate pulse.

Analysis: Apoplexy due to yin blockage is usually caused by stagnation of dampness of phlegm. Sudden collapse, unconsciousness, closed mouth and lockjaw, firm clasping of fists and stiff and inflexible body and limbs are due to stagnation of phlegmatic dampness in combination with pathogenic wind, which invades into the upper orifices, bringing about internal blockage of meridians and collaterals; preference for lying down quietly and no restlessness is due to the fact that phlegmatic dampness is yin pathogen, pertaining to quietness; cold limbs, pale complexion and pale darkish mouth and lips are due to failure of yang qi to disperse because of blockage of phlegmatic dampness in meridians and collaterals; greasy whitish fur and sunken, slippery and moderate pulse are signs of failure to disperse internal blockage of phlegmatic dampness.

Prescription: Resolve phlegm, calm endogenous wind and wake up consciousness with pungent-and-warm natured medicinal herbs.

Formulas: Suhexiang Wan (Pill) for Emergency taken by drenching or nasal feeding (nasogastric gavage) to wake up consciousness and Ditan Tang (Decoction) for subsequent use. In the formulas, Banxia (*Rhizoma Pinelliae*), Juhong (*Exocarpium Citri Rubrum*), Fuling (*Poriae Cocos*) and Zhuru (*Caulis Bambusae in Taenia*) have an action of drying dampness and resolving phlegm; Shichangpu (*Rhizoma Acori Tatarinowii*) and Dannanxing (*Rhizoma Arisaematis Cum Bile*) can wake up consciousness and eliminate phlegm; Zhishi (*Fructus Aurantii Immaturus*) can descend qi to guide wind and phlegm downward. Tianma (*Rhizoma Gastrodiae*) and Gouteng (*Ramulus Uncariae Cum Uncis*) can be combined to suppress the liver and calm endogenous wind.

2. 脱证
29.2.2　Apoplexy due to depletion

【症状】突然昏仆，不省人事，目合口张，鼻鼾息微，手撒肢冷，汗多，大小便自遗，肢体软瘫，舌萎，脉象细弱，或脉微欲绝。

【分析】阳浮于上，阴竭于下，有阴阳离决之势。正气虚脱，心神涣散，神不自主，故见突然昏仆、不省人事、目合口张、鼻鼾、舌萎、大小便失禁等五脏元气败绝之危症。呼吸低微、汗出不止、四肢厥冷、脉象微弱，为阳气暴脱、阴精欲绝之兆。

【治法】益气温阳，救阴固脱。

【方药】立即用大剂参附汤合生脉散，以回阳救逆。方取人参、麦冬、五味子大补气阴，附子回阳救逆。如汗多不止，可加黄芪、生牡蛎、生龙骨、山茱萸，以敛阴固脱。也可用参附制剂静脉滴注。如见病人面赤足冷，虚烦不安，脉大无根，这是由于真阴亏损，阳无所附，虚阳上越之脱证前兆，可用地黄饮子加减，以滋肾阴，扶肾阳，开窍化痰，使阴精充足，阳气归根，自无虚阳上越之虞。

Clinical manifestations: Sudden syncope, unconsciousness, closed eyes and open mouth, weak breath with stertor, tremor of hands and cold limbs, profuse sweating, incontinence of urination and defecation, flaccidity of body and limbs, atrophy of tongue as well as thin and weak pulse or indistinct and even insensible pulse.

Analysis: Up-floating of yang and exhaustion of yin cause the condition of yin-yang disassociation. Depletion of healthy qi and disturbance of mind result in the critical syndrome of depletion of primordial qi in the zang organs with such manifestations as sudden syncope, unconsciousness, closed eyes and open mouth, weak breath with stertor, atrophy of tongue and incontinence of urination and defecation. Weak breath, profuse cold sweating, cold limbs and weak pulse are signs of depletion of yang qi and declination of yin and essence.

Prescription: Supplement qi by warming yang and rescue yin to relieve depletion.

Formulas: Large dosage of Shen Fu Tang (Decoction) combined with Shengmai San (Powder) for emergent use so as to restore yang by saving from collapse. In the formula, Renshen (*Radix Ginseng*), Maidong (*Radix Ophiopogonis*) and Wuweizi (*Fructus Schisandrae Chinensis*) have an action of supplementing qi and yin; Fuzi (*Radix Aconiti Lateralis Preparata*) can restore yang to save from collapse. For profuse sweating, Huangqi (*Radix Astragali seu Hedysari*), Shengmuli (*Concha Ostreae*), Shenglonggu (*Os Draconis*) and Shanzhuyu (*Fructus Corni*) can astringe yin to relieve depletion. Shen Fu Tang can be made into infusion and used as intravenous dripping injection. For signs of depletion syndrome with symptoms such as flushed complexion and cold limbs, dysphoria and restlessness as well as large pulse due to deficiency of kidney yin, up-floating of deficient yang, Dihuang Yinzi Jiajian (Decoction) may be adopted to moisten kidney yin and strengthen kidney yang, waking up consciousness and resolving phlegm so that yin essence could be sufficient and yang qi could be returned to the root. As a result, the syndrome of up-floating of yang could disappear.

（三）后遗症
29.3　Sequelae

脑中风经过抢救之后，神志清醒，但多数留有后遗症，如半身不遂、口眼㖞斜、语言不利等。这时需要中药与针灸、推拿按摩配合治疗，并适度体育锻炼，以提高治疗效果。

After being rescued, consciousness of patients who suffer from cerebral apoplexy can get restored. However, in most cases, the patients could have sequelae, for instance, hemiplegia, facial distortion, slurred speech, etc. Therefore, TCM treatment by means of Chinese medicinal herbs is not enough, acupuncture and moxibustion, massage as well as appropriate exercises should be taken so as to achieve better curative effect.

1. 半身不遂
29.3.1　Hemiplegia

【症状】一侧肢体不能自主活动，或偏身麻木，感觉丧失；或肢体强痉而屈伸不利；有的肢体软瘫；舌质偏暗，或夹有紫斑，舌苔偏腻，脉象弦滑，或滑缓无力。

【分析】风痰流注经络，血脉痹阻，经隧不通，气不能行，血不能濡，故肢体废而不用。凡肢体强痉不能屈伸者，为阴血亏虚，风阳内动所致；肢体软瘫，为气血亏虚，血不濡养所致；偏身麻木者，为气血失养，血脉涩滞所致；舌质为瘀血象，紫斑为血瘀之重症；苔腻为痰阻；脉象弦滑，为痰湿内蕴，而滑缓为气血流通不畅之象。

【治法】补气活血，通经活络。

【方药】补阳还五汤加减。方取大剂量黄芪，以补气回阳；桃仁、红花、当归、赤芍、川芎，为活血养血之药；地龙为通经活络之要药，具有贯通血脉的作用。临床常加桑枝、桂枝、鸡血藤、牛膝等，以增强通经活络的功效。如手足瘀肿者，可加茯苓、猪苓、薏苡仁、防己等淡渗利湿。

Clinical manifestations: Failure of the arm, leg, and trunk on the same side of the body to move by itself, or numbness or loss of sense of the arm, leg, and trunk on the same side of the body; or inflexibility of the joints due to stiffness and convulsion of the body or limbs; flaccidity or paralysis of the body and limbs in some cases, darkish tongue with purplish spots, greasy fur as well as taut and slippery pulse or slippery, moderate and weak pulse.

Analysis：Migration of pathogenic wind and phlegm into the meridians and collaterals and obstruction of blood vessels result in qi obstructed in the meridians and failure of blood to nourish the whole body, which gives rise to disabled body and limbs. Inflexible joints and stiffness and convulsion of the body or limbs are caused by asthenia of yin and blood and endogenous wind transformed from hyperactive liver yang；flaccidity or paralysis of the body and limbs are due to asthenic qi and blood and failure of blood to nourish the body；numbness of the same side of the body is caused by malnutrition of qi and blood as well as obstructive and unsmooth blood circulation；darkish tongue indicates blood stasis, purplish spots on the tongue suggest severe blood stasis；greasy fur is a sign of internal obstruction of damp phlegm, taut and slippery pulse signifies internal retention of damp phlegm, while slippery and moderate pulse is a sign of unsmooth circulation of qi and blood.

Prescription：Supplement qi, activate blood and dredge the meridians and collaterals.

Formulas：Buyang Huanwu Tang Jiajian (Modified Buyang Huanwu Decoction). In the formula, Huangqi (*Radix Astragali seu Hedysari*) is used in large amount to supplement qi and restore yang；Taoren (*Semen Persicae*), Honghua (*Flos Carthami*), Danggui (*Radix Angelicae Sinensis*), Chishao (*Radix Paeoniae Rubra*) and Chuanxiong (*Rhizoma Ligustici Chuanxiong*) have the action of activating blood and nourishing blood；Dilong (*Lumbricus*), with the effect of dredging blood vessels, is used as the principal drug to activate the meridians and collaterals. Clinically, Sangzhi (*Ramulus Mori*), Guizhi (*Ramulus Cinnamomi*), Jixueteng (*Caulis Spatholobi*) and Niuxi (*Radix Achyranthis Bidentatae*) can be added to strengthen the effect of activating the meridians and collaterals. For swollen hands and feet due to blood stasis, Fuling (*Poriae Cocos*), Zhuling (*Polyporus Umbellatus*), Yiyiren (*Semen Coicis*) and Fangji (*Radix Stephaniae Tetrandrae*) can be combined to induce diuresis with its bland flavor.

2. 语言不利
29.3.2 Slurred speech

【症状】舌体欠灵活，语言不清，或欲言不能，舌形多偏斜，舌苔白腻，脉象弦滑。

【分析】中风不语，为风痰与瘀血滞于舌本所致，与心脉、脾脉、肾脉等络脉不和有关。由于风痰、瘀血阻于舌本，所以舌形偏斜不能正常伸出；舌苔白腻，为风痰之象；脉象弦滑，为瘀血作祟之征。

【治法】祛风除痰，通络开窍。

【方药】资寿解语汤加减。资寿解语汤由白附子、石菖蒲、远志、天麻、全蝎、羌活、胆南星、木香、甘草组成。方中天麻、白附子、全蝎平肝熄风除痰，胆南星豁痰宁心，石菖蒲芳香开窍，远志交通心肾，羌活祛风通络，甘草调和诸药。病邪偏于心脉者，加珍珠母、琥珀；偏于脾脉者，加苍术、半夏、陈皮；偏于肾脉者，加地黄、山茱萸。

Clinical manifestations: Inflexible movement of the tongue, unclear speech, or inability to speak, deviated tongue, greasy whitish fur as well as taut and slippery pulse.

Analysis: Aphasia from apoplexy is caused by wind, phlegm and blood stasis stagnated at the root of the tongue, which is related to disharmony of collaterals of the heart, spleen and kidney. Deviated tongue is due to obstruction of wind, phlegm and blood stasis at the root of tongue; greasy whitish fur is a sign of wind phlegm; taut and slippery pulse is caused by blood stasis.

Prescription: Expel wind and eliminate phlegm and activate blood vessels to wake up consciousness.

Formulas: Zishou Jieyu Tang Jiajian (Modified Zishou Jieyu Decoction). Zishou Jieyu Tang consists of Baifuzi (*Rhizoma Typhonii*), Shichangpu (*Rhizoma Acori Tatarinowii*), Yuanzhi (*Radix Polygalae*), Tianma (*Rhizoma Gastrodiae*), Quanxie (*Scorpio*), Qianghuo (*Rhizoma et Radix Notopterygii*), Dannanxing (*Rhizoma Arisaematis Cum Bile*), Muxiang (*Radix Aucklandiae*) and Gancao (*Radix Glycyrrhizae*). In the formula, Tianma, Baifuzi and Quanxie have an action of calming the liver, suppressing endogenous wind and eliminating phlegm; Dannanxing can dispel phlegm and tranquilize the heart; Shichangpu has an action of waking up consciousness with its aromatic flavor; Yuanzhi can restore the normal coordination between the heart and kidney; Qianghuo can dispel wind and dredge blood vessels, and Gancao has an action of reconciling the above medicinal herbs. For the symptom of pathogenic factors gathering in heart meridians, Zhenzhumu (*Concha Margaritifera*) and Hupo (*Succinum*) can be added; for accumulation of pathogenic factors in spleen meridians, Cangzhu (*Rhizoma Atractylodis*), Banxia (*Rhizoma Pinelliae*) and Chenpi (*Pericarpium Citri Reticulatae*) should be added; for pathogenic factors in kidney meridians, Dihuang (*Radix Rehmanniae Recens*) and Shanzhuyu (*Fructus Corni*) should be combined.

3. 口眼㖞斜
29.3.3 Facial distortion

【症状】口眼㖞斜多伴随在其他后遗症中，但也有仅见口眼㖞斜者。

【分析】口眼㖞斜与风痰阻于经络有关，特别是阳明经之络脉。手阳明经脉与足阳明经脉，其起始部位都在面部，一个在目下，一个在鼻旁，阳明经脉又主津液之输布，以及水谷营卫之运行，一旦受风邪所扰，就会形成风痰而干扰脑窍，使面部经脉阻塞、拘紧，出现口眼㖞斜等症。

【治法】除风、豁痰、通络。

【方药】牵正散加减。方中白附子祛风、通络、化痰；僵蚕、全蝎熄风、化痰、镇痉。本方用散剂吞服，较汤剂效果好。口眼瞤动者，可加天麻、钩藤、石决明以平肝熄风。

Clinical manifestations: Facial distortion is usually complicated with other sequelae. However, in some cases, it can appear by itself.

Analysis: Facial distortion is related to obstruction of wind phlegm in meridians and collaterals, especially the collaterals of yangming meridian. Meridians of hand yangming and foot yangming originate from the face, the former starting from beneath the eyes, and the latter from the nose. Yangming meridian dominates distribution of body fluid and transportation of food, nutrition and defensive qi. Disturbance of wind phlegm into the cerebral orifice results in obstructed meridians of the face and spasm, which brings about facial distortion.

Prescription: Dispel wind, eliminate phlegm and dredge collaterals.

Formulas: Qianzheng San Jiajian (Modified Qianzheng Powder). In the formula, Baifuzi (*Rhizoma Typhonii*) has an action of dispelling wind, dredging the collaterals and resolving phlegm; Jiangcan (*Bombyx Batryticatus*) and Quanxie (*Scorpio*) can calm wind, resolve phlegm and suppress convulsion. Oral use of powder made from this formula is much better than the decoction. For convulsive eyes and mouth, Tianma (*Rhizoma Gastrodiae*), Gouteng (*Ramulus Uncariae Cum Uncis*) and Shijueming (*Concha Haliotidis*) should be combined to calm the liver and suppress wind.

三十、失眠

30　Insomnia

〔**概说**〕　Summary

失眠在中医古籍中被称为"不得眠""不得卧""目不瞑"等。

失眠的临床表现不一，有入睡困难者，有眠而易醒者，有醒后不能再入眠者，亦有时寐时醒者，严重者整夜不能入眠。

形成失眠的原因很多。思虑不遂，内伤心脾，阳不交阴；心肾不交，阴虚火旺；怒气伤肝，肝阳扰动；胃气不和，阳明脉逆；心胆气虚，神不守舍，等等，均可引起失眠。在辨证上，大致分虚实两证，但在具体辨证时，还要注意病变的部位、致病因素等。

In TCM classic works, insomnia is regarded as "failure to fall asleep" "inability to sleep", or "failure to rest", etc.

Clinical manifestations of insomnia are various, for instance, difficulty in falling asleep, shallow sleep with susceptibility to being waken up, disturbed sleep, even in some severe cases, inability to sleep all night.

There are many factors that contribute to insomnia, including excess thinking of unfulfilled wish impairing the heart and spleen and failure of yang to enter into yin; yin asthenia and fire exuberance due to imbalance between the heart and kidney; hyperactive liver yang disturbing the mind because of impairment of rage in the liver; adverse yangming meridian resulting from disharmony of stomach qi; failure of the heart to house the mind because of qi asthenia of the heart and gallbladder. Syndrome differentiation of insomnia can be classified into asthenia and sthenia. However, in clinical practice, attention should be paid to the location of the pathological change and factors that cause diseases.

〔辨证论治〕 Syndrome differentiation and treatment

（一）实证
30.1 Sthenia syndrome

1. 肝郁化火

30.1.1 Transforming of fire due to liver qi stagnation

【症状】不眠，急躁易怒，不思饮食，目赤口苦，口渴喜饮，大便秘结，小便黄赤，舌红，苔黄，脉象弦数。

【分析】本证多因恼怒伤肝，肝气郁结，郁久化火，上扰心神所致。肝气犯胃，则不思饮食；肝郁化火，肝火乘胃，胃热则口渴喜饮；肝火偏旺，则急躁易怒；火热上扰，则目赤口苦；大便秘结，小便黄赤，舌红、苔黄、脉象弦数，均为化火之象。

【治法】疏肝泻热，佐以安神。

【方药】龙胆泻肝汤加味。方中龙胆草、栀子、黄芩清肝泻火；泽泻、木通、车前子清泻肝热；当归、生地黄养血和肝；柴胡舒达肝气；甘草和中。临床常加生龙骨、生牡蛎、茯神镇静安神。若胸胁苦满，可加郁金、川楝子、香附解郁疏肝。

Clinical manifestations: Sleeplessness, restlessness with susceptibility to rage, poor appetite, flushed eyes and bitter taste, thirst with desire to drink, dry feces, yellowish and brownish urine, reddish tongue with yellowish fur as well as taut and fast pulse.

Analysis: This syndrome is usually caused by impairment of the liver due to rage and transformation of fire from liver qi stagnation, which disturbs the mind. Poor appetite is due to liver qi attacking the stomach; fire transformed from liver qi stagnation attacks the stomach, resulting in stomach heat, which brings about thirst with desire to drink; restlessness with susceptibility to rage is due to hyperactivity of liver fire; flushed eyes and bitter taste of the mouth are due to up-disturbance of fire and heat; dry feces, yellowish and brownish urine, reddish tongue with yellowish fur and taut and fast pulse are signs of transformation of fire.

Prescription: Soothe the liver and purge heat in combination with tranquilizing the mind.

Formulas: Longdan Xiegan Tang Jiawei (Modified Longdan Xiegan Decoction). In the formula, Longdancao (*Radix Gentianae*), Zhizi (*Fructus Gardeniae*) and Huangqin (*Radix Scutellariae*) have an action of clearing the liver and purging fire; Zexie (*Rhizoma Alismatis*), Mutong (*Caulis Akebiae*) and Cheqianzi (*Semen Plantaginis*) can purge heat from the liver; Danggui (*Radix Angelicae Sinensis*) and Shengdihuang (*Radix Rehmanniae Recens*) can nourish blood and reconcile the liver; Chaihu (*Radix Bupleuri*) has the action of soothing qi of the liver; Gancao (*Radix Glycyrrhizae*) can harmonize middle energizer. Clinically, Shenglonggu (*Os Draconis*), Shengmuli (*Concha Ostreae*), and Fushen

(*Sclerotium Poriae Circum Radicem*) are usually combined to tranquilize the mind. For distention and fullness of the chest and hypochondrium, Yujin (*Radix Curcumae*), Chuanlianzi (*Fructus Meliae Toosendan*) and Xiangfu (*Rhizoma Cyperi*) can be added to relieve qi stagnation and soothe the liver.

2. 痰热内扰
30.1.2　Internal disturbance of phlegmatic heat

【症状】不眠，头重胸闷，厌食嗳气，吞酸恶心，心烦口苦，目眩，舌苔黄腻，脉象滑数。

【分析】本证多由饮食不节，积食生痰，因痰生热，痰热上扰，而致不眠。痰湿积于胸中，故胸闷；清阳被蒙，故头重目眩；痰湿停滞，中焦不开，故不思饮食；胃失和降，则嗳气吞酸；舌苔黄腻，脉象滑数，为痰热之征。

【治法】化痰清热，和中安神。

【方药】黄连温胆汤加味。方取陈皮、半夏、枳实、竹茹理气化痰，和胃降逆；茯苓宁心安神；甘草和中；另加黄连、栀子清心除烦。若痰食积滞，可加神曲、麦芽、山楂消食化痰，起到和胃安神的效果。

Clinical manifestations: Sleeplessness, heavy sensation of the head and chest oppression, anorexia and belching, acid regurgitation and nausea, vexation and bitter taste in the mouth, dizziness, greasy yellowish fur as well as slippery and fast pulse.

Analysis: The syndrome is caused by improper diet. Insomnia is due to phlegm generated from food retention transforming into heat and disturbing upward. Chest oppression is due to accumulation of damp phlegm in the chest; heavy sensation of the head and dizziness are caused by lucid yang being blocked by phlegm; anorexia is due to retention of damp phlegm in middle energizer; belching and acid regurgitation are caused by dysfunction of the stomach in descending qi; greasy yellowish fur and slippery and fast pulse are signs of phlegmatic heat.

Prescription: Resolve phlegm, clear away heat, harmonize middle energizer and tranquilize the mind.

Formulas: Huanglian Wendan Tang Jiawei (Modified Huanglian Wendan Decoction). In the formula, Chenpi (*Pericarpium Citri Reticulatae*), Banxia (*Rhizoma Pinelliae*), Zhishi (*Fructus Aurantii Immaturus*) and Zhuru (*Caulis Bambusae in Taenia*) have an action of regulating qi, resolving phlegm, reconciling the stomach and descending adverse flow of qi; Fuling (*Poriae Cocos*) can calm the heart and tranquilize the mind; Gancao (*Radix Glycyrrhizae*) may harmonize middle energizer; Huanglian (*Rhizoma Coptidis*) and Zhizi (*Fructus Gardeniae*) can be added to clear away heart fire and relieve vexation. For accumulation of phlegm and food retention, Shenqu (*Massa Medicata Fermentata*), Maiya (*Fructus Hordei Germinatus*) and Shanzha (*Fructus Crataegi*) can be added to eliminate food retention and resolve phlegm so as to achieve the effect of regulating the stomach and tranquilizing the mind.

（二）虚证

30.2 Asthenia syndrome

1. 阴虚火旺

30.2.1 Yin asthenia and fire exuberance

【症状】心烦不眠，心悸不安，头晕，耳鸣，健忘，五心烦热，口干津少，时有梦遗，月经量少而色赤，舌红，脉数。

【分析】肾阴不足，不能上济心火，心火独旺，火性炎上，扰乱心神，故心烦不眠、心悸不安；肾阴亏虚，髓海不足，则头晕、耳鸣、健忘；阴亏，故口干津少；男子阴虚火旺，时时扰动精室，则有梦遗；女子阴虚火旺，血源渐亏，故经量少而色赤；其他均为阴虚火旺之象。

【治法】滋阴降火，养心安神。

【方药】黄连阿胶汤或朱砂安神丸，随证选用。黄连阿胶汤重在滋阴清火，适用于心烦不眠，心悸不安者。若面红微热，头晕耳鸣，可加生牡蛎、龟板、磁石等，以重镇潜阳，阳入于阴，则可安眠。朱砂安神丸亦以黄连为主药，作用与黄连阿胶汤相似，方中有酸枣仁、柏子仁，其安神作用更为显著。

Clinical manifestations：Vexation and sleeplessness, palpitation and restlessness, vertigo, tinnitus, forgetfulness, feverish sensation over the palms, soles and chest, dry mouth with scanty fluid, occasional nocturnal emission, scanty brownish menstrual blood, reddish tongue as well as fast pulse.

Analysis：Failure of insufficient kidney yin to coordinate heart fire causes disturbance of the mind by flaring-up of hyperactive fire, which, in turn, gives rise to vexation and sleeplessness, palpitation and restlessness; vertigo, tinnitus and forgetfulness are due to deficiency of kidney yin and insufficiency of marrow; dry mouth with scanty fluid is due to yin asthenia; occasional nocturnal emission in male is due to yin asthenia and fire exuberance, which disturbs sperm house; scanty brownish menstrual blood in female is due to yin asthenia and fire exuberance and deficiency of blood; feverish sensation over the palms, soles and chest, reddish tongue and fast pulse are signs of yin asthenia and fire exuberance.

Prescription：Nourish yin, purge fire, replenish the heart and tranquilize the mind.

Formulas：Huanglian Ejiao Tang（Decoction）or Zhusha Anshen Wan（Pill）can be chosen according to different syndromes. For vexation, sleeplessness, restlessness and palpitation, Huanglian Ejiao Tang can nourish yin by clearing away fire. For flushed complexion, mild fever, dizziness and tinnitus, Shengmuli（*Concha Ostreae*）, Guiban（*Plastrum Testudinis*）and Cishi（*Magnetitum*）can be added to suppress hyperactive yang to help yang communicate with yin and the patient could fall into sleep. Zhusha Anshen Wan is based on Huanglian, and it has the similar action to Huanglian Ejiao Tang. In the formula, Suanzaoren（*Semen Ziziphi Spinosae*）and Baiziren（*Semen Platycladi*）can have obvious action of tranquilizing the mind.

2. 心脾两虚
30.2.2 Asthenia of the heart and spleen

【症状】多梦易醒，心悸健忘，头晕目眩，神疲体倦，饮食无味，面色少华，舌淡苔薄，脉象细弱。

【分析】心主血脉，脾主气血，心脾亏虚，血不养心，神不守舍，故多梦易醒、健忘心悸；心脾亏虚，不能上奉于脑，则头晕目眩、精神疲倦；血虚不能上荣于面，故面色少华；脾虚则运化力差，故饮食无味；气血亏虚，故脉细弱，舌淡红而薄。

【治法】补益心脾，以生气血。

【方药】归脾汤主之。方中人参、白术、黄芪、甘草补气健脾；远志、酸枣仁、茯神、龙眼肉补心益脾，安神定志；当归滋阴养血；木香行气舒脾，使之补而不滞。诸药合用，养血以宁心神，健脾以资化源。如心血不足，可加熟地黄、白芍、阿胶以养心血；不眠严重者，可加柏子仁、五味子以助养心安神。

Clinical manifestations: Dreaminess with susceptibility to waking up, palpitation and forgetfulness, vertigo and dizziness, dispiritedness and lassitude, poor appetite, lusterless or sallow complexion, pale tongue with thin fur as well as thin and feeble pulse.

Analysis: The heart governs blood vessels and the spleen dominates qi and blood circulation. Dreaminess with susceptibility to waking up, palpitation and forgetfulness are due to failure of blood to nourish the heart and inability of the heart to house the mind because of asthenic heart and spleen; vertigo and dizziness, dispiritedness and lassitude are due to dysfunction of asthenic heart and spleen in transporting nutrition to the brain; lusterless or sallow complexion is due to failure of asthenic blood to nourish the face; poor appetite is caused by dysfunction of the spleen in transportation and transformation; pale tongue with thin fur and thin and feeble pulse indicate asthenia of qi and blood.

Prescription: Tonify the heart and spleen to promote production of qi and blood.

Formulas: Guipi Tang (Decoction). In the formula, Renshen (*Radix Ginseng*), Baizhu (*Rhizoma Atractylodis Macrocephalae*), Huangqi (*Radix Astragali seu Hedysari*) and Gancao (*Radix Glycyrrhizae*) have an action of supplementing qi and invigorating the spleen; Yuanzhi (*Radix Polygalae*), Suanzaoren (*Semen Ziziphi Spinosae*), Fushen (*Sclerotium Poriae Circum Radicem*) and Longyanrou (*Arillus Longan*) can nourish the heart and spleen, tranquilize the mind and calm emotion; Danggui (*Radix Angelicae Sinensis*) has an action of nourishing yin and blood; Muxiang (*Radix Aucklandiae*) has an effect of activating qi and soothing the spleen to avoid qi stagnation. Combined together, the formula can nourish blood to tranquilize the heart and mind, and invigorate the spleen to promote transformation. For insufficient heart blood, Shudihuang (*Radix Rehmanniae Preparata*), Baishao (*Radix Paeoniae Alba*) and Ejiao (*Colla Corii Asini*) can be added to nourish heart blood; for severe insomnia, Baiziren (*Semen Platycladi*) and Wuweizi (*Fructus Schisandrae Chinensis*) may be combined to help nourish the heart and tranquilize the mind.

3. 心胆气虚
30.2.3 Qi asthenia of the heart and gallbladder

【症状】不眠多梦，易于惊醒，胆怯心悸，遇事易惊，气短怠倦，小便清长，舌质淡，脉象弦细。

【分析】心虚则心神不安，胆虚则善恐易惊，故多梦易醒；心悸善惊，气短怠倦，小便清长，以及舌脉象，均为气虚失养所致。

【治法】益气镇惊，安神定志。

【方药】安神定志丸。方中人参益气；龙齿镇惊；茯苓、茯神、石菖蒲补气益胆安神。若血虚阳浮，虚烦不眠，可改用酸枣仁汤治之。

Clinical manifestations：Insomnia and dreaminess, susceptibility to being disturbed in sleep；timidity and palpitation, susceptibility to fright；short breath and lassitude；thin clear urine；light-colored tongue as well as taut and thin pulse.

Analysis：Asthenic heart results in unease of the heart and mind, asthenic gallbladder brings about susceptibility to fright, which give rise to insomnia and dreaminess；timidity and palpitation, short breath and lassitude, thin clear urine, light-colored tongue and taut and thin pulse are signs of malnutrition due to qi asthenia.

Prescription：Benefit qi, relieve fright and tranquilize the mind and emotion.

Formulas：Anshen Dingzhi Wan （Pill）. In the formula, Renshen （*Radix Ginseng*）can benefit qi；Longchi （*Dens Draconis*）has an action of relieving fright；Fuling （*Poriae Cocos*）, Fushen （*Sclerotium Poriae Circum Radicem*）and Shichangpu （*Rhizoma Acori Tatarinowii*）can tonify qi and benefit the gallbladder to tranquilize the mind. For asthenic blood and floating yang, dysphoria and insomnia, Suanzaoren Tang can be used to remove Anshen Dingzhi Wan.

三十一、风湿性关节炎
31 Rheumatoid arthritis

〔**概说**〕 Summary

类风湿性关节炎到目前为止，医学界认为是一种原因不明的自身免疫性全身风湿病，病理改变以关节滑膜炎症为主，其关节炎具有对称性、多发性、反复发作的特点。此外，还伴有低热、消瘦、淋巴结肿大等全身症状。

类风湿性关节炎归属于中医学"顽痹""尪痹""骨痹""肾痹"等范畴。认为正气虚弱，感受外邪为其主要发病因素，而正气虚弱以肝肾虚为主，尤以肾虚显著。其证候正虚与邪实交错，风湿与寒毒、湿热互结，故治疗上常常顾此失彼，即单纯祛邪或单纯扶正都难以取效。呈现病程缠绵，治疗棘手，难以速效。对此，辨证论治显得更为重要。目前，中医药及针灸治疗具有一定优势，并且有广阔的发展前途。

Rheumatoid arthritis has been regarded as a systemic autoimmune rheumatic disease with unknown causes up to now. Its pathogenic change mainly involves inflammation of synovial membrane of the joints, characterized by symmetrical, multiple and recurrent outbreak. Furthermore, rheumatoid arthritis is complicated with systemic symptoms such as mild fever, emaciation, swollen lymph nodes and so on.

In TCM, rheumatoid arthritis falls into the scopes of " obstinate arthralgia " " arthromyodynia " " bone arthralgia " and " kidney arthralgia ". Causes for it is probably invasion of exogenous pathogenic factors because of deficient healthy qi, which is mainly marked by asthenic liver and kidney, in particular, asthenic kidney. The syndromes of rheumatoid arthritis include alternate asthenia of healthy qi and sthenic pathogenic factors, inter-coagulation of rheumatism and severe pathogenic cold and damp heat. Therefore, treatment for it usually neglects some aspects, that is, only dispelling pathogenic factors or simply strengthening healthy qi cannot achieve effective result. And difficulty will arise due to prolonged course of the disease. Consequently, it is necessary to treat rheumatoid arthritis based on syndrome differentiation. At present, treatment for the disease by means of Chinese medicine and acupuncture has certain advantages and it will display its broad development prospect.

〔辨证论治〕 Syndrome differentiation and treatment

（一）急性期
31.1 Acute stage

1. 湿热阻络
31.1.1 Obstruction of damp heat in the collaterals

【症状】关节肿胀，疼痛重着，活动不利，身热不扬，身困乏力，大便溏薄，小便短赤，舌苔黄腻，脉象濡滑而数。

【分析】湿热之邪，留而不去，着于关节，故关节肿胀，且疼痛重着；热被湿困，则身热不扬；湿性重着，使其气血流通不畅，故身困乏力；湿热下迫，则大便溏薄，小便短赤；舌苔黄腻与脉象濡滑，为湿热交困的明证。辨别此证，舌苔与脉象显得非常重要，若是舌苔薄白不腻，脉象沉细，则非湿热之证，应考虑其他证候。

【治法】清热利湿，通络止痛。

【方药】四妙散加味。四妙散即苍术、黄柏、薏苡仁、牛膝。方中苍术、黄柏为其主药，苍术燥湿健脾，黄柏清热燥湿，两药配合起来，虽苦寒而不伤脾胃；薏苡仁为利水渗湿之妙品，生用既渗湿又清热，且除湿的作用大于清热，是湿热痹病的必用之药；牛膝有川牛膝与怀牛膝之分，川牛膝祛湿、化瘀作用比较大，而怀牛膝偏于补肾，所以此方要用川牛膝。一般可以加入桑枝祛风通络止痛，忍冬藤清热通络止痛；湿邪偏盛者，加防己、白术、茯苓以健脾利湿除痹；热邪偏盛者，加牡丹皮、生石膏、赤芍以清热活瘀止痛。

Clinical manifestations：Swollen joints with pain and heavy sensation, inflexibility of the joints with movement, mild fever, exhaustion and lack of energy, loose stool, scanty brownish urine, greasy yellowish fur as well as soft, slippery and fast pulse.

Analysis：Swollen joints with pain and heavy sensation is due to retention of pathogenic damp and heat factors in the joints; mild fever is due to heat being constrained by dampness; exhaustion and lack of energy are caused by unsmooth qi and blood circulation because of severe dampness; loose stool and scanty brownish urine are due to down migration of damp heat; greasy yellowish fur and soft and slippery pulse are obvious signs of obstruction of dampness and heat. In order to differentiate this syndrome, it is very essential to inspect tongue fur and pulse condition. Thin whitish tongue fur as well as sunken and thin pulse indicates that the syndrome is not damp heat, it must be other syndrome.

Prescription：Clear away heat, induce diuresis and dredge collaterals to stop pain.

Formulas：Simiao San Jiawei (Modified Simiao Powder). Simiao San is made up of Cangzhu (*Rhizoma Atractylodis*), Huangbo (*Cortex Phellodendri*), Yiyiren (*Semen Coicis*) and Niuxi (*Radix Achyranthis Bidentatae*). In the recipe, Cangzhu and Huangbo are used as principal drug, Cangzhu can dry dampness and invigorate the spleen, Huangbo has an action of clearing away heat and drying dampness, combined together, though bitter and cold in nature, they cannot impair the spleen and stomach; Yiyiren is the best for inducing diuresis and resolving dampness, and raw Yiyiren can be used to resolve dampness and clear away heat, and its action of resolving dampness is much stronger than that of clearing heat, so it is the essential medicine for Bi-syndrome (arthralgia) induced by damp heat; Niuxi can be divided into Chuanniuxi (produced in Sichuan Province) and Huainiuxi (produced in Henan Province). The former has stronger action of dispelling dampness and dissolving blood stasis, while the main action of the latter is to tonify the kidney, therefore, Chuanniuxi should be adopted in the formula. Sangzhi (*Ramulus Mori*) can be added to dispel wind and dredge collaterals so as to stop pain, Rendongteng (*Caulis Lonicerae*) has an action of clearing away heat and dredging collaterals to stop pain; for exuberance of damp pathogen, Fangji (*Radix Stephaniae Tetrandrae*), Baizhu (*Rhizoma Atractylodis Macrocephalae*) and Fuling (*Poriae Cocos*) can be combined to invigorate the spleen, induce diuresis and remove Bi-syndrome; for exuberance of heat pathogen, Mudanpi (*Cortex Moutan Radicis*), Shengshigao (*Gypsum Fibrosum*) and Chishao (*Radix Paeoniae Rubra*) should be added to activate blood by removing stasis to stop pain.

2. 热毒炽盛

31.1.2 Superabundance of toxic heat pathogen

【症状】关节红肿灼热，疼痛剧烈，日轻夜重，冷敷则舒，壮热烦渴，舌红少津，脉象弦数。

【分析】热毒浸淫，或湿邪蕴结从热而化，则关节红肿灼热；热为阳邪，表示病势进展，故疼痛剧烈，白天热邪可以透出，到了夜间热邪不得透发，故疼痛日轻夜重；冷敷则有利于遏制热邪的弛张，故疼痛减轻；内热炽盛，故壮热烦渴；舌红少津，热毒伤津也；脉象弦数，热邪未减也。总之，本证表现出病势进展之象。

【治法】清热解毒，凉血止痛。

【方药】白虎汤合生地四藤汤（自拟方）。白虎汤由生石膏、知母、粳米、甘草组成；生地四藤汤由生地黄、忍冬藤、络石藤、夜交藤、石楠藤组成。白虎汤有清热解毒、透热外发的作用；生地黄清热凉血解毒，为治疗风湿性关节炎热毒内侵证的主要药物；"四藤"合用，具有清热解毒、凉血活血、通络止痛之效。若大便干燥，可加大黄泻下解毒；伤津甚者，可加石斛、沙参、麦冬、玄参养阴生津，凉血退热。

Clinical manifestations: Swollen joints with acute scorching pain, alleviation of pain during the day and aggravation at night, comfort from pain after cold compression, high fever with polydipsia, reddish tongue with scanty fur and taut and fast pulse.

Analysis: Swollen joints with severe scorching pain are due to invasion and spreading of toxic heat pathogen, or due to heat transformed from accumulated pathogenic dampness; heat is yang pathogen, indicating advanced course of the disease, which results in acute scorching pain; heat pathogen can be erupted during the day, but it could not be let out at night, therefore, pain is alleviated during the day and aggravated at night; cold compression is helpful to restrain heat pathogen from spreading, therefore, pain could get relieved after being compressed with cold; high fever with polydipsia is due to superabundance of endogenous heat; reddish tongue with scanty fur indicates toxic heat pathogen impairing body fluid; taut and fast pulse suggests unrelieved heat pathogen. Manifestations of this syndrome indicate advanced course of the disease.

Prescription: Clear away toxic heat pathogen, cool blood and stop pain.

Formulas: Baihu Tang (Decoction) combined with Shengdi Siteng Tang (Decoction) (designed by the author of the book). Baihu Tang is made up of Shengshigao (*Gypsum Fibrosum*), Zhimu (*Rhizoma Anemarrhenae*), Jingmi (*Semen Oryzae Sativae*) and Gancao (*Radix Glycyrrhizae*); and Shengdi Siteng Tang is composed of Shengdihuang (*Radix Rehmanniae Recens*), Rendongteng (*Caulis Lonicerae*), Luoshiteng (*Caulis Trachelospermi*), Yejiaoteng (*Caulis Polygoni Multiflori*) and Shinanteng (*Photinia serrulata Lindl*). Baihu Tang has an action of clearing away toxic heat pathogen and letting out heat; Shengdihuang is an important drug for treating internal invasion of toxic heat pathogen of rheumatoid arthritis with its function of clearing away toxic heat pathogen and cooling blood; the combination of Rendongteng, Luoshiteng, Yejiaoteng and Shinanteng can clear away heat, relieve toxic heat pathogen, cool blood, activate blood, dredge collaterals and stop pain. For dry feces, Dahuang can be added to purge heat and relieve toxic heat; for severe impairment of body fluid, Shihu (*Herba Dendrobii*), Shashen (*Radix Adenophorae*), Maidong (*Radix Ophiopogonis*) and Xuanshen (*Radix Scrophulariae*) should be added to nourish yin, promote inducing fluid and cool blood by eliminating heat.

（二）慢性期
31. 2　Chronic stage

1. 阴虚痹阻
31.2.1　Obstruction of blood vessels due to yin asthenia

【症状】关节疼痛，时轻时重，局部肿胀变形，不得屈伸，腰膝酸软，头晕耳鸣，周身筋脉拘紧，形体消瘦，持续低热，口干咽燥，烦热盗汗，舌质红赤，苔少，脉象弦细或细数。

【分析】此证病程日久，为慢性难愈期。由于正气不支，关节疼痛难以缓解，变得局部肿胀变形，随着天气的变化或药物的治疗，疼痛时轻时重；气血郁滞过重，则不得屈伸；腰膝酸软、头晕耳鸣，都是肾虚所致；由于阴虚，筋脉也变得拘紧不舒；肾阴日渐亏耗，所以会出现持续低热，口干咽燥，烦热盗汗；"阳主气，阴主形"，阴血不足，形体也日渐消瘦；阴血不能充盈，上不能润泽口舌，故舌质红赤，舌苔也少而干；脉象也不那么充盈，变得弦细或细数无力。呈现一派正虚邪胜的状态。

【治法】滋肾养阴，通络止痛。

【方药】虎潜丸加减。本方是在大补阴丸的基础上加入一些药，主要是补肝肾的。熟地黄、龟板、白芍是用来补肝肾阴精的，知母、黄柏是滋阴降火的；锁阳是补益阴精的，但它温而不燥，不像其他补阴药偏寒偏凉；陈皮、干姜是健脾的，同时对大寒的知母、黄柏有反佐的含义，还能振奋脾阳，加强运化，使其滋阴的药物更好地发挥作用；虎骨是强筋壮骨的药，还是一味追风的药，就是除筋骨中的风，这种"风"是肝肾阴虚引起的，现在用狗骨代替。

Clinical manifestations: Occasional alleviation and aggravation of sore joints, failure to stretch and twist regional deformed joints with swellings, aching and weakness of the loins and knees, vertigo and tinnitus, spasm of the tendons and blood vessels of the whole body, emaciation, continuous mild fever, dry mouth and throat, dysphoria and night sweating, reddish tongue with scanty fur as well as taut and thin pulse or thin and fast pulse.

Analysis: Prolonged duration of the syndrome indicates the disease is difficult to be cured. Regional deformed joints with swellings result from unrelieved pain of joints because of insufficient healthy qi, alleviation or aggravation of pain is caused by change of weather or medication; failure to stretch or twist the joints is due to worsening qi stagnation and blood stasis; aching and weakness of the loins and knees as well as vertigo and tinnitus are caused by asthenia of the kidney; spasm of the tendons and blood vessels are due to yin asthenia; continuous mild fever, dry mouth and throat, dysphoria and night sweating are due to insufficiency and gradual consumption of kidney yin; "yang governs qi and yin dominates the body", insufficiency of yin and blood brings about emaciated body; reddish tongue with dry scanty fur is due to failure of insufficient yin and blood to moisten the mouth and tongue; taut and thin pulse or thin and fast weak pulse is a sign of asthenia of healthy qi and exuberance of pathogenic factors.

Prescription: Nourish the kidney and yin and dredge blood vessels to stop pain.

Formulas: Huqian Wan Jiajian (Modified Huqian Pill). The formula is the combination of Large Buyin Wan with some medicinal herbs with the action of tonifying the liver and kidney. Shudihuang (*Radix Rehmanniae Preparata*), Guiban (*Plastrum Testudinis*) and Baishao (*Radix Paeoniae Alba*) can tonify yin and essence in the liver and kidney, Zhimu (*Rhizoma Anemarrhenae*) and Huangbo (*Cortex Phellodendri*) have an action of moistening yin and descending fire; warm but not dry natured Suoyang (*Herba Cynomorii*) may supplement yin and essence, for it is not as cold and cool as other yin-tonifying medicinal herbs; Chenpi (*Pericarpium Citri Reticulatae*) and Ganjiang (*Rhizoma Zingiberis*) have an action of invigorating the spleen, in the meantime, they could restrain the action of severe cold-natured Zhimu and Huangbo by strengthening the function of spleen yang in transportation and transformation in order to bring the action of other medicinal herbs of nourishing yin into full play; Hugu (tiger-bone) can strengthen the tendons and bones, and it can dispel wind from them, the "wind" here is generated from yin asthenia of the liver and kidney. Nowadays, Hugu is replaced by Gougu (dog-bone) nowadays.

2. 瘀血痹阻
31.2.2 Obstruction of blood stasis

【症状】痹症反复发作，疼痛剧烈，痛处重着不移，骨关节变形、僵硬，不可屈伸，舌质多有紫暗瘀斑，脉象细涩。

【分析】疾病由经入络，由气入血，停滞日久，便成瘀血痹阻证。由于正气不支，可以反复发作；瘀血不散，则疼痛剧烈，由于瘀血着于局部，所以痛处比较固定；瘀血集结，可使关节变形、僵硬，严重者不难屈伸；舌质紫暗与脉象细涩，是瘀血之明证。

【治法】活血化瘀，通络止痛。

【方药】活络效灵丹加味。活络效灵丹由四味药组成，方中当归、丹参养血活血，并有化瘀血的作用；乳香、没药为活血止痛之良药，常常配合使用，乳香对风湿痛效果较好，而没药的活血化瘀作用比乳香强一点，但它们的作用差异不是太大，所以配合使用的机会多一些。另外，可以加搜风通络药，如全蝎、蜈蚣、地龙等；祛湿通痹药，如牛膝、秦艽、羌活、独活等；也可以加辛润通络药，如细辛、白芥子、生麻黄等。

Clinical manifestations：Recurrent outbreak of Bi-syndrome（arthralgia）, acute pain with fixed position, deformed and stiff joints, failure to stretch and twist, darkish tongue with purplish petechia and thin and astringent pulse.

Analysis：Transmission of the disease from meridians into collaterals, from qi into blood, and prolonged stagnation of pathogens in blood vessels results in obstruction of blood stasis. Recurrent outbreak of Bi-syndrome is due to insufficient healthy qi；acute pain is due to failure to scatter blood stasis, pain with fixed position is due to blood stasis being confined to certain region；deformed and stiff joints even with failure to stretch and twist are due to blood stasis；darkish tongue with purplish petechiae and thin and astringent pulse are obvious signs of blood stasis.

Prescription：Activate blood, dissolve stasis and eliminate obstruction of blood vessels to stop pain.

Formulas：Huoluo Xiaoling Dan Jiawei（Modified Huoluo Xiaoling Pill）. In the formula, Danggui（*Radix Angelicae Sinensis*）and Danshen（*Radix Salviae Miltiorrhizae*）can have an action of nourishing blood, activating blood circulation and dissolving blood stasis；Ruxiang（*Olibanum*）and Moyao（*Myrrha*）are effective for activating blood and stopping pain. Combined together, Ruxiang could have a better action for rheumatalgia, the effect of Moyao in activating blood and dissolving blood stasis is stronger than that of Ruxiang, yet the difference between them is not obvious, therefore it is possible to combine them together. Besides, medicinal herbs for removing wind and eliminating obstructed blood vessels such as Quanxie（*Scorpio*）, Wugong（*Scolopendra*）and Dilong（*Lumbricus*）as well as medicine for dispelling dampness and dredging obstructed blood vessels such as Niuxi（*Radix Achyranthis Bidentatae*）, Qinjiao（*Radix Gentianae Macrophyllae*）, Qianghuo（*Rhizoma et Radix Notopterygii*）and Duhuo（*Radix Angelicae Pubescentis*）can be combined, or pungent-flavored medicinal herbs for moistening and dredging collaterals such as Xixin（*Herba Asari*）, Baijiezi（*Semen Sinapis Albae*）and Shengmahuang（*Herba Ephedrae*）can be combined.

3. 肾虚寒湿

31.2.3　Asthenia of kidney due to cold and dampness

【症状】痹症日久，关节畸形，其疼痛重着并肿胀，肢体沉重，活动不利，喜温怕冷，遇寒遇劳尤甚，腰膝酸困，舌质淡暗，脉象沉细。

【分析】痹症日久，肾气愈虚，寒湿流注不去，则疼痛日渐加重；寒湿为有形之邪，凝结关节，则关节变形肿胀；寒湿重着，故肢体沉重，活动不利；寒湿为阴邪，故遇寒加重，遇热减轻；寒湿之邪，最易伤及肾气，"腰为肾之府"，又主骨，肾腰被寒湿所困，故腰膝酸困；阳气不能温运血脉，故舌质淡暗，脉象沉细。

【治法】温肾散寒，通络止痛。

【方药】尪痹冲剂。此方为中华中医药学会内科分会痹证学组协定处方。方中以附子、骨碎补、仙灵脾、补骨脂、羊胫骨等补肝肾、强筋骨、益元气、填精髓；独活、桂枝、防风、威灵仙等散风除湿、通经活络、蠲痹痛；知母、白芍、生地黄、熟地黄等养血营筋，并兼制其他药物刚燥之弊。诸药合用，共奏补益肝肾、活血通络、蠲痹止痛之效。关节畸形者，加全蝎、地鳖虫、白芥子、僵蚕以搜风通络，化瘀止痛；疼痛剧烈者，可以加重附子的用量。

Clinical manifestations: Prolonged duration of Bi-syndrome (arthralgia), deformed swollen joints with heavy sensation and pain, heaviness of the body, inflexible movement, preference for warmth and aversion to cold, aggravation of the symptoms with cold and overstrain, aching and tiredness of the loins and knees, pale darkish tongue as well as sunken and thin pulse.

Analysis: Gradual aggravation of pain is due to downward migration of cold and dampness resulting from prolonged duration of Bi-syndrome (arthromyodynia) and asthenia of kidney qi; cold and dampness are tangible pathogens, coagulation of cold and dampness in the joints gives rise to deformed swollen joints; heaviness of the body and inflexible movement are due to heaviness and turbidity of cold and dampness; cold and dampness are yin pathogens, which gives rise to aggravation of pain with cold and alleviation with warmth; cold and dampness pathogens are susceptible to impairing kidney qi, the loins are the residence of the kidney, which dominates bones, aching and tiredness of the loins and knees are due to obstruction of cold and dampness; pale darkish tongue and sunken and thin pulse are due to failure of yang qi to warm and transport blood.

Prescription: Warm the kidney, disperse cold and dredge collaterals to stop pain.

Formulas: Wangbi Granules. This formula is designed by the academic branch of Bi-syndrome (arthralgia) under the department of internal medicine of China association of traditional Chinese medicine and pharmacy. In the formula, Fuzi (*Radix Aconiti Lateralis Preparata*), Gusuibu (*Rhizoma Drynariae*), Xianlingpi (*Herba Epimedii*), Buguzhi (*Fructus Psoraleae*) and Yangjinggu (shin bone of goat or sheep) can supplement the liver and kidney, strengthen the tendons and bones, benefit primordial qi, and enrich marrow; Duhuo (*Radix Angelicae Pubescentis*), Guizhi (*Ramulus Cinnamomi*), Fangfeng (*Radix Saposhnikoviae*) and Weilingxian (*Radix Clematidis*) have an action of dispersing wind, dispelling dampness, dredging meridians and collaterals as well as eliminating pain casused by Bi-syndrome (arthralgia); Zhimu (*Rhizoma Anemarrhenae*), Baishao (*Radix Paeoniae Alba*), Shengdihuang (*Radix Rehmanniae Recens*) and Shudihuang (*Radix Rehmanniae Preparata*) can nourish blood and tendons and avoid dryness of other medicinal herbs. Combined together, all medicinal herbs can bring tonifying the liver and kidney, activating blood, dredging blood vessels as well as eliminating pain of Bi-syndrome (arthralgia) into full play; for deformed joints, Quanxie (*Scorpio*), Tubiechong (*Eupolyphaga Seu Steleophaga*), Baijiezi (*Semen Sinapis Albae*) and Jiangcan (*Bombyx Batryticatus*) can be combined to remove wind, dredge blood vessels and dissolve stasis to stop pain; for acute pain, the amount of Fuzi can be increased.

三十二、痛经

32 Dysmenorrhea

〔概说〕 Summary

妇女正值经期或行经前后，出现周期性小腹疼痛，或痛引腰骶，甚则剧痛昏厥者，称为"痛经"，亦称"经行腹痛"。本病以青年女性较为常见。

痛经是常见的妇科病，以情志所伤、起居不慎或六淫所害为致病因素。气滞血瘀所致者，为"不通则痛"；胞宫失养所致者，为"不荣则痛"；寒邪内伤所致者，为"寒凝则痛"；湿热下注所致者，为"湿聚则痛"。总之，在治疗痛经时，要注意致病因素，以及证候变化，对于难以缓解的痛经，还要进行全身检查和妇科检查，以便明确病因，进行有的放矢的治疗。

Dysmenorrhea is a gynecological condition of periodic pain over the lower abdomen or pain involving the waist and sacrum. In some cases, acute pain can even cause syncope during menstruation, or before or after menstruation. Dysmenorrhea is usually defined as "abdominal pain with menstruation". The disease is commonly seen in young women.

Dysmenorrhea is a common gynecological disease caused by emotional impairment, improper living style or the six climatic pathogenic factors that cause disease such as wind, cold, summer heat, dampness, dryness and fire. In some cases, the disease may be caused by qi stagnation and blood stasis, known as "stagnation of qi and blood bringing about dysmenorrhea", or caused by malnutrition of the uterus, known as "malnutrition resulting in dysmenorrhea", or it is due to internal impairment because of retention of cold pathogens, which is named as "cold retention causing dysmenorrhea", or caused by downward migration of damp-heat, which is defined as "accumulation of dampness bringing about dysmenorrhea". In a word, in treating dysmenorrhea, much stress should be attached to the factors that cause the disease as well as syndrome changes. For unrelieved dysmenorrhea, overall physical checkup and gynecological examination should be taken for the sake of discerning its etiology and taking the most effective therapeutic principles accordingly.

〔辨证论治〕 Syndrome differentiation and treatment

1. 气滞血瘀

32.1 Qi stagnation and blood stasis

【症状】每于经前一二日或经期小腹胀痛，拒按，常伴有胸胁、乳房胀痛，或经量少，或经行不畅，经色紫暗有块，血块排出后痛减，经期过后疼痛消失。舌质紫暗或

369

有瘀点，脉象弦滑。

【分析】肝为血海，又主疏泄，肝气条达，则血海通调。若情志不遂，肝气怫郁，冲任气血郁滞，气血流通就会不通畅，故经期或行经时小腹胀痛、拒按；气血郁滞，故行经不畅，经色紫暗有块；待经块排出后，瘀血得解，腹痛自然减轻；胸胁、乳房为肝经经络行走之路，肝气郁滞，其经行之路自然不通畅，而发生胀痛；其舌象与脉搏为郁滞之征。

【治法】理气化瘀止痛。

【方药】膈下逐瘀汤加味。方中枳壳、香附、乌药理气疏肝，当归养血和血，川芎、赤芍、桃仁、红花、牡丹皮活血化瘀，延胡索、五灵脂化瘀止痛，甘草缓急调和诸药。若行经时，前后二阴下坠胀痛者，加川楝子、柴胡；若肝郁伐脾，腹胀纳少，加陈皮、麦芽、谷芽；若肝气犯胃，呕恶吞酸，加黄连、吴茱萸；若出现口苦、咽干、苔黄，为肝郁化热之象，加栀子、夏枯草。

Clinical manifestations: Distending pain over the lower abdomen, unpressable and accompanied with distending pain over the chest, hypochondrium as well as the breast one or two days before menstruation or during menstruation, or unsmooth menstruation with dark purplish menstrual blood mingled with clots, alleviation of pain after discharge of clots, disappearance of the pain after menstruation, dark purplish tongue with petechiae and taut and slippery pulse.

Analysis: The liver stores blood and it dominates dispersion of qi. Free flow of liver qi results in regulated blood circulation. Emotional upset causes stagnation of liver qi; stagnation of qi and blood in conception vessel and thoroughfare vessel brings about inhibited qi and blood circulation, which gives rise to distending pain over the lower abdomen unpressable during menstruation; unsmooth menstruation with dark purplish menstrual blood mingled with clots is due to qi and blood stagnation; after discharge of clots, blood stasis has been relieved, therefore, abdominal pain is alleviated, too; the chest, hypochondrium and breast are the passage of liver meridians and collaterals, qi stagnation in liver meridians results in inhibited menstruation and distending pain; dark purplish tongue with petechiae and taut and slippery pulse are signs of qi stagnation and blood stasis.

Prescription: Regulate qi and dissolve blood stasis to stop pain.

Formulas: Gexia Zhuyu Tang Jiawei (Modified Gexia Zhuyu Decoction). In the formula, Zhiqiao (*Fructus Aurantii*), Xiangfu (*Rhizoma Cyperi*) and Wuyao (*Radix Linderae*) can regulate qi and soothe the liver, Danggui (*Radix Angelicae Sinensis*) can nourish blood and regulate blood, Chuanxiong (*Rhizoma Ligustici Chuanxiong*), Chishao (*Radix Paeoniae Rubra*), Taoren (*Semen Persicae*), Honghua (*Flos Carthami*) and Mudanpi (*Cortex Moutan Radicis*) have an action of activating blood and dissolving blood stastis, Yanhusuo (*Rhizoma Corydalis*) and Wulingzhi (*Faeces Togopteri*) could dissolve stasis and stop pain, Gancao (*Radix Glycyrrhizae*) may relieve spasm and pain and reconcile the above medicinal herbs. For prolapse, distention and pain over external genitalia and anus during menstruation, Chuanlianzi (*Fructus Meliae Toosendan*) and Chaihu (*Radix Bupleuri*) could be added；for oppressed liver qi attacking the spleen，abdominal distention and poor appetite，Chenpi（*Pericarpium Citri Reticulatae*）, Maiya（*Fructus Hordei Germinatus*）and Guya（*Fructus Setariae Germinatus*）could be combined；for liver qi attacking the stomach, vomiting，nausea and acid regurgitation，Huanglian（*Rhizoma Coptidis*）and Wuzhuyu （*Fructus Evodiae*）may be added；for heat transformed from liver qi stagnation with symptoms such as bitter taste，dry mouth and yellowish fur，Zhizi（*Fructus Gardeniae*）and Xiakuxao （*Spica Prunellae*）can be combined.

2. 阳虚内寒
32.2 Yang asthenia due to internal retention of cold

【症状】经期或经后小腹冷痛，喜按，得热则减，经色暗淡，经量少，腰腿酸软，舌苔白润，脉象沉细。

【分析】肾为冲任之本，又主一身之阳气，肾阳虚弱，冲任失于温煦，胞宫自然寒凉，故经期或经后小腹冷痛，经量少而色暗淡；寒得热则减，故喜按喜温热；"腰为肾之府"，又主下焦，肾阳不足，故腰痛酸软；舌苔白润、脉象沉细，为虚寒之象。

【治法】温经暖宫止痛。

【方药】温经汤加味。温经汤为《金匮要略》之名方，为治疗妇科疾病的常用方。方中吴茱萸、肉桂温经散寒，兼通血脉而止痛；当归、川芎养血活血而调经；麦冬、阿胶滋阴养血；牡丹皮化瘀行血；芍药、甘草缓急止痛；人参益气温中；生姜、半夏散寒和中。在运用中，常加附子、艾叶、小茴香以增强温肾暖宫、散寒止痛之效。若手足不温，面色青白，舌质淡嫩，可去麦冬、阿胶，以防阴柔碍阳。

Clinical manifestations：Cold pain over the lower abdomen during or after menstruation, preference for pressure，alleviation of pain with warmth，pale darkish and scanty menstrual blood，aching and weakness of the loins and knees，whitish and moist tongue fur as well as sunken and thin pulse.

Analysis：The kidney is the origin of conception vessel and thoroughfare vessel, dominating yang qi of the whole body. Asthenia of kidney yang and loss of warmth of conception vessel and thoroughfare vessel result in cold and coolness of the uterus，which, gives rise to cold pain over the lower abdomen during or after menstruation and pale darkish scanty menstrual blood；preference for pressure and warmth is due to alleviation of cold with warmth；"the loins are the residence of the kidney"，they pertain to lower energizer, asthenia of kidney yang brings about aching and weakness of the loins and knees；whitish and moist tongue fur and sunken and thin pulse are signs of asthenia and cold.

Prescription：Warm the meridians and uterus and stop pain.

Formulas：Wenjing Tang Jiawei（Modified Wenjing Decoction）. Wenjing Tang is a famous formula quoted from *Jingui Yaolue*（*Synopsis of Golden Chamber*）, it is also a common recipe for gynecological disease，of which，Wuzhuyu（*Fructus Evodiae*）and Rougui（*Cortex Cinnamomi*）can warm the meridians，disperse cold and dredge blood vessels to stop pain；

Danggui (*Radix Angelicae Sinensis*) and Chuanxiong (*Rhizoma Ligustici Chuanxiong*) can nourish blood and regulate menstruation by activating blood; Maidong (*Radix Ophiopogonis*) and Ejiao (*Colla Corii Asini*) can nourish yin and nourish blood; Mudanpi (*Cortex Moutan Radicis*) has an action of dissolving stasis and blood, Chishao (*Radix Paeoniae Rubra*) and Gancao (*Radix Glycyrrhizae*) can relieve spasm and stop pain; Renshen (*Fructus Foeniculi*) can benefit qi and warm middle energizer; Shengjiang (*Rhizoma Zingiberis Recens*) and Banxia (*Rhizoma Pinelliae*) have the function of dispelling cold and reconciling middle energizer. In clinical practice, Fuzi (*Radix Aconiti Lateralis Preparata*), Aiye (*Folium Artemisiae Argyi*) and Xiaohuixiang (*Fructus Foeniculi*) could be added to strengthen the effect of warming the kidney and uterus so as to dispel cold and stop pain. For cold hands and feet, cyanic and whitish complexion as well as pale tender tongue, Maidong and Ejiao can be removed from the formula to prevent tenderness of yin from restraining yang.

3. 寒湿凝滞
32.3 Coagulation of cold and dampness

【症状】经前数日或经期小腹冷痛，得热痛减，按之痛甚，经量少，经色暗黑有块，形寒肢冷，舌苔白腻，脉象沉紧。

【分析】寒湿之邪重浊而沉凝，客于胞宫，与经血相搏，可使经血运行不畅，故于经前或经期小腹冷痛；血被寒凝，则经色暗黑有块；寒客经络，故形寒肢冷；热则寒气散，故痛减；舌苔白腻与脉象沉紧，为寒湿内闭之象。

【治法】温经散寒，除湿止痛。

【方药】少腹逐瘀汤加减。此方为温宫散寒之要方。方中肉桂、小茴香、干姜温经散寒除湿；当归、赤芍、川芎养血活血化瘀；延胡索、五灵脂、蒲黄、没药化瘀止痛。全方温经散寒、除湿止痛。可加苍术燥湿化浊，茯苓健脾渗湿。若寒湿郁闭于内，可加炮附子温壮阳气以通血脉。

Clinical manifestations: Cold pain over the lower abdomen several days before or during menstruation, alleviation of pain with warmth, aggravation of it with pressure, scanty darkish menstrual blood mingled with clots, cold body and limbs; greasy whitish fur as well as sunken and tense pulse.

Analysis: Heaviness and turbidity of pathogenic cold and dampness invade the uterus and struggle with menstrual blood, resulting in unsmooth menstrual blood circulation and cold pain over the lower abdomen before or during menstruation; darkish menstrual blood mingled with clots is due to coagulation of blood with cold; cold body and limbs are caused by cold attacking the meridians and collaterals; alleviation of pain with warmth is due to cold and qi being dispersed by warmth; whitish greasy fur and sunken and tense pulse are signs of internal blockage of cold and dampness.

Prescription: Warm meridians, disperse cold and eliminate dampness to stop pain.

Formulas: Shaofu Zhuyu Tang Jiajian (Modified Shaofu Zhuyu Decoction), which is a principal formula for warming the uterus and dispersing cold. In the formula, Rougui (*Cortex Cinnamomi*), Xiaohuixiang (*Fructus Foeniculi*) and Ganjiang (*Rhizoma Zingiberis*) can warm the meridians, disperse cold and eliminate dampness; Danggui (*Radix Angelicae Sinensis*), Chishao (*Radix Paeoniae Rubra*) and Chuanxiong (*Rhizoma Ligustici Chuanxiong*) can nourish blood, activate blood and dissolve stasis; Yanhusuo (*Rhizoma Corydalis*), Wulingzhi (*Faeces Togopteri*), Puhuang (*Pollen Typhae*) and Moyao (*Myrrha*) could dissolve stasis and stop pain. The whole formula has the action of warming meridians, dispersing cold and eliminating dampness to stop pain. Cangzhu (*Rhizoma Atractylodis*) can be added to dry dampness and resolve turbidity, Fuling (*Poriae Cocos*) may be combined to invigorate the spleen and resolve dampness. For internal blockage of cold and dampness, soaked Fuzi (*Radix Aconiti Lateralis Preparata*) may be combined to warm yang and strengthen qi to dredge blood vessels.

4. 湿热下注
32.4 Downward migration of dampness and heat

【症状】经前小腹疼痛拒按，行经时有灼热感，经来疼痛明显，经色暗红，质稠有块，带下黄稠，有低热起伏，小便短赤，舌苔黄腻，脉象弦滑而数。

【分析】湿热之证，有外感与内蕴之分，但与体质有密切关系。本证为湿热下注所致。湿热之邪，下注胞宫，与血相搏，故小腹疼痛拒按，且经血有块；经来湿热浸淫，故有灼热感；湿热下注不散，故带下黄稠，小便短赤；湿热之邪，缠绵难愈，故有低热起伏；其舌苔与脉象，为湿热之征。

【治法】清热除湿，化瘀止痛。

【方药】清热调血汤加味。清热调血汤为《古今医鉴》之方。方以牡丹皮清热凉血散瘀；生地黄清热凉血；黄连清热燥湿；当归、白芍养血活血；川芎、红花、桃仁、莪术活血化瘀；香附、延胡索行气止痛。另加红藤、薏苡仁、败酱草清热解毒，除湿消瘀。

Clinical manifestations: Unpressable pain over the lower abdomen before menstruation, scorching sensation and obvious pain during menstruation, thick and dark reddish menstrual blood mingled with clots, thick yellowish leucorrhea, occasional mild fever, scanty brownish urine, yellowish greasy fur as well as taut, slippery and fast pulse.

Analysis: Syndrome of dampness and heat is classified into exogenous damp-heat and internal damp-heat, both of them are connected with constitution. This syndrome is caused by downward migration of dampness and heat. Migration of pathogenic dampness and heat factors into the uterus causes struggle with blood, giving rise to unpressable pain over the lower abdomen as well as menstrual blood with clots; scorching sensation during menstruation is due to invasion and spreading of dampness and heat; thick yellowish leucorrhea and scanty brownish urine are due to downward migration of unscattered dampness and heat; occasional mild fever is caused by prolonged stagnation of pathogenic dampness and heat factors with difficulty to be cured; yellowish greasy fur and taut, slippery and fast pulse are signs of the syndrome of dampness and heat.

Prescription: Clear away heat, dispel dampness and dissolve stasis to stop pain.

Formulas: Qingre Tiaoxue Tang Jiawei (Modified Qingre Tiaoxue Decoction). Qingre Tiaoxue Tang is a formula quoted from *Gujin Yijian* (*The Ancient and Modern Medicine*). In the formula, Mudanpi (*Cortex Moutan Radicis*) can clear away heat, cool blood and disperse stasis; Shengdihuang (*Radix Rehmanniae Recens*) has an action of clearing away heat and cooling blood; Huanglian (*Rhizoma Coptidis*) can clear away heat and dry dampness; Danggui (*Radix Angelicae Sinensis*) and Baishao (*Radix Paeoniae Alba*) may nourish blood and activate blood; Chuanxiong (*Rhizoma Ligustici Chuanxiong*), Honghua (*Flos Carthami*), Taoren (*Semen Persicae*) and Ezhu (*Rhizoma Curcumae*) can nourish blood, activate blood and dissolve stasis; Xiangfu (*Rhizoma Cyperi*) and Yanhusuo (*Rhizoma Corydalis*) can activate qi and stop pain. Hongteng (*Caulis Sargentodoxae*), Yiyiren (*Semen Coicis*) and Baijiangcao (*Herba Patriniae*) can be added to clear away heat and resolve toxic pathogen so as to eliminate dampness and stasis.

5. 气血虚弱
32.5 Qi and blood asthenia

【症状】经后一二日或经期小腹隐隐作痛，或小腹及阴部有空坠感，喜揉按，月经量少，色淡质薄，面色无华，神气疲倦，食少便溏，舌质淡红，脉象细弱。

【分析】气血不足，冲任空虚，经后血海更虚，血虚濡养不足，气虚运行无力，血脉行迟，故小腹隐隐作痛；喜揉按为虚证之特点；血虚精血不荣，则经色淡而质薄，面色无华；气血失于濡养，则神气自然疲倦；脾胃气虚，则食少便溏；舌淡脉、脉象细弱，为气血虚弱之征。

【治法】益气补血止痛。

【方药】圣愈汤加减。圣愈汤为《兰室秘藏》方，即参芪四物汤（减白芍），方由人参、黄芪、熟地黄、当归、川芎、生地黄六味组成。人参、黄芪大补元气；四物汤（加入白芍）养血和血；另加香附、延胡索调气止痛。若血虚甚，可加鸡血藤、酸枣仁、大枣以补血安神；若腰膝酸痛明显，可加菟丝子、续断、桑寄生以补肾壮腰。

Clinical Manifestations: Dull pain over the lower abdomen one or two days after menstruation or during menstruation, or vacuous pain with prolapsing sensation over the lower abdomen as well as vagina, preference for pressing, scanty menstruation, pale and thin menstrual blood, lusterless complexion, dispiritedness and exhaustion, reduced appetite and loose stool, pale reddish tongue as well as thin and weak pulse.

Analysis: Insufficient qi and blood results in weakness of the thoroughfare and conception vessels and even vacuity of the thoroughfare vessel sea of blood after menstruation. Blood asthenia causes insufficient nutrition and qi asthenia results in weakness as well as slow and tardy circulation of blood, which gives rise to dull pain over the lower abdomen; preference for pressing is a feature of asthenia syndrome; pale and thin menstrual blood and lusterless complexion are caused by blood asthenia and failure of essence and blood to nourish the face; dispiritedness and exhaustion are due to loss of nutrition of qi and blood; reduced appetite and loose stool are due to qi asthenia of the spleen and stomach; pale reddish tongue and thin and weak pulse are signs of qi and blood asthenia.

Prescription: Supplement qi and blood and arrest pain.

Formulas: Shengyu Tang Jiajian (Modified Shengyu Decoction). Shengyu Tang is a formula quoted from *Lanshi Micang* (*A Secret Book Kept in Orchid Chamber*), namely, removing Baishao (*Radix Paeoniae Alba*) from Shen Qi Siwu Tang. The formula is made up of Renshen (*Fructus Foeniculi*), Huangqi (*Radix Astragali seu Hedysari*), Shudihuang (*Radix Rehmanniae Preparata*), Danggui (*Radix Angelicae Sinensis*), Chuanxiong (*Rhizoma Ligustici Chuanxiong*) and Shengdihuang (*Radix Rehmanniae Recens*). Among them, Renshen and Huangqi can tonify primordial qi, Siwu Tang combined with Baishao has an action of nourishing blood and harmonizing blood; Xiangfu (*Rhizoma Cyperi*) and Yanhusuo (*Rhizoma Corydalis*) can be added to regulate qi circulation so as to arrest pain. For blood asthenia, Jixueteng (*Caulis Spatholobi*), Suanzaoren (*Semen Ziziphi Spinosae*) and Dazao (*Fructus Jujubae*) can be combined to supplement blood and tranquilize the mind; for obvious aching and pain over the loins and knees, Tusizi (*Semen Cuscutae*), Xuduan (*Radix Dipsaci*) and Sangjisheng (*Herba Taxilli*) can be added to supplement the kidney and strengthen the loins.

6. 肝肾亏损
32.6 Deficiency of the liver and kidney

【症状】经行后一二日小腹绵绵作痛，腰部酸胀，经色暗淡，量少，经质稀薄，或有潮热、耳鸣，舌苔薄白而干或薄黄，脉象细弱。

【分析】肝肾不足，精血亏损，血海空虚，胞脉失养，故行经之后，小腹隐隐作痛，且经量少而质稀薄；"阴虚则内热"，故有潮热、耳鸣；肾虚其府失养，故腰部酸胀；其舌苔薄白而干或薄黄，脉象细弱，为精血亏虚之象。

【治法】益肾养肝止痛。

【方药】调肝汤加减。调肝汤为清代傅青主所创。方中当归、白芍养血柔肝；山茱萸养肝填精；巴戟天温肾益冲任；阿胶滋阴养血；山药健脾和中。另加杜仲、续断、桑寄生益肾壮腰；若肝气不调，可加川楝子、小茴香、橘核疏肝理气止痛。

Clinical manifestations: Lingering dull pain over the lower abdomen one or two days after menstruation, aching and distending sensation over the loins, dark reddish menstrual blood, scanty menstruation with pale and thin menstrual blood; or accompanied with tidal fever, tinnitus, thin, dry and whitish tongue fur or thin, dry and yellowish fur as well as thin and weak pulse.

Analysis: Asthenia of the liver and kidney causes deficiency of kidney essence and blood as well as emptiness of thoroughfare vessel, which results in malnutrition of the vessels of the uterus and dull pain over the lower abdomen after menstruation as well as scanty and thin menstrual blood; tidal fever and tinnitus are due to "yin asthenia generating endogenous heat"; aching and distending sensation over the loins are due to kidney asthenia and failure to nourish its residence; thin and dry tongue fur or thin yellowish fur as well as thin and weak pulse are signs of asthenia of kidney essence and blood.

Prescription: Strengthen the kidney and nourish the liver to stop pain.

Formulas: Tiaogan Tang Jiajian (Modified Tiaogan Decoction). Tiaogan Tang is designed by Fu Qingzhu from the Qing Dynasty, of which, Danggui (*Radix Angelicae Sinensis*) and Baishao (*Radix Paeoniae Alba*) can nourish blood and soften the liver; Shanzhuyu (*Fructus Corni*) has an action of nourishing the liver and enriching kidney essence; Bajitian (*Radix Morindae Officinalis*) could warm the kidney and strengthen thoroughfare and conception vessels; Ejiao (*Colla Corii Asini*) can tonify yin and nourish blood; Shanyao (*Rhizoma Dioscoreae*) has an action of invigorating the spleen and harmonizing middle energizer. Duzhong (*Cortex Eucommiae*), Xuduan (*Radix Dipsaci*) and Sangjisheng (*Herba Taxilli*) can be added to supplement the kidney and strengthen the loins; for failure to regulate liver qi, Chuanlianzi (*Fructus Meliae Toosendan*), Xiaohuixiang (*Fructus Foeniculi*) and Juhe (*Semen Citri Reticulatae*) could be combined to soothe the liver and regulate qi to stop pain.

三十三、带下

33　Leukorrheal disease

〔概说〕Summary

带下有白带、黄带、赤带、青带、黑带、赤白带等。

带下是指从女子阴部内流出一种黏滞的物质，绵绵如带，临床以白带为多，故本文主要叙述白带，兼及黄带、赤白带等。

中医学认为，白带多是脾虚证，也有肝气郁结而致者。病程日久也有肾虚不能温化，水湿下注而出现者。其治疗不外乎健脾、燥湿、温肾、气化、清热等。

Leukorrheal disease includes abnormal discharge of whitish, or yellowish, or reddish, or blackish, or greenish leucorrhea as well as reddish mingled with whitish leucorrhea and so on.

Morbid leukorrhea is a kind of mucous and sticky vaginal excreta like a strip. Whitish leucorrhea is commonly seen in clinical practice, so it is the focus of this chapter. Other morbid leucorrhea such as yellowish, or reddish mingled with whitish leucorrhea can also be involved.

In terms of TCM, profuse leucorrhea indicates asthenia of the spleen, or it is caused by stagnation of liver qi. Prolonged course of the disease probably results from failure of asthenic kidney in warming and transformation and downward migration of dampness. Therapeutic methods for leucorrhea involves invigorating the spleen, drying dampness, warming the kidney, transforming qi, clearing away heat, etc.

〔辨证论治〕 Syndrome differentiation and treatment

1. 脾虚
33.1 Leukorrhea due to asthenic spleen

【症状】带下量多，色白或淡黄，质黏稠，无臭气，绵绵不断，面色㿠白或萎黄，四肢不温，精神疲倦，纳少便溏，足背浮肿，舌淡苔白或腻，脉象缓弱。

【分析】脾主运化，若脾气虚弱，失却运化之力，水湿下陷而为带下；脾虚中阳不振，则面色㿠白或萎黄；脾阳不能达于四肢，故四肢不温；湿浊困于中焦，则纳呆；水湿下注，则足背浮肿，大便稀薄；舌淡苔白或腻，脉象缓弱，为脾虚阳气不振之象。

【治法】健脾益气，升阳除湿。

【方药】完带汤。完带汤为治疗脾虚带下的主方。方中重用白术、山药以健脾束带；人参、甘草补气扶中；苍术健脾燥湿；柴胡、白芍、陈皮疏肝解郁，理气升阳；车前子利水除湿；黑荆芥穗入于血分祛风胜湿。全方脾、胃、肝同治，具有健脾益气，除湿止带之功。若肾虚腰痛，加杜仲、菟丝子；若带下日久，可加金樱子、芡实、乌贼骨等，以固涩止带；若湿浊化热，夹有黄带，可加知母、黄柏清热除湿。

Clinical manifestations: Profuse discharge of whitish or pale yellowish leucorrhea with mucous and thick texture, no odor, lingering duration, pale or sallow complexion, cold limbs, dispiritedness, poor appetite and loose stool, dropsy over the dorsum of the feet, pale tongue with greasy whitish fur as well as moderate and weak pulse.

Analysis: The spleen dominates transportation and transformation of food, deficiency and weakness of splenic qi results in dysfunction of the spleen in transportation and transformation, which gives rise to leucorrhea due to downward migration of dampness; pale or sallow complexion is due to weakness of yang qi in middle energizer because of asthenic spleen; cold limbs are caused by failure of yang qi in the spleen to reach the limbs; poor appetite is due to retention of dampness and turbidity in middle energizer; dropsy over the dorsum of the feet and loose stool are caused by downward migration of dampness; pale tongue with greasy whitish fur and moderate and weak pulse are signs of weakness of yang qi because of asthenic spleen.

Prescription: Supplement the spleen, benefit qi, invigorate splenic yang and eliminate dampness.

Formulas: Wandai Tang (Decoction). It is an essential formula for leukorrhea due to asthenic spleen. In the formula, Baizhu (*Rhizoma Atractylodis Macrocephalae*) and Shanyao (*Rhizoma Dioscoreae*) can tonify the spleen to control leucorrhea; Renshen (*Fructus Foeniculi*) and Gancao (*Radix Glycyrrhizae*) can supplement qi to strengthen middle energizer; Cangzhu (*Rhizoma Atractylodis*) has an action of invigorating the spleen to dry dampness; Chaihu (*Radix Bupleuri*), Baishao (*Radix Paeoniae Alba*) and Chenpi (*Pericarpium Citri Reticulatae*) can soothe the liver, relieve qi stagnation, regulate qi and invigorate yang; Cheqianzi (*Semen Plantaginis*) has an function of inducing diuresis and eliminating dampness; black Jingjiesui (*Spica Schizonepetae*) can expel wind and dampness by transmitting into blood phase. The whole formula can treat the spleen, stomach and liver simultaneously with the action of tonifying the spleen, benefiting qi as well as eliminating dampness and leukorrhea. For aching loins due to asthenic kidney, Duzhong (*Cortex Eucommiae*) and Tusizi (*Semen Cuscutae*) can be added; for prolonged leucorrhea, Jinyingzi (*Fructus Rosae Laevigatae*), Qianshi (*Semen Euryales*) and Wuzeigu (*Sepium*) can be combined to astringe and arrest leucorrhea; for heat transformed from dampness and turbidity as well as leucorrhea mingled with yellowish color, Zhimu (*Rhizoma Anemarrhenae*) and Huangbo (*Cortex Phellodendri*) should be added to clear away heat and dispel dampness.

2. 肾虚
33.2 Leukorrhea due to asthenia of the kidney

（1）肾阴虚
【症状】带下赤白，质黏无臭，阴部灼热，头昏目眩，或面部烘热，五心烦热，失眠多梦，大便不爽，小便黄赤，舌红少苔，脉象细数。
【分析】肾阴不足，相火偏旺，损伤血络，故带下赤白、质黏，阴部灼热；阴虚不能潜阳，相火上炎，故头昏目眩，面部烘热，五心烦热；肾阴虚亏，不能上济心火，则失眠多梦；阴虚失于濡润，则大便不爽，小便黄赤；舌红少苔、脉象细数，为阴虚火旺之象。
【治法】滋肾养阴，清热止带。
【方药】知柏地黄汤加减。知柏地黄汤见"慢性肾小球肾炎"。临床应用时，可加芡实、金樱子，补肾固涩止带。

（1）Leukorrhea due to asthenia of kidney yin

Clinical manifestations: Reddish and whitish leucorrhea, odorless and sticky texture, scorching sensation over the vagina, vertigo and dizziness, or mild feverish sensation over the face, dysphoria and feverish sensation over the chest, palms and soles, insomnia and dreaminess, unsmooth defecation, yellowish and brownish urine, reddish tongue with scanty fur as well as thin and fast pulse.

Analysis: Insufficiency of kidney yin results in hyperactive ministerial fire (fire in lower energizer) impairing blood vessels, which gives rise to reddish, whitish, sticky and odorless leucorrhea as well as scorching sensation over the vagina; vertigo and dizziness, or mild feverish sensation over the face, chest, palms and soles are due to up-flaming of ministerial fire because of failure of asthenic yin to suppress yang; insomnia and dreaminess are due to failure of asthenic kidney yin to arrest heart fire; unsmooth defecation and yellowish and brownish urine are due to loss of moisture due to asthenic yin; reddish tongue with scanty fur and thin and fast pulse are signs of hyperactive fire due to yin asthenia.

Prescription: Nourish the kidney and yin and clear away heat to stop leucorrhea.

Formulas: Zhi Bo Dihuang Tang Jiajian (Modified Zhi Bo Dihuang Decoction). The formula has been discussed in the chapter of *Chronic Glomerulonephritis*. Clinically, Qianshi (*Semen Euryales*) and Jinyingzi (*Fructus Rosae Laevigatae*) can be added to tonify the kidney and astringe leucorrhea.

（2）肾阳虚

【症状】白带清冷，量多，质稀薄，淋漓不断，腰酸如折，小腹冷痛，小便频数清长，夜间尤甚，大便溏薄，舌质淡红，脉象沉迟。

【分析】肾阳不足，阳虚内寒，带脉失约，任脉不固，故带下清冷，量多，质稀薄，且淋沥不断；"腰为肾之府"，肾虚失养，故腰酸如折；小腹为胞宫所居之地，胞脉系于肾，肾阳虚弱，不能温煦胞宫，故小腹冷痛；肾虚于下，不能温暖下焦，故小便频数清长，夜间尤甚；脾阳虚弱，则大便溏薄；舌质淡红，脉象沉迟，为肾阳不足之征。

【治法】温肾培元，固涩止带。

【方药】内补丸。方中以鹿茸、肉苁蓉温肾阳，生精髓；菟丝子补肝肾，固任脉；黄芪补气；肉桂、附子温命火，补真火；潼蒺藜温肾止腰痛；白蒺藜疏肝祛风；紫菀温肺益肾；桑螵蛸收涩固精。全方具有温肾壮阳、益精固涩之力。若便溏者，去肉苁蓉，加补骨脂、肉豆蔻。

（2）Leukorrhea due to asthenic kidney yang

Clinical manifestations: Clear leucorrhea with cold sensation, profuse and dripping leucorrhea with thin texture, aching loins with the sensation like being broken, cold pain over the lower abdomen, frequent urination with clear and profuse discharge, aggravation of urination at night, thin and loose stool, pale reddish tongue as well as sunken and moderate pulse.

Analysis: Insufficiency of kidney yang causes asthenic yang and internal cold, which resulting in loss of control of belt vessel and weakness of conception vessel, thus, giving rise to clear leucorrhea with cold sensation, and profuse, thin and dripping leucorrhea; "the loins are the house of the kidney", aching loins with the sensation like being broken is due to malnutrition because of asthenic kidney; the lower abdomen is the residence of the uterus, blood vessels of the uterus are connected with the kidney, cold pain over the lower abdomen is due to failure of asthenic kidney yang to warm the uterus; frequent urination with clear and profuse discharge and aggravation at night are due to failure of asthenic kidney to warm lower energizer; thin and loose stool is due to asthenia of splenic yang; pale reddish tongue and sunken and slow pulse are indications of insufficient kidney yang.

Prescription: Warm the kidney to supplement primordial qi and stop leucorrhea with astringent medicinal herbs.

Formulas：Neibu Wan（Pill）. In the formula，Lurong（*Cornu Cervi Pantotrichum*）and Roucongrong（*Herba Cistanches*）have an action of warming kidney yang and generating kidney essence and marrow；Tusizi（*Semen Cuscutae*）can supplement the kidney and strengthen conception vessel；Huangqi（*Radix Astragali seu Hedysari*）can supplement qi；Rougui（*Cortex Cinnamomi*）and Fuzi（*Radix Aconiti Lateralis Preparata*）have an action of warming the fire in Mingmen（the gate of vitality）as well as fire in the kidney；Tongjili（*Semen Astragali Complanati*）can warm the kidney to stop pain in the loins，Baijili（*Tribulus Terrestris*）may soothe the liver and expel wind；Ziwan（*Radix Asteris*）has an action of warming the lung and supplementing the kidney；Sangpiaoxiao（*Ootheca Mantidis*）can control nocturnal emission with its astringent action. The whole recipe can warm the kidney，strengthen kidney yang and benefit essence. For loose stool，Roucongrong can be removed，Buguzhi（*Fructus Psoraleae*）and Roudoukou（*Semen Myristicae*）may be added.

3. 湿热
33.3 Leukorrhea due to damp heat

【症状】带下量多，色黄或黄白相兼，质黏腻，有秽浊之气，或带下如豆腐渣样，食欲不振，口腻，阴痒，小便黄少，舌苔厚腻，脉象濡数。

【分析】湿热蕴积于下焦，任、带二脉受损，故带下量多，色黄或黄白相兼；若湿浊偏重，则带下如豆腐渣样，阴痒；湿热下注，元气秽浊，则有难闻之气；湿热内阻，脾胃不和，则食欲不振；湿热伤津，故小便黄少；舌苔厚腻与脉象濡数，均为湿热之征。

【治法】清利湿热。

【方药】止带汤。方中以茯苓、猪苓、泽泻、车前子利水除湿；茵陈、黄柏、栀子、牡丹皮清热泻火解毒；牛膝引药下行。若带下色黄、秽浊难闻，阴痒，可用龙胆泻肝汤治疗。

Clinical manifestations：Profuse leucorrhea，yellowish color or yellowish mingled with white color，sticky and greasy texture with foul odor，or leucorrhea like residue of soybean curb，poor appetite，greasy taste of the mouth，pruritus vulvae，scanty and yellowish urine，thick greasy fur as well as soft and fast pulse.

Analysis：Profuse leucorrhea with yellowish color or yellowish mingled with white color is due to accumulation of dampness and heat in lower energizer which impairs belt vessel and conception vessels；leucorrhea like residue of soybean curb and pruritus vulvae are caused by severe turbidity of dampness；foul odor is due to foul and turbid primordial qi because of downward migration of dampness and heat；poor appetite is caused by internal retention of dampness and heat and disharmony of the spleen and stomach；scanty and yellowish urine is due to damp-heat impairing body fluid；thick greasy fur and soft and fast pulse are signs of dampness and heat.

Prescription：Eliminate dampness and heat.

Formulas：Zhidai Tang (Decoction). In the formula, Fuling (*Poriae Cocos*), Zhuling (*Polyporus Umbellatus*), Zexie (*Rhizoma Alismatis*) and Cheqianzi (*Semen Plantaginis*) can induce diuresis and eliminate dampness; Yinchen (*Herba Artemisiae Scopariae*), Huangbo (*Cortex Phellodendri*), Zhizi (*Fructus Gardeniae*) and Mudanpi (*Cortex Moutan Radicis*) have an action of purging fire and relieving toxic pathogens; Niuxi (*Radix Achyranthis Bidentatae*) can guide medicine downward. For yellowish leucorrhea with foul odor and pruritus vulvae, Longdan Xiegan Tang can be combined.

4. 热毒
33.4 Leukorrhea due to heat toxin

【症状】带下量多，或赤白相兼，或五色杂下，质黏腻，或如脓样，有臭气，阴痒，烦热口渴，午后尤甚，小腹作痛，大便干结，小便黄少，舌质红，苔黄干，脉象濡数。

【分析】热毒损伤任、带二脉，气血俱伤，故带下赤白，或五色杂下，量多；热毒蕴结不解，故有带下臭气，阴痒；热毒伤津，则烦热口渴，午后尤甚；热毒纠结于下，则小腹作痛；热毒伤津，大便干结，小便黄少；舌红、苔黄、脉数，均为热毒之征。

【治法】清热解毒。

【方药】五味消毒饮加减。方中蒲公英、金银花、野菊花、紫花地丁、天葵子，均为清热解毒之品；加白花蛇舌草既能清热解毒，又能利湿；椿皮在清热利湿中有止血作用；加白术健脾利湿。若脾胃虚弱，健运不及，可加黄芪益气健脾。

Clinical manifestations：Profuse leucorrhea, or reddish mingled with whitish leucorrhea, or leucorrhea with various colors with sticky greasy texture, or leucorrhea like pus with foul odor and pruritus vulvae, dysphoria and thirst, aggravated thirst in the afternoon, lower abdominal pain, dry feces and scanty yellowish urine, reddish tongue with yellowish dry fur as well as soft and fast pulse.

Analysis：Reddish mingled with whitish leucorrhea, or profuse leucorrhea with various color is due to impairment of qi and blood because of heat toxin impairing thoroughfare and conception vessels; leucorrhea with foul odor and pruritus vulvae are due to unrelieved stagnation of heat toxic pathogens; dysphoria and thirst with aggravation in the afternoon are due to heat toxin impairing body fluid; lower abdominal pain is caused by downward invasion of heat toxin; dry feces and scanty yellowish urine are due to heat toxin impairing body fluid; reddish tongue with yellowish fur as well as fast pulse are signs of heat toxin.

Prescription：Clear away heat and toxin.

Formulas：Wuwei Xiaodu Yin Jiajian (Modified Wuwei Xiaodu Decoction). In the formula, Pugongying (*Herba Taraxaci*), Jinyinhua (*Flos Lonicerae*), Yejuhua (*Flos Chrysanthemi Indici*), Zihuadiding (*Herba Violae*) and Tiankuizi (*Radix Semiaquilegiae*) are medicinal herbs to clear away heat and relieve toxic pathogens; Baihuasheshecao (*Herba Hedyotidis*) can be added to clear away heat, relieve toxic pathogens and remove dampness through diuresis；Chunpi（*Cortex Ailanthi*）has an action of stopping bleeding as well as clearing away heat and removing dampness；Baizhu（*Rhizoma Atractylodis Macrocephalae*）can be added to invigorate the spleen and resolve dampness. For dysfunction of asthenic spleen and stomach in transportation，Huangqi（*Radix Astragali seu Hedysari*）should be added to supplement qi and invigorate the spleen.

三十四、产后缺乳

34 Hypogalactia after childbirth

〔**概说**〕 Summary

产后缺乳是指产后乳汁甚少或全无乳汁。

引起产后缺乳的原因一般有两种，一是产后气血虚弱，一是产后肝郁气滞。前者为气血虚弱，难以产乳；后者为乳络郁滞，难以出乳。中医对产后缺乳有着良好的治疗效果，且无副作用，深受产妇喜爱。

Hypogalactia is a condition in which secretion of milk in nursing mothers is insufficient to meet the demands of their babies or failure of secreting breast milk after childbirth.

Hypogalactia can be attributed to asthenia of qi and blood after childbirth and qi stagnation due to qi depression of the liver. The former case is caused by failure of asthenic qi and blood to excrete milk，while the latter is due to stagnation of breast collaterals. TCM therapeutic methods for hypogalactia could achieve a good curative effect without any side effect，which，therefore，have been accepted and loved by delivery women.

〔**辨证论治**〕 Syndrome differentiation and treatment

1. 气血虚弱

34.1 Asthenia of qi and blood

【症状】产后乳汁分泌少，面色苍白，食欲不振，气短，乏力，便溏，乳房柔软无胀痛，舌淡苔少，脉象虚细。

【分析】产后气血虚弱，或脾胃虚弱，或分娩时失血过多，气血不足，势必影响乳汁分泌。气血不足以荣面，故面色苍白；脾胃虚弱，难以运化水谷，故食欲不振；中气不足，则气短、乏力；脾虚湿浊不化，故便溏；因无气滞血瘀，故乳房柔软无胀痛；舌淡苔少、脉象虚细，为脾胃气虚虚弱之表现。

【治法】补气养血，佐以通乳。

【方药】八珍汤加减。八珍汤由四君子汤和四物汤两方组成，为补益气血之首选方，且对中焦亦有健脾益胃的作用。方中四君子汤为补气之首方，四物汤为补血之首方，两方组合，气血兼顾，非常适合产后补虚之用。可加生麦芽开胃醒脾下乳，丝瓜络、路路通通络行乳。

Clinical manifestations：Insufficient excretion of milk following childbirth, pale complexion, poor appetite, short breath, lack of energy, loose stool, softness of the breasts without distending pain, pale tongue with scanty fur as well as weak and thin pulse.

Analysis：Asthenia of qi and blood after childbirth, or asthenic spleen and stomach, or excessive loss of blood during delivery causes deficient qi and blood, which, must have an effect on milk excretion. Pale complexion is due to failure of insufficient qi and blood to nourish the face; poor appetite is due to dysfunction of asthenic spleen and stomach in food transportation and transformation; short breath and lack of energy are caused by insufficiency of qi in middle energizer; loose stool is due to failure of asthenic spleen to transform dampness and turbidity; softness of the breast without distending pain is due to non-existence of qi stagnation and blood stasis; pale tongue with scanty fur and weak and thin pulse are presentations of qi asthenia of the spleen and stomach.

Prescription：Supplement qi, nourish blood and dredge breast collaterals for promoting secretion of milk.

Formulas：Bazhen Tang Jiajian (Modified Bazhen Decoction). Bazhen Tang is made up of Sijunzi Tang and Siwu Tang, the first choice for supplement qi and blood, which is beneficial for invigorating the function of middle energizer. Sijunzi Tang is the best choice for supplementing qi, and Siwu Tang is the best formula for tonifying blood, combined together, they are very suitable for treating asthenia syndrome after childbirth. Shengmaiya (*Fructus Hordei Germinatus*) could be added to stimulate appetite and refresh the spleen to promote excretion of milk, Sigualuo (*Retinervus Luffae Fructus*) and Lulutong (*Fructus Liquidambaris*) can be combined to dredge collaterals so as to activate excretion of milk.

2. 肝郁气滞

34.2　Qi stagnation due to liver depression

【症状】产后乳汁不行，乳房胀满、疼痛或有肿块，食少，胸闷，呃逆，便干，舌红苔薄黄，脉象弦滑。

【分析】产后情志抑郁，肝气不舒，气机不畅，影响乳汁生化，因而乳汁不行。乳房为肝经循行部位，肝郁气滞，则胸闷、乳房胀痛，或有肿块；肝郁影响脾胃的纳谷与运化，故食少，呃逆，便干；舌红苔薄黄，脉象弦滑，为肝郁化热之象。

【治法】疏肝通络，佐以通乳。

【方药】涌泉散加减。涌泉散为治疗乳汁不通之名方，组成为白丁香、王不留行、天花粉、漏芦、白僵蚕，猪蹄汤煎服。白丁香现在一般不用；王不留行、漏芦、猪蹄汤，具有通络下乳的作用；天花粉润燥泻火，白僵蚕化痰祛风；猪蹄汤具有补气养血、通络下乳的作用，一般都要选用。在应用处方时，可以进行调整，王不留行、漏芦、天花粉、柴胡、生麦芽、通草、猪蹄汤煎药服用；若乳房牵扯胸胁疼痛，可加郁金、香附疏肝散结。

Clinical manifestations：Failure to secrete milk after childbirth, distending pain, fullness or swollen lumps of the breasts, reduced appetite, chest oppression, hiccup, dry feces, reddish tongue with thin yellowish fur as well as taut and slippery pulse.

Analysis：Qi stagnation due to liver depression following childbirth results in disorder of qi circulation, which affects production and excretion of milk, thus, leading to failure of producing milk. The breasts are the area the liver meridians pass through, qi stagnation due to liver depression brings about distending pain, fullness or swollen lumps of the breasts; reduced appetite, chest oppression, hiccup and dry feces are due to dysfunction of the spleen and stomach in receiving food as well as transporting and transforming food because of qi depression of the liver; reddish tongue with thin yellowish fur and taut and slippery pulse are signs of transformation of heat from qi depression in the liver.

Prescription：Soothe the liver, dredge collaterals and promote secretion of milk.

Formulas：Yongquan San Jiajian (Modified Yongquan Powder). Yongquan San is a famous recipe for treating failure of production and secretion of milk, which consists of Baidingxiang (*Syringa Oblatavar Alba*); Wangbuliuxing (*Semen Vaccariae*), Tianhuafen (*Radix Trichosanthis*), Loulu (*Radix Rhapontici*), Baijiangcan (*Bombyx Batryticatus*) and soup made with pig's feet, with all ingredients decocted together. Baidingxiang is not used nowadays; Wangbuliuxing, Loulu and soup made with pig's feet have the action of dredging collaterals to promote secretion of milk; Tianhuafen can moisten dryness and purge fire, Baijiangcan may resolve phlegm and dispel wind; soup made with pig's feet can supplement qi to nourish blood, and dredge collaterals to promote secretion of milk. In clinical practice, the recipe can be replaced by the combination of Wangbuliuxing, Loulu, Tianhuafen, Chaihu (*Radix Bupleuri*), Shengmaiya (*Fructus Hordei Germinatus*), Tongcao (*Medulla Tetrapanacis*) and soup made with pig's feet; for pain in the breasts involving the chest and hypochondrium, Yujin (*Radix Curcumae*) and Xiangfu (*Rhizoma Cyperi*) can be combined to soothe the liver and disperse lumps.

三十五、产后发热

35 Puerperal fever

〔概说〕 Summary

产褥期内出现发热持续不退，或突然高热寒战，并称为"产后发热"。如产后一二日内，出现轻微发热，并无其他症状者，这是由于阴血骤虚，阳气浮越，阴阳暂时不平衡所致，为正常生理现象。

中医学认为，产后发热，主要是产时感染邪毒，正邪交争；或产后阴血骤虚，阴不协阳，阳气浮越；或瘀血内阻，气机壅滞所致。常见证候有感染邪毒发热、血瘀发热、外感发热、血虚发热等。

At the stage of puerperium, a syndrome with symptoms such as prolonged fever, or sudden high fever with shiver may arise, known as "puerperal fever". Mild fever after delivery without other symptoms is caused by abrupt asthenia of yin and blood, outward floating of yang qi as well as temporary imbalance of yin and yang, so the disease is regarded as a normal physiological phenomenon.

In terms of TCM, puerperal fever is mainly caused by infection of toxic pathogens and struggle between healthy qi and pathogens, or by abrupt asthenia of yin and blood, which results in failure of yin to harmonize yang and outward floating of yang qi, or by internal obstruction of blood stasis as well as qi stagnation. The disease includes the following common syndromes such as fever due to infection of toxic pathogens, fever due to blood stasis, fever caused by exogenous pathogens as well as fever caused by blood asthenia.

〔辨证论治〕 Syndrome differentiation and treatment

1. 感染邪毒
35.1 Fever due to infection of toxic pathogens

【症状】高热寒战，小腹剧痛拒按，恶露或多或少，色紫暗如败酱，有臭气，烦躁口渴，尿少色黄，大便燥结，舌红苔黄，脉数有力。

【分析】产后感染邪毒，直犯胞宫，正邪交争剧烈，故高热寒战；邪毒入于胞宫，与瘀血相搏，故小腹剧痛拒按；依据瘀血之多少，恶露或多或少；瘀血不散，色紫如败酱，并有臭气；热盛于内，伤及津液，则烦躁口渴，大便燥结，尿少色黄；舌红苔黄、脉数有力，为邪毒感染内结之征。

【治法】清热解毒，凉血化瘀。

【方药】解毒活血汤加减。解毒活血汤为王清任《医林改错》中的主要方剂。方中连翘、葛根、柴胡、甘草清热解毒，升散退热；生地黄、赤芍、当归养血、凉血；红花、桃仁活血化瘀；枳壳散结消滞；赤芍配甘草可以缓急止痛。加入金银花、益母草可以加强活血解毒之力。若小腹剧痛，恶露不尽，可以改用大黄牡丹皮汤（《金匮要略》）。方中大黄、芒硝清热解毒，软坚散结；牡丹皮清热凉血；桃仁活血散淤滞；冬瓜子清热解毒，排脓消痈；加红藤、败酱草，以增强清热解毒之力。

Clinical manifestations: High fever with shiver, unpressable pain over the lower abdomen, more or less lochia with dark purplish color like Baijiang (*Herba Patriniae*), foul odor, restlessness and thirst, scanty yellowish urine, constipation, reddish tongue with yellowish fur as well as fast and powerful pulse.

Analysis: After delivery, exogeonous toxic pathogens attacking the uterus causes acute struggle between healthy qi and pathogenic factors, which brings about high fever and shiver; invasion of toxic pathogens into the uterus causes its struggle with blood stasis, therefore, resulting in unpressable pain over the lower abdomen; the amount of lochia depends on the amount of blood stasis; foul-odor lochia with dark purplish color like Baijiangcao is due to undispersed stasis of blood; restlessness, thirst, constipation and scanty yellowish urine are due to exuberant internal heat impairing body fluid; reddish tongue with yellowish fur and fast and powerful pulse indicate internal accumulation of infective toxic pathogens.

Prescription: Clear away heat, relieve toxic pathogens and cool blood to dissolve blood stasis.

Formulas: Jiedu Huoxue Tang Jiajian (Modified Jiedu Huoxue Decoction). Jiedu Huoxue Tang is an essential formula from Wang Qingren's *Yilin Gaicuo* (*Correction on Errors in Medical Classics*). In the formula, Lianqiao (*Fructus Forsythiae*), Gegen (*Radix Puerariae*), Chaihu (*Radix Bupleuri*), and Gancao (*Radix Glycyrrhizae*) can clear away heat and relieve toxin; Shengdihuang (*Radix Rehmanniae Recens*), Chishao (*Radix Paeoniae Rubra*) and Danggui (*Radix Angelicae Sinensis*) can nourish blood and cool blood; Honghua (*Flos Carthami*) and Taoren (*Semen Persicae*) have an action of invigorating blood circulation and dissolving blood stasis; Zhiqiao (*Fructus Aurantii*) can disperse lumps and eliminate qi stagnation; Chishao combined with Gancao may relieve spasm and arrest pain. Jinyinhua (*Flos Lonicerae*) and Yimucao (*Herba Leonuri*) can be added to strengthen the function of invigorating blood circulation and relieving toxin. For acute pain over the lower abdomen and endless lochia, the formula can be changed into Dahuang Mudanpi Tang, which is quoted from *Jingui Yaolue* (*Synopsis of Golden Chamber*). In the formula, Dahuang (*Radix et Rhizoma Rhei*) and Mangxiao (*Natrii Sulfas*) can clear away heat and relieve toxin, soften dry feces and scatter lumps, Mudanpi (*Cortex Moutan Radicis*) can purge fire and cool blood; Taoren has an action of invigorating blood to disperse stagnated qi; Dongguazi (*Semen Benincasae*) could clear away heat, relieve toxic pathogens and eliminate pus and carbuncle; Hongteng (*Caulis Sargentodoxae*) and Baijiangcao (*Herba Patriniae*) can be added to strengthen the action of clearing away heat and relieving toxic pathogens.

2. 血瘀发热
35.2　Fever due to blood stasis

【症状】产后寒热时作，恶露不下，或恶露甚少，色紫暗有块，小腹疼痛拒按，口干不欲饮，舌质紫暗有瘀斑，脉象弦涩。

【分析】产后恶露不下，或下而甚少，以致瘀血内阻，营卫失调，故寒热时作；气机不畅，瘀血停滞，故小腹疼痛拒按，色紫暗有块；瘀血内停，津液不能上潮，故口干不欲饮；舌质紫暗或有瘀斑，脉象弦涩，为血瘀之征。

【治法】活血化瘀。

【方药】生化汤加减。生化汤为治疗产后恶露停滞的主要方药。方中以当归补血活血，化瘀生新，为君药。川芎活血行气，桃仁活血祛瘀，均为臣药。炮姜入血散寒，温经止痛；黄酒温通血脉，以助药力；加入童便，取其益阳化瘀，并引败血下行。三药共为佐药。炙甘草调和诸药，为使药。合用之，共奏养血化瘀、温经止痛之效。若产后吃寒凉食品，腹内结块痛甚，可加肉桂于生化汤内；血块未消，不可加人参、黄芪，以免留瘀。

Clinical manifestations：Occasional alternation of aversion to cold with fever following childbirth，scanty lochia or lochiostasis，dark purplish lochia mingled with clots，unpressable pain over the lower abdomen，dry mouth without desire for drink，dark purplish tongue with petechia as well as taut and astringent pulse.

Analysis：Scanty lochia or lochiostasis following childbirth causes internal obstruction of blood stasis and imbalance between nutrient qi and defensive qi，which gives rise to occasional alternation of cold and fever；unpressable pain over the lower abdomen and dark purplish lochia mingled with clots are due to qi disorder and retention of blood stasis；dry mouth without desire for drink is due to failure of body fluid to flow upward resulting from internal retention of blood stasis；dark purplish tongue with petechiae and taut and astringent pulse are indications of blood stasis.

Prescription：Activate blood circulation and resolve stasis.

Formulas：Shenghua Tang Jiajian (Modified Shenghua Decoction). Shenghua Tang is an essential recipe for stagnation of lochia, of which, Danggui (*Radix Angelicae Sinensis*) is used as sovereign drug with its action of supplementing blood to activate blood circulation and dissolving blood stasis to improve production of new blood. Chuanxiong (*Rhizoma Ligustici Chuanxiong*) has an function of activating circulation of blood and qi, Taoren (*Semen Persicae*) can improve blood circulation and dispel stasis, both of them are used as ministerial drug. Paojiang (*Rhizoma Zingiberis Preparata*) can transmit into blood to disperse cold and warm meridians to stop pain；Huangjiu (yellow rice wine or millet wine) can warm and dredge blood vessels to help induce the function of medicinal herbs；Tongbian (urine of boys under ten years old) can be added to benefit yang qi and resolve blood stasis and guide poisoned blood to flow downward. The above three are used as adjuvant drug. Zhigancao (*Radix Glycyrrhizae Preparata*) is used as courier drug to harmonize the above medicinal herbs. Combined together, all ingredients of the recipe could bring nourishing blood to resolve blood stasis and warming the meridians to arrest pain into full play. For worsening pain due to lumps in the abdomen because of intake of cold food, Rougui (*Cortex Cinnamomi*) can be added to the recipe；for undispersed blood clots, Renshen (*Radix Ginseng*) and Huangqi (*Radix Astragali seu Hedysari*) must not be added in case that blood stasis remains in blood vessels.

3. 外感发热
35.3 Fever due to exogenous pathogenic factors

【症状】产后恶寒发热，头痛，肢体疼痛，无汗，流清涕，咳嗽，舌苔薄白，脉象浮数。

【分析】产后气血虚弱，卫外能力降低，恶寒侵入，正邪交争，故恶寒发热；外感之邪，上犯足太阳之表，足太阳之经脉，络于头目项背，故头痛、肢体疼痛；腠理为恶寒所困，故无汗；邪犯于肺，故咳嗽、流清涕；舌苔薄白，脉浮数，为风寒犯表之征。

【治法】养血祛风。

【方药】荆防四物汤。方中四物汤（川芎、当归、白芍、熟地黄）养血，兼以活血；荆芥、防风祛风解表；可加苏叶疏风解表。若症见寒热往来、口苦、咽干、呕吐，舌苔白润，脉象弦者，为少阳病证，可改用小柴胡汤。

Clinical manifestations: Aversion to cold and fever following childbirth, headache, painful sensation of the limbs and body, no sweating, stuffy nose with clear snivel, cough, thin and whitish tongue fur as well as floating and fast pulse.

Analysis: Asthenia of qi and blood after childbirth results in declined ability of defensive qi in protecting the superficies from internal invasion of pathogenic cold factors, which causes the struggle between healthy qi and pathogenic factors, thus, giving rise to aversion to cold and fever; upward invasion of exogenous pathogenic factors into superficies of foot taiyang meridians associated with collaterals that run through the head, eyes, neck as well as the back, brings about headache and painful limbs and body; no sweating are due to obstruction of cold in muscular interstices; cough and stuffy nose with clear snivel are due to exogenous pathogens attacking the lung; thin whitish tongue fur and floating and fast pulse are signs of pathogenic wind and cold factors attacking the superficies.

Prescription: Nourish blood and dispel wind.

Formulas: Jing Fang Siwu Tang (Decoction). In the formula, Siwu Tang consisting of Chuanxiong (*Rhizoma Ligustici Chuanxiong*), Danggui (*Radix Angelicae Sinensis*), Baishao (*Radix Paeoniae Alba*) and Shudihuang (*Radix Rehmanniae Preparata*), can nourish blood and invigorate blood circulation; Jingjie (*Herba Schizonepetae*) and Fangfeng (*Radix Saposhnikoviae*) can dispel wind pathogen and relieve superficial syndrome; Suye (*Folium Perillae*) could be added to expel wind to relieve superficial syndrome. For syndrome of shaoyang with symptoms such as bitter taste of the mouth, dry throat, vomiting, moist whitish tongue fur as well as taut pulse, Small Chaihu Tang can be used to replace the above formula.

4. 血虚发热
35.4 Fever due to blood asthenia

【症状】产后失血过多，身有微热，自汗，头晕目眩，心悸少眠，腹痛绵绵，手足麻木，舌淡红，苔薄白，脉象虚而微数。

【分析】产后失血伤津，阴不敛阳，虚阳外越，故有微热自汗；血虚清窍失养，故头晕目眩；血不养心，则心悸少眠；胞脉失养，则腹痛绵绵；血虚不能濡养四肢，则手足麻木；舌淡红、苔薄、脉象虚数，为血虚之征。

【治法】补益气血。

【方药】八珍汤去川芎，加黄芪补气。方中以四物汤补血，四君子汤补气。若有热象，可加知母、地骨皮以滋阴清热；若胃口不开，可加焦三仙健脾开胃消食；食积易于化热，可加连翘清热散结。

Clinical manifestations：Excessive loss of blood after childbirth, mild fever, spontaneous sweating, dizziness and vertigo, palpitation and insomnia, lingering abdominal pain, numbness of hands and feet, pale reddish tongue with thin whitish fur as well as indistinct and fast pulse.

Analysis：Loss of blood after childbirth causes impairment of body fluid, and failure of yin to restrict yang resulting in outward floating of deficient yang, which gives rise to mild fever and spontaneous sweating; dizziness and vertigo are due to malnutrition of the upper orifices because of blood asthenia; palpitation and insomnia are due to failure of blood to nourish the heart; lingering abdominal pain is caused by malnutrition of vessels of the uterus; numbness of hands and feet is due to failure of asthenic blood to nourish the limbs; pale reddish tongue with thin whitish fur and indistinct and fast pulse are indications of blood asthenia.

Prescription：Supplement qi and benefit blood.

Formulas：Modified Bazhen Tang (Decoction) by removing Chuanxiong (*Rhizoma Ligustici Chuanxiong*) and adding Huangqi (*Radix Astragali seu Hedysari*). In the formula, Siwu Tang can tonify blood, Sijunzi Tang can supplement qi. For the symptom of fever, Zhimu (*Rhizoma Anemarrhenae*) and Digupi (*Cortex Lycii*) can be added to nourish yin and clear away heat; for poor appetite, stir-baked Maiya (*Fructus Hordei Germinatus*), stir-baked Shanzha (*Fructus Crataegi*) and stir-baked Shenqu (*Massa Medicata Fermentata*) can be added to invigorate the spleen, promote appetite and help digestion; because food retention can transform into heat, Lianqiao (*Fructus Forsythiae*) can be added to clear away heat and disperse lumps.

三十六、急性乳腺炎
36　Acute mastitis

〔**概说**〕Summary

急性乳腺炎是发生于乳房的一种急性化脓性疾病。多发生于哺乳期妇女，以初产妇多见，好发于产后3~4周，是乳房疾病中的常见病。

急性乳腺炎属于中医学"乳漏""乳痈""外吹""内吹""乳疽"等病范畴。其成因有乳汁淤积、肝郁胃热等因素。辨证论治不以具体证候分类，而以初起、成脓、溃后为界。治疗上有内治与外治之分，治疗效果比较满意。

Acute mastitis is a rapid infection of abscess in the breasts, usually seen in lactating mothers, particularly the first-delivery women, 3~4 weeks after childbirth. Acute mastitis is regarded as a common sickness of mammary gland disease.

In TCM, acute mastitis pertains to "galactorrhea" "mammary abscess in puerperium" "mastitis during pregnancy" "intramammary abscess", as well as "breast cellulitis" etc. The causes for the disease are milk stagnation and liver depression with gastric heat. Treatment for the disease should not be based on its detailed syndromes but the stages of initial onset, transformation of pus as well as the period that follows ulceration, including internal and external treatment. TCM therapeutic methods for the disease could achieve a satisfactory curative effect.

〔辨证论治〕 Syndrome differentiation and treatment

1. 初起
36.1　The stage of initial onset

【症状】乳房肿胀疼痛，皮肤微红或不红，肿块或有或无，乳汁分泌不畅，伴有恶寒发热、头痛、胸闷，舌苔薄黄或黄腻，脉象弦数。

【分析】产后不知调养，郁怒不解，致使肝脉不通，乳汁不出，阳明血热沸腾，故热化为脓，引起乳房肿胀疼痛，皮肤微红；内结不散，则形成肿块；肝与胆相表里，肝郁则胆经郁热不解，故有少阳经症状，如恶寒发热、头痛、胸闷等；舌苔黄腻与脉象弦数，为热郁于内的表象。

【治法】疏肝清热，通乳消肿。

【方药】瓜蒌牛蒡汤加味。瓜蒌牛蒡汤出自《医宗金鉴》，由瓜蒌、牛蒡子、天花粉、黄芩、陈皮、生栀子、皂角刺、金银花、青皮、柴胡、连翘、甘草组成。方中金银花、连翘、黄芩、牛蒡子、生栀子、甘草清肝经之热；陈皮、青皮、柴胡疏肝之络；皂角刺、天花粉、瓜蒌通乳消肿。乳汁不通，可加穿山甲、王不留行、漏芦、木通；肝气郁结，可加橘叶、川楝子；恶露不尽，可加当归、益母草、川芎；热盛，可加生石膏、知母；肿痛甚，可加乳香、没药；回乳，可加焦山楂、炒麦芽。

Clinical manifestations: Swelling and distending pain of the breasts, slight reddish or no red color of the breasts, visible or invisible swelling lumps, unsmooth secretion of milk, accompanied with aversion to cold, fever, headache, chest oppression, thin yellowish tongue fur as well as greasy yellowish fur as well as taut and fast pulse.

Analysis: Failure to recuperate and unrelieved anger and depression cause stagnation of liver meridians and failure to excrete milk. Hot or even boiling blood in yangming meridian brings about pus transformed from heat, swelling and distending pain of the breasts and slight red breast; swelling lumps are due to undispersed internal heat accumulation; the liver is internally and externally connected with the gallbladder, liver depression causes unrelieved stagnation of heat in gallbladder meridian, which gives rise to syndrome of shaoyang meridian with symptoms such as aversion to cold, fever, headache and chest oppression; greasy yellowish fur and taut and fast pulse are signs of accumulation of internal heat.

Prescription: Soothe the liver, clear away heat, dredge collaterals of the breasts and eliminate swelling lumps.

Formulas: Gualou Niubang Tang Jiawei (Modified Gualou Niubang Decoction). The formula is quoted from *Yizong Jinjian* (*Golden Mirror of Medicine*), consisting of Gualou (*Fructus Trichosanthis*), Niubangzi (*Fructus Arctii*), Tianhuafen (*Radix Trichosanthis*), Huangqin (*Radix Scutellariae*), Chenpi (*Pericarpium Citri Reticulatae*), Shengzhizi (*Fructus Gardeniae*), Zaojiaoci (*Spina Gleditsiae*), Jinyinhua (*Flos Lonicerae*), Qingpi (*Pericarpium Citri Reticulatae Viride*), Chaihu (*Radix Bupleuri*), Lianqiao (*Fructus Forsythiae*) and Gancao (*Radix Glycyrrhizae*). In the formula, Jinyinhua, Lianqiao, Huangqin, Niubangzi, Shengzhizi and Gancao can purge heat in the liver meridians; Chenpi, Qingpi and Chaihu could soothe collaterals of the liver; Zaojiaoci, Tianhuafen and Gualou have an action of dredging collaterals of the breast and eliminating swellings. For failure to dredge collaterals of the breast, Chuanshanjia (*Squama Manis*), Wangbuliuxing (*Semen Vaccariae*), Loulu (*Radix Rhapontici*) and Mutong (*Caulis Akebiae*) can be added; for liver depression, Juye (tangerine leaf) and Chuanlianzi (*Fructus Meliae Toosendan*) can be combined; for endless lochia, Danggui (*Radix Angelicae Sinensis*), Yimucao (*Herba Leonuri*) and Chuanxiong (*Rhizoma Ligustici Chuanxiong*) can be added; for exuberant heat, Shengshigao (*Gypsum Fibrosum*) and Zhimu (*Rhizoma Anemarrhenae*) can be combined; for worsening swellings and pain, Ruxiang (*Olibanum*) and Moyao (*Myrrha*) should be added; and stir-baked Shanzha (*Fructus Crataegi*) and stir-baked Maiya (*Fructus Hordei Germinatus*) can be combined to eliminate secretion of milk.

2. 成脓
36.2 The stage of transformation of pus

【症状】肿块逐渐增大，皮色焮红，疼痛加重，壮热不退，口渴引饮，舌苔黄腻，脉象弦数，此为化脓之势。若壮热、疼痛十余日不退，硬块中央变软，按之有波动感，是成脓阶段。

【分析】成脓为热毒壅盛阶段。热毒盛，故肿块增大，皮色焮红，疼痛加重，壮热不退；热盛伤阴，则口渴引饮；若壮热、疼痛不退，硬块中央变软，说明热毒伤血，血化为脓，成脓则有波动感，这是成脓的指征。成脓期为热毒渐盛阶段，故舌苔黄腻、脉象弦数，为阳证、热证之象。

【治法】清热解毒，托里透脓。

【方药】透脓散加味。透脓散出自《外科正宗》，由当归、黄芪、炒穿山甲、川芎、皂角刺组成，以托里透脓为主要功效。黄芪、当归补气养血，以托里为主；炒穿山甲、川芎、皂角刺以透脓为主。但此方清热解毒不足，故加金银花、连翘、蒲公英以清热解毒。如此，扶正与祛邪相结合，补气养血与清热解毒相配伍，治疗效果更为快捷。

Clinical manifestations: Gradual enlargement of swellings, red swollen skin, aggravation of pain, unrelieved high fever, thirst with desire to drink, greasy yellowish fur and taut and fast pulse indicating the tendency to transform into pus. Unrelieved high fever and pain lasting more than ten days and softening lumps in the center with a wavy shaking sense indicate the disease has developed into the stage of pus transformation.

Analysis: Transformation of pus is the stage of exuberance of toxic heat. Enlargement of swellings, red swollen skin, aggravation of pain and unrelieved high fever are caused by exuberant toxic heat; thirst with desire for drink is due to hyperactive heat impairing yin fluid; unrelieved high fever, pain and softening lumps in the center indicate toxic heat pathogen impairing blood, and pus transformed from blood with a wavy shaking sense shows transformation of pus, a stage of hyperactive toxic heat, thus, bringing about greasy yellowish fur and taut and fast pulse, which are also signs of yang and heat syndromes.

Prescription: Clear away heat, relieve toxin, drain toxin and draw pus.

Formulas: Tounong San Jiawei (Modified Tounong Powder). The formula is quoted from *Waike Zhengzong* (*Orthodox Manual of External Diseases*), consisting of Danggui (*Radix Angelicae Sinensis*), Huangqi (*Radix Astragali seu Hedysari*), stir-baked Chuanshanjia (*Squama Manis*), Chuanxiong (*Rhizoma Ligustici Chuanxiong*) and Zaojiaoci (*Spina Gleditsiae*). The main function of the formula is to drain internal toxin and draw pus, in which, Huangqi and Danggui, with an action of draining internal toxin, can supplement qi and nourish blood; stir-baked Chuanshanjia, Chuanxiong and Zaojiaoci have an action of drawing pus; because of its limited function of clearing away heat and relieving toxin, Jinyinhua (*Flos Lonicerae*), Lianqiao (*Fructus Forsythiae*) and Pugongying (*Herba Taraxaci*) are added to reinforce the action of clearing away heat and relieving toxin. Through the combination of strengthening healthy qi with eliminating pathogenic factors supplementing qi and nourishing blood with clearing away heat and relieving toxin, the formula could achieve a better curative effect.

3. 溃后
36.3　The stage after ulceration

【症状】乳房破溃出脓后，一般热退、肿消，逐渐愈合。若破溃后，脓出不畅，胀痛不减，身热不退，属脓液波及其他乳络，为"传囊"之变。若破溃后，乳汁从疮口溢出，形成乳漏，其愈合较慢。

【分析】乳房破溃后，一般应该热退、肿消，说明疾患逐渐愈合，是正常演变过程。若破溃后，仍然脓出不畅，胀痛不减，身热不退，说明脓毒并未减少，而且还有波及其他乳络之兆，此谓"传囊"，即形成囊状之物，不易治愈；若破溃后，乳汁继续从疮口流出，这是正气虚弱，不能拖毒外出，疗程自然会延长难愈。

【治法】溃后热退身凉，胀痛逐渐消退，治宜排脓托毒；若溃后身热不退，胀痛不减，为余毒未尽，而成"传囊"之势，此时可参照初起、成脓期治法。

【方药】四妙散加味。四妙散出自《外科精要》，由炙黄芪、当归、金银花、炙甘草四味组成。黄芪、当归补气养血，为扶正托里之要药；金银花、炙甘草，为清热解毒之配伍。可加皂角刺、川芎以增加排脓之力。

Clinical manifestations：Generally, after ulceration and drawing pus, fever can be relieved, swellings can disappear, and the breasts will get healed. Unsmooth process of drawing pus with unrelieved distending pain and fever suggests pus permeating into other collaterals of the breasts and "acute mastitis transmitting into other region". With the diabrosis of ulceration of the breasts, milk spills out of sores, which is known as "mammary fistula", and the process of healing will be much slower.

Analysis：In general, with the diabrosis of ulceration of the breasts, fever will be relieved, and swellings will disappear, indicating gradual tendency of healing, a normal process of evolution. Unsmooth process of drawing pus with unrelieved distending pain and fever suggests that unreduced poisonous pus involves other collaterals of the breasts, which is known as "transmission of acute mastitis into other region", namely, the permeated pus forming into cyst-like tissue, which is hard to be cured; if milk still flows out of sores, it signifies asthenia of healthy qi failing to drain heat toxin, in which case, the treating process will be prolonged.

Prescription：For alleviation of fever and gradual disappearance of distending pain after ulceration, drain pus and draw toxin; as for unrelieved fever and distending pain which indicates that unrelieved residual toxin tends to transmit into other region, the treatment should be based on the therapeutic methods for the stage of initial onset as well as those for the stage of pus transformation.

Formulas：Simiao San Jiawei (Modified Simiao Powder). Simiao San is quoted from *Waike Jingyao* (*Essence of External Diseases*), consisting of honey-fried Huangqi (*Radix Astragali seu Hedysari*), Danggui (*Radix Angelicae Sinensis*), Jinyinhua (*Flos Lonicerae*) and Zhigancao (*Radix Glycyrrhizae Preparata*). In the formula, Huangqi and Danggui, with the action of supplementing qi and nourishing blood, are used as essential medicinal herbs to strengthen healthy qi and draw internal toxin out; Jinyinhua and Zhigancao are the herbs for clearing away heat and relieving toxin; Zaojiaoci (*Spina Gleditsiae*) and Chuanxiong (*Rhizoma Ligustici Chuanxiong*) can be added to reinforce the action of draining pus.

附：外治法

①乳房按摩：乳汁不通，局部胀痛，可行乳房按摩，使其乳汁疏通。在按摩前，先在乳房上涂上少许润滑油，用五指由乳房四周轻轻向乳头方向按摩，但不宜用力挤压或旋转按压，而是沿着乳络方向施以正压，将淤积的乳汁逐步推出。在按摩的时候，可以轻揪乳头数次，以扩张乳头部的乳络。若在按摩前做热敷，效果更好。

②外敷法：取如意金黄散、玉露散或双柏散，用水或鲜菊花叶、鲜蒲公英等捣汁调敷患处。或用仙人掌去刺捣烂外敷。

③针刺法：取肩井、膻中、足三里穴强刺激。留针 15 分钟，每日 1 次。发热者，加曲池穴。

以上用于病患初起。若成脓，则可切开引流。

External therapies：

a. Massage on the breasts

Massage on the breasts can be applied to the syndrome of failure to dredge collaterals of the breasts and regional distending pain so as to improve excretion of milk.

The massage method：Coat a little lubricative oil on the breasts, then massage with five fingers from the root of the breasts through the nipples slightly. Massage operators should not squeeze the breasts with strength, nor press the breasts in a swirl, but press the breasts in the direction of the collaterals to push stagnated milk out little by little. During the process, nipples can be pulled up slightly for several times so as to expand the collaterals around the nipples. A better therapeutic effect could be achieved if hot compression on the breasts is applied before the massage.

b. External compression with Chinese medicinal herbs

Mix water or fresh leaves of Juhua (*Flos Chrysanthemi*) and fresh Pugongying (*Herba Taraxaci*) with Ruyi Jinhuang San (Powder), Yulu San (Powder) or Shuangbo San (Powder) in a hard container and squeeze them with force continuously until the mixture turns into thick juice or paste, and coat the paste onto the infected region of the breasts. Or just squeeze cactus into juice and coat it on the wounded area of the breast.

c. Acupuncture

Prescription：Jianjing (GB 21), Danzhong (CV 17) and Zusanli (ST 36) are needled with strong stimulation. The needles are retained for 15 minutes, and such needling should be adopted once a day. For complication with fever, Quchi (LI 11) should be added.

The above therapeutic methods are used for the initial onset of acute mastitis. If pus has been transformed, the ulcerated region can be cut apart to drain pus.

三十七、乳腺增生

37　Hyperplasia of mammary glands

〔概说〕　Summary

乳腺增生病是乳房部一种非炎症性疾病，其特点是：乳房肿块，经前胀痛加重，经后减轻。好发于 30~40 岁女性，是妇科常见病之一。

乳腺增生病，属于中医学"乳癖"范畴。多由于郁怒伤肝，肝郁气滞；思虑伤脾，脾失健运，痰湿内生，以致肝脾两伤，痰气互结，郁滞而成块。或因冲任失调，阳虚痰湿内结所致。治疗以疏肝为主，兼以化痰散结、温阳化痰为辅。

Hyperplasia of mammary glands is an uninflamed disease, characterized by swollen lumps in one or both breasts, aggravation of distending pain in the breasts before menstruation, and alleviation after menstruation. As a common gynecopathy disease, it usually occurs among women aged from 30 to 40.

Hyperplasia of mammary glands pertains to the conception of "lumps in breasts" in TCM, usually caused by liver depression and qi stagnation which impairs the liver, dysfunction of the spleen in transportation because of overthinking impairing the spleen, resulting in internal retention of phlegmatic dampness, which, in turn, causes impairment of the liver and spleen, coagulation of phlegm and qi, and stagnated qi forming into lumps; or it is caused by dysfunction of thoroughfare and conception vessels, yang asthenia and internal accumulation of phlegmatic dampness. Treatment for it is marked by soothing the liver, resolving phlegm, dispersing lumps as well as warming yang.

〔辨证论治〕 Syndrome differentiation and treatment

1. 肝郁痰凝
37.1 Liver depression and coagulation of phlegm

【症状】双侧乳房出现大小不一的肿块，伴有心烦易怒，失眠多梦，情绪急躁，乳房胀痛，不思饮食，舌苔薄白，脉象弦滑。

【分析】乳房分布着胃、胆、肝三经经脉。若情绪不稳定，肝气不舒，肝胆之经脉郁滞，久之就会出现肿块，或大或小；肝郁化火，则会见心烦易怒，失眠多梦；乳络不通，则乳房胀痛；肝郁伤脾，湿浊生痰，则不思饮食，并见薄白舌苔；脉象弦滑，为肝郁伤脾之象。

【治法】疏肝解郁，化痰散结。

【方药】逍遥蒌贝散。此方由逍遥散化裁而成。方中保留逍遥散中的当归、白芍、柴胡以疏肝养血，茯苓、白术健脾渗湿。另加入瓜蒌、贝母、半夏化痰散结；生牡蛎软坚散结；胆南星辅助半夏燥湿化痰；山慈姑消毒散结。为逍遥散的变化方，除具有逍遥散的疏肝解郁作用外，所加之药多为化痰散结、软坚消毒之品，变单纯的疏肝解郁为兼有消散肿块功效的方剂。

Clinical manifestations: Lumps in various size in both breasts, accompanied with vexation, susceptibility to rage, insomnia, dreaminess, dysphoria, distending pain over the breasts, anorexia, thin and whitish fur as well as taut and slippery pulse.

Analysis: Meridians of the stomach, gallbladder and liver run through the breasts. Emotional upset, liver qi depression and prolonged stagnation of liver and gallbladder meridians give rise to swollen lumps or nodules with different size; vexation, susceptibility to rage, insomnia and dreaminess are due to fire transformed from liver depression; distending pain over the breasts is due to stagnation of collaterals in the breasts; anorexia and thin whitish fur are due to impairment of the spleen because of liver depression and generation of phlegm from turbid dampness; taut and slippery pulse indicates liver depression impairing the spleen.

Prescription: Soothe the liver to relieve stagnation and resolve phlegm to disperse lumps.

Formulas：Xiaoyao Lou Bei San （Powder）. The formula is changed from Xiaoyao San, in which, Danggui （*Radix Angelicae Sinensis*）, Baishao （*Radix Paeoniae Alba*） and Chaihu （*Radix Bupleuri*） can soothe the liver and nourish blood, Fuling （*Herba Menthae*） and Baizhu （*Rhizoma Atractylodis Macrocephalae*） have an action of invigorating the spleen and resolving dampness. Gualou （*Fructus Trichosanthis*）, Beimu （*Bulbus Fritillaria*） and Banxia （*Rhizoma Pinelliae*） can be added to resolve phlegm and disperse lumps；Shengmuli （*Concha Ostreae*） has an action of softening hard lumps and dispersing nodules；Dannanxing （*Rhizoma Arisaematis Cum Bile*） can help Banxia improve the action of drying dampness and resolving phlegm；Shancigu （*Pseudobulbus Cremastrae seu Pleiones*） has an action of eliminating toxin and dispersing lumps. In addition to the single action of soothing the liver and relieving stagnation of the original formula, the additional ingredients have the function of resolving phlegm, dispersing lumps, softening hard lumps and eliminating toxin.

2. 冲任失调
37.2 Maladjustment of thoroughfare and conception vessels

【症状】双侧乳房相继出现大小不一的肿块，伴有月经不调，腰膝酸软，经水少而色淡，或经闭，舌质淡红，苔薄白，脉象弦细。

【分析】冲任二脉，主妇女之阴血的调达，若冲任二脉失调，就会使肝经脉络失和，除有乳房肿块外，兼有月经不调，腰膝酸软；阴血亏虚，经水自然减少而色淡，甚至经闭；舌质淡红，为阴虚不足之象，苔薄白为气不化湿；脉象弦细，为肝气郁结之征。

【治法】调理冲任，温阳化痰。

【方药】二仙汤合苓桂术甘汤。二仙汤为调节妇女阴阳失调的创新方剂，方中以当归养血疏肝，巴戟天温阳补肾，知母、黄柏滋阴降火，仙茅、仙灵脾温阳通络；苓桂术甘汤具有健脾化痰、除湿通络的作用。两方合用，可以调理冲任的气血阴阳，温阳和中，健脾化痰。如果有阴虚火旺之征，可以加入二至丸（女贞子、旱莲草）滋阴清热，并抑制仙茅、仙灵脾过燥之性。

Clinical manifestations：Lumps with various size in both breasts, accompanied with irregular menstruation, aching and weakness of the loins and knees, pale and scanty menstrual blood, or amenorrhea, pale reddish tongue with thin whitish fur as well as taut and thin pulse.

Analysis：Thoroughfare and conception vessels dominate dispersion and distribution of yin blood, maladjustment of thoroughfare and conception vessels results in disharmony of collaterals of liver meridians, lumps in the breasts, irregular menstruation as well as aching and weakness of the loins and knees; pale and scanty menstrual blood, or even amenorrhea, is due to deficiency of yin and blood; pale reddish tongue is a sign of deficient yin; thin and whitish fur is caused by failure of qi to resolve dampness; taut and thin pulse indicates qi stagnation in the liver.

Prescription: Regulate thoroughfare and conception vessels, warm yang and resolve phlegm.

Formulas: Erxian Tang (Decoction) combined with Ling Gui Zhu Gan Tang (Decoction). The former is an innovated formula for regulating imbalance between yin and yang in female patients, in which, Danggui (*Radix Angelicae Sinensis*) can nourish blood and soothe the liver, Bajitian (*Radix Morindae Officinalis*) has an action of warming yang and supplementing the kidney, Zhimu (*Rhizoma Anemarrhenae*) and Huangbo (Cortex Phellodendri) can nourish yin and descend fire, Xianmao (*Rhizoma Curculigins*) and Xianlingpi (*Herba Epimedii*) could warm yang and dredge collaterals; the latter formula has an action of invigorating the spleen to resolve phlegm, eliminating dampness and dredging blood vessels. Combined together, both formulas can regulate qi, blood, yin and yang in thoroughfare and conception vessels, warm yang and harmonize middle energizer, invigorate the spleen and resolve phlegm. For hyperactive fire due to yin asthenia, Erzhi Wan (Pill), including Nuzhenzi (*Fructus Ligustri Lucidi*) and Hanliancao (*Eclipta Alba*), can be added to nourish yin and clear away heat, furthermore, they could restrain the excessive dry nature of Xianmao and Xianlingpi.

三十八、小儿急性上呼吸道感染
38 Acute infantile upper respiratory tract infection

〔**概说**〕 Summary

小儿急性上呼吸道感染，是指鼻、鼻咽和咽部的急性炎症病变，发病时以发热、怕冷、鼻塞、流涕、咳嗽、头痛等为主症。鼻咽部感染可涉及邻近器官，如喉、气管、口腔、鼻窦、中耳、眼及颈淋巴等。在秋冬和冬春天气多变时发病率较高。

小儿上呼吸道感染，属于中医学"伤风""感冒""咳嗽"等病证范畴。中医学认为，小儿脏腑娇嫩，每遇风寒，易患伤风、感冒，且得病之后，容易出现兼证，如夹痰、夹滞、夹惊等，故应予特别关注。

Acute infantile upper respiratory tract infection is a rapid inflammation of the nose, nasopharynx and pharynx, characterized by fever, aversion to cold, stuffy nose with snivel, cough and headache. Infection of the nasopharynx can involve its adjacent organs, such as the larynx, tracheal sac, oral cavity, nasal sinus, auris media, eyes as well as lymphatic system in the neck. The period from autumn through winter and that from winter to spring are the time of high incidence of the disease.

In TCM, acute infantile upper respiratory tract infection pertains to "catching cold" "common cold" and "cough". TCM holds that zang-fu organs of the infants are tender and delicate, attack of wind and cold will bring about susceptibility to catching cold or common cold, which could give rise to complicated syndromes such as complication with phlegm, food retention, as well as convulsion, therefore, much stress should be attached to the disease.

〔辨证论治〕 Syndrome differentiation and treatment

1. 风寒
38.1　Syndrome of wind-cold

【症状】发热、怕冷、无汗，鼻塞、流清涕，喷嚏、咳嗽、喉痒，舌苔薄白，脉浮。

【分析】风寒外袭，卫阳不固，必然发热、怕冷、无汗；肺气不得宣发，则会出现不同程度的鼻塞、咳嗽、流清涕、喷嚏、喉痒等；舌苔薄白与脉浮，为风寒外袭之象。

【治法】辛温解表。

【方药】荆防败毒散加减。荆防败毒散是由人参败毒散去人参加荆芥、防风而成。方以荆芥、防风、羌活、独活辛温发散，通治一身上下之风寒湿邪；川芎活血祛风；柴胡解散半表半里之邪；枳壳降气；桔梗开肺；前胡祛痰；茯苓渗湿；甘草调和诸药。头痛加白芷；咳嗽加杏仁；纳呆加厚朴花；若汗出怕风，可加桂枝汤以调和营卫。

Clinical manifestations: Fever, aversion to cold, no sweating, stuffy nose with clear snivel, sneeze, cough, itchy throat, thin and whitish fur as well as floating pulse.

Analysis: Fever, aversion to cold and no sweating are due to failure of defensive yang to protect the superficies because of attack of exogenous wind cold on the superficies; stuffy nose with clear snivel, sneeze, cough and itchy throat are caused by failure of lung qi to disperse; thin whitish fur and floating pulse are signs of wind cold attacking the superficies.

Prescription: Relieve the superficial syndrome with pungent-and-warm natured medicinal herbs.

Formulas: Jing Fang Baidu San Jiajian (Modified Jing Fang Baidu Powder). Jing Fang Baidu San is the combination of Jingjie (*Herba Schizonepetae*) and Fangfeng (*Radix Saposhnikoviae*) with Renshen Baidu San by removing Renshen (*Radix Ginseng*) from it. In the formula, Jingjie, Fangfeng, Qianghuo (*Rhizoma et Radix Notopterygii*) and Duhuo (*Radix Angelicae Pubescentis*), pungent and warm in nature, have an action of dispelling wind, cold and dampness pathogens; Chuanxiong (*Rhizoma Ligustici Chuanxiong*) can invigorate blood circulation and dispel wind; Chaihu (*Radix Bupleuri*) could relieve and disperse pathogenic factors in the region of semi-interior and semi-exterior, Zhiqiao (*Fructus Aurantii*) can descend qi; Jiegeng (*Radix Platycodonis*) could disperse lung qi and resolve phlegm; Qianhu (*Radix Peucedani*) has an action of expelling phlegm; Fuling can eliminate dampness; Gancao could harmonize the above medicinal herbs. For headache, Baizhi (*Radix Angelicae Dahuricae*) should be combined; for cough, Xingren (*Semen Armeniacae Amarum*) can be added; for anorexia, Houpohua (*Flos Magnoliae Officinalis*) should be combined; for the symptoms of sweating and aversion to wind, Guizhi Tang (Decoction) can be added to regulate nutrient qi and defensive qi.

2. 风热

38.2 syndrome of wind-heat

【症状】高热、稍怕冷、微汗出，头痛、鼻塞、流脓涕，喷嚏、咳嗽、咽部红肿疼痛，舌苔薄白或微黄而干，脉象浮数。

【分析】外感风热，与卫阳相搏，则高热，但怕冷不甚，汗出不多，故高热不退；热扰于上，则头痛；肺气不利，则鼻塞、喷嚏；热伤肺阴，则咳嗽，流脓涕；热郁于呼吸之道，故咽部红肿疼痛；舌苔薄白少津，脉象浮数，为热邪袭表之象。

【治法】辛凉解表。

【方药】桑菊饮或银翘散为主方。咳嗽重者用桑菊饮，发热重者用银翘散。

桑菊饮以桑叶清透肺络之热、菊花清散上焦风热，并作君药；臣以薄荷辛散肺热，桔梗、杏仁一升一降，以利肺气之开合；连翘清透膈上之热，芦根清热生津止渴，用为佐药；甘草调和诸药，为使药。诸药合用，有疏散风热、宣肺止咳之效。

银翘散用金银花、连翘为君药，既有辛凉透邪清热之效，又有芳香辟秽解毒之功；臣药以荆芥穗、淡豆豉、牛蒡子开皮毛而逐邪；桔梗宣肺利咽，甘草清热解毒，竹叶清上焦热，芦根清热生津，皆是佐使药。

以上二方为温热病初期辛凉解表之首选良方。二方均有连翘、桔梗、甘草、薄荷、芦根。但桑菊饮有桑叶、菊花、杏仁，肃肺止咳力大；银翘散有金银花、荆芥穗、淡豆豉、牛蒡子、竹叶，解表清热力强。桑菊饮为"辛凉轻剂"，银翘散为"辛凉平剂"。

Clinical manifestations: High fever, slight aversion to cold, mild sweating, headache, stuffy nose with thick snivel, sneeze, cough, swollen and painful throat, thin and whitish fur or slight yellowish dry fur as well as floating and fast pulse.

Analysis: High fever with slight aversion to cold is due to struggle of exogenous wind heat pathogens with defensive yang qi; unrelieved high fever is due to mild sweating because of slight aversion to cold; headache is due to up-disturbance of pathogenic heat factor; stuffy nose and sneeze are due to disorder of lung qi; cough and runny thick snivel are caused by heat impairing lung yin; swollen and painful throat is due to heat stagnation in the respiratory tract; thin and whitish fur with scanty fluid and floating and fast pulse indicate pathogenic heat factors attacking the superficies.

Prescription: Relieve superficial syndrome with pungent-cool natured medicinal herbs.

Formulas: Sang Ju Yin (Decoction) used as the principal recipe for severe cough, or Yinqiao San (Powder) used as the essential formula for high fever.

In Sang Ju Yin, Sangye (*Folium Mori*) has an action of clearing away heat from the lung collaterals, Juhua (*Florist's chrysanthemum*) can purge and disperse wind heat from upper energizer, both of them are used as sovereign drug. Bohe (*Herba Menthae*), pungent in nature, has an action of dispersing heat in the lung, Jiegeng (*Radix Platycodi*) can lift qi, and Xingren (*Semen Armeniacae Amarum*) could descend qi. The three herbs are used as ministerial drug, and the latter two can help improve circulation of lung qi. Lianqiao (*Fructus Forsythiae*) can eliminate heat from the region above the diaphragm, Lugen (*Rhizoma Phragmitis*) can clear away heat and produce fluid to stop thirst. They both are used as adjuvant drug. Gancao (*Radix Glycyrrhizae*) is used as courier drug to harmonize the above medicinal herbs. Combined together, the herbs in the formula could achieve the effect of expelling wind heat and dispersing the lung to stop cough.

In Yinqiao San, Jinyinhua (*Flos Lonicerae*) and Lianqiao, pungent and aromatic in flavor and cool in nature, are used as sovereign drug to let out heat, eliminate foul odor and relieve toxin; Jingjiesui (*Spica Schizonepetae*), Dandouchi (*Semen Sojae Preperatum*) and Niubangzi (*Fructus Arctii*) are used as ministerial drug to eliminate pathogenic factors from the superficies by helping open hair pores of the skin; Jiegeng (*Radix Platycodonis*) can disperse lung qi and relieve sore throat, Gancao (*Radix Glycyrrhizae*) could clear away heat and relieve toxin, Zhuye (*Herba Lophatheri*) can clear away heat from upper energizer, Lugen (*Rhizoma Phragmitis*) has an action of clearing away heat and promote production of body fluid, the four herbs are used as courier drug.

Both formulas are the best choices for eliminating the superficial syndromes of the primary stage of warm febrile disease. Though both of them contain Lianqiao, Jiegeng, Gancao, Bohe, and Lugen, Sang Ju Yin, as a mild "pungent-cool formula", has a stronger action of dispersing lung qi and stopping cough, for it includes Sangye, Juhua and Xingren; Yinqiao San is a moderate "pungent-cool formula", with a stronger function of clearing away heat and relieving the superficies, for it contains Jinyinhua, Jingjiesui, Dandouchi, Niubangzi and Zhuye.

3. 兼夹症
38.3 Complicated syndromes

(1) 夹痰

症见咳嗽剧烈，痰声呼呼，甚则气急鼻煽，脉象浮数。治疗以宣肺解表，清热化痰。方选三拗汤，或麻杏石甘汤加味。

(1) Syndrome complicated with retention of phlegm

Clinical manifestations: Severe cough, wheeze accompanied with phlegm even with dyspnea and flaring of nares due to short breath as well as floating and fast pulse.

Prescription and formulas: Disperse the lung, relieve the superficial syndromes, clear away heat and resolve phlegm. San'ao Tang (Decoction) or Mahuang Xingren Shigao Gancao Tang Jiewei (Modified Mahuang Xingren Shigao Gancao Decoction).

(2) 夹滞

症见脘腹胀满，食欲减退，呕吐酸腐，口气秽臭，腹痛便泻，舌苔厚腻，或白或黄，脉滑数。治以健脾消食，和中化滞。方选保和丸，便秘者用凉膈散。

(2) Syndrome complicated with food retention

Clinical manifestations: Distention and fullness in the epigastrium and abdomen, reduced appetite, vomiting and acid regurgitation, eructation with foul and fetid odor, abdominal pain with diarrhea, thick greasy fur with whitish or yellowish color as well as slippery and fast pulse.

Prescription: Invigorate the spleen and harmonize middle energizer to eliminate food retention.

Formulas: Baohe Wan (Pill), or Liangge San (Powder) for constipation.

(3) 夹惊

症见烦躁不安，睡卧不宁，惊惕抽搐，脉象弦数。治以清热化痰，熄风镇惊，方选小儿回春丹。

(3) Syndrome complicated with fright

Clinical manifestations: Restlessness and vexation, disturbed sleep, tremor and convulsion as well as taut and fast pulse.

Prescription: Clear away heat, resolve phlegm, suppress endogenous wind and arrest convulsion.

Formulas: Xiao'er Huichun Dan (Pill).

三十九、小儿消化不良
39 Infantile indigestion

〔概说〕 Summary

小儿消化不良是指因小儿内伤乳食过久，停聚不化，气滞不行所形成的一种慢性消化功能紊乱的综合征。临床上以不思乳食、食而不化、腹部胀满、形体消瘦、大便不调等为特征。

小儿消化不良属于中医学"积滞"范畴。它是由于喂养不当，饮食过量或无定时，或过食难以消化之物，或断奶时突然改变饮食等，致使脾胃受伤，受纳运化失职，升降失序，而成积滞。如果治疗不当，日久可致骨质疏松、佝偻病、眼干燥症及贫血等。因此，科学喂养是预防此病的主要措施。

Infantile indigestion is a disease of a chronic dysfunction of digestive system due to prolonged internal damage caused by infantile dyspepsia, unresolved food retention and failure to promote qi circulation. Clinically, it is marked by anorexia, failure to resolve food retention, abdominal distention and fullness, emaciation and irregular defecation.

In TCM, infantile indigestion pertains to "food retention", it is caused by improper feeding, excessive intake of food or unfixed feeding time, or excessive intake of indigestive food, or sudden change of food after weaning, resulting in impairment of the spleen and stomach, dysfunction in receiving, transporting and transforming food, disordered lifting and descending qi, which gives rise to food retention. Prolonged improper treatment could cause rarefaction of bone, rhachitis, scheroma as well as anemia. Therefore, feeding infants with scientific and reasonable methods is very essential to prevent this disease.

〔辨证论治〕 Syndrome differentiation and treatment

1. 乳食壅积

39.1　Retention of food

【症状】呕吐乳片或酸馊残渣，腹胀、腹痛拒按，夜睡不安，啼哭，伴有低热，不思饮食，大便臭秽，腹痛欲泻，泻后痛减。舌苔厚腻，脉滑。

【分析】此证主要是伤于乳食，乳食积滞所引起。乳食停滞，不能消化，故呕吐乳片或酸馊残渣；乳食停于脾胃，不能正常运化，故腹痛、腹胀且拒按；"胃不和则卧不安"，故有夜睡不安，啼哭不止；乳食停滞，积而生热，故见低热；胃纳失职，则不欲饮食；积滞日久，大便臭秽，时有欲泻除积之感，泻后积滞排出，故腹痛减轻；舌苔厚腻、脉滑，为食滞之征。

【治法】消食导滞。

【方药】保和丸加减。保和丸为治疗乳积、食积的主要方剂。方中以山楂味酸性温为君药，可消一切饮食积滞，尤善消肉食油腻之积。以神曲消食健脾，更化饮食陈腐之积；莱菔子下气消食，长于消谷面之积，共为臣药。三味同用，消各种饮食之积。佐以半夏、陈皮行气化滞，和胃止呕；茯苓健脾利湿，和中止泻；食积易于化热，故以连翘清热散结。诸药配伍，可使乳食之积化解，胃气因和。大便秘结，可加大黄消食导滞；呕吐乳片，可加黄连、竹茹清热和胃止呕。

Clinical manifestations: Vomiting of milk, or vomiting of indigestive food with decayed and fetid odor, abdominal distention, unpressable abdominal pain, disturbed sleep and crying at night, accompanied with mild fever, anorexia, stool with foul odor, abdominal pain with a desire of diarrhea; alleviation of pain after defecation; thick greasy fur as well as slippery pulse.

Analysis: This syndrome is mainly caused by internal impairment due to dyspepsia, which results in retention of indigestive food. Vomiting of milk, or vomiting of indigestive food with decayed and fetid odor is due to food retention and infantile dyspepsia; abdominal distention and unpressable pain are caused by dysfunction of the spleen and stomach because of food retention; disturbed sleep and non-stop crying at night are due to failure to descend stomach qi; mild fever is due to generation of heat from retention of infantile food; anorexia is caused by dysfunction of the stomach in receiving food; stool with foul odor as well as occasional desire of defecation is due to prolonged food retention; alleviation of pain after defecation is due to discharge of food retention. Thick greasy fur and slippery pulse are signs of food retention.

Prescription: Eliminate food retention and dredge retention.

Formulas: Baohe Wan Jiajian (Modified Baohe Pill). Baohe Wan is a principal recipe for infantile food retention as well as food accumulation. In the formula, Shanzha (*Fructus Crataegi*), sour in flavor and warm in nature, is used as sovereign drug to eliminate various food retention, in particular, retention of meat and greasy food. Shenqu (*Massa Medicata Fermentata*) can invigorate the spleen by eliminating food retention and resolve accumulation of decayed food; Laifuzi (*Semen Raphani*) can descend stomach qi and eliminate food retention, especially it can eliminate accumulation of food of cereal and flour, both of them are used as ministerial drug. Combined together, the three can eliminate all kinds of food retention. Banxia (*Rhizoma Pinelliae*) and Chenpi (*Pericarpium Citri Reticulatae*) are used as adjuvant drug to activate qi, resolve stagnation, regulate the stomach and stop vomiting; Fuling (*Poriae Cocos*) can invigorate the spleen, remove dampness by inducing diuresis and harmonize middle energizer to stop diarrhea; prolonged food retention is prone to generating endogenous heat, so Lianqiao (*Fructus Forsythiae*) can be combined to disperse stagnation by clearing away heat. The combination of all medicinal herbs can resolve infantile indigestion of food, as a result, stomach qi can be regulated. For dry feces, Dahuang (*Radix et Rhizoma Rhei*) can be added to eliminate food retention and dredge stagnation; for vomiting milk, Huanglian (*Rhizoma Coptidis*) and Zhuru (*Caulis Bambusae in Taenia*) can be combined to clear away heat, regulate stomach qi and stop vomiting.

2. 脾胃虚弱
39.2 Asthenia of the spleen and stomach

【症状】面色萎黄，困倦无力，不思饮食，呕吐不化，食则胀饱，腹满喜按，大便不化，唇舌淡白，苔白腻，脉沉细而滑。

【分析】脾胃虚弱，受纳与运化能力均弱，受纳力差，则不思饮食，运化力差，则食则胀饱；脾胃虚弱，生化气血自然减少，故面色萎黄，困倦无力；虚则喜按，大便自有不消化食物；营卫不足，则唇舌淡白；胃内有不消化食物，故苔白腻；气血不能充盈，则脉沉细而滑。

【治法】健脾和胃。

【方药】七味白术散加味。七味白术散以健脾理气、和胃宽中见长。方以补气健脾之四君子汤为主方；藿香辛、温，芳香化浊祛湿而和中止呕；木香辛、苦、温，行气止痛；葛根甘、辛、平，鼓舞胃气上行而止泻。全方对脾胃虚弱而致食积中焦，有良好效果。食滞明显的，可加鸡内金、神曲、麦芽等；腹胀明显者，可加青皮、陈皮；四肢不温者，可加干姜、桂枝。

Clinical manifestations: Sallow complexion, lassitude and lack of energy, anorexia, vomiting undigested food, distention and full sensation of the stomach after intake of a little amount of food, preference for pressing, stool with undigested food, pale lips and tongue, greasy whitish fur as well as sunken, thin and slippery pulse.

Analysis: Asthenic spleen and stomach results in weakness to receive food, which, gives rise to anorexia and dysfunction in transportation and transformation, thus, bringing about distention and full sensation after intaking a little amount of food; sallow complexion, lassitude and lack of energy are due to reduced qi and blood generated and transformed from food because of asthenia of the spleen and stomach; asthenia indicates preference for pressing as well as stool with undigested food; pale lips and tongue are caused by insufficiency of nutrient qi and defensive qi; greasy whitish fur is due to retention of undigested food in the stomach; sunken, thin and slippery pulse is due to failure of qi and blood to fill up blood vessels.

Prescription: Invigorate the spleen and harmonize the stomach.

Formulas: Qiwei Baizhu San Jiawei (Modified Qiwei Baizhu Powder). Qiwei Baizhu San is good at invigorating the spleen, regulating qi, harmonizing the stomach and soothing middle energizer. In the formula, Sijunzi Tang, with the action of tonifying qi and invigorating the spleen, is used as the principal recipe; Huoxiang (*Herba Agastachis*), pungent and aromatic in flavor and warm in nature, can regulate middle energizer and stop vomiting by resolving turbidity and dispelling dampness; Muxiang (*Radix Aucklandiae*), pungent and bitter in flavor and warm in nature, could promote qi circulation and arrest pain; Gegen (*Radix Puerariae*), with its sweet and bland taste and pungent flavor, could guide stomach qi to flow upward so as to stop diarrhea. The whole formula could achieve a good effect for food retention in middle energizer because of asthenic spleen and stomach. For obvious food retention, Jineijin (*Endothelium Corneum Gigeriae Galli*), Shenqu (*Massa Medicata Fermentata*) and Maiya (*Fructus Hordei Germinatus*) can be combined; for obvious abdominal distention, Qingpi (*Pericarpium Citri Reticulatae Viride*) and Chenpi (*Pericarpium Citri Reticulatae*) should be added; for cold limbs, Ganjiang (*Rhizoma Zingiberis*) and Guizhi (*Ramulus Cinnamomi*) can be combined.

四十、荨麻疹
40 Nettle-rash

〔概说〕 Summary

荨麻疹是由于皮肤黏膜小血管扩张及渗透性增加而出现的一种局限性水肿反应。临床表现为皮肤黏膜突然出现风团，剧痒，有急性和慢性之分。其急性期与进食某种食物，如鱼虾、海鲜类食物，或服用某些药物，或对寒冷敏感有关；而慢性期的病因尚不明确，可以迁延数月、数年而不愈。

荨麻疹属于中医学"瘾疹"等病范畴。中医学认为此病是由于感受风寒湿邪，或饮食不慎，异物伤及胃肠所致。治疗上，中医对慢性期病症效果较好，而对急性期可以采用针灸疗法选穴治之。

Nettle-rash is an edematous reaction limited to some area of the skin caused by expansion and pervasive increase of mucous membrane of small blood vessels located in the inner layers of the skin. Clinical manifestation of nettle-rash is marked by sudden outbreak of wheal with an itching sensation, and it can be divided into acute and chronic type of nettle-rash. Seafood, especially fishes, shrimp and shellfish, or medications, or allergic reactions to cold can cause acute nettle-rash, while chronic nettle-rash has unknown causes, and it can last several months or years.

Nettle-rash pertains to "urticaria" in term of TCM. The disease is caused by exogenous wind cold or dampness, or improper diet, or impairment of the stomach and even the intestines by foreign objects. TCM therapeutic methods for treating chronic type of nettle-rash could achieve a better effect, as for acute type, body acupuncture can be applied.

〔辨证论治〕 Syndrome differentiation and treatment

1. 风寒
40.1 Syndrome of wind-cold

【症状】发病急骤，皮疹色淡红，浸淫冷水或吹风受寒后发病或加剧，得暖则消，舌质淡，苔白，脉象浮紧。

【分析】骤然寒冷之风或冷水浸淫，皮肤之营卫不能适应，则局部起疹，皮疹淡红色，得温则寒散，故可减轻；舌质淡红、苔白、脉象浮紧，均为风寒袭表之征。

【治法】疏风散寒。

【方药】麻黄桂枝各半汤。此方出自《伤寒论》一书，方由麻黄、桂枝、白芍、杏仁、甘草、生姜、大枣组成，是由麻黄汤与桂枝汤各取三分之一，合而服之。由于风寒郁于肌表，营卫失和，阳气怫郁不得外越，是可汗而不大汗，故取麻黄桂枝各半汤，以立和解之法，小发其汗，以祛肌表之邪，而又不伤其营卫之气。前人说这是"阴阳和法"。

Clinical manifestations: Sudden outbreak, pale reddish rash, aggravation or onset of rash after being soaked in cold water or after being attacked by wind cold, disappearance with warmth, pale tongue with whitish fur as well as floating and tense pulse.

Analysis: Sudden attack of cold wind or being soaked in cold water, to which nutrient qi and defensive qi of the skin cannot adapt, giving rise to regional outbreak of nettle-rash with pale reddish color; alleviation of nettle-rash is due to the fact that skin has acquired warmth which dispels cold; pale tongue with whitish fur and floating and tense pulse are signs of wind cold attacking the superficies.

Prescription: Dispel wind and disperse cold.

Formulas: Mahuang Guizhi Geban Tang (Semi-decoction of Mahuang and Guizhi). The formula is quoted from *Shanghan Lun*（*Treatise on Febrile Diseases*）, consisting of Mahuang （*Herba Ephedrae*）, Guizhi（*Ramulus Cinnamomi*）, Baishao（*Radix Paeoniae Alba*）, Xingren（*Semen Armeniacae Amarum*）, Gancao（*Radix Glycyrrhizae*）, Shengjiang （*Rhizoma Zingiberis Recens*）and Dazao（*Fructus Jujubae*）. It is the combination of one third of Mahuang Tang（Decoction）and that of Guizhi Tang. Stagnation of wind and cold in the superficies and disharmony of nutrient qi and defensive qi cause failure of yang qi to move outward, which can be relieved by sweating, while profuse sweating should be prevented. Therefore, Mahuang Guizhi Geban Tang can be applied to harmonize the syndrome, mild sweating could dispel superficial pathogens without impairing nutrient qi and defensive qi, so it is regarded as "a treating method of harmonizing yin and yang" by ancient TCM practitioners.

2. 风热
40.2　Syndrome of wind-heat

【症状】发病急骤，风团色红，剧痒，遇热加重，得冷则轻，口渴心烦，舌红，苔黄，脉象浮数。

【分析】风热郁于肌表，不得外越，营卫因而不得宣通，郁而不发，故形成风团剧痒，遇热则热毒内攻，故风团加重，遇冷则热邪缓解，故有所减轻；风热不除，耗伤津液，故口苦，心烦；舌红、苔黄、脉象浮数，为风热袭表之象。

【治法】清热疏风。

【方药】消风散加减。消风散出自《外科正宗》，是治疗荨麻疹常用之方。方取当归、生地黄、胡麻养血润燥；知母、石膏、木通清热解毒；荆芥、防风、蝉蜕、牛蒡子除风解毒；苦参、苍术燥湿解毒；甘草和中解毒。全方综合诸药之特性，以祛风、清热、燥湿、养血、润燥于一方，为治疗荨麻疹风热证候之主方。若皮肤瘙痒甚者，可加穿山龙、徐长卿以祛风止痒。

Clinical manifestations：Sudden outbreak, reddish wheal of rash, acute itching sensation, aggravation with heat and alleviation with cold, polydypsia, reddish tongue with yellowish fur as well as floating and fast pulse.

Analysis：Failure of stagnated wind and heat in the superficial skin to let out results in inability to disperse stagnation of nutrient qi and defensive qi, thus, bringing about wheal of rash with acute itching sensation, aggravation with heat is due to internal invasion of toxic heat, alleviation with cold is due to relieved pathogenic heat factors when encountering cold； bitter taste and polydypsia are caused by unrelieved wind heat consuming and impairing body fluid； reddish tongue with yellowish fur and floating and fast pulse indicate wind heat attacking the superficies of the skin.

Prescription：Clear away heat and dispel wind pathogens.

Formulas：Xiaofeng San Jiajian（Modified Xiaofeng Powder）. The formula, quoted from *Waike Zhengzong*（*Orthodox Manual of External Diseases*）, is used as a common recipe for treating nettle-rash, in which, Danggui（*Radix Angelicae Sinensis*）, Shengdihuang（*Radix*

Rehmanniae Recens）and Huma（*Sesamum Indicum*）can nourish blood and moisten dryness；Zhimu（*Rhizoma Anemarrhenae*），Shigao（*Gypsum Fibrosum*）and Mutong（*Caulis Akebiae*）can eliminate heat toxin；Jingjie（*Herba Schizonepetae*），Fangfeng（*Radix Saposhnikoviae*），Chantui（*Periostracum Cicadae*）and Niubangzi（*Fructus Arctii*）have an action of dispelling wind and relieving toxic pathogens；Kushen（*Radix Sophorae Flavescentis*）and Cangzhu（*Rhizoma Atractylodis*）can dry dampness and relieve toxic pathogens；Gancao（*Radix Glycyrrhizae*）could regulate middle energizer and relieve toxin. The whole formula combines the function of dispelling wind，clearing away heat，drying dampness，nourishing blood and moistening dryness together，so it is used as the principal recipe for treating nettle-rash. For acute itchy skin，Chuanshanlong（*Ningpo Yam Rhizome*）and Xuchangqing（*Radix Cynanchi Paniculati*）can be added to dispel wind and relieve itching sensation.

3. 风湿热

40.3　Syndrome of wind，dampness and heat

【症状】夏秋季多发，风团色红，常数日不愈，口苦而黏，不欲饮食，尿黄，舌红，苔黄腻，脉象弦滑。

【分析】夏秋季节，天热地湿，湿热交蒸，人在其中，若感受风湿热毒，不能消散，发于肌表，则为荨麻疹。风湿热为阳邪，故风团色红；湿邪缠绵，故数日难愈；湿热蕴于中焦，使其脾胃失和，故食欲不振，口苦而黏；湿热下注，则尿黄；其舌苔与脉象，为湿热蕴结之征。

【治法】散风化湿清热。

【方药】消风导赤汤。此方出自《医宗金鉴》，由牛蒡子、黄连、白鲜皮、生地黄、茯苓、薄荷、金银花、灯芯草、木通、甘草组成。方取牛蒡子、白鲜皮、薄荷散风；金银花、黄连、灯芯草清热解毒；茯苓、木通化湿；生地黄凉血清热；甘草和中解毒。具体应用时，可加冬瓜皮、赤小豆、薏苡仁以加强健脾化湿作用，亦可加地肤子、苦参以除湿止痒。

Clinical manifestations：Frequent outbreak of nettle-rash in summer and autumn，reddish wheal of rash unhealed after several days，bitter and sticky taste of the mouth，anorexia，yellowish urine，reddish tongue with greasy yellowish fur as well as taut and slippery pulse.

Analysis：Summer and autumn are the seasons of heat and dampness，alternate fumigation of exogenous heat and dampness，attack of unscattered exogenous wind，dampness and heat pathogens on the superficies of skin brings about nettle-rash. Reddish color of wheal of rash is due to the fact that wind，dampness and heat are pathogenic yang factors；rash unhealed after several days is due to lingering dampness pathogen；anorexia，bitter and sticky taste of the mouth are due to disharmony of the spleen and stomach because of accumulation of heat and dampness in middle energizer；yellowish urine is caused by downward migration of heat and dampness；reddish tongue with greasy yellowish fur as well as taut and slippery pulse are signs of coagulation of heat and dampness.

Prescription: Dispel wind, resolve dampness and clear away heat.

Formulas: Xiaofeng Daochi Tang (Decoction). The formula, quoted from *Yizong Jinjian* (*Golden Mirror of Medicine*), consists of Niubangzi (*Fructus Arctii*), Huanglian (*Rhizoma Coptidis*), Baixianpi (*Cortex Dictamni*), Shengdihuang (*Radix Rehmanniae*), Fuling (*Poriae Cocos*), Bohe (*Herba Menthae*), Jinyinhua (*Flos Lonicerae*), Dengxincao (*Medulla Junci*), Mutong (*Caulis Akebiae*) and Gancao (*Radix Glycyrrhizae*). Among them, Niubangzi, Baixianpi and Bohe can dispel wind; Jinyinhua, Huanlian and Dengxin cao have an action of eliminating heat toxin; Fuling and Mutong can resolve dampness; Shengdihuang may cool blood and clear away heat; Gancao could regulate middle energizer and eliminate toxic pathogens. In clinical practice, Dongguapi (*Exocarpium Benincasae*), Chixiaodou (*Semen Phaseoli*) and Yiyiren (*Semen Coicis*) can be added to strengthen the action of invigorating the spleen and resolving dampness; Difuzi (*Fructus Kochiae*) and Kushen (*Radix Sophorae Flavescentis*) can be combined to eliminate dampness and itching sensation.

4. 阴血亏损
40.4 Deficiency of yin and blood

【症状】皮疹反复发作，迁延日久，午后或夜间加重，心烦易怒，手足心热，口干，舌质红少津，脉象沉细或细数。

【分析】阴血亏损，"阴虚生内热"，可使旧疾反复发作；午后或夜间为阴，阴不主事，故其时加重；内热干扰，故心烦易怒；阴血不足以养，故手足心热，口干；阴津内耗，则舌红少津，脉象沉细或呈细数之象。

【治法】滋阴养血散风。

【方药】当归饮子。此方出自《外科正宗》，方由荆防四物汤加味组成。四物汤为滋阴养血之剂，荆芥、防风散风；另加黄芪补气，何首乌滋阴，白蒺藜除风，甘草和中。是治疗血虚生风证候的主要方剂。具体应用时，可加地肤子、白鲜皮以除风止痒。

Clinical manifestations: Frequent outbreak of nettle-rash lasting for several days, aggravation in the afternoon or at night, vexation with susceptibility to rage, feverish sensation over the palms and soles, dry mouth, reddish tongue with scanty fur as well as sunken and thin pulse or thin and fast pulse.

Analysis: "Asthenia of yin generates endogenous heat", deficiency of yin and blood can cause frequent outbreak of unhealed diseases; the period between afternoon and night pertains to yin, which fails to dominate at that time, therefore, the disease is aggravated; vexation with susceptibility to rage is due to disturbance of endogenous heat; feverish sensation over the palms and soles and dry mouth are due to failure of insufficient yin and blood to nourish the body; reddish tongue with scanty fur and sunken and thin pulse or thin and fast pulse indicate internal consumption of yin fluid.

Prescription: Nourish yin and blood and dispel wind pathogen.

Formulas：Danggui Yinzi（Decoction）. The formula, quoted from *Waike Zhengzong*（*Orthodox Manual of External Diseases*）, consists of modified Jingfang Siwu Tang. Siwu Tang is a recipe for nourishing yin and blood, Jingjie（*Herba Schizonepetae*）and Fangfeng（*Radix Saposhnikoviae*）can disperse pathogenic wind；Huangqi（*Radix Astragali seu Hedysari*）can be added to replenish qi, Heshouwu（*Radix Polygoni Multiflori*）could be used to nourish yin, Baijili（*Fructus Tribuli*）has an action of eliminating wind, Gancao（*Radix Glycyrrhizae*）can harmonize middle energizer. The recipe is an essential one for treating the syndrome of generation of endogenous wind from asthenic blood. In clinical practice, Difuzi（*Fructus Kochiae*）and Baixianpi（*Cortex Dictamni*）could be combined to dispel wind and stop itching sensation.

四十一、湿疹

41 Eczema

〔**概说**〕 Summary

湿疹是一种急性、亚急性或慢性炎症性皮肤病。临床表现为皮损多形性、多渗出、剧烈瘙痒、反复发作和趋向慢性化。其病因多与变态反应有关。有急性期、亚急性期、慢性期等不同分类。

湿疹属于中医学"浸淫疮""旋耳疮""绣球风""四弯风"等病范畴。急性期以湿热为主；亚急性期多与脾虚不运，湿邪留恋有关；慢性期因病久伤血，血虚生风生燥，肌肤失去濡养而致。

Eczema is a term for different types of inflammatory skin disease including acute, subacute or chronic types. The clinical manifestation of eczema is marked by various forms of skin trauma, fluid oozing, intense itching sensation, frequent recurrence as well as a tendency to turn into chronic dermatitis. Pathogenesis for eczema is related to allergic reaction. It can be divided into acute, subacute and chronic stages.

Eczema pertains to "acute eczema" "eczema of the ear" "skin diseases of the scrota" and "ectopic eczema" in terms of TCM. Acute stage of eczema is characterized by dampness and heat. Subacute eczema is connected with dysfunction of asthenic spleen and retention of pathogenic dampness factor；chronic eczema is usually caused by impairment of blood because of prolonged process of diseases, generation of wind and dryness from asthenic blood as well as malnutrition of the skin.

湿疹急性期起病较快，常对称发生，可发于身体任何部位，亦可泛发全身，但以面部的前额、眼皮、颊部、耳部、口周围及肘窝、腘窝、手部、小腿、外阴、肛门周围等处多见。初起皮肤潮红、肿胀、瘙痒，面积大小不一，边界不清。继而出现丘疹、丘疱疹、水疱，群集或密集成片，常因搔抓，水疱破裂，形成糜烂、流滋、结痂，最后痂盖脱落，露出光滑红色皮肤，并有少量的脱屑，乃至痊愈。

亚急性湿疹是从急性发展迁延而来，急性期的红肿、水疱减轻，流滋减少，尚有红斑、丘疹、脱屑。一般无全身不适，或有胸闷、纳呆、便溏、苔腻、脉滑等。

湿疹慢性期乃由急性和亚急性反复发作而成。其特征是皮肤增厚，触之较硬，呈暗红或紫褐色，表面粗糙，皮纹显著或出现苔藓样变，常伴有少量抓痕、血痂、鳞屑及色素沉着，间有糜烂和流滋。瘙痒剧烈，尤以夜间或情绪紧张时更甚。病程较长，可拖延数月或数年。

Acute stage：This stage is characterized by sudden onset of eczema, symmetrically distribution in some area of the body, even all over the whole body. However, it can often be seen in the forehead, the eyelid, the cheek, the area around the ears and mouth, the chelidon and popliteal fossa, the hands, the shanks, the genital area and anus. At the beginning, the following symptoms may appear, such as flushed skin, swellings and pruritus in different size and without clear boundary. Afterwards, papulae, papulo-vesicles and blisters might appear in large patches or densely. Usually, because of scratching, the blisters can break up, then, fluid may ooze from ulcerated blisters, and scabs. At last, scabs will become crusty scale and fall off layer by layer until the slippery, tender and reddish skin comes out. The process is accompanied with a little amount of desquamation till the disease is cured.

Subacute stage：Eczema develops from the acute stage. With the decrease of swollen patches, blisters and alleviation of fluid oozing at the stage of acute eczema, some reddish patches, papulae and desquamation still remain. In general, the process is not accompanied with discomfort all over the body, but with symptoms such as occasional chest oppression, anorexia, loose stool, greasy fur as well as slippery pulse.

Chronic stage：Eczema evolves from recurrent outbreaks of acute dermatitis and subacute dermatitis, characterized by thickening of skin, hard sensation of skin when being touched, dark reddish, purplish or brownish color, scaly skin, remarkable dermatoglyphics, or lichenification. It is usually accompanied with scratching marks, bloody scabs, crusty scales as well as pathologic pigmentation, or accompanied with occasional ulceration and fluid oozing, severe itching, aggravation of itching especially at night or in stressed-out situation. The course of the disease is long and in some cases, it can last several months or years.

〔辨证论治〕 Syndrome differentiation and treatment

湿疹辨证分为湿热证和血虚风燥证。

Syndromes of eczema can be divided into syndrome of dampness and heat and syndrome of asthenic blood and wind dryness.

1. 湿热

41.1 Syndrome of dampness and heat

【症状】多见于急性期。表现为皮肤潮红、肿胀、糜烂、流滋、浸淫成片，结痂，瘙痒不甚，或伴有大便秘结，小便短赤，苔黄腻，脉象滑数。

【分析】湿热浸淫，湿毒与热毒互结，患处皮肤气血不和，郁结不散，故而潮红、肿胀、糜烂、流滋；因非风毒所致，故瘙痒不甚；湿热内结，则大便秘结，小便短赤；湿热上蒸，故苔黄腻，脉象滑数。

【治法】清热利湿。

【方药】龙胆泻肝汤、萆薢渗湿汤合二妙丸。龙胆泻肝汤为清热利湿之主方，尤以清泻肝胆湿热最为见长；萆薢渗湿汤为《疡科心得集》方，其作用为清利下焦湿热；二妙丸由苍术、黄柏组成，作用为清热化湿。三方合用，具有很强的清泻湿热功效。发于上部者，加桑叶、菊花、蝉蜕；发于中部者，加龙胆草、黄芩；发于下部者，加车前子、泽泻；瘙痒甚者，加地肤子、白鲜皮、徐长卿；局部焮红热盛者，加生地黄、赤芍、牡丹皮；便秘者，加生大黄（后下）；便溏者，加山药、焦扁豆。

Clinical manifestations： （The following symptoms are usually manifested at the stage of acute eczema.） Flushed and swollen skin, ulcerated blisters with fluid oozing, eczema spreading into patches and crusty scales, mild itching, or accompanied with constipation, scanty and brownish urine, yellowish greasy fur as well as slippery and fast pulse.

Analysis： Spreading of dampness and heat and coagulation of pathogenic dampness and heat toxin result in stagnation of unscattered qi and blood due to disharmony of qi and blood on the infected skin, which brings about flushed and swollen skin, ulcerated blisters with fluid oozing. The syndrome is not caused by pathogenic wind toxin, so itching is not severe. Dry feces and scanty brownish urine are due to coagulation of pathogenic dampness and heat； yellowish greasy fur and slippery and fast pulse are caused by up-fumigating of dampness and heat.

Prescription： Clear away heat and remove dampness by inducing diuresis.

Formulas： Longdan Xiegan Tang （Decoction） combined with Bixie Shenshi Tang （Decoction） and Ermiao Wan （Pill）. Longdan Xiegan Tang is an essential formula for clearing away heat and removing dampness, in particular, for purging damp-heat from the liver and gallbladder； Bixie Shenshi Tang is quoted from *Yangke Xinde Ji* （*Experience Gained in Treating External Diseases*）, and it has a strong action of clearing away damp heat in lower energizer； Ermiao Wan is made up of Cangzhu （*Rhizoma Atractylodis*） and Huangbo （*Cortex Phellodendri*）, having an action of purging heat and resolving dampness. Combined together, the three formulas can eliminate damp-heat. For eczema in the upper part of the body, Sangye （*Folium Mori*）, Juhua （*Flos Chrysanthemi*） and Chantui （*Periostracum Cicadae*） can be added； for eczema in the middle, Longdancao （*Radix Geutianae*） and Huangqin （*Radix Scutellariae*） should be added； for eczema in the lower, Cheqianzi （*Semen Plantaginis*） and Zexie （*Rhizoma Alismatis*） can be combined； for severe itching, Difuzi （*Fructus Kochiae*），

Baixianpi (*Cortex Dictamni*) and Xuchangqing (*Radix Cynanchi Paniculati*) could be added; for regional swellings and hyperactive heat, Shengdihuang (*Radix Rehmanniae Recens*), Chishao (*Radix Paeoniae Rubra*) and Mudanpi (*Cortex Moutan Radicis*) could be combined; for constipation, Shengdahuang (*Radix et Rhizoma Rhei*) (decocted later) should be added; for loose stool, Shanyao (*Rhizoma Dioscoreae*) and stir-baked Biandou (*Semen Dolichoris Album*) could be added.

2. 血虚风燥
41.2　Syndrome of blood asthenia and wind dryness

【症状】常见于慢性湿疹。反复发作，病程较长，皮损颜色暗淡，浸润肥厚，苔藓样变，色素沉着，血痂，脱屑，舌苔淡白，脉象濡细。

【分析】湿疹日久，形成慢性，必然使皮肤受损，呈现皮色暗淡；由于浸润时间长，故浸润皮肤肥厚；局部色素沉着；日久则形成血痂、脱屑；舌苔淡白，脉象濡数，为湿热之象。

【治法】养血祛风，清热利湿。

【方药】四物汤合萆薢渗湿汤。瘙痒不能安睡者，加珍珠母、生牡蛎（均先煎），夜交藤、酸枣仁；腰膝酸软者，加狗脊、仙灵脾、菟丝子；皮肤粗糙肥厚者，加丹参、益母草、鸡血藤。

Clinical manifestations: (The following symptoms are usually manifested at the stage of chronic eczema.) Recurrent outbreak, long course of the disease, skin lesion with dark color, thickening skin due to spreading of eczema, lichenification, pigmentation, bloody scab, crusty scales, pale whitish fur as well as soft and thin pulse.

Analysis: Prolonged course of eczema develops into chronic disease, which must bring about skin lesion with dark coloration; prolonged spreading of eczema causes thickening skin and regional pigmentation, bloody scab, crusty scales; pale whitish fur and soft and thin pulse are indication of dampness and heat.

Prescription: Nourish blood, expel wind, purge heat and remove dampness by inducing diuresis.

Formulas: Siwu Tang (Deccotion) combined with Bixie Shenshi Tang (Deccotion). For failure to fall asleep due to itchy skin, Zhenzhumu (*Concha Margaritifera*), Shengmuli (*Concha Ostreae*) (both of them should be decocted first), Yejiaoteng (*Caulis Polygoni Multiflori*) and Suanzaoren (*Semen Ziziphi Spinosae*) can be added; for aching and weakness of the loins and knees, Gouji (*Rhizoma Cibotii*), Xianlingpi (*Herba Epimedii*) and Tusizi (*Semen Cuscutae*) can be added; for scaly and thickening skin, Danshen (*Radix Salviae Miltiorrhizae*), Yimucao (*Herba Leonuri*) and Jixueteng (*Spatholobi*) could be combined.

此外，湿疹的治疗，还可以配合针灸、外敷、中成药等治疗，以提高治疗效果。

In addition to the above prescriptions, acupuncture, external compression as well as

Chinese-patent drug can be applied in treating the disease for the sake of improving curative effect.

四十二、神经性皮炎
42　Neurodermatitis

〔**概说**〕　Summary

神经性皮炎，又称慢性单纯性苔藓，病因尚未清楚。一般认为可能由皮质抑制和兴奋功能紊乱所致。而情绪、局部刺激和辛辣酒类可诱发并加重本病。临床以剧烈瘙痒或皮肤苔藓样病变为其特点。

神经性皮炎属于中医学"牛皮癣"等病证范畴。由于本病状如牛领之皮，厚而且坚，故名"牛皮癣"。基本损害多是圆形或多角形的扁平丘疹融合成片，搔抓后皮肤肥厚，皮沟加深，皮嵴隆起，极易形成苔藓化，这是本病的重要指征。牛皮癣的形成因素与外因的风湿热侵袭有关，并与情绪不安，肝血不足，血虚生风，皮肤失去濡养有着密不可分的关系。治疗上扶正与祛邪并重，以滋阴养血为主，祛风渗湿清热为辅，标本并治，方可取得预期效果。

Neurodermatitis is also known as "chronic lichen simplex" with unknown pathogenesis. It is generally believed that the disease is probably caused by cortical inhibition and dysfunction of excitable cells of the skin. Stress, depression, stimulus in some specific area, alcoholism as well as pungent or hot food can trigger and even aggravate the disease. Clinical manifestation of neurodermatitis is marked by severe itching of the skin or lichenification.

In TCM, neurodermatitis pertains to "psoriasis", the term derives from the similarity of lesioned skin to the cow leather, for both of them are thick and hard. Basically, the disease is characterized by skin damage with round or polygonal patches of flat papulae, thickening skin, deepening grooves of skin, raised dermal ridges as well as susceptibility to lichenification. Factors that contribute to the onset of psoriasis may be associated with invasion of wind, dampness and heat, emotional upset, insufficient liver blood, endogenous wind generated from asthenic blood as well as malnutrition of the skin. Based on the principle of "laying equal stress on strengthening healthy qi and dispelling pathogenic factors", treatment for it should focus on nourishing yin and blood, with expelling wind, resolving dampness and clearing away heat being the assistant therapeutic methods. Only in this way, could the symptoms and root cause be addressed, and the expected curative effect be achieved.

〔辨证论治〕 Syndrome differentiation and treatment

1. 风湿热
42.1　Syndrome of wind, dampness and heat

【症状】局部除有成片丘疹肥厚外，并伴有部分皮损潮红、糜烂、湿润和血痂，苔黄或黄腻，脉象濡数。

【分析】风湿热邪侵犯肌表，损伤皮肤，除有丘疹外，还会使皮损表现出潮红、糜烂、湿润、血痂等，依次为不同程度的损害。但以湿热比较明显，所以会有苔黄或黄腻、脉数之征。

【治法】疏风清热利湿。

【方药】消风散加减。（消风散方义见"荨麻疹"篇。）常加白鲜皮、苦参、皂角刺，以增强疏风清热止痒之效。

Clinical manifestations: Patches of thickening papulae in some region, partial lesion with reddish skin, ulceration, moisture and scabs mingled with blood, yellowish tongue fur or yellowish greasy fur as well as soft and fast pulse.

Analysis: Pathogenic wind, dampness and heat factors invade the superficies of the skin, causing skin damage to different degree, such as papulae, flushed skin, ulceration, moisture as well as bloody scabs. Yellowish fur or yellowish greasy fur and fast pulse are due to obvious dampness and heat.

Prescription: Dispel wind, clear away heat and remove dampness by inducing diuresis.

Formulas: Xiaofeng San Jiajian (Modified Xiaofeng Powder). (It has been discussed in the chapter of *Nettle-rash*). Baixianpi (*Cortex Dictamni*), Kushen (*Radix Sophorae Flavescentis*) and Zaojiaoci (*Spina Gleditsiae*) can be added to the formula to reinforce the effect of dispelling wind, clearing away heat and arresting itching.

2. 血虚风燥
42.2　Syndrome of asthenic blood and wind dryness

【症状】病程较长，局部干燥、肥厚、脱屑，状如牛领之皮，苔薄，脉象濡细。

【分析】此证病程较长，血分受损，出现血虚生风化燥之象。燥性必干，故皮肤干燥、肥厚、脱屑，其状如牛领之皮；津液伤，则苔薄；脉濡细，为血分受伤之象。

【治法】养血祛风润燥。

【方药】四物汤加减。（四物汤方义见"头痛"篇。）常加荆芥、防风、白蒺藜，以祛风止痒。

Clinical manifestations: Prolonged course of the disease, regional dryness, thickening skin with crusty scales, skin like the leather of cow neck, thin tongue fur as well as soft and thin pulse.

Analysis：Asthenic blood generating endogenous wind and transforming into dryness is caused by impairment of blood phase resulting from prolonged course of the disease. Dry and thickening skin and crusty scales like cow leather are caused by dry nature of dryness；thin tongue fur is due to impairment of body fluid，soft and thin pulse indicates impairment of blood phase.

Prescription：Nourish blood，dispel wind and moisten dryness.

Formulas：Siwu Tang Jiajian（Modified Siwu Decoction）.（The formula has been introduced in the chapter of *Headache*.）Jingjie（*Herba Schizonepetae*），Fangfeng（*Radix Saposhnikoviae*）and Baijili（*Tribulus Territris*）can be added to dispel wind and arrest itching sensation.

以上两个证候，如果遇到情绪波动，病情加重，均可在原方中加入珍珠母（先煎）、代赭石（先煎）、生牡蛎（先煎）、五味子、夜交藤等。

In the above syndromes, Zhenzhumu（*Concha Margaritifera*）（decocted first），Daizheshi（*Haematitum*）（decocted first），Shengmuli（*Concha Ostreae*）（decocted first），Wuweizi（*Fructus Schisandrae Chinensis*）and Yejiaoteng（*Caulis Polygoni Multiflori*）can be added to the original formulas to treat aggravation of the disease due to mood instability.

附：其他疗法

①苦参陈醋饮：苦参 200 克，陈醋 500 毫升，浸泡 5 天后，用浸泡药液外擦皮损处，每日 2~3 次。

②针刺法：播散型者，取曲池、血海、大椎、足三里、合谷、三阴交等穴，隔日 1 次。

③艾灸法：小块肥厚皮损，可用艾卷灸患处，每次 15~30 分钟，每日 1 次。

④梅花针法：苔藓化明显者，可用七星针在患处来回移动击刺，每日 1 次。

Other therapeutic methods on the syndromes

a. Kushen Chencu Yin（Decoction）：200 g of Kushen（*Radix Sophorae Flavescentis*），500 mL of Chencu（mature vinegar），soak Kushen in Chencu for five days，then coat the vinegar onto the wounded area for 2 or 3 times a day.

b. Body acupuncture：For the type of diffusive neurodermatitis，needle Quchi（LI 11），Xuehai（SP 10），Dazhui（GV 14），Zusanli（ST 36），Hegu（LI 4）and Sanyinjiao（SP 6），once every other day.

c. Moxibustion：For small patches of thickening skin damage，moxa roll can be applied to burn on the affected skin，15~30 minutes each time，once each day.

d. Plum-blossom needle therapy：For obvious lichenification，the technique of seven-star needle can be applied to stimulate and pierce the affected skin back and forth，once each day.

四十三、寻常痤疮
43　Acne vulgaris

〔**概说**〕　Summary

　　寻常痤疮好发于颜面、胸、背等处，一般认为是青春发育期体内雄激素过多、皮脂溢出、毛囊口堵塞，并发细菌、真菌感染所致。皮损初起为粉刺，可发展为丘疹、脓疱、结节、囊肿、瘢痕等。本病好发于青春发育期的男女，青春期后大多数病人能自愈或缓解。但成年后，亦有发病者。

　　本病属于中医学"肺风粉刺"范畴。发病机制与肺经风热、肠胃湿热、脾失健运有关。除用必要的药物治疗外，注意饮食调节，不食或少食油腻及辛辣食物，多吃新鲜水果和蔬菜，对缩短疗程也是不可或缺的。

　　Acne vulgaris usually appears in the area of the face, chest, and back. It typically occurs at youth because of excess sebum secretion triggered by increased androgen levels, sebum overflow, blocked pores, as well as complicated infection of bacteria and fungi. Initially, skin lesion starts with appearance of comedo, which can evolve into papulae, pustules, nodules, cysts as well as scabs. It is commonly seen in adolescents. After the period, patients can be healed or the disease can get alleviated. However it could occur in adulthood too.

　　Acne vulgaris pertains to "acne due to pulmonary wind" in TCM. Pathogenesis for it is associated with wind heat in lung meridian, stagnation of dampness and heat in the intestines and stomach and dysfunction of the spleen. In addition to necessary medication, much stress should be attached to proper dietary, for instance, fatty or pungent and hot food should be avoided and eating fresh fruits and vegetables should be encouraged, for they are indispensable to shorten the course of treatment.

〔**辨证论治**〕　Syndrome differentiation and treatment

1. 肺经风热
43.1　Syndrome of wind and heat in lung meridian

　　【症状】颜面潮红，粉刺焮热、疼痛，或有脓疱，舌质红赤，苔薄黄，脉象细数。

　　【分析】肺经风热证，多发于鼻子周围，鼻子及其周围属于肺经。肺经风热熏蒸，蕴阻肌肤，难以透发，遂发粉刺。热毒蕴结，则焮热疼痛；若热毒与湿浊蕴结，则发为脓疱；风热不散，故舌脉呈阳热之象。

　　【治法】疏风宣肺清热。

　　【方药】枇杷清肺饮加减。枇杷清肺饮出自《医宗金鉴》，由人参、枇杷叶、黄连、黄柏、桑白皮、甘草组成。人参扶助正气；枇杷叶与桑白皮为清肺热之要药，有宣肺散热作用；黄连、黄柏清热解毒；甘草和中解毒。热势甚者，加连翘、白花蛇舌草。

Clinical manifestations：Flushed complexion, swelling and heat sensation of the acnes, pain, or outbreak of pustules, reddish tongue with thin yellowish fur as well as thin and fast pulse.

Analysis：Syndrome of wind heat in lung meridian usually occurs at the area around the nose which pertains to lung meridian. Accumulation of steaming wind and heat in lung meridian obstructs the skin from letting out heat, thus, bringing about acnes. Burning sensation and pain are due to accumulation of heat toxin; outbreak of pustules is caused by coagulation of heat toxin and dampness and turbidity; the pulse condition of yang and heat indicates undispersed wind and heat.

Prescription：Dispel wind, disperse lung qi and clear away heat.

Formulas：Pipa Qingfei Yin Jiajian (Modified Pipa Qingfei Decoction). The formula is quoted from *Yizong Jinjian* (*Golden Mirror of Medicine*), consisting of Renshen (*Radix Ginseng*), Pipaye (*Folium Eriobotryae*), Huanglian (*Rhizoma Coptidis*), Huangbo (*Cortex Phellodendri*), Sangbaipi (*Cortex Mori*) and Gancao (*Radix Glycyrrhizae*). Renshen has an action of strengthening healthy qi; Pipaye and Sangbaipi are the essential medicinal herbs for clearing away heat and dispersing lung heat; Huanglian and Huangbo could relieve heat and toxin; Gancao has an action of harmonizing middle energizer and relieving toxin. For severe fever, Lianqiao (*Fructus Forsythiae*) and Baihuasheshecao (*Hedyotis Diffusa*) can be combined.

2. 肠胃湿热

43.2 Syndrome of dampness and heat in the intestines and stomach

【症状】皮疹红肿疼痛，伴有便秘，小便短赤，纳呆腹胀，舌苔黄腻，脉象滑数。

【分析】多由于过食辛辣油腻之品，生湿生热，结于肠胃，不能下达，反而上逆，阻于面部肌肤而成。腑气不通，故大便秘结，腹胀，小便短赤；胃气不降，故胃纳不振；湿热熏蒸，则舌苔黄腻，脉象滑数。

【治法】清热化湿通腑。

【方药】清胃散加减。清胃散出自《兰室秘藏》，由生地黄、当归、牡丹皮、黄连、升麻组成。面部为足阳明胃经与手阳明大肠经经脉所过，故取清胃之黄连、牡丹皮清阳明经之热；当归、生地黄养胃阴；升麻为阳明经之引经药，可使诸药到达阳明经所过之面部，使其发挥治疗作用。具体应用时，可加知母、生石膏清热泻火；加茵陈、大黄清泻胃肠之积热。

Clinical manifestations：Swollen and painful papulae, accompanied with constipation, scanty brownish urine, anorexia, abdominal pain, yellowish greasy fur as well as slippery and fast pulse.

Analysis：The syndrome is mainly caused by accumulation of dampness and heat in the intestines and stomach generated from excessive intake of pungent and fatty food, which fails to move downward, thus, moving adversely upward and getting obstructed on the surface of facial skin. Constipation, abdominal pain and scanty brownish urine are due to stagnation of intestinal qi; anorexia is due to failure of stomach qi to descend; yellowish greasy fur and slippery and fast pulse indicate fumigation of dampness and heat.

Prescription: Clear away heat, resolve dampness and dispel intestinal qi.

Formulas: Qingwei San Jiajian (Modified Qingwei Powder). It is quoted from *Lanshi Micang* (*Secret Book of Orchid Chamber*), consisting of Shengdihuang (*Radix Rehmanniae Recens*), Danggui (*Radix Angelicae Sinensis*), Mudanpi (*Cortex Moutan Radicis*), Huanglian (*Rhizoma Coptidis*) and Shengma (*Rhizoma Cimicifugae*). The face is the area stomach meridian of foot yangming and large intestine meridian of hand yangming pass through, so Huanglian and Mudanpi are used to purge heat from yangming meridian; Danggui and Shengdihuang can nourish stomach yin; Shengma is used as meridian-ushering drug to help the above drug reach the face where yangming meridian pass, so as to bring their effect into full play. In clinical practice, Zhimu (*Rhizoma Anemarrhenae*) and Shengshigao (*Gypsum Fibrosum*) can be combined to purge heat and fire; Yinchen (*Herba Artemisiae Scopariae*) and Dahuang (*Radix et Rhizoma Rhei*) can be combined to clear away accumulation of heat from the stomach and intestines.

3. 脾失健运
43.3 Syndrome of dysfunction of the spleen in transportation

【症状】皮疹色红不鲜，反复发作，或结成囊肿，或伴有纳呆，便溏，神疲乏力，舌苔薄白，脉象濡滑。

【分析】由于脾失运化之力，水湿内停，日久成痰，湿郁化热，湿热夹痰，凝滞肌肤，而成痤疮。热毒不重，故疹色不鲜；湿聚日久，会成囊肿；脾失健运，则有便溏、纳呆之苦；脾主四肢，脾不运化水谷，则四肢不得营养，故神疲乏力；舌苔薄白与脉象濡滑，为脾虚湿聚之象。

【治法】健脾化湿。

【方药】参苓白术散加减。（参苓白术散见"慢性腹泻"篇。）食欲不振，加焦三仙；大便稀薄，可加车前子、猪苓等。

Clinical manifestations: Dark reddish papulae with frequent outbreak, or formation of cyst, or accompanied with anorexia, loose stool, dispiritedness, thin whitish fur as well as soft and slippery pulse.

Analysis: Dysfunction of the spleen results in internal retention of dampness, which transforms into phlegm and heat, formation of acne is due to stagnation of coagulated dampness, heat and phlegm in the skin. Dark reddish papulae is due to unserious heat toxin; formation of cyst is due to prolonged accumulation of dampness; loose stool and anorexia are caused by dysfunction of the spleen in transporting food; the spleen dominates the limbs, failure of the spleen in transporting and transforming food results in malnutrition of the limbs, bringing about dispiritedness; thin whitish fur and soft and slippery pulse indicate retention of dampness due to asthenic spleen.

Prescription: Invigorate the spleen and resolve dampness.

Formulas: Shen Ling Baizhu San Jiajian (Modified Shen Ling Baizhu Powder). (It has been discussed in the chapter of *Chronic Diarrhea*.) For poor appetite, stir-baked Maiya (*Fructus Hordei Germinatus*), stir-baked Shanzha (*Fructus Crataegi*) and stir-baked Shenqu (*Massa Medicata Fermentata*) can be added; for loose and thin stool, Cheqianzi (*Semen Plantaginis*) and Zhuling (*Polyporus Umbellatus*) can be combined with the formula.

以上不论何种证候，凡口渴唇燥者，可加玄参、天冬、麦冬、天花粉；结节囊肿者，可加莪术、夏枯草、海藻、牡蛎；女子月经不调者，可加当归、白芍、益母草。

In any one of the above three syndromes, for thirst and dry lips, Xuanshen (*Radix Scrophulariae*), Tiandong (*Radix Asparagi*), Maidong (*Radix Ophiopogonis*) and Tianhuafen (*Radix Trichosanthis*) can be added; for nodules and cysts, Ezhu (*Rhizoma Curcumae*), Xiakucao (*Spica Prunellae*), Haizao (*Sargassum*) and Muli (*Concha Ostreae*) can be combined; for irregular menstruation, Danggui (*Radix Angelicae Sinensis*), Baishao (*Radix Paeoniae Alba*) and Yimucao (*Herba Leonuri*) can be added.

另外，可用温水、硫黄香皂洗脸。禁止用手挤压。少吃油腻及辛辣食物，多吃新鲜蔬菜或水果。

Furthermore, patients should wash their faces with warm water and sulfur soap. Squeezing acne with hands and pungent or fatty food should be avoided, and intake of fresh fruits and vegetables are encouraged.

四十四、斑秃

44 Alopecia areata

〔概说〕 Summary

斑秃，又称圆形斑秃，俗称"鬼剃头"。起病突然，病人多在无意中发现头发脱落，呈圆形或不规则形，小如指甲，大如钱币或更大，数目不等。一般无自觉症状，少数病人头发会全部脱落，称全秃；严重者眉毛、胡须、腋毛、阴毛等全部脱落，称普秃。

由于本病起病突然，头发脱落，头皮油光发亮，故中医称"油风"。

中医学认为本病与肝气怫郁，耗伤阴血，气滞血瘀有关。肝藏血，发为血之余，肾主骨，其荣在发，肝肾不足，则导致脱发；而气滞血瘀，毛发无所养，亦可导致脱发。

斑秃有自愈趋向，但很易再行脱落，以致病程可达数月或数年。治愈后，头发日渐变粗、变黑、变硬，最后与健康头发无异。

Alopecia areata, known as "round spot baldness", has got its popular Chinese name "alopecia" (mysterious shaving of head). It is a condition in which hair fall out suddenly from several patches of the scalp, of which, patients may be unaware. The patches can take many shapes, usually they are round or irregular, in some cases, they are as small as fingernail, or as big as coins, or even bigger. In some cases, complete loss of hair occurs, known as "total alopecia". If all body hair, including eyebrow, beard, armpit hair, even pubic hair, is lost, the symptom is called as "universal alopecia".

Because of sudden outbreak of the disease, hair falls out and the scalp becomes oily and shiny, so it is known as "oily wind".

In TCM, alopecia areata is associated with qi stagnation and blood stasis due to depression of qi in the liver impairing yin and blood. The liver stores blood, hair is the rest part of blood. The kidney dominates bone, manifesting its condition by hair. Insufficiency of the liver and kidney results in loss of hair; qi stagnation and blood stasis cause malnutrition of hair, which could lead to hair loss.

Alopecia areata can be healed itself, but the new hair is easy to fall out again. Most people who have one such episode will have more episodes of hair loss, and the course of the disease can last for several months even several years. After being cured, the new hair may get thicker, blacker and harder. Finally, it could even become the same as healthy hair.

〔辨证论治〕 Syndrome differentiation and treatment

1. 血虚风燥
44.1 Syndrome of asthenic blood and dry wind

【症状】脱发时间较短，有轻度瘙痒感，伴有头昏、失眠，舌苔薄白，脉象细数。

【分析】体质本虚，血虚不能濡养皮肤，以致毛孔开张，风邪乘虚而入，风盛血燥，发失所养，而呈片状脱落；风邪客于营卫，或有轻度皮肤瘙痒；风邪上扰，则有头昏、失眠之苦；舌苔薄白，为风邪在表之象；脉象细数，为风盛之征。

【治法】养血祛风。

【方药】神应养真汤加减。神应养真汤出自《外科正宗》，由四物汤加天麻、羌活、木瓜、菟丝子组成。此方是在养血活血的基础上，加入祛风的天麻、羌活，补肾的菟丝子，舒筋的木瓜，具有养血祛风、活血生发的功效。具体应用时，可以加入何首乌、黑芝麻，以增加养血的功效。若瘙痒甚者，可加地肤子、白鲜皮以祛风止痒。

Clinical manifestations: Hair loss for a short time, slight itching, accompanied with vertigo, insomnia, thin whitish fur as well as thin and fast pulse.

Analysis: Asthenic constitution results in failure of asthenic blood to nourish the skin, leading to opening of hair pores and internal invasion of wind pathogen, exuberant wind and dry blood result in malnutrition of hair falling out in patches; slight itching is due to wind pathogen attacking nutrient qi and defensive qi; vertigo and insomnia are due to up-attack of wind pathogen; thin whitish fur indicates pathogenic wind factor is on the surface; thin and fast pulse is the sign of exuberant wind pathogen.

Prescription: Nourish blood and dispel wind pathogen.

Formulas: Shenying Yangzhen Tang Jiajian (Modified Shenying Yangzhen Decoction). Shenying Yangzhen Tang is quoted from *Waike Zhengzong* (*Orthodox Manual of External Diseases*), consisting of Siwu Tang, Tianma (*Rhizoma Gastrodiae*), Qianghuo (*Rhizoma et Radix Notopterygii*), Mugua (*Fructus Chaenomelis*) and Tusizi (*Semen Cuscutae*). Based on the function of nourishing blood and activating blood of Siwu Tang, this formula is combined with medicinal herbs such as Tianma and Qianghuo to strengthen the action of dispelling wind, Tusizi is added to replenish the kidney, and Mugua is added to relax tendons. Therefore, the newly combined formula has the action of nourishing blood, dispelling wind and activating blood to promote multiplying hair. In clinical practice, Heshouwu (*Radix Polygoni Multiflori*) and Heizhima (*Semen Sesami Nigri*) can be added to improve the effect of nourishing blood. For severe itching, Difuzi (*Fructus Kochiae*) and Baixianpi (*Cortex Dictamni*) may be added to dispel wind and stop itching.

2. 气滞血瘀
44.2 Syndrome of qi stagnation and blood stasis

【症状】病程时间较长，伴有头痛，胸胁疼痛，夜眠难安，或有外伤史，舌质有瘀点，脉象沉涩。

【分析】患病时间长，由表入里，由气入血，使其气血运行不畅，毛发失其所养，则毛发脱落；头部络脉不通，则见头痛；气滞血瘀多由肝气郁滞所致，故胸胁疼痛；心脉不通，则夜眠难安；若有外伤史，瘀血更为明显，舌质瘀点，明显沉涩，为气滞血瘀之象。

【治法】理气活血。

【方药】逍遥散合通窍活血汤。逍遥散为疏肝解郁、理气活血的要方，它是在养血的基础上，加入疏肝的柴胡、薄荷、陈皮、枳壳等，具有养血活血、疏肝理气的功效；通窍活血汤（方义见"头痛"篇）是头部活血化瘀的主要方剂，应用范围比较广泛，用于此是借其对头部络脉的通络化瘀作用，以使其发根祛瘀生新，促其新发的生长。

Clinical manifestations: Prolonged course, accompanied with headache, pain in the chest and hypochondrium, disturbed sleep at night, or accompanied with trauma, petechiae on the tongue as well as sunken and astringent pulse.

Analysis: Prolonged course of the disease indicates pathogens have transmitted from the exterior to the interior, and from qi phase to blood phase, causing inhibited qi and blood circulation, failure to nourish body hair, which brings about loss of hair; headache is due to stagnation of collaterals of the head; pain in the chest and hypochondrium is due to qi stagnation and blood stasis caused by qi depression in the liver; disturbed sleep at night is due to failure to dredge heart vessels; trauma causes more serious blood stasis, petechiae on the tongue and sunken and astringent pulse are obvious signs of qi stagnation and blood stasis.

Prescription: Regulate qi and promote blood circulation.

Formulas: Xiaoyao San (Powder) combined with Tongqiao Huoxue Tang (Decoction). Xiaoyao San is an essential recipe for soothing the liver, relieving depression and activating blood by regulating qi, and it is the combination of herbs with the action of nourishing blood with Chaihu (*Radix Bupleuri*), Bohe (*Herba Menthae*), Chenpi (*Pericarpium Citri Reticulatae*) and Zhiqiao (*Fructus Aurantii*), which have the effect of nourishing blood, activating blood circulation, soothing the liver and regulating qi; Tongqiao Huoxue Tang (it has been discussed in the chapter of *Headache*), is a principal formula for activating blood and resolving stasis in the head, and it can be applied widely. Here it is used to dredge the collaterals of the head and invigorate blood circulation to improve the growth of new hair by eliminating stasis of blood in the area of hair root.

3. 肝肾不足
44.3　Syndrome of deficiency of the liver and kidney

【症状】病程较长，呈现全秃或普秃，多伴有头昏、耳鸣、失眠，舌苔剥落，脉象沉细。

【分析】病程较长，损伤肝肾之阴，使其肝血不足，肾阴亏耗，血不足以养发，精不足以生发，故脱发严重，且多伴有头昏、耳鸣、失眠等；由于阴血亏耗，所以舌苔剥落如地图样，脉象也显得细弱无力。

【治法】补益肝肾。

【方药】七宝美髯丹加减。七宝美髯丹出自《邵应节方》，由何首乌、菟丝子、牛膝、茯苓、补骨脂、枸杞子、当归组成。其方有补肾的何首乌、菟丝子、牛膝、补骨脂，补肝的枸杞子、当归，以及祛湿浊的茯苓，是补益肝肾的代表方剂。肝血足，肾精充，则头发自然生长。本方只是补益方剂，见效非一日之功，需坚持服用。若有头昏，可加菊花、旱莲草以清头目；夜眠不安，可加夜交藤、五味子以滋阴安神。

Clinical manifestations: Prolonged course of the disease, total or universe alopecia, usually accompanied with vertigo, tinnitus, insomnia, exfoliated fur as well as sunken and thin pulse.

Analysis: Prolonged course of the disease impairs yin of the liver and kidney, causing insufficiency of liver blood, consumption of kidney yin, and failure of deficient blood to nourish hair as well as failure of insufficient kidney essence to produce hair, which brings about serious hair loss, vertigo, tinnitus and insomnia. Exfoliated fur like a map and sunken and thin pulse are due to asthenia of yin and blood.

Prescription: Qibao Meiran Dan Jiajian (Modified Qibao Meiran Pill). Qibao Meiran

Dan is quoted from *Shao Yingjie Fang* (*Collected formulas of Shao Yingjie*), consisting of Heshouwu (*Radix Polygoni Multiflori*), Tusizi (*Semen Cuscutae*), Niuxi (*Radix Achyranthis Bidentatae*); and Fuling (*Poriae Cocos*), Buguzhi (*Fructus Psoraleae*), Gouqizi (*Fructus Lycii*) and Danggui (*Radix Angelicae Sinensis*). Of them, Heshouwu, Tusizi, Niuxi and Buguzhi can supplement the kidney; Gouqizi and Danggui have an action of tonifying the liver; and Fuling could dispel dampness and turbidity. The whole formula is a typical one for benefiting the liver and kidney. Sufficiency of liver blood and kidney essence can surely improve the growth of hair. Because it is just a formula for benefiting and supplementing the liver and kidney, its curative effect could only be achieved by insisting on taking the drug for a long time. For vertigo, Juhua (*Flos Chrysanthemi*) and Hanliancao (*Eclipta alba*) can be added to clear away heat in the head and eyes; for disturbed night sleep, Yejiaoteng (*Caulis Polygoni Multiflori*) and Wuweizi (*Fructus Schisandrae Chinensis*) could be combined to nourish yin and tranquilize the mind.

四十五、过敏性鼻炎
45　Allergic rhinitis

〔**概说**〕 Summary

过敏性鼻炎，即变态反应性鼻炎，与变态反应体质、精神因素、内分泌失调有关。由于鼻黏膜有特殊敏感反应，当外界各种致敏原，如冷热变化、化学气体、刺激性气味、烟尘、花粉等刺激时，即会引发本病。主要症状为发作鼻痒、喷嚏、流清涕等。

过敏性鼻炎，属于中医学"鼻鼽"或"鼽嚏"等，其发病机制与肺、脾、肾气虚有密切关系。脾气虚，则肺气虚；而气之根在于肾，肾气虚则摄纳无权，气不归原，阳气外散，风邪得以入侵于内，发为本病。病虽发于肺，但与脾肾二经有着不可分离的关系。

Allergic rhinitis, as an allergic reactive disease, is associated with allergic reactive constitution, psychic factors as well as endocrine dyscrasia. Nasal mucosa can react to some particular allergic substances. It occurs when nasal mucosa is allergic to the outside allergen triggered by change of temperature, chemicals, stimulating odor, dust as well as pollen. The main clinical manifestations include rhinocnesmus (itchy nose), sneeze and running clear snivel.

In TCM, allergic rhinitis pertains to "nasal discharge" or "sneezing". Pathogenesis for it is closely connected with qi asthenia of the lung, spleen and kidney. Asthenia of splenic qi results in asthenic lung qi; the root of qi lies in the kidney, asthenic kidney qi gives rise to failure in receiving and inability of qi to return to its source, causing yang qi to scatter on the exterior, while wind pathogen invades the interior. Finally, allergic rhinitis has been developed. Though the disease originates from the lung, it is closely related to the spleen and kidney meridians.

〔辨证论治〕 Syndrome differentiation and treatment

1. 肺气虚
45.1　Syndrome of asthenic lung qi

【症状】鼻腔发痒，随之喷嚏频作，鼻塞，流清涕，全身困倦，或有自汗，面色㿠白，舌淡苔薄白，脉象虚弱。

【分析】鼻为肺之窍，肺气虚，风寒之邪乘虚而入，故鼻腔发痒；肺气不利，则鼻塞；风邪内伤于肺，正邪交争，格邪外出，故喷嚏频作；寒邪外遏，肺气不能摄津，津水外溢，则清涕外流；肺主一身之卫气，卫气被遏，故全身困倦，或有自汗；气虚则血不荣面，故面色㿠白；风寒外袭，则舌淡苔薄白，脉象呈虚弱之象。

【治法】温养肺气，外散风寒。

【方药】玉屏风散合苍耳子散。玉屏风散的组成为黄芪、白术、防风，具有温养肺卫、外散风寒，并预防风寒内入的功效；苍耳子散的组成为白芷、薄荷、辛夷、苍耳子，为治疗鼻炎（鼻鼽）的主要对证方剂，具有外散风寒、内通鼻腔的作用。二方合用，固本与祛邪并施，疗效快捷。

Clinical manifestations: Itchy nasal cavity, frequent sneeze, stuffy nose with clear snivel, tiredness and lassitude, or spontaneous sweating, pale complexion, pale tongue with thin whitish fur as well as feeble pulse.

Analysis: The nose is the orifice of the lung, asthenic lung qi causes invasion of wind and cold pathogens, resulting in itchy nose; stuffy nose is due to disorder of lung qi; frequent sneeze is due to wind pathogen impairing the lung, the struggle between healthy qi and pathogenic factors forces the latter to be expelled out; clear snivel is caused by cold pathogen being restrained outside and failure of lung qi to receive fluid, causing outflowing of fluid; the lung dominates defensive qi of the whole body, tiredness of the body and spontaneous sweating are due to defensive qi being refrained; pale complexion is due to asthenic qi and failure of blood to nourish the face; pale tongue with thin whitish fur is caused by wind cold attacking the superficies, and weak pulse is a sign of asthenia.

Prescription: Warm and nourish lung qi and expel wind cold.

Formulas: Yupingfeng San (Powder) combined with Cang'erzi San (Powder). The former includes Huangqi (*Radix Astragali seu Hedysari*), Baizhu (*Rhizoma Atractylodis Macrocephalae*) and Fangfeng (*Radix Saposhnikoviae*), having an action of warming and nourishing the lung, expelling wind cold outward, and preventing wind cold from invading the interior; the latter, consisting of Baizhi (*Radix Angelicae Dahuricae*), Bohe (*Herba Menthae*), Xinyi (*Flos Magnoliae*) and Cang'erzi (*Fructus Xanthii*), is used as a principal formula for treating allergic rhinitis with its action of dispersing wind cold externally and dredging nasal cavity internally. Combined together, the whole formula could consolidate the root and expel pathogenic factors, so it can achieve a quick curative effect.

2. 脾肺气虚
45.2 Syndrome of qi asthenia of the lung and spleen

【症状】鼻塞，鼻流清涕，并有纳呆，腹胀，便溏，肢体困倦，舌质淡红、舌苔淡白，脉象濡弱。

【分析】脾肺为母子关系。可以由母及子，也可由子及母，出现脾肺两虚证。肺虚失其卫外作用，故有鼻塞、流清涕等症；脾气虚弱，不能运化，则影响纳谷、运化等，故有纳呆、腹胀、便溏；脾主四肢，水谷之营养缺乏，故肢体困倦；其舌脉均呈现虚弱之象。

【治法】健脾补肺。

【方药】四君子汤加减。四君子汤为补气之首方，即可补脾气，又可益肺气，可以加入黄芪、诃子、辛夷，以增强固表卫外、通窍止涕的功效。

Clinical manifestations: Stuffy nose with clear snivel, anorexia, abdominal distention, loose stool, tiredness of the body, pale reddish tongue with pale whitish fur as well as soft and feeble pulse.

Analysis: The relationship between the lung and spleen are like that of a mother and her son, the syndrome of asthenia of the lung and spleen can be caused by mother (the spleen) who infects her child (the lung), or by child (the lung) who infects his mother (the spleen). Stuffy nose with clear snivel is due to failure of asthenic lung to defend the superficies; anorexia, abdominal distention and loose stool are due to failure of asthenic splenic qi to transport and transform food; the spleen dominates the limbs, tiredness of the body is caused by malnutrition; pale reddish tongue, pale whitish fur and soft and weak pulse are signs of asthenia.

Prescription: Invigorate the spleen and tonify the lung.

Formulas: Sijunzi Tang Jiajian (Modified Sijunzi Decoction). Sijunzi Tang is the most suitable formula for supplementing qi, for it could not only supplement splenic qi, but it can also benefit lung qi; Huangqi (*Radix Astragali seu Hedysari*), Hezi (*Fructus Chebulae*) and Xinyi (*Flos Magnoliae Liliflorae*) can be combined to strengthen the effect of consolidating the superficies and dredging the orifices to stop snivel.

3. 肺肾虚
45.3 Syndrome of asthenic lung and kindey

【症状】鼻塞，流清涕，伴有腰膝酸软、形寒肢冷、夜尿多等症，舌淡苔白，脉象沉细。

【分析】肺肾亦为母子关系，肺为肾之母，而肾为肺之子。肺肾虚证，为母病及子；但亦有肾气虚，未能康复，子病及母者。肺气虚，风寒外袭，则鼻塞，流清涕；肾气虚，则腰膝酸软；肾为气之根，肺为气之主，肺肾气虚，卫阳必疲惫，故形寒肢冷；肾气虚而气化能力弱，故夜尿增多；舌淡苔白、脉象沉细，为脏腑气虚之象。

【治法】温肺益肾。

【方药】温肺止流丹加减。温肺止流丹出自《疡医大全》，由人参、荆芥、细辛、诃子、桔梗、甘草、鱼脑石组成。方中人参补气温阳；荆芥、细辛，辛温散风寒而除外邪；诃子敛肺利咽；桔梗、甘草，为甘桔汤，为肃肺利咽之常用对药；鱼脑石，为石首鱼（黄鱼）头骨中的耳石，一般在 5~6 月鱼汛期收集，具有消炎、通淋、化石的作用，此处取其消炎功效，内服 3~10 克，一般研末服用。

Clinical manifestations：Stuffy nose with clear snivel, aching and weakness of the loins and knees, cold body and limbs, frequent urination at night, pale tongue with whitish fur as well as sunken and thin pulse.

Analysis：The relationship between the lung and the kidney is like mother and son, the lung being the mother, while the kidney is the child. Asthenia of the lung and kidney is caused by the lung, but in some cases, the syndrome can be caused by qi asthenia of the kidney, involving the lung. Stuffy nose with clear snivel is due to wind cold attacking the superficies because of asthenic lung qi; aching and weakness of the loins and knees is due to qi asthenia of the kidney; the kidney is the root of qi, and the lung is the governor of qi, qi asthenia in the lung and kidney causes exhaustion of defensive yang, giving rise to cold body and limbs; frequent urination at night is due to weakness in transformation of qi because of asthenic kidney qi; pale tongue with whitish fur and sunken and thin pulse are signs of qi asthenia in zang-fu organs.

Precription：Warm the lung and benefit the kidney.

Formulas：Wenfei Zhiliu Dan Jiajian (Modified Wenfei Zhiliu Pill). Wenfei Zhiliu Dan is quoted from *Yangyi Daquan* (*Complete Book of External diseases*). The formula is made up of Renshen (*Radix Ginseng*), Jingjie (*Herba Schizonepetae*), Xixin (*Herba Asari*), Hezi (*Fructus Chebulae*), Jiegeng (*Radix Platycodonis*), Gancao (*Radix Glycyrrhizae*) and Yunaoshi (*Asteriscus Pseudosciaenae*). Among them, Renshen can supplement qi and warm yang; Jingjie and Xixin, pungent and warm in nature, can disperse wind cold and eliminate exogenous pathogens; Hezi astringes the lung and clear the throat; Jiegeng and Gancao constitute Gan Jie Tang (Decoction), a common recipe for depurating the lung and relieving sore throat; Yunaoshi, the ear crystal in the head of corvine collected in the fishing season from May to June, has an action of reducing inflammation, eliminating stranguria and resolving calculus, here it is used to reduce inflammation by grinding it into powder and taking orally 3~10 g each day.

四十六、慢性咽炎

46　Chronic pharyngitis

〔概说〕 Summary

慢性咽炎为咽部黏膜、黏膜下及淋巴组织的炎性病变。急性咽炎多与急性鼻炎、扁桃体炎、喉痒并存；而慢性咽炎为咽部的弥漫性炎症，一般病程较长，难以治愈。

咽炎，归于中医学"喉痹"范畴。慢性咽炎为"虚火喉痹"或"阴虚喉痹"。临床表现为咽部有异物感，作痒作痛，干燥灼热，常有黏膜分泌物附于咽后壁不易清除，夜间尤甚，时时"吭吭"作声，意欲清除而后快。虽属小恙，但常常影响生活与工作，故不可轻视。

Chronic pharyngitis refers to inflammatory pathological changes of the mucous membranes of the pharynx and the lymphoid tissue below mucous coat. Acute pharyngitis is usually accompanied with acute rhinitis, amygdalitis and itchy larynx, while chronic pharyngitis is a type of diffusive inflammation in the pharynx with a long course, so it is difficult to cure.

In terms of TCM, pharyngitis pertains to "throat obstruction", and chronic pharyngitis belongs to "throat obstruction due to asthenic fire" or "throat obstruction due to yin asthenia". Clinical manifestations of chronic pharyngitis are as follows: foreign body sensation, itching and pain, dry and scorching sensation, posterior pharyngeal wall stuck with mucous secretion which is difficult to be cleared away, worsening at night, discomfort of the throat with a desire to clear it. Although it is not a severe disease, chronic pharyngitis can affect life and work, so much stress should be attached to it.

〔辨证论治〕 Syndrome differentiation and treatment

1. 肺阴虚

46.1　Yin asthenia of the lung

【症状】咽部不适，微痛，干痒，常有"吭""咯"之声，并时有咳嗽，多于早晨轻而午后重，舌质红赤，苔少，脉象细数。

【分析】虚火上炎，阴津不足，故咽部不适，微痛，干痒，肺失清肃，故有"吭""咯"之声；早晨阳气轻，故病轻，午后阳气重，故病重；舌质与脉象，为阴虚火旺之征。

【治法】养阴清肺。

【方药】养阴清肺汤。养阴清肺汤出自《重楼玉钥》，由生地黄、麦冬、白芍、牡丹皮、贝母、玄参、薄荷、甘草组成。方以生地黄养肾阴，麦冬养肺阴，玄参清火解毒，牡丹皮凉血消肿，贝母润肺化痰，白芍敛阴泻热，薄荷散邪利咽，甘草和药解毒。

全方滋肺阴，又养肾阴，有凉血之品，又有化痰之药。临证可加射干、牛蒡子，以利于咽部异物的清除。

Clinical manifestations：Discomfort of the pharynx, slight pain, dry and itching sensation, frequent cough, alleviation of the disease in the morning and aggravation in the afternoon, reddish tongue with scanty fur as well as thin and fast pulse.

Analysis：Discomfort of the pharynx, slight pain, dry and itching sensation are due to up-flaming of asthenic fire and insufficient yin fluid; frequent cough is due to dysfunction of the lung in depuration; alleviation of the disease in the morning is due to deficiency of yang qi in the morning; aggravation in the afternoon is due to sufficiency of yang qi; reddish tongue with scanty fur and thin and fast pulse are signs of yin asthenia and fire exuberance.

Prescription：Nourish yin and clear away heat from the lung.

Formulas：Yangyin Qingfei Tang (Decoction). The formula is quoted from *Chonglou Yuyao* (*Jade Key to the Secluded Chamber*), consisting of Shengdihuang (*Radix Rehmanniae Recens*), Maidong (*Radix Ophiopogonis*), Baishao (*Radix Paeoniae Alba*), Mudanpi (*Cortex Moutan Radicis*), Beimu (*Bulbus Fritillaria*), Xuanshen (*Radix Scrophulariae*), Bohe (*Herba Menthae*) and Gancao (*Radix Glycyrrhizae*). Among them, Shengdihuang can promote production of kidney yin, Maidong can nourish lung yin, Xuanshen has an action of relieving fire and toxin, Mudanpi could cool blood and eliminate swellings; Beimu may moisten the lung and resolve phlegm, Baishao can astringe yin and purge heat, Bohe can disperse pathogens and relieve sore throat, and Gancao may harmonize the above medicinal herbs and relieve toxin. Therefore, the whole formula has the action of nourishing lung yin and kidney yin, cooling blood and resolving phlegm. In clinical practice, Shegan (*Rhizoma Belamcandae*) and Niubangzi (*Fructus Arctii*) could be added to help remove foreign body in the pharynx.

2. 肾阴虚
46.2 Yin asthenia of the kidney

【症状】咽部不适，干痒，五心烦热，时有盗汗，口咽干燥，咳声低怯，夜间难眠，舌质红赤，苔薄少津，脉象细数。

【分析】发生于咽部，必然有咽部不适之苦，如口咽干燥、干痒等；但肾阴不足，"阴虚生内热"，故有五心烦热，时时盗汗，阴津亏耗，故咳声低怯；夜间阴虚更甚，故夜间难眠；其舌脉为阴虚火旺之象。

【治法】滋肾泻火。

【方药】知柏地黄丸加减。知柏地黄丸，即六味地黄丸加知母、黄柏。六味地黄丸为滋补肾阴之主方。知母生津润燥、清热泻火，黄柏以清热泻火为其特长，两药配合，为滋阴泻火之最佳配对。还可加入麦冬、天冬、沙参，增加滋养肺阴的药力。

Clinical manifestations：Discomfort of the pharynx, dry and itchy sensation, feverish sensation and dysphoria over the soles, palms and chest, frequent night sweating, dry mouth and throat, cough with low voice, insomnia at night, reddish tongue, thin fur with scanty fluid as well as thin and fast pulse.

Analysis: Chronic pharyngitis occurs in the pharynx, leading to discomfort of the pharynx such as dry mouth and throat as well as dry and itchy sensation; feverish sensation and dysphoria over the soles, palms and chest and frequent night sweating are due to insufficiency of kidney yin, "asthenia of yin generates endogenous heat"; cough with low voice is caused by deficiency and consumption of yin fluid; insomnia at night is due to severe yin asthenia at night; reddish tongue, thin fur with scanty fluid and thin and fast pulse indicate yin asthenia and fire exuberance.

Prescription: Nourish yin and purge fire.

Formulas: Zhi Bo Dihuang Wan Jiajian (Modified Zhi Bo Dihuang Pill). The formula is made up of Liuwei Dihuang Wan combined with Zhimu (*Rhizoma Anemarrhenae*) and Huangbo (*Cortex Phellodendri*). Liuwei Dihuang Wan is a main recipe for nourishing and tonifying kidney yin. Zhimu can promote production of fluid, moisten dryness and purge heat and fire, Huangbo is skilled in clearing away heat and fire, combined together, the formula is the best one for nourishing yin and purging fire. Maidong (*Radix Ophiopogonis*), Tiandong (*Radix Asparagi*) and Shashen (*Radix Adenophorae*) can be added to strengthen the effect of nourishing lung yin.

四十七、复发性口腔溃疡
47　Recurrent oral ulcer

〔**概说**〕 Summary

复发性口腔溃疡是口腔黏膜反复发作的局部溃疡性疾病，又称复发性阿弗他口炎、复发性阿弗他溃疡、复发性口疮等。其发病原因比较复杂，具有长期反复发作的慢性病程，长达数月、数年，乃至十几年、几十年之久。有家族史者占24%~45%。

复发性口腔溃疡，属于中医"口舌生疮""口疮"等。认为与脾胃积热、心火上炎、阴虚火旺等有关，但亦有阳虚所致者。中医治疗效果较使用抗生素满意。

Recurrent oral ulcer refers to a regional ulceration of oral mucosa with repeated onset, and it is also termed as "recurrent aphthous stomatitis" "recurrent aphthous ulceration" or "recurring oral aphthae" and so on. The disease is a pathological condition characterized by a chronic course, which typically lasts for several months, years, and even several decades. The cause for it is relatively complex. About 24% ~ 45% of people with it have a positive family disease history, suggesting that some people are genetically predisposed to suffering from oral ulceration.

Recurrent oral ulcer pertains to "mouth ulcer" and "canker sore" in TCM. And it is regarded to be associated with accumulated heat in the spleen and stomach, up-flaming of the heart fire, as well as yin asthenia and hyperactive fire. However, it is considered to be caused by yang asthenia, too. The curative effect of the disease by means of TCM therapeutic methods is much better than that of antibiotics.

〔辨证论治〕 Syndrome differentiation and treatment

1. 脾胃积热
47.1 Accumulation of heat in the spleen and stomach

【症状】溃疡数目多而密集，周边充血，中心区表面有淡黄色假膜，灼痛明显，口渴口臭，唇红干燥，大便秘结，舌质红，苔黄，脉数而有力。

【分析】脾胃与口腔有着密切关联，若脾胃积热不除，就会熏蒸于上，出现口腔溃疡。积热日久，溃疡数目多而密集；热盛则灼痛明显，口渴口臭；口唇属于脾经，脾经积热，则唇红干燥；积热伤阴，则大便秘结；舌质红、苔黄、脉数，为内热炽盛之象。

【治法】清热泻火，凉血通腑。

【方药】清胃散加减。清胃散为治疗脾胃积热常用方剂。方中黄连苦寒清热，为主药；生地黄凉血滋阴，牡丹皮凉血清热，共为臣药；并佐当归养血和血；升麻散火解毒，与黄连相配，使上炎之火得散，内郁之热得降，并为阳明引经药。五味药配伍，可使上炎之热从泻火而降，血热从甘凉滋阴清除。若大便秘结，可加大黄导热下行；若口渴甚，可加麦冬、玄参滋阴生水。

Clinical manifestations: Plenty of densely distributed ulcers in the oral cavity, erythematous "congestion" surrounding the ulcers, with the central area covered with a pale yellowish fibrinous membrane, obvious scorching pain, thirst and foul odor of the mouth, dry reddish lips, dry feces, reddish tongue with yellowish fur as well as fast and powerful pulse.

Analysis: The oral cavity is closely connected with the spleen and stomach, formation of ulcers is due to failure to get rid of accumulated heat in the spleen and stomach, which fumigates and steams upward. Plenty of densely distributed ulcers in the oral cavity are caused by prolonged accumulation of heat; obvious scorching pain and thirst and foul odor of the mouth are due to hyperactive heat; the mouth and lips are connected with the spleen meridian, accumulation of heat in spleen meridian causes dry reddish lips; dry feces is due to accumulated heat impairing yin fluid; reddish tongue with yellowish fur and fast pulse are signs of hyperactivity of endogenous heat.

Prescription: Purge fire and heat, cool blood and dredge stagnated qi in fu organs.

Formulas: Qingwei San Jiajian (Modified Qingwei Powder). Qingwei San is a common formula used for treating heat accumulation in the spleen and stomach, in which, Huanglian (*Rhizoma Coptidis*), bitter and cold in nature, is used as principal drug to clear away heat; Shengdihuang (*Radix Rehmanniae Recens*) could cool blood and nourish yin, Mudanpi

(*Cortex Moutan Radicis*) can cool blood and clear away heat, both of them are used as ministerial drug; Danggui (*Radix Angelicae Sinensis*) is combined as adjuvant drug to nourish blood and harmonize blood; Shengma (*Rhizoma Cimicifugae*), together with Huanglian, is used as ushering drug of yangming meridian to disperse up-flaring fire and descend internal stagnation of heat. The combination of the above herbs can purge fire to descend up-flaring heat and eliminate blood heat by nourishing yin with sweet-cool natured drug. For dry feces, Dahuang (*Radix et Rhizoma Rhei*) can be added to guide heat to flow downward; for severe thirst, Maidong (*Radix Ophiopogonis*) and Xuanshen (*Radix Scrophulariae*) can be combined to nourish yin so as to promote production of fluid.

2. 心火上炎
47.2　Up-flaring of heart fire

【症状】口舌生疮，溃疡面积小而数目多，多位于舌尖和舌前部或舌侧缘，溃疡周围充血明显，灼痛剧烈，口渴，急躁心烦，夜眠不安，小便短赤，舌尖红、舌苔薄黄，脉数。

【分析】"舌为心之苗"，即心开窍于舌。心火上炎，舌必生疮，且溃疡数目多，主要见于舌尖及舌前部，或舌侧缘；热盛则痛甚；若热盛伤阴，则口渴、心烦，夜眠不安；心与小肠经脉相通，心热移于小肠，则小便短赤；心火上炎于所属部位，故舌尖红、苔薄黄；脉数者，心火上炎之象也。

【治法】清心降火，凉血利尿。

【方药】导赤散合泻心汤。导赤散为清心养阴、利水通淋之主方。方中生地黄凉血滋阴以制心火；木通上清心经之热，下则清利小肠，利水通淋。生甘草清热解毒，调和诸药；竹叶清心除烦。全方配伍，清心与养阴并顾，使上炎之火，导热下行。泻心汤由大黄、黄连、黄芩三味组成，具有泻火解毒、燥湿泻痞的作用，意在加强泻心火的功效。患有慢性泄泻者不宜用此方。

Clinical manifestations: Sores and ulceration in the mouth and tongue with small size but large number, most sores and ulcers distributed on the tips, front part or lateral margin of the tongue, obvious erythematous "congestion" surrounding the ulcers and apparent scorching pain, thirst, vexation, disturbed night sleep; scanty brownish urine, reddish tongue tip with thin yellowish fur as well as fast pulse.

Analysis: "The tongue serves as the mirror of the heart", which means the heart opens at the tongue. Up-flaring of heart fire results in sores and ulceration in the mouth and tongue with small size but large number distributed on the tips, front part or lateral margin of the tongue; thirst, vexation and disturbed night sleep are caused by hyperactive heat impairing yin fluid of the body; the heart is connected with the small intestine meridian, scanty brownish urine is due to heat in the heart transmitting to the small intestine; reddish tongue tip with thin yellowish fur is due to heart fire flaring upward to its corresponding region—the tongue; fast pulse is a sign of up-flaring of heart fire.

Prescription：Clear away heat and descend fire from the heart, cool blood and induce diuresis.

Formulas：Daochi San (Powder) combined with Xiexin Tang (Decoction). The former is an essential formula for clearing away heat of the heart, nourishing yin, inducing diuresis and eliminating stranguria. In the formula, Shengdihuang (*Radix Rehmanniae Recens*) can restrain heart fire with its function of cooling blood and moistening yin; Mutong (*Caulis Akebiae*) can move upward to eliminate heat in heart meridian, and flow downward to clear away heat in the small intestine, induce diuresis and remove stranguria; Shenggancao (*Radix Glycyrrhizae*) has an action of relieving heat and toxin and harmonizing the above medicinal herbs; Zhuye (*Folium Lophatheri*) could eliminate heart fire and vexation. Combined together, the whole formula could clear away heart fire and nourish yin, descend up-flaring fire. The latter, consisting of Dahuang (*Radix et Rhizoma Rhei*), Huanglian (*Rhizoma Coptidis*) and Huangqin (*Radix Scutellariae*), has an action of purging fire and relieving toxin, drying dampness and discharging distending lumps, here, the recipe is used to strengthen the function of purging heart fire, yet it is not suitable for those patients with chronic diarrhea.

3. 阴虚火旺
47.3　Hyperactive fire due to yin asthenia

【症状】口舌生疮，多发于舌根、舌尖、舌下，溃疡数目少，灼痛轻微，口干口燥，头晕耳鸣，失眠多梦，五心烦热，尿黄便干，舌苔薄黄，脉象细数。

【分析】阴虚火旺与体质有着密切关系。此类证候的体质偏于消瘦，阴虚于下，火旺于上，阴虚多指肾阴虚，火旺多指心火旺。火旺于上，则心之苗——舌，就会发生口疮，且多见于舌根、舌下、舌尖，并有口干、口燥等火旺之症；阴虚于下，即肾水不足，则会出现头晕耳鸣、失眠多梦、五心烦热等症；阴虚则便干，心热移于小肠，则尿黄；舌苔薄黄，脉象细数，为阴虚火旺之象。

【治法】滋阴降火。

【方药】知柏地黄汤加减。（知柏地黄汤方义见"慢性肾小球肾炎"篇。）失眠多梦，可加酸枣仁、柏子仁养阴安神；头晕耳鸣，可加女贞子、旱莲草滋阴清热；舌根黄腻苔，可加生薏苡仁、赤小豆淡渗利湿。若单纯口疮，疼痛不减，舌苔白腻，可改用三才封髓丹治疗，方用砂仁培土伏火，黄柏清降相火（即上焦虚火），甘草和中解毒，天冬滋阴，生地黄生水，西洋参滋阴清热。舌苔中部白腻者，可加干姜，温化中焦之湿。

Clinical manifestations：Sores and ulceration appearing on the root, the tip of the tongue or the area below the tongue, ulcers in small number, slight scorching pain, dry mouth and thirst, vertigo and tinnitus, insomnia and dreaminess, feverish sensation and dysphoria over the palms, soles and the chest, brownish urine and dry feces, thin yellowish fur as well as thin and fast pulse.

Analysis: Hyperactive fire due to yin asthenia is closely related to a patient's constitution. The patient with the constitution of yin asthenia and fire exuberance tends to be thin and slim. Yin asthenia refers to asthenia of kidney yin, and fire exuberance signifies hyperactivity of heart fire. Hyperactive fire tending to move upward causes ulcers forming on the tongue, the mirror of the heart, usually ulcers are distributed on the root and tip of the tongue or beneath the tongue and accompanied with dry mouth and thirst; asthenic yin here refers to insufficiency of kidney yin, bringing about vertigo, tinnitus, insomnia and dreaminess, feverish sensation and dysphoria over the palms, soles and the chest; dry feces is due to yin asthenia, brownish urine indicates heat in the heart transmitting to the small intestine; thin yellowish fur as well as thin and fast pulse suggests yin asthenia and fire exuberance.

Prescription: Nourish yin and descend fire.

Formulas: Zhi Bo Dihuang Tang Jiajian (Modified Zhi Bo Dihuang Decoction). (The formula has been discussed in the chapter of *Chronic Glomerular nephritis.*) For insomnia and dreaminess, Suanzaoren (*Semen Ziziphi Spinosae*) and Baiziren (*Semen Platycladi*) can be added to nourish yin and tranquilize the mind; for vertigo and tinnitus, Nuzhenzi (*Fructus Ligustri Lucidi*) and Hanliancao (*Eclipta Alba*) can be combined to nourish yin and clear away heat; for greasy yellowish fur on the root of the tongue, Shengyiyiren (*Semen Coicis*) and Chixiaodou (*Semen Phaseoli*) could be added to promate diuresis with their bland taste. For oral ulcer with unalleviated pain and whitish greasy fur, Sancai Fengsui Dan (Pill) can be used to replace Zhi Bo Dihuang Tang, of which, Sharen (*Fructus Amomi Villosi*) could strengthen earth (the spleen) and suppress fire, Huangbo (*Cortex Phellodendri*) can purge ministerial fire (fire in lower energizer), Gancao (*Radix Glycyrrhizae*) could harmonize middle energizer and relieve toxin, Tiandong (*Radix Asparagi*) has an action of nourishing yin and Shengdihuang (*Radix Rehmanniae Recens*) may improve the producton of fluid, Xiyangshen (*Radix Panacis Quinquefolii*) could nourish yin and clear away heat. For greasy whitish fur on the centre of the tongue, Ganjiang (*Rhizoma Zingiberis*) can be combined to resolve dampness in middle energizer by warming.

4. 脾肾阳虚
47.4 Yang asthenia of the spleen and kidney

【症状】口舌生疮，溃疡少而分散，表面暗紫，周围苍白，疼痛轻微，面色㿠白，形寒肢冷，下利清谷，小腹冷痛，小便多，舌质淡红，苔薄白，脉象沉弱。

【分析】脾肾阳虚，亦可发生口疮。但其特点为：口疮表面暗紫，疼痛不重；形体一派阳虚寒象，如面色㿠白，形寒肢冷，下利清谷，小腹冷痛等；脾肾阳虚，还可出现小便清长、量多等。舌质淡红、苔薄白、脉象沉弱，为阳气虚弱之象。由于阴寒内盛，阳气不能内潜，浮越于上，故发生类似"火性炎上"口疮之疾。

【治法】温补脾肾，散寒化湿。

【方药】桂附地黄汤加减。桂附地黄汤即金匮肾气丸，为补益肾气的代表方剂。其方义见"支气管哮喘"篇。本方是在滋阴的基础上寓有扶阳的作用，为中医方剂学温补肾气之祖。肾阴充足，自能涵养阳气，加之附子、桂枝能温阳济阴，"阴平阳秘"，口疮自然痊愈。

Clinical manifestations：Sores and ulceration scattered in the mouth in a small number, dark purplish surface of ulcers with pale whitish color in the center, slight pain, pale complexion, cold limbs and body, discharge with undigested food, cold pain over the lower abdomen, profuse urine, pale reddish tongue with thin whitish fur as well as sunken and weak pulse.

Analysis：Yang asthenia of the spleen and kidney can cause oral ulcers, which is characterized by dark purplish surface of ulcers, unserious pain and signs of yang asthenic cold constitution such as pale complexion, cold limbs and body, discharge with undigested food, cold and pain over the lower abdomen; thin clear profuse urine is due to yang asthenia in the spleen and kidney, pale reddish tongue with thin whitish fur and sunken and weak pulse indicate asthenia of yang and qi. Exuberance of yin and cold results in yang and qi floating outward because of failure to accumulate internally, which gives rise to oral ulcers because of "up-flaring fire".

Prescription：Warm and tonify the spleen and kidney, dispel cold and resolve dampness.

Formulas：Guifu Dihuang Tang Jiajian（Modified Guifu Dihuang Decoction）. The formula is also known as Jingui Shenqi Wan（Pill）, a typical recipe for supplementing kidney qi and it has been introduced in *Bronchia Asthma*. Based on the action of nourishing yin, the formula has obtained the effect of strengthening yang, and it is regarded as the first recipe of warming and tonifying kidney qi. Sufficiency of kidney yin can surely nourish yang qi, coupled with the action of warming yang and supplementing yin of Fuzi（*Radix Aconiti Lateralis Preparata*）and Guizhi（*Ramulus Cinnamomi*）, "yin and yang can be kept in a relative balance", therefore, oral ulcer will surely be healed.

四十八、急性扁桃体炎

48　Acute amygdalitis

〔**概说**〕 Summary

急性扁桃体炎是腭扁桃体的一种非特异性急性炎症。可分为充血性和化脓性两种，常伴有一定程度的咽黏膜及咽淋巴组织炎症。本病多见于儿童及青年，季节交替、气温变化时容易发病，而劳碌、受凉、潮湿、烟酒刺激等，常为本病的诱发因素。

本病属中医"乳蛾"，急性扁桃体炎则属"风热乳蛾"。中医学认为，咽喉为呼吸饮食之门户，故有"肺胃之门"之称。故急性扁桃体炎与肺胃关系密切。致病因素有风热外袭、过食辛辣等。由于风热、辛辣之毒搏于咽喉，灼腐肌膜，而发为本病。

Acute amygdalitis is a non-specific acute inflammation of the amygdale, which can be divided into congestive and purulent types. It is usually complicated with inflammation of mucosa of the pharynx and lymphatic tissues. Acute amygdalitis is commonly seen in children and young people and it can be triggered by change of seasons and temperature, overstrain, catching cold, humid weather as well as stimulation such as smoking and alcoholism.

In terms of TCM, amygdalitis pertains to "nippled moth", acute amygdalitis is "nippled moth due to wind and heat". The pharynx is the door for breathing and eating, therefore, it is called "the door of the lung and stomach", indicating the close relationship between acute amygdalitis and the lung and stomach. The factors that cause the disease includes wind heat attacking superficies of the body, excessive intake of pungent and spicy food and so on. Attack of pathogenic toxin of wind and heat as well as pungent toxin in the pharynx and throat results in scorching and decaying sarolemma and develops into acute amygdalitis.

〔辨证论治〕 Syndrome differentiation and treatment

1. 肺经风热
48.1 Wind and heat in lung meridian

【症状】咽喉疼痛逐渐加重，吞咽不利，咽喉有干燥灼热感，喉核红肿，连及周围咽部，并兼见发热恶寒，头痛，鼻塞，咳嗽有痰，身体困倦，舌质红赤，苔薄白或微黄，脉象浮数。

【分析】肺经蕴热，加之感受风热，搏结于喉核，故见咽部红肿疼痛，吞咽不利；风热在表，以致营卫不和，故见发热恶寒，头痛，鼻塞；肺气失宣，故咳嗽有痰；营卫被风热所困，故身体困倦；舌质红赤，苔薄白或微黄，脉象浮数，为风热在表的征象。

【治法】疏风清热，解毒利咽。

【方药】疏风清肺利咽汤（经验方）。方由荆芥、防风、牛蒡子、射干、黄芩、金银花、桔梗、山豆根、玄参、浙贝母、甘草组成。方中荆芥、防风疏散风邪；金银花、黄芩、山豆根、玄参清热解毒；牛蒡子、射干清利咽喉；浙贝母清热化痰；桔梗、甘草缓解咽喉之急。若口干口苦，可加北沙参、麦冬以滋阴润肺。

Clinical manifestations: Worsening pain in the laryngopharynx, unsmooth swallowing, dry and scorching sensation of the region, swollen node of the throat involving its surroundings, and complicated with fever, aversion to cold, headache, stuffy nose, cough with sputum, tiredness and fatigue, reddish tongue, thin whitish fur or slight yellowish fur as well as floating and fast pulse.

Analysis: Accumulated heat in lung meridian together with invasion of exogenous wind and heat obstructing in the node of the throat gives rise to swollen laryngopharynx and unsmooth swallowing; fever, aversion to cold, headache and stuffy nose are caused by disharmony of defensive qi and nutrient qi because of wind and heat attacking the superficies; cough with sputum is due to failure to disperse lung qi; tiredness and fatigue are due to nutrient qi and defensive qi being obstructed by wind heat; reddish tongue with thin whitish fur or slight yellowish fur and floating and fast pulse indicate wind and heat attacking the superficies.

Prescription: Dispel wind, clear away heat and relieve toxin and sore throat.

Formulas: Shufeng Qingfei Liyan Tang (Decoction). The formula has been regarded as an empirical one, made up of Jingjie (*Herba Schizonepetae*), Fangfeng (*Radix Saposhnikoviae*), Niubangzi (*Fructus Arctii*), Shegan (*Rhizoma Belamcandae*), Huangqin (*Radix Scutellariae*), Jinyinhua (*Flos Lonicerae*), Jiegeng (*Radix Platycodonis*), Shandougen (*Radix Sophorae Tonkinensis*), Xuanshen (*Radix Scrophulariae*), Zhebeimu (*Bulbus Fritillaria*) and Gancao (*Radix Glycyrrhizae*). Among the medicinal herbs, Jingjie and Fangfeng could dispel wind pathogen; Jinyinhua, Huangqin, Sandougen and Xuanshen have an action of clearing away heat and relieving toxin; Niubangzi and Shegan could clear away heat from the throat; Zhebeimu could purge heat and resolve phlegm; Jiegeng and Gancao have an action of relieving pain in the throat. For dry mouth and bitter taste, Beishashen (*Radix Glehniae*) and Maidong (*Radix Ophiopogonis*) can be combined to nourish yin and moisten the lung.

2. 肺胃热盛
48.2 Exuberance of heat in the lung and stomach

【症状】咽部疼痛剧烈，痛连耳根及颌下，吞咽困难，咽部有堵塞感，或有声嘶；全身可见高热，口渴引饮，咳嗽脓黄痰，口臭，腹胀，大便秘结，小便黄赤，舌质红赤，苔黄腻，脉象洪大而数。

【分析】热盛为火，火毒蒸腾，灼伤肌膜，故咽喉部疼痛剧烈，痛甚则连及周围组织；胃热上炎，故吞咽困难，且咽部有堵塞感，伤津则声音嘶哑；阳热火毒，攻于全身，故有高热、口渴；肺热则咳嗽脓黄痰；胃热则口臭、腹胀；大肠热盛，则大便秘结；膀胱热盛，则小便黄赤；其舌质与脉象均为阳热炽盛之征。

【治法】泻热解毒，清利咽喉。

【方药】普济消毒饮加减。普济消毒饮出自《东垣试效方》，为疏风散邪、清热解毒之要方，广泛应用于急性温热病。方中以黄芩、黄连清降头面之火，为君药；牛蒡子、连翘、薄荷、僵蚕疏散头面风热，为臣药；玄参、马勃、板蓝根加强清热解毒作用；配以甘草、桔梗清利咽喉；陈皮理气疏散郁结；升麻、柴胡可使诸药上行，以利于头面热毒的清解。咽喉干痛者，可加北沙参、麦冬、生地黄，以增水制火。

Clinical manifestations: Acute pain in the pharynx, even involving the root of the ears and the jaw; difficulty in swallowing and sensation of being obstructed in the pharynx or hoarse voice, high fever and thirst with desire to drink, cough with yellow sputum mingled with pus, foul odor of the mouth, abdominal distention, dry feces, brownish urine, reddish tongue as well as full and fast pulse.

Analysis: Transformation of fire from hyperactive heat and fumigation of fire toxin scorching sarolemma result in acute pain in the pharynx, even involving the root of the ears and the jaw; difficulty in swallowing and sensation of being obstructed in the pharynx are due to impairment of body fluid because of up-flaring of heat in the stomach, thus, causing hoarse voice; high fever and thirst with desire to drink are caused by invasion of fire toxin, yang and heat; cough with yellow sputum mingled with pus is due to heat in the lung; foul odor of the mouth and abdominal distention are caused by hyperactive heat in the stomach; dry feces is due to exuberance of heat in the large intestine; brownish urine is due to hyperactivity of heat in the bladder, reddish tongue and full and fast pulse indicate superabundance of yang and heat.

Prescription: Purge heat and toxin and relieve sore throat.

Formulas: Puji Xiaodu Yin Jiajian (Modified Puji Xiaodu Decoction). The formula is quoted from *Dongyuan Shixiao Fang* (*Effective formulas by Dongyuan's Trial*), an essential one for dispelling wind, eliminating pathogens and relieving heat and toxin, and it is widely applied in treating acute exogenous febrile disease. In the formula, Huangqin (*Radix Scutellariae*) and Huanglian (*Rhizoma Coptidis*) are used as sovereign drug to descend fire form the head; Niubangzi (*Fructus Arctii*), Lianqiao (*Fructus Forsythiae*), Bohe (*Herba Menthae*) and Jiangcan (*Bombyx Batryticatus*) are used as ministerial drug to dispel wind heat from the head; Xuanshen (*Radix Scrophulariae*), Mabo (*Lasiosphaera seu Calvatia*) and Banlangen (*Radix Isatidis*) could strengthen the action of relieving heat and toxin; Gancao (*Radix Glycyrrhizae*) and Jiegeng (*Radix Platycodonis*) are combined to relieve sore throat; Chenpi (*Pericarpium Citri Reticulatae*) can regulate qi and eliminate nodules and lumps; Shengma (*Rhizoma Cimicifugae*) and Chaihu (*Radix Bupleuri*) could guide all the drug to move upward so as to help relieve heat and toxin from the head. For dry and sore throat, Beishashen (*Radix Glehniae*), Maidong (*Radix Ophiopogonis*) and Shengdihuang (*Radix Rehmanniae Recens*) can be combined to promote the production of body fluid to restrain fire.

四十九、流行性腮腺炎
49 Epidemic parotitis

〔概说〕 Summary

流行性腮腺炎，是由流行性腮腺炎病毒所引起的一种急性传染病。多发于冬春两季，以 5~10 岁小儿多见，青春发育期以后的病人可能并发睾丸炎或卵巢炎，个别病人可并发脑膜脑炎。患本病后，一般可获得终身免疫。

该病以发病急骤、腮腺肿胀为特点。中医学称本病为"痄腮"，由风温邪毒所致。邪毒通过飞沫从口鼻而入，邪毒阻滞于少阳经络，郁结不散，足少阳经脉绕耳而行，故表现为两耳下腮部漫肿坚硬作痛。少阳与厥阴相表里，足厥阴（肝经）经脉绕阴器，若病毒传至足厥阴肝经，则年龄较大患儿可并发睾丸炎或卵巢炎。若病毒炽盛，病毒内陷心包，则可并发脑膜炎，甚至出现昏迷或惊厥。中医治疗此病具有独特优势，中药内服与外敷，加上针灸，效果更为显著。

Epidemic parotitis is an acute infectious disease caused by parotitis virus. Winter and spring are the seasons of high incidence of the disease, which usually occurs in children from 5 to 10 years old. Outbreak of parotitis after the period of adolescency can result in complicated disease of orchitis, or ovaritis, and in a few cases, meningoencephalitis may follow. After the illness, one can acquire lifelong immunity to parotitis.

Epidemic parotitis is characterized by sudden outbreak and swollen parotid gland and it is known as "mumps" in TCM caused by pathogenic tonic wind-warm pathogens. When an infected person coughs or sneezes, the droplets of pathogenic toxin aerosolize and enter the eyes, nose, or mouth of another person. Failure to disperse stagnation of pathogenic toxin obstructed in shaoyang meridian and collaterals causes foot shaoyang meridian to travel around the ears, thus, bringing about hard and painful swollen lumps over the regions from the ears to the jaw. Shaoyang and jueyin form an interior-and-exterior relationship, liver meridian of foot jueyin travels through the external genitals, if parotitis virus transmits into liver meridian of foot jueyin, elder patients can contract parotitis complicated with orchitis, or ovaritis. Exuberance of parotitis virus could cause it to be trapped in the pericardium, triggering the complicated syndrome of meningoencephalitis, even coma or convulsion. Treatment for the disease by means of TCM therapeutic methods has its specific advantages, remarkable curative effect could be achieved by means of intake of Chinese medicinal herbs and external application as well as acupuncture.

〔辨证论治〕 Syndrome differentiation and treatment

1. 温毒袭表
49.1　Warm toxin attacking the superficies

【症状】恶寒发热，咽干津少，腮部（一侧或两侧）漫肿疼痛，舌红，苔黄或薄白干，脉象浮数。

【分析】温毒袭表，肌表被郁，故恶寒发热；温毒为阳邪，易伤阴耗津，故咽干津少；温毒滞留于少阳经脉，气血不畅，气滞血瘀，故腮部肿胀；温毒为阳邪，毒邪上浮，故舌脉均呈阳热毒邪不散之象。

【治法】清热解毒，散结消肿。

【方药】五味消毒饮加减。方中金银花清热透表，紫花地丁、野菊花、蒲公英清热解毒；天葵子凉血化瘀散结；另加板蓝根专于攻毒，薄荷透热外出，夏枯草清热散结。大便秘结，可加大黄轻泻，以导热下行。

Clinical manifestations: Fever and aversion to cold, dry throat with scanty fluid, pain and dispersive swellings on one or both sides of the cheeks, reddish tongue with yellowish fur or thin whitish fur, as well as floating and fast pulse.

Analysis: Fever and aversion to cold are due to warm toxin attacking the superficies; warm toxin belongs to yang pathogen, with susceptibility to impairing body fluid, thus, giving rise to dry throat with scanty fluid; pain and dispersive swellings of the cheeks are caused by qi stagnation and blood stasis, which results from unsmooth circulation of qi and blood because of warm toxin stagnating in shaoyang meridian; warm toxin belongs to yang pathogen, up-floating of toxic pathogen results in failure to eliminate yang, heat and toxic pathogen with such symptoms as reddish tongue with yellowish fur or thin whitish fur as well as floating and fast pulse.

Prescription: Eliminate heat and toxin and disperse swelling lumps.

Formulas: Wuwei Xiaodu Yin Jiajian (Modified Wuwei Xiaodu Decoction). In the formula, Jinyinhua (*Flos Lonicerae*) can clear away heat and let out the superficies; Zihuadiding (*Herba Violae*), Yejuhua (*Flos Chrysanthemi Indici*) and Pugongying (*Herba Taraxaci*) can relieve heat and toxin; Tiankuizi (*Radix Semiaquilegiae*) has an action of resolving blood stasis and dispersing lumps by cooling blood; Banlangen (*Radix Isatidis*) can be added to eliminate toxin, Bohe (*Herba Menthae*) could be added to let out heat, Xiakucao (*Spica Prunellae*) can be added to clear away heat and disperse lumps. As for dry feces, Dahuang (*Radix et Rhizoma Rhei*) can be used as a laxation to descend heat.

2. 热毒壅滞
49.2 Stagnation of exuberance of heat toxin

【症状】壮热烦渴，头痛呕吐，腮肿硬痛，咽红肿痛，舌红苔黄，脉象滑数。

【分析】邪热入里，热毒炽盛，伤津耗液，故壮热烦渴；火扰清阳，犯及胃腑，故头痛呕吐；热毒结聚少阳、阳明之经络，故腮肿硬痛，咽红肿痛；舌红苔黄，脉象滑数，均为热毒壅盛之象。

【治法】清热解毒，软坚散结。

【方药】普济消毒饮加减。（普济消毒饮方义见"急性扁桃体炎"篇。）软坚散结，可加夏枯草、海藻、僵蚕等；口渴甚者，可加北沙参、玄参、天花粉等；大便秘结，可加大黄（后下）、芒硝（冲服）等。

Clinical manifestations: High fever with polydipsia, headache and vomiting, hard and painful swollen cheeks, swollen and sore throat, reddish tongue with yellowish fur as well as slippery and fast pulse.

Analysis: High fever with polydipsia is caused by invasion of pathogenic heat into the interior, resulting in exuberant heat toxin impairing body fluid; headache and vomiting are due to fire disturbing lucid yang, which involves the stomach; hard and painful swollen cheeks and swollen and sore throat are caused by accumulation of heat and toxin in the meridians of shaoyang and yangming; reddish tongue with yellowish fur as well as slippery and fast pulse indicate exuberance of heat and toxin.

Prescription：Eliminate heat and toxin, soften dryness and disperse lumps.

Formulas：Puji Xiaodu Yin Jiajian (Modified Puji Xiaodu Decoction). (The formula has been introduced in the chapter of *Acute Amygdalitis*.) Xiakucao (*Spica Prunellae*), Haizao (*Sargassum*) and Jiangcan (*Bombyx Batryticatus*) can be added to strengthen the function of softening dryness and dispersing lumps; for aggravation of thirst, Beishashen (*Radix Glehniae*), Xuanshen (*Radix Scrophulariae*) and Tianhuafen (*Radix Trichosanthis*) could be added; for dry feces, Dahuang (*Radix et Rhizoma Rhei*) (decocted later) and Mangxiao (*Natrii Sulfas*) (used as infusion taken orally) should be combined.

3. 痰湿阻塞
49.3　Obstruction of damp phlegm

【症状】本病热退后，神情呆滞，痰鸣涎多，肢体活动不灵，舌质淡暗或紫暗，舌体胖大而润，芒硝细涩。

【分析】热退后气血亏耗，不可能很快恢复，心神失养，故神情呆滞；痰湿阻塞，故痰鸣涎多；气血亏虚，痰湿阻滞经络，故肢体活动不灵；舌体与脉象，均为痰湿瘀血阻滞经络之象。

【治法】益气活血，化痰通络。

【方药】菖蒲郁金汤加减。方选石菖蒲、郁金、丹参行气活血，开窍安神；远志、胆南星化痰安神定志；黄芪、白术、茯苓益气利湿；地龙通经络以治肢体屈伸不利；葛根解肌缓急。

Clinical manifestations：Dull facial expression after decline of high fever, sputum rale and profuse saliva, inflexibility of the limbs, light darkish or dark purplish tongue, bulgy moistening tongue as well as thin and astringent pulse.

Analysis：After the decline of high fever, asthenic qi and blood cannot be restored quickly, causing malnutrition of the heart and mind, which gives rise to dull facial expression; sputum rale and profuse saliva are caused by obstruction of dampness and phlegm; inflexibility of the limbs is due to asthenia of qi and blood, dampness and phlegm obstructing meridians and collaterals; light darkish or dark purplish tongue, bulgy and moistening tongue and thin and astringent pulse indicate obstruction of dampness and phlegm in meridians and collaterals.

Prescription：Benefit qi, invigorate blood circulation, resolve phlegm and dredge collaterals.

Formulas：Changpu Yujin Tang Jiajian (Modified Changpu Yujin Decoction). In the formula, Shichangpu (*Rhizoma Acori Tatarinowii*), Yujin (*Radix Curcumae*), Danshen (*Radix Salviae Miltiorrhizae*) can activate qi and invigorate blood, induce resuscitation of consciousness and tranquilize the mind; Yuanzhi (*Radix Polygalae*) and Dannanxing (*Rhizoma Arisaematis Cum Bile*) could resolve phlegm and tranquilize the mind; Huangqi

（*Radix Astragali seu Hedysari*）, Baizhu（*Rhizoma Atractylodis Macrocephalae*）and Fuling （*Poriae Cocos*）have an action of benefiting qi and resolving dampness by inducing diuresis; Dilong（*Lumbricus*）could dredge meridians and collaterals to eliminate inflexibility of the limbs; Gegen（*Radix Puerariae*）can expel pathogenic factors from the muscles and skin to relieve spasm.

4. 瘀血留聚
49.4 Retention of blood stasis

【症状】两腮肿胀迟迟不散，压之疼痛，舌质暗或有瘀点，舌苔薄白，脉象细涩。

【分析】邪毒久羁少阳，气血运行不畅，瘀血留聚，故两腮硬肿迟迟不散，压之疼痛；舌质暗或有瘀点，以及脉象细涩，均属瘀血留聚之象。

【治法】行气活血，软坚散结。

【方药】桃红四物汤加减。方取四物汤加桃仁、红花，养血活血。可加入橘核、枳实、夏枯草行气散结；加黄芪补气，以助行气之力；或加三棱、莪术，以增强活血化瘀的作用。

Clinical manifestations: Undispersed swollen lumps of the cheeks, pain sensation with pressure, darkish tongue or spotted with petechiae, thin whitish fur as well as thin and astringent pulse.

Analysis: Prolonged retention of pathogenic toxin in shaoyang meridian results in unsmooth circulation of qi and blood and blood stasis, causing failure to disperse hard lumps of the cheeks and pain sensation with pressure; darkish tongue or tongue spotted with petechiae, thin whitish fur and thin and astringent pulse are signs of retention of blood stasis.

Prescription: Activate qi and invigorate blood circulation, soften dryness and disperse lumps.

Formulas: Tao Hong Siwu Tang Jiajian（Modified Tao Hong Siwu Decoction）. The formula is the combination of Siwu Tang（Decoction）with Taoren（*Semen Persicae*）and Honghua（*Flos Carthami*）which are added to nourish blood and activate blood. Juhe （*Semen Citri Reticulatae*）, Zhishi（*Fructus Aurantii Immaturus*）and Xiakucao（*Spica Prunellae*）can be added to activate qi and disperse lumps; Huangqi（*Radix Astragali seu Hedysari*）could be added to strengthen the action of activating qi; Sanling（*Rhizoma Sparganii*）and Ezhu（*Rhizoma Curcumae*）can be combined to reinforce the action of invigorating blood circulation and dissolving blood stasis.

五十、急性中耳炎

50　Acute tympanitis

〔**概说**〕 Summary

　　急性中耳炎是中耳黏膜的急性化脓性疾病。若治疗不及时或治之不当，可演变为慢性中耳炎或急性乳突炎及各种严重并发症。

　　急性中耳炎归属中医"脓耳""聤耳""耳疳""耳痈"等范畴。认为与风湿热搏结，气血凝滞，经络闭塞，肝胆湿热壅盛，肾元亏虚等有关。治疗上注重病因辨证与脏腑辨证相结合，特别是在急性期，以清泻肝胆之湿热为要务。单纯的补益法不宜急用、多用。

　　Acute tympanitis is an acute purulent condition of inflammatory mucosa of the eardrum. Delayed or improper treatment of the disease can cause it to develop into chronic tympanitis or acute mastoiditis, even various severe complicated diseases.

　　In terms of TCM, acute tympanitis pertains to "pyotorrhea" "suppurative otitis media" "acute otitis media" "pyoauricular disease" and so on. It is generally believed that acute tympanitis is related to coagulation of wind, dampness and heat, qi stagnation and blood stasis, obstruction of meridians and collaterals, exuberance of dampness and heat in the liver and gallbladder as well as asthenia of kidney qi. As far as treatment is concerned, much stress should be placed on the integration of syndrome differentiation of etiology and of zang-fu organs, in particular, at the acute stage of the disease, purging dampness and heat from the liver and gallbladder is taken as the most important therapeutic methods. However, simple treating methods such as supplementing and benefiting should not be adopted widely and in some urgent cases.

〔**辨证论治**〕 Syndrome differentiation and treatment

　　急性中耳炎初起多属实证、热证，以脓耳为其主要特征。多因风热之邪侵袭，致使肝胆火盛，结聚耳窍所致。

　　The initial stage of acute tympanitis belongs to sthenia and heat syndromes, and characterized by pyotorrhea. Usually it is caused by invasion of pathogenic wind and heat factors, resulting in coagulation of exuberant fire in the ear orifice transmitted from the liver and gallbladder.

1. 肝胆火热

50.1 Exuberance of fire and heat in the liver and gallbladder

【症状】起病较急，耳内疼痛，伴有发热恶寒，头痛，鼻塞，流涕，口苦，咽干，小便黄赤，大便秘结，舌红苔黄，脉象弦数。

【分析】风热侵袭肝胆之经，正邪交争，故有发热恶寒、口苦咽干等胆经症状；足少阳胆经"起于目锐眦，上抵头角，下耳后……其支者，从耳后入耳中，出走耳前……"风热伤及胆经，故耳内疼痛；小便黄赤、大便秘结，为热毒下注之象；舌红苔黄、脉象弦数，为风热侵袭肝胆经脉，火热炽盛之征。

【治法】清泻肝胆之火。

【方药】龙胆泻肝汤加减。龙胆泻肝汤为清泻肝胆之火的首选方剂。（其方义见"慢性肝炎"篇。）耳内疼痛明显不减者，可加夏枯草、郁金清热散结止痛；大便秘结甚者，可加大黄（后下）、芒硝（冲服）。

Clinical manifestations：Sudden outbreak，sore ears，accompanied with fever，aversion to cold，headache，stuffy nose，runny nose with snivel，bitter taste of the mouth，dry throat，brownish urine，dry feces，reddish tongue with yellowish fur as well as taut and fast pulse.

Analysis：Attack of wind heat in meridians of the liver and gallbladder causes struggle between healthy qi and pathogenic factors，which brings about fever，aversion to cold，bitter taste of the mouth and dry throat；gallbladder meridian of foot Shaoyang "starts from the inner canthus，reaches the head，then passes through the back of the ears... and the branches of the meridian travel through the back of the ears into the interior of the ears，then arrives at the front of the ears..." Sore ears are caused by wind heat impairing the gallbladder meridian；brownish urine and dry feces indicate down migration of heat toxin；reddish tongue with yellowish fur and taut and fast pulse are signs of exuberant fire and heat.

Prescription：Purge fire from the liver and gallbladder.

Formulas：Longdan Xiegan Tang Jiajian（Modified Longdan Xiegan Decoction）. The formula is the first choice for purging fire from the liver and gallbladder，which has been discussed in the chapter of *Chronic Hepatitis*. For unalleviated pain in the ears，Xiakucao（*Spica Prunellae*）and Yujin（*Radix Curcumae*）can be added to relieve heat，disperse lumps and stop pain；for dry feces，Dahuang（*Radix et Rhizoma Rhei*）（decocted later）and Mangxiao（*Natrii Sulfas*）（used as infusion for oral taking）should be combined.

2. 热毒结脓

50.2 Heat toxin generating purulence

【症状】起病较急，耳内疼痛，并见耳鸣，听力障碍，耳内发胀；耳痛逐渐加重，或跳痛，或如锥刺痛，疼痛连及头部，剧痛之后，鼓膜穿孔，流出脓液，脓流之后，疼痛减轻，其他症状也随之减缓。

【分析】风热之邪，侵袭耳窍，固结不散，故耳内疼痛、耳鸣、听力出现障碍；热邪盛则疼痛加重；热毒伤及耳膜，继而化腐成脓；若兼有湿邪，脓量较多；脓流出之后，热毒外泄，故其症状自然减轻。

【治法】疏散风热，解毒消肿。

【方药】蔓荆子散加减。蔓荆子散出自《东垣十书》，由蔓荆子、生地黄、赤芍、甘菊、桑白皮、木通、麦冬、升麻、前胡、茯苓、炙甘草组成。本方蔓荆子、甘菊、升麻体轻气清上浮，善于疏散风热，清利头目；生地黄、赤芍、麦冬养阴凉血；木通、茯苓、桑白皮清热利水，祛湿；前胡助蔓荆子宣散，助桑白皮化痰；炙甘草和解诸药之性。鼓膜穿孔，耳脓流出后，热势减轻，治疗上可改为渗湿解毒、活血排脓，方用仙方活命饮加减，可加入车前子、地肤子、苦参等渗湿解毒之品。

Clinical manifestations: Sudden outbreak, sore ears, accompanied with tinnitus, hearing disorder, distending ears; aggravation of earache with symptoms as jumping pain and piercing pain involving the head, tympanic membrane perforation and oozing of pus with acute pain, alleviation of pain after oozing of pus, and then other symptoms relieved.

Analysis: Undispersed coagulation of wind and heat resulting from invasion of wind and heat pathogens into the external acoustic meatus causes sore ears, tinnitus as well as hearing disorder; aggravation of earache is due to hyperactivity of heat toxin; heat toxin impairing tympanic membrane, which, in turn, develops into purulence; if it is complicated with pathogenic dampness factor, the amount of purulence will increase; heat toxin can be eliminated with oozing of pus, therefore, the symptoms can surely get alleviated.

Prescription: Dispel wind and heat, relieve toxin and swelling.

Formulas: Manjingzi San Jiajian (Modified Manjingzi Powder). The formula is quoted from *Dongyuan Shishu* (*A Series of medical books*). And it consists of Manjingzi (*Fructus Viticis*), Shengdihuang (*Radix Rehmanniae Recens*), Chishao (*Radix Paeoniae Rubra*) Ganju (*Flores Chamomillae*), Sangbaipi (*Cortex Mori*), Mutong (*Caulis Akebiae*), Maidong (*Radix Ophiopogonis*), Shengma (*Rhizoma Cimicifugae*), Qianhu (*Radix Peucedani*), Fuling (*Poriae Cocos*) and Zhigancao (*Radix Glycyrrhizae Preparata*). In the formula, Manjingzi, Ganju and Shengma are light, clearing and lifting in nature, so they have the action of dispelling wind and heat and clearing away heat from the head; Shengdihuang, Chishao and Maidong can nourish yin and cool blood; Mutong, Fuling and Sangbaipi could eliminate heat and resolve dampness; Qianhu could assist Manjingzi to disperse heat, and it can help Sangbaipi resolve phlegm; Zhigancao has the action of harmonizing the above drug. For alleviation of heat because of tympanic membrane perforation and oozing of pus, the prescription can be replaced by resolving dampness and toxin, invigorating blood and eliminating pus. Therefore, the recipe of Xianfang Huoming Yin Jiajian (Modified Xianfang Huoming Decoction) can be adopted. Cheqianzi (*Semen Plantaginis*), Difuzi (*Fructus Kochiae*) and Kushen (*Radix Sophorae Flavescentis*) can be combined to resolve dampness and relieve toxin.

五十一、耳鸣、耳聋

51 Tinnitus and deafness

〔**概说**〕 Summary

耳鸣是指病人自觉耳内鸣响，妨碍听觉，或若蝉鸣，或若钟鸣，或若流水声，或若火熇熇（hehe，火势很盛）然，或若敲鼓声，或若风吹耳，等等。

耳聋是指不同程度的听力减低，轻者耳失聪敏，听力不真，称为重听；重者全然不闻外声，则为全聋。

古代中医学认为，耳鸣与耳聋不可截然分开，"耳鸣者，聋之渐也"，"诸般耳聋，未有不先鸣者"。耳者，肾之外窍，但又与肝经、脾经有着密切关系。治疗耳鸣与耳聋，关键在于抢时间，早发现，早治疗，做到"未病先防"，中药与针灸并用，预期效果较好。

Tinitus refers to noise in the ears like chirping of a cicada, or bell ringing, or tidal sound of water flowing, or hyperactive burning fire, or like beating a drum, or the sound of wind passing through the ears, and so on.

Deafness means decline of hearing to some extent. As for unserious syndrome, the patient loses sagacity or the sound they hear is unreal, it is known as diplacusis. For severe syndrome, the patient cannot feel any outside sound, which is known as complete deafness.

Ancient TCM experts hold that tinnitus and deafness cannot be differentiated clearly. "Tinnitus can change gradually into deafness" "Each case of deafness comes from tinnitus". The ear is the external orifice of the kidney; yet it is closely connected with meridians of the liver and spleen. The key to treating them is to grasp the time, that is, treating the diseases as soon as possible and trying to prevent the disease before it comes into being. In addition, application of Chinese medicinal herbs together with acupuncture can ensure a better and desirable effect.

〔**辨证论治**〕 Syndrome differentiation and treatment

1. 肝火上扰

51.1 Up-disturbance of liver fire

【症状】两耳蝉鸣，如风雷声，耳聋时轻时重，每遇情绪激动时，耳鸣、耳聋突发加重，伴有头晕、头痛、面红目赤，或伴心烦不宁，大便秘结，小便黄赤，舌红苔黄，脉象弦数有力。

【分析】怒则伤肝，肝胆之气上逆，犯于清窍，故突发耳鸣，听觉失灵；火盛炎上，故头痛、头晕，面红面赤，或心烦不宁；火盛伤阴，故大便秘结，小便黄赤；舌红苔黄，脉象弦数，均为肝胆火盛之象。

【治法】清肝泻热，开郁通窍。

【方药】龙胆泻肝汤加减。方中以龙胆草、栀子、黄芩、柴胡清泻肝胆，苦寒直折火势为主药；辅以木通、车前子、泽泻等利水及导热下行；佐以当归、生地黄养血凉血，以帮助主药泻火；甘草和中解毒，调和诸药。可加石菖蒲、蔓荆子祛风开窍；若热势重，可加大黄、芦荟、青黛，以增强清肝泻火的作用。

Clinical manifestations：Noise in the ears like chirping of a cicada, or like the sound of wind-thunder storm, occasional alleviation or aggravation of deafness, sudden worsening tinnitus and deafness accompanied with vertigo, headache, flushed complexion and eyes, or complicated with vexation and restlessness, dry faces, brownish urine, reddish tongue with yellowish fur as well as taut, fast and powerful pulse.

Analysis：Rage impairs the liver. Adverse flow of qi in the liver and gallbladder attacking the upper orifice causes sudden outbreak of tinnitus and disorder of hearing; up-flaring of exuberant fire results in vertigo, headache, flushed complexion and eyes, or complicated by vexation and restlessness; dry feces and brownish urine are due to hyperactive fire impairing yin fluid; reddish tongue with yellowish fur as well as taut, fast and powerful pulse indicates exuberant fire in the liver and gallbladder.

Prescription：Clear away heat from the liver, disperse stagnated qi and wake up consciousness.

Formulas：Longdan Xiegan Tang Jiajian (Modified Longdan Xiegan Decoction). In this formula, Longdancao (*Radix Geutianae*), Zhizi (*Fructus Gardeniae*), Huangqin (*Radix Scutellariae*) and Chaihu (*Radix Bupleuri*), cold and bitter in nature, are used as principal drug to purge fire and heat from the liver and gallbladder; Mutong (*Caulis Akebiae*), Cheqianzi (*Semen Plantaginis*) and Zexie (*Rhizoma Alismatis*) are used as adjuvant drug to induce diuresis to remove dampness and guide heat to move downward; Danggui (*Radix Angelicae Sinensis*) and Shengdihuang (*Radix Rehmanniae Recens*) are applied to assist the principal drug to purge fire with their action of nourishing and cooling blood; Gancao (*Radix Glycyrrhizae*) has an effect of regulating middle energizer, relieving toxin and reconciling the above herbs. Shichangpu (*Rhizoma Acori Tatarinowii*) and Manjingzi (*Fructus Viticis*) can be added to dispel wind and wake up consciousness; for exuberant heat of the liver, Dahuang (*Radix et Rhizoma Rhei*), Luhui (*Aloe*) and Qingdai (*Indigo Naturalis*) could be combined to strengthen the action of purging fire from the liver.

2. 痰火郁结
51.2　Stagnation of phlegmatic fire

【症状】两耳蝉鸣不断，或"呼呼"作响，时而闭塞如聋，头昏头重，胸闷脘闷，咳嗽痰涎多，口苦，二便不畅，舌红，苔黄腻，脉象弦滑。

【分析】痰火上扰，气道不通，故耳鸣不断，时而闭塞如聋；痰火蒙蔽清窍，故头昏头重；痰火郁结，宗气不畅，则胸闷脘闷；痰火上涌，则咳嗽痰涎多；"火性炎上"，故口苦；痰火伤及胃肠之津，故二便不畅；舌红、苔黄腻、脉弦数，为痰火之征。

【治法】清火化痰，和胃降浊。

【方药】黄连温胆汤加减。黄连温胆汤即温胆汤加黄连，温胆汤为清胆和胃之化痰方，加入黄连，起到清火降浊作用。临证使用，加入石菖蒲开窍，芦根清胃化痰，白芥子通络，其效果更好。

Clinical manifestations：Non-stop noises in the ears like chirping of a cicada, or like the sound of wind passing through the ears, occasional loss of hearing, dizziness and heavy sensation of the head, oppression of the chest and epigastrium, cough with profuse saliva and sputum, bitter taste of the mouth, unsmooth of defecation and urination, reddish tongue with greasy yellowish fur as well as taut and slippery pulse.

Analysis：Non-stop tinnitus or occasional loss of hearing is caused by obstruction of air passage because of upward disturbance of phlegmatic fire; dizziness and heavy sensation of the head are due to phlegmatic fire blocking the upper orifice; oppression of the chest and epigastrium is caused by disorder of thoracic qi because of stagnation of phlegmatic fire; cough with profuse saliva and sputum results from upsurge of phlegmatic fire; bitter taste of the mouth is due to "up-flaring nature" of fire; unsmooth of defecation and urination is caused by phlegmatic fire impairing fluid of the stomach and intestines; reddish tongue with greasy yellowish fur as well as taut and slippery pulse indicates phlegmatic fire.

Prescription：Clear away fire, resolve phlegm, harmonize the stomach and descend turbid qi.

Formulas：Huanglian Wendan Tang Jiajian (Modified Huanglian Wendan Decoction). The formula is made up of Wendan Tang (Decoction) and Huanglian. The former is a formula for resolving phlegm by clearing away heat from the gallbladder and regulating the stomach. Huanglian (*Rhizoma Coptidis*) is combined to clear away fire and descend turbid qi. In some specific cases, Shichangpu (*Rhizoma Acori Tatarinowii*) can be added to induce resuscitation, Lugen (*Rhizoma Phragmitis*) may be combined to clear away fire from the stomach so as to resolve phlegm, and Baijiezi (*Semen Sinapis Albae*) has a better effect of dredging collaterals.

3. 肾精亏耗
51.3 Deficiency and exhaustion of kidney essence

【症状】耳内常闻蝉鸣之声，由微到重，夜间尤甚，以致虚烦不眠，兼见头晕目暗，腰膝酸软，遗精，盗汗，舌质红，苔少，脉象细弱。

【分析】肾精亏虚，不能上荣于清窍，以致耳鸣、耳聋，由轻到重；夜间阴液不能充盈，故夜间尤甚，且虚烦不眠；肾主骨而生髓，脑为髓海，肾亏则脑髓空虚，故头晕目暗；"腰为肾之府"，肾亏则髓不能充于骨，故腰膝酸软；肾精亏耗，相火妄动，则遗精、盗汗；精血不足，故舌红少苔，脉来细弱，若细而兼数，可知阴虚相火亢盛。

【治法】补肾益精，滋阴潜阳。

【方药】耳聋左慈丸加减。耳聋左慈丸出自《广温热论》，方由熟地黄、山药、山茱萸、牡丹皮、茯苓、泽泻、五味子、磁石组成。即在六味地黄丸滋阴补肾的基础上，加入五味子补肾纳气，磁石潜阳降火。

若兼见下肢寒冷，阳痿，舌质淡嫩，脉细弱，为肾阳虚证，治以温补肾阳，方用补骨脂丸，方出《中医内科学讲义》，方中以补骨脂、葫芦巴、杜仲、菟丝子填精益肾，肉桂、花椒温阳散寒，熟地黄、当归、川芎补血，石菖蒲、白芷、白蒺藜通窍行气，磁石镇纳浮阳。

Clinical manifestations: Noise in the ears like chirping of a cicada ranging from low to loudness, aggravated tinnitus at night causes dysphoria and insomnia, complicated with vertigo and dizziness, aching sensation of the loins and knees, seminal emission, night sweating, reddish tongue with scanty fur as well as thin weak pulse.

Analysis: Tinnitus and deafness ranging from low to loudness are caused by failure of deficient kidney essence to nourish the upper orifices; aggravated tinnitus and deafness at night causing dysphoria and insomnia are due to failure to enrich yin fluid at night; the kidney dominates the bones and produces marrow, and the brain is the sea of marrow, asthenia of the kidney results in insufficient marrow of the brain, giving rise to vertigo and dizziness; "the loins is the house of the kidney", deficiency of the kidney causes failure of marrow to enrich the bones, bringing about aching sensation of the loins and knees; seminal emission and night sweating are due to deficient and exhausted kidney essence, which gives rise to hyperactive fire of lower energizer; reddish tongue with scanty fur as well as thin and weak pulse indicates insufficiency of essence and blood, and thin and fast pulse suggests yin asthenia and hyperactivity of ministerial fire.

Prescription: Supplement the kidney and essence, nourish yin and suppress yang.

Formulas: Erlong Zuoci Wan Jiajian (Modified Erlong Zuoci Pill). The formula is quoted from *Guang Wenre Lun* (*Treatise on Universal Exogenous Febrile Disease*), consisting of Shudihuang (*Radix Rehmanniae Preparata*), Shanyao (*Rhizoma Dioscoreae*), Shanzhuyu (*Fructus Corni*), Mudanpi (*Cortex Moutan Radicis*), Fuling (*Poriae Cocos*), Zexie (*Rhizoma Alismatis*), Wuweizi (*Fructus Schisandrae Chinensis*) and Cishi (*Magnetitum*). In other words, based on Liuwei Dihuang Wan (Pill) which has the function of nourishing yin and tonifying kidney, the formula is combined with Wuweizi to tonify the kidney and strengthen reception of qi and with Cishi to suppress yang and descend fire.

For the complicated syndrome of yang asthenia of the kidney with the following symptoms such as cold lower limbs, impotence, pale and tender tongue as well as thin and weak pulse, prescription of warming and tonifying kidney yang should be adopted, and its formula should be Buguzhi Wan (Pill) quoted from *Zhongyi Neikexue Jiangyi* (*Lectures on Internal Medicine of Chinese Traditional Medicine*). In the formula, Buguzhi (*Fructus Psoraleae*), Huluba (*Semen Trigonellae*), Duzhong (*Cortex Eucommiae*) and Tusizi (*Semen Cuscutae*) have an action of enriching kidney essence and tonifying the kidney; Rougui (*Cortex Cinnamomi*) and

Huajiao（*Capsicum Annuum*）can warm yang and disperse cold；Shudihuang（*Radix Rehmanniae Preparata*），Danggui（*Radix Angelicae Sinensis*）and Chuanxiong（*Rhizoma Ligustici Chuanxiong*）could supplement blood；Shichangpu（*Rhizoma Acori Tatarinowii*），Baizhi（*Radix Angelicae Dahuricae*）and Baijili（*Tribulus Terrestris*）may dredge the orifices to activate qi circulation；Cishi（*Magnetitum*）has an action of tranquilizing the mind，improving reception of qi and suppressing floating of yang.

4. 脾胃虚弱

51.4 Asthenia of the spleen and stomach

【症状】耳鸣耳聋，劳碌更甚，或下蹲时较甚，耳内有突然空虚或发凉的感觉，纳少，食后腹胀，大便溏薄，面色萎黄，唇舌淡红，苔薄白，脉象虚弱。

【分析】脾胃为气血生化之源，脾胃虚弱则清气不能上升，耳部经脉空虚，故耳鸣耳聋发作；蹲下时，气血趋下，脑部气血不足，或劳碌耗气耗血，故耳鸣、耳聋更甚，并有突然空虚或发凉的感觉；脾胃虚弱，纳谷与运化无力，故纳呆，食后腹胀；清气不升，故大便溏薄；气血不能荣于面，故面色萎黄，唇舌淡红，苔薄白；气为血之帅，气弱血少，故脉来虚弱无力。

【治法】健脾益气升阳。

【方药】补中益气汤或益气聪明汤加减。补中益气汤为补益脾胃之气首选之方（具体方义见"胃下垂"篇），用于此，主要是取其升清降浊的功效。益气聪明汤出自《证治准绳》，方由蔓荆子、黄芪、党参、黄柏、白芍、炙甘草、升麻、葛根组成。此方黄芪、党参健脾益气，为主药；升麻、葛根、蔓荆子轻清之品，升提清阳之气，以达清窍；黄柏清泻相火，不使虚火上扰清窍；白芍滋阴，收敛耗散之气。若加石菖蒲开窍之品，效果更好。

Clinical manifestation：Tinnitus and deafness，aggravation with overstrain or in crouching position，sudden vacuous or cooling sensation of the ears，poor appetite，abdominal distention after meals，thin loose stool，sallow complexion，pale reddish tongue and lips，thin whitish fur as well as weak pulse.

Analysis：The spleen and stomach are the origin where qi and blood are generated and transformed. Asthenia of the spleen and stomach results in failure to lift lucid yang qi and emptiness of the ear meridians，causing outbreak of tinnitus and deafness；aggravation of tinnitus and deafness in crouching position with sudden vacuous or cool sensation of the ears is due to down-flow of qi and blood in crouching position causing by insufficiency of qi and blood in the brain；aggravation of tinnitus and deafness with overstrain results from consuming large amount of qi and blood because of overstrain；poor appetite and abdominal distention after meals are due to asthenic spleen and stomach，causing failure to transport and transform food；thin loose stool is due to failure to lift yang qi；sallow complexion，pale reddish tongue and lips and thin whitish fur indicate failure of qi and blood to nourish the face；qi is the commander of blood，asthenic qi leads to scanty blood，giving rise to weak pulse.

Prescription: Invigorate the spleen, benefit qi and lift yang.

Formulas: Buzhong Yiqi Tang or Yiqi Congming Tang Jiajian (Modified Buzhong Yiqi Decoction or Yiqi Congming Decoction). The former is the best choice for supplementing qi in the spleen and stomach (it has been discussed in the chapter of *Gastroptosis*). Here, it is used to lift lucid yang and descend turbid qi. The latter, quoted from *Zhengzhi Zhunsheng* (*Standards for Diagnosis and Treatment*), consists of Manjingzi (*Fructus Viticis*), Huangqi (*Radix Astragali seu Hedysari*), Dangshen (*Radix Codonopsis*), Huangbo (*Cortex Phellodendri*), Baishao (*Radix Paeoniae Alba*), Zhigancao (*Radix Glycyrrhizae Preparata*), Shengma (*Rhizoma Cimicifugae*) and Gegen (*Radix Puerariae*). Among them, Huangqi and Dangshen are used as principal drug to invigorate the spleen and benefit qi; Shengma, Gegen and Manjingzi are light and clear, so they are used to lift lucid yang qi and help them reach the upper orifice; Huangbo can purge fire from lower energizer to prevent asthenic fire from disturbing the upper orifice; Baishao has an action of nourishing yin and astringing consumed qi; Shichangpu should be added to awake consciousness to ensure a better curative effect.

附录一   常见舌诊图谱

Appendix I   Atlas of tongue diagnosis

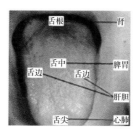

舌与脏腑关系
Relations between the tongue
and zang-fu organs

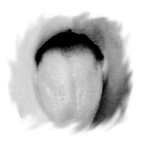

正常舌象
Normal tongue

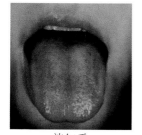

淡红舌
Pale reddish tongue

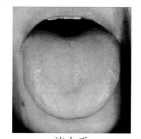

淡白舌
Pale tongue

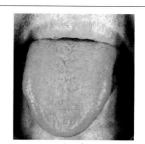

红舌
Reddish tongue

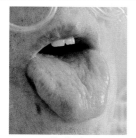

淡紫舌
Pale purplish tongue

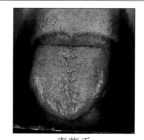

青紫舌
Cyanotic and purplish tongue

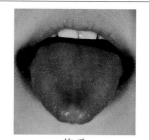

绛舌
Deep-reddish tongue

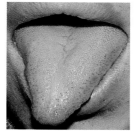

老舌
Tough tongue

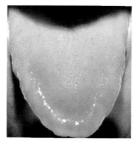

嫩舌
Tender tongue

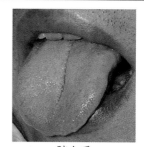

胖大舌
Enlarged tongue

451

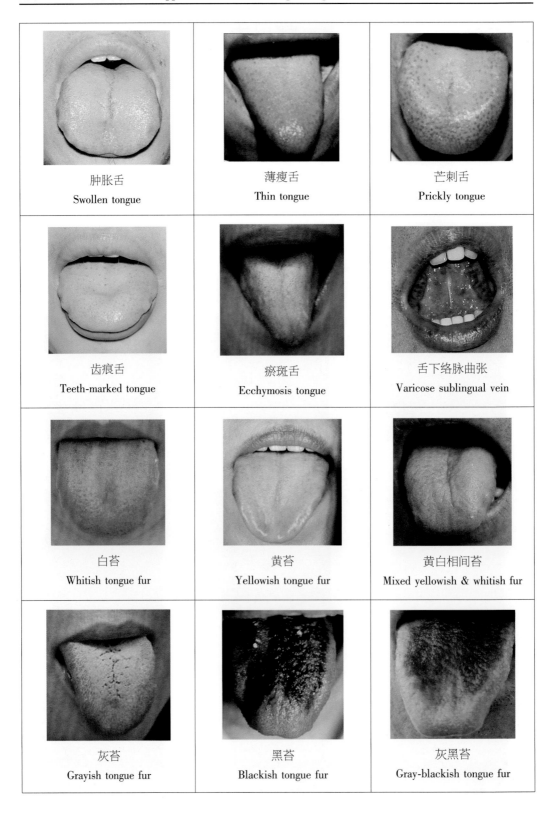

肿胀舌
Swollen tongue

薄瘦舌
Thin tongue

芒刺舌
Prickly tongue

齿痕舌
Teeth-marked tongue

瘀斑舌
Ecchymosis tongue

舌下络脉曲张
Varicose sublingual vein

白苔
Whitish tongue fur

黄苔
Yellowish tongue fur

黄白相间苔
Mixed yellowish & whitish fur

灰苔
Grayish tongue fur

黑苔
Blackish tongue fur

灰黑苔
Gray-blackish tongue fur

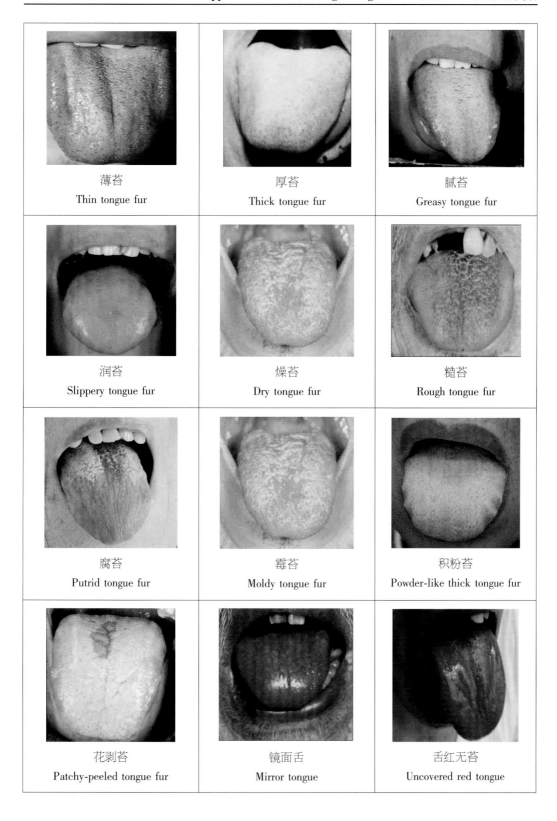

薄苔
Thin tongue fur

厚苔
Thick tongue fur

腻苔
Greasy tongue fur

润苔
Slippery tongue fur

燥苔
Dry tongue fur

糙苔
Rough tongue fur

腐苔
Putrid tongue fur

霉苔
Moldy tongue fur

积粉苔
Powder-like thick tongue fur

花剥苔
Patchy-peeled tongue fur

镜面舌
Mirror tongue

舌红无苔
Uncovered red tongue

附录二　常见脉象示意图

Appendix Ⅱ　Diagram of common pulse type

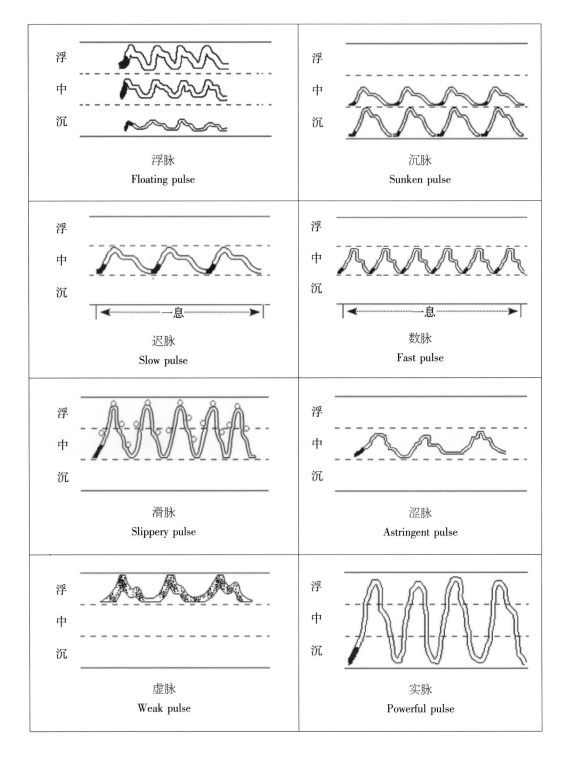

浮脉
Floating pulse

沉脉
Sunken pulse

迟脉
Slow pulse

数脉
Fast pulse

滑脉
Slippery pulse

涩脉
Astringent pulse

虚脉
Weak pulse

实脉
Powerful pulse

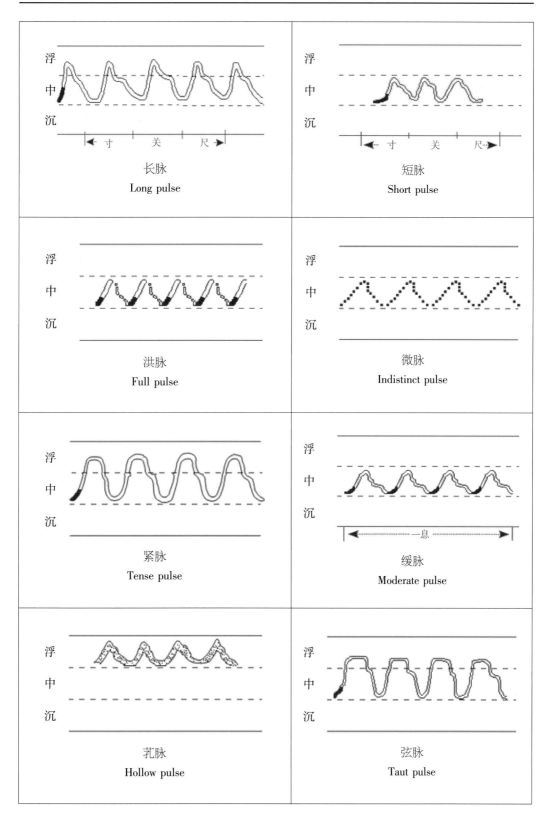

长脉
Long pulse

短脉
Short pulse

洪脉
Full pulse

微脉
Indistinct pulse

紧脉
Tense pulse

缓脉
Moderate pulse

芤脉
Hollow pulse

弦脉
Taut pulse

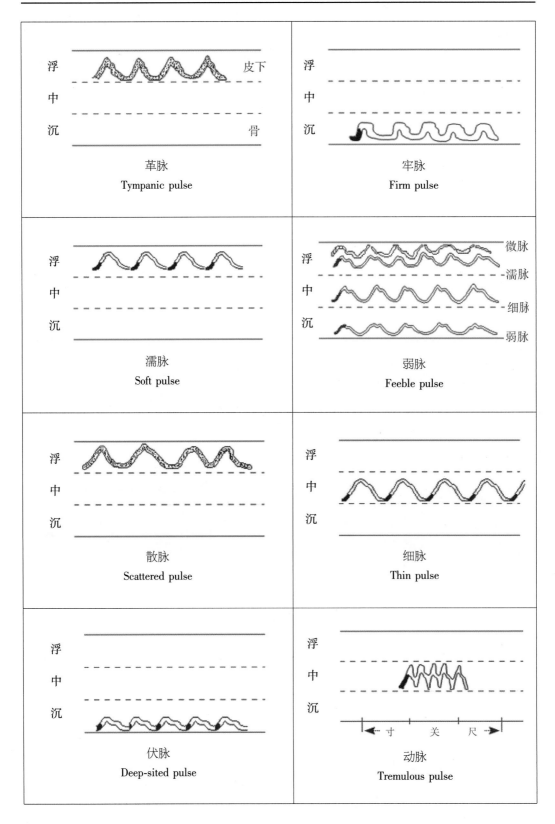

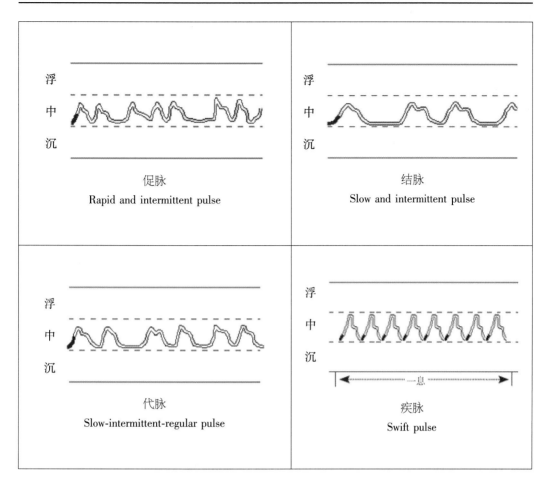

促脉
Rapid and intermittent pulse

结脉
Slow and intermittent pulse

代脉
Slow-intermittent-regular pulse

疾脉
Swift pulse